Color Atlas of Demonstrations in Surgical Pathology

Royal College of Surgeons of Edinburgh

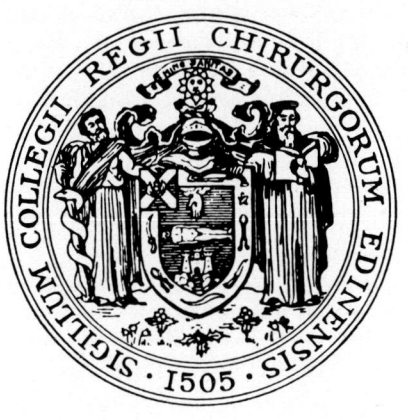

Volume 1
The Alimentary System

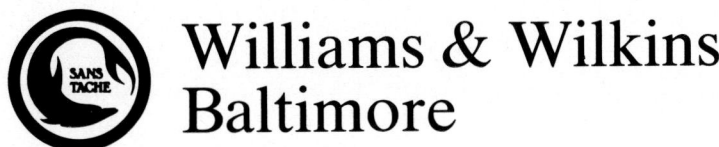

Williams & Wilkins
Baltimore

Copyright © The Royal College of Surgeons of Edinburgh, 1983
Copyright © Wolfe Medical Publications Ltd, 1983
Published by Wolfe Medical Publications Ltd, 1983
Printed by George Philip Printers Ltd, London
Colour separations by Excel Lithoplates Ltd, Slough

This book is the first in a short series produced by the
Royal College of Surgeons of Edinburgh.
For further information regarding forthcoming volumes
please see the last page of this volume.

Library of Congress Cataloging in Publication Data

Surgical pathology.

  Includes index.
  Contents: v. 1. Alimentary system.
  1. Pathology, Surgical. 2. Royal College of Surgeons of
Edinburgh. I. Fraser, James, Sir. II. Mekie, D. E. C. III. Royal
College of Surgeons of Edinburgh. [DNLM: 1. Pathology,
Surgical–Atlases. WO 517 R888s]
RD57.S86 1983   617'.07   83–14589
ISBN 0–683–07401–6 (v.1)

Contents

Foreword

The quality of the clinical practice of surgery, the art of teaching and the development of research are unquestionably dependent upon sure foundations in the basic sciences of anatomy, physiology and biochemistry and the ability to apply them. The understanding of surgical disease and its pattern of evolution depends upon this fundamental knowledge together with a full appreciation of pathology, including dynamic or 'living' pathology as Moynihan called it. This new series on Surgical Pathology is based on the unique collection of specimens from the Museum of the Royal College of Surgeons of Edinburgh which houses one of the largest and most historic collections of surgical pathological specimens in the United Kingdom. This material is now presented in a synoptic and illustrative form which makes understanding and learning easy. It has evolved from the development of a series of demonstration boards which have been on permanent display singly or in groups in the hall over the past few years. This method of presentation was originally devised in the Wellcome Museum for Tropical Diseases in London and adapted to our needs by the then Conservator, Professor D.E.C. Mekie, and his colleagues. They have met with considerable acceptance from postgraduate students and other visitors and it was this that inspired their publication. I am proud to be associated with this important publication which has been authorised by the College.

John Gillingham C.B.E.
PRESIDENT.
6 October 1982

5

Acknowledgements

The Editors have been aided in their task of co-ordinating the contributions received and arranging the layout of the material. This has been achieved with the aid of a team to whom tribute is paid for their great contribution and advice.

Mr A.N. Smith has been our adviser for the whole field of alimentary diseases. Dr N. MacLean has prepared the histopathological studies and captions. Dr M.O. Wright has contributed much of the script dealing with physiology. Dr W.A. Copland has advised on radiology. Mr I.S. Kirkland has given guidance on lesions which are peculiar to paediatric surgery. Our thanks are also due to Mr I.S. Kirkland, Dr N. MacLean and Mr A.I.S. Macpherson for the great assistance they have given in the preparation of the final manuscript. The photography has been undertaken by Mr M. McKenzie the College photographic technician and we acknowledge especially his meticulous care in securing reproductions of highest quality, often a difficult task. Mrs Violet Tansey has assisted in the editorial work and has undertaken the whole of the typescript. She has cheerfully endured the many revisions and without her this work could not have been undertaken.

Editors

Professor D.E.C. Mekie O.B.E.
Sir James Fraser Bt

Editorial board

Professor F.J. Gillingham C.B.E. – Chairman
  (Neuropathology)
Professor G. Chisholm
  (Urology)
Mr I.S. Kirkland
  (Paediatrics)
Mr D.W. Lamb
  (Orthopaedics)
Mr A.I.S. Macpherson
  (General surgery)
Mr R.J.M. McCormack
  (Thoracic surgery)
Mr B. Nolan
  (Peripheral vascular system)
Dr A.A. Shivas
  (Conservator)
Mr A.N. Smith
  (Alimentary system)
Professor D.J. Wheatley
  (Cardiology)

Contributors

Mr J.R. Anderson	*Belfast*
Mr J. Cook	*Edinburgh*
Mr A.C.B. Dean	*Edinburgh*
Mr A.A. Gunn	*Edinburgh*
Mr I.S. Kirkland	*Edinburgh*
Mr R.J.M. McCormack	*Edinburgh*
Mr I.F. MacLaren	*Edinburgh*
Dr N. Maclean	*Edinburgh*
Mr A.I.S. Macpherson	*Edinburgh*
Tan Sri G.B. Ong	*Hong Kong*
Mr A.H. McLean Ross	*Edinburgh*
Mr W.G. Scobie	*Edinburgh*
Mr I.S.R. Sinclair	*Edinburgh*
Mr A.N. Smith	*Edinburgh*
Mr J.W.W. Thomson	*Edinburgh*
Dr M.O. Wright	*Edinburgh*
Datuk Yeoh Bok Choon	*Malaysia*

Introduction

An essential requirement for the surgeon is a knowledge of the pathology of lesions encountered in practice to the point where the individual tissue changes can be visualised, and an ability to recognise with accuracy the nature and character of lesions when exposed at operation. Such knowledge may be partly achieved from textbooks but a full visual concept can only be adequately acquired by the study of specimens whether as seen fresh in the operating room, exposed at post mortem examination or as found in museums. The Museum of the Royal College of Surgeons of Edinburgh was commenced in 1807 for this very purpose and has continued to grow and evolve to meet new concepts. It is now chiefly used by postgraduate students preparing for the Fellowship examinations and research workers.

It is essential as well as convenient that these two methods of approach should be conducted simultaneously. In recent years, therefore, the College Museum collection has been supplemented by a series of demonstrations on which photographs together with histological, radiological and clinical illustrations and diagrams are associated with an appropriate text. The text has been in synoptic form and arranged schematically to indicate logical lines of learning. The text covered essential related embryology, anatomy and physiology together with an account of the aetiology and nature of the lesion as would be found in larger textbooks. The demonstrations have thus integrated the visual advantages of the study of specimens with the systematic approach of the textbooks.

This work is based on these demonstrations which have been revised and expanded to meet the needs of postgraduate students preparing for Fellowship examinations or for more advanced higher diplomas. This revision has been undertaken by individual contributors who possess expertise in the different fields. The demonstrations are identified by the alpha-numeric index of the museum catalogue.

Saliva

In addition to secreting the enzyme amylase which is concerned with the breakdown of starch, the saliva plays an important part in maintaining a constant pH in the oral cavity. Saliva is slightly acid in reaction (pH 6.3 to 6.8) and the acidity is controlled by the CO_2 content and shows little variation. The pH within the oral cavity is maintained by the secretion of saliva which amounts to 1000 to 1500 ml daily. The intake of acid or alkali into the mouth is controlled with great rapidity by the salivary flow.

Constituents:
1 Water (99.5%)
2 Salts (0.2%)
   Sodium and potassium chloride
   Sodium bicarbonate
   Acid and alkaline sodium phosphates
   Calcium carbonate and calcium phosphate
   Potassium sulphocyanate
3 Gases – CO_2, O_2
4 Organic substances
   Ptyalin (salivary amylase) and maltase
   Serum albumin and globulin
   Urea, uric acid, creatine and amino-acids
   Mucin

There is a distinction between the secretion of the parotid, submaxillary and sublingual glands. The latter two have a very high mucin content. The parotid secretes little mucin.

Pathology

Salivary calculi are found predominantly in adult male patients and are rare in the edentulous. The calculi may result from a pre-existing infection, desquamated cells having formed a nucleus for crystallisation. The deposition of crystalline salts about a tooth-brush bristle or a small nodule of tooth-paste which has entered the salivary duct has been recorded.

1

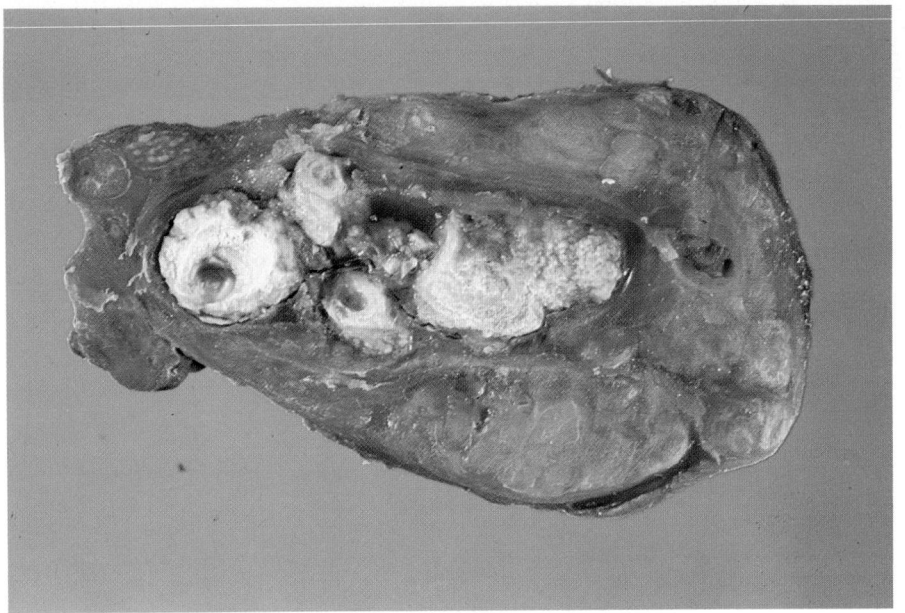

G.C.9715

Two forms of calculi are described:
1 Amorphous, multiple deposits in the substance of the gland.
2 A cigar-shaped calculus within the main duct, sometimes solitary.

1 From a male aged 75 years. Over a period of 3 years, calculus formation had occurred, first in the right and later in the left submandibular gland.

A stone in a duct causes obstruction when the salivary secretion is stimulated after eating. Due to accumulation of secretion in the duct and gland swelling occurs but usually subsides before the next meal. This is associated with discomfort or pain. The majority of calculi are found in the submandibular salivary gland and duct. This is attributed to the high mucin content secretion of this gland. The calculi consist of calcium salts and are therefore radio-opaque.

2

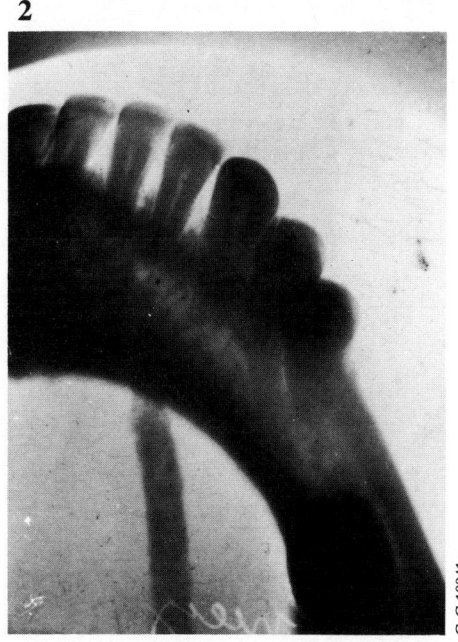

3

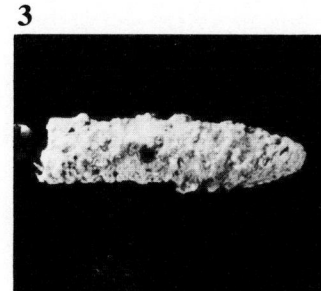

2 and **3** From a male aged 36 years. A palpable calculus approximately 2cm long was present in the submandibular duct. The calculus was clearly seen in the X-ray.

Sialectasis

The salivary duct may be obstructed either by stone or by stenosis of the duct following inflammation. If persistent this may lead to dilatation of the salivary ducts and acini – sialectasis. The lesion can be demonstrated by sialography.

4a

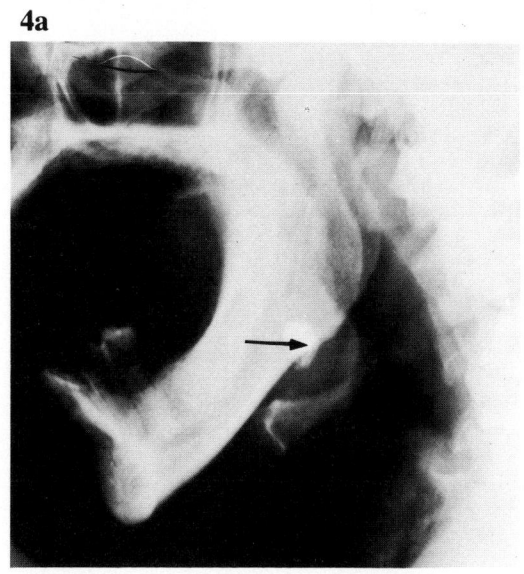

4b

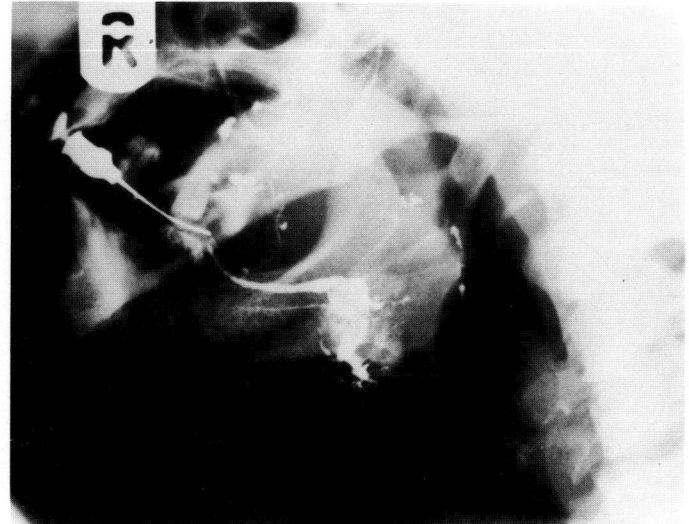

4a and **4b** From a male aged 45 years. History of recurrent swelling of the right submandibular gland over a period of years. Plain X-ray demonstrates (**a**) the presence of a calculus. Sialography demonstrates (**b**) dilatation of the main ducts in the gland substance.

The clinical enlargement of a salivary gland(s) may be attributable to a variety of lesions which may be acute or chronic. The differential diagnosis of those which run a chronic course may be difficult.

Mikulicz – Sjögren disease

An inflammatory disease, possibly auto-immune, occurring most frequently in females with rheumatoid arthritis. It may cause swelling of the salivary and lacrimal glands and results in dryness of the mouth and conjunctivae, the 'sicca syndrome'.

Benign lymphoepithelial lesion

This is a somewhat similar lesion where glandular enlargement is unaccompanied by the 'sicca syndrome'.
  Both these conditions may cause sufficient salivary gland enlargement to arouse suspicion of malignancy but histologically the three main features are:
  1 Lymphocytic infiltration.
  2 Atrophy of glandular tissue.
  3 Proliferation of duct epithelium sometimes leading to formation of myoepithelial islands.

Heerfordt's disease

Sarcoidosis involving the parotid and uveal tracts giving rise to the clinical condition known as uveo-parotid fever. The swelling of the parotid glands may be substantial and may be associated with facial palsy but unlike that of mumps is painless.

Parotid gland – Sarcoidosis

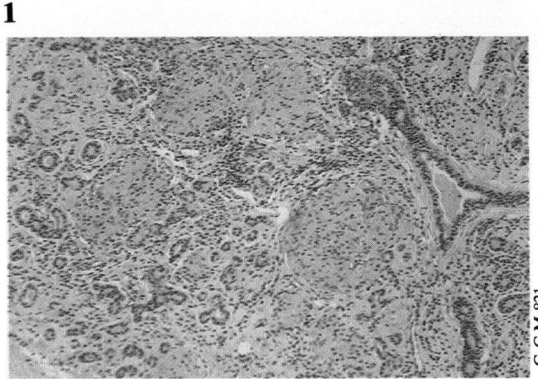

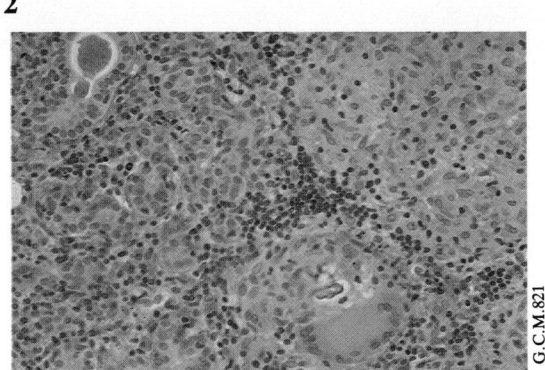

1 Several follicles of epithelioid cells are present. The inflammation has resulted in atrophy of acinar tissue and fibrosis. Ducts are well-preserved or even hyperplastic. *(H&E ×80)*

2 This field includes a follicle composed of epithelioid cells with pale elongated nuclei, and a multinucleated giant cell containing a small calcified 'Shaumann body'. The duct epithelium and myoepithelium is hyperplastic and lymphocytes surround the follicle and giant cell. *(H&E ×200)*

Infection

Enlargement of the salivary glands may also be attributable to chronic infection. This may arise from oral sepsis and spread from the primary source by lymphatic channels to lymph nodes which exist within the gland capsule.

Tuberculosis involving the salivary gland is rare but well recognised.

Malignant lymphoma

This neoplasm occurs most often in the parotid and less frequently in the submandibular gland.

The tumour is usually unilateral and of slow growth. The lesion is commonly solitary but may be part of a diffuse lymphomatosis.

Microscopically the tumour may be nodular or diffuse and the lymphocytes are well differentiated.

Secondary malignant disease

Tumours of the oral cavity may spread by periductal lymphatics to nodes which are adjacent to or lie within the substance of the gland and present as hard, fixed tumours.

Post irradiation fibrosis

Following irradiation for tumours of the mouth the salivary glands may be within the field of irradiation and thereafter undergo a loss of their parenchymal elements followed by fibrosis. The epithelium lining the ducts of the gland undergoes a squamous metaplasia. The condition is sometimes mistaken for secondary carcinoma.

Other rare tumours of the salivary gland include haemangioma, lipoma and neurilemmoma.

N. Maclean

Anatomy

Structure

The normal salivary gland is composed of lobules with stroma, ducts and glands.

Ducts – lined by cubical or columnar epithelium becoming stratified near the mouth.

Glands – formed of serous or mucous cells or both.
  Parotid – serous.
  Submandibular – serous predominantly and mucous.
  Sublingual – mucous predominantly and serous.

↓

Serous cells – secrete a watery fluid containing salts and proteins.
Mucous cells – a viscid mucin.
Duct cells – concentrate and modify these secretions.

Serous cells are rich in ribosomes and endoplasmic reticulum which stain darkly with haematoxylin. Mucous cells are pale. Myoepithelial cells are stellate, lying flattened between epithelium and basement membranes of glands and ducts.

↓

Also found:
(a) In the mucosa of the salivary ducts are a variable number of mucin-secreting cells (goblet cells).
(b) Eosinophilic (oxyphil) cells are a constant feature and increase in number with advancing age (oncocytes).
(c) Rarely some parenchymal cells show the features and formation of sebaceous glands.

1

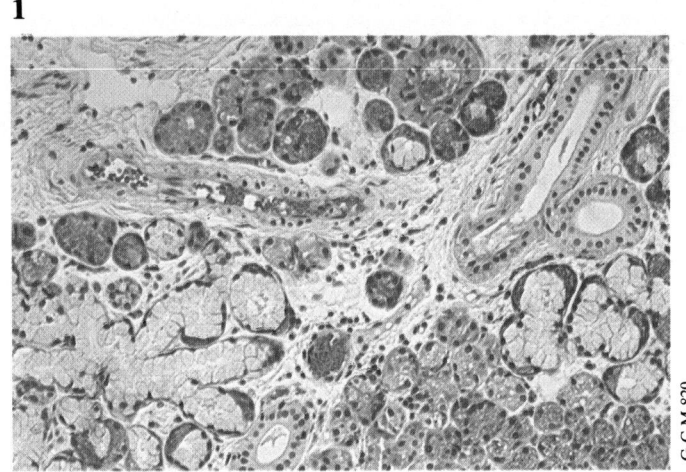

1 Submandibular gland showing ducts, artery, stroma, pale mucous glands and dark serous glands. *(H&E ×175)*

2

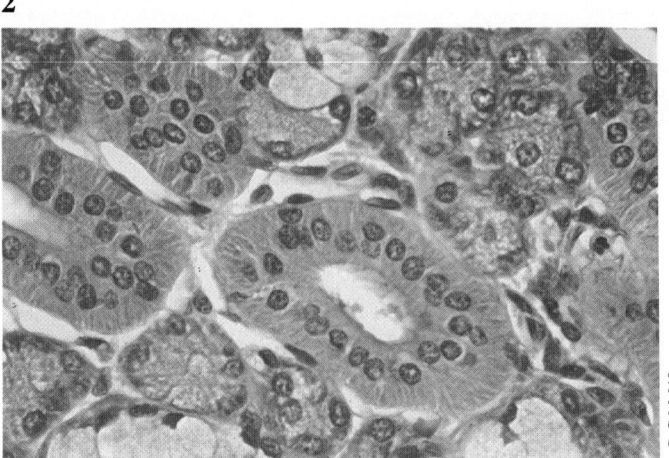

2 Section of a parotid gland showing dark, serous cells, columnar duct cells and flattened nuclei of myoepithelial cells. *(H&E ×480)*

Development

The salivary glands develop by the downgrowth of epithelial buds from the stomatodaeum and receive a capsule from the surrounding mesoderm. The parotid gland is encapsulated late and may show wider ramification. Parotid elements may thereby show a close association with the cervical lymph chain. Lymph nodes may lie within the parotid tissue or adjacent lymph nodes may show isolated islets of parotid gland tissue (heterotopic salivary gland).

Classification

Adenomas   Pleomorphic (Approximately 70% of all salivary gland tumours).
Monomorphic: Adenolymphoma, oxyphil, basal cell, others.

Mucoepidermoid tumours

Acinic cell tumours

Carcinomas   Adenocystic, Adenocarcinoma, Squamous, Undifferentiated.
Carcinoma arising in pleomorphic adenoma.

Incidence

These tumours are relatively uncommon (10 to 12/1 000 000 of population) and the relative incidence in the salivary gland varies:

Parotid	65–75%	Sublingual	1%
Submandibular	10–20%	Minor glands	10%

The minor or anomalous salivary glands are found beneath the mucosa of the palate and tongue.

The benign tumours may develop at any age (6 to 80 years). Malignant lesions usually appear between 50 and 60 years.

Malignancy

10 to 15% of tumours in the parotid gland are malignant. In other glands approximately 30% are malignant.

Pleomorphic adenoma

This tumour, which contains apparently both epithelial and chondromatous elements, is now held to be solely of epithelial origin – an adenoma. The matrix contains chondroitin, a mucopolysaccharide, which is responsible for the cartilaginous appearance. Some authorities assert that myoepithelium plays an important part in tumour development and suggest it is from the myoepithelial cells that the matrix and 'cartilage' develop. Older views that the tumour was either in the nature of a teratoma or a hamartoma are wholly abandoned.

Pathology

A pleomorphic adenoma is almost invariably solitary. It forms an irregularly lobulated, roughly globular mass possessing a capsule of varying thickness. On section, fibrous strands traverse the variegated surface of the tumour thus delineating lobules. Some of these are fleshy and others cystic, myxomatous or cartilaginous. The ratio of component parts varies.

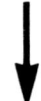

The tumour expands by phases of focal growth producing nodular extensions into the capsule. Since the capsule is seldom complete, in some areas tumour abuts on, or is in continuity with normal glandular tissue. Nodules which may be found exterior to the capsule and may appear to be satellite tumours, can be shown by serial sectioning to be extensions of the main tumour and not independent neoplasms.

Operative enucleation of the tumour or failure to excise a rim of normal gland outside the capsule is frequently responsible for leaving satellite nodules *in situ*. This accounts for the frequency and the multiplicity of recurrent nodules after such operations.

3

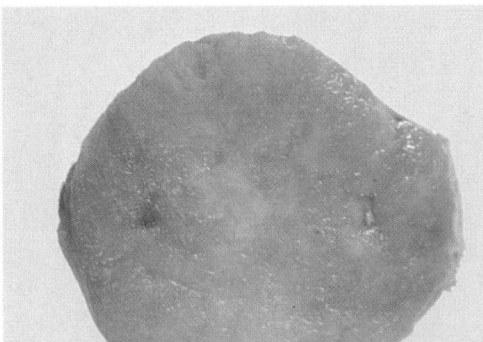

G.C.14912

3 The middle-aged woman from whom the tumour was excised stated that a small painless nodule which had been present on the right side of her neck for most of her life, had been increasing in size for two months.

The spherical nodule measured about 2cm in diameter, was firm and had a fibro-cartilaginous appearance and consistency centrally.

3a

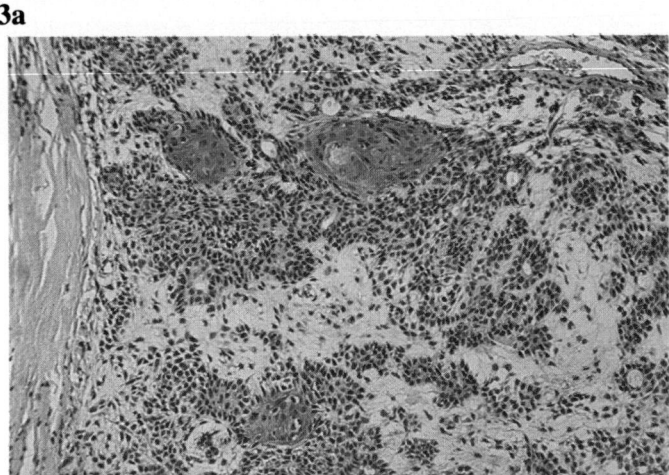

3a Microscopic field of above tumour including a small part of the capsule (left). Masses of basal cells are set in a myxoid stroma containing myoepithelial cells. Squamous cell nests can also be seen. Characteristic chondroid nodules were present in other fields. *(H&E ×125)*

Histology

Complex and variable.

(a) Epithelial element. The cells may be arranged in sheets, or lie sparsely in a 'mucoid' or 'chondromyxomatous' matrix. In the peripheral parts of the tumour, adenomatous or tubular formation is common. Occasional squamous metaplasia is observed.

(b) The matrix. Areas of mucoid, myxoid or chondromatous appearance are a major feature. In the mucoid and myxoid areas myoepithelial cells are present. They may appear as dense sheets or thin strands of cells and may resemble chondrocytes, basal epithelial cells or spindle cells. Clear cells and other forms also occur. The cartilaginous areas may calcify or ossify.

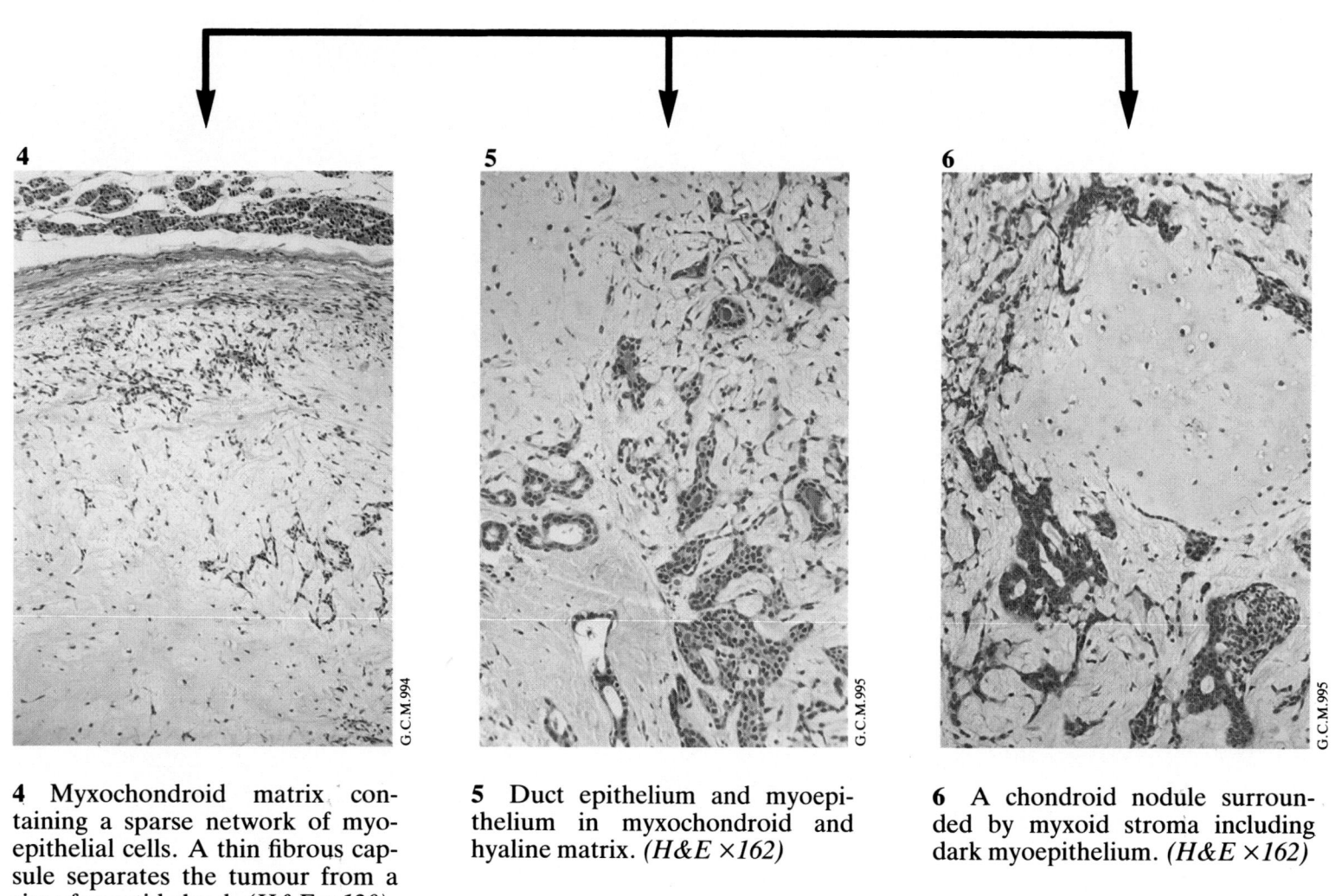

4 Myxochondroid matrix containing a sparse network of myoepithelial cells. A thin fibrous capsule separates the tumour from a rim of parotid gland. *(H&E ×120)*

5 Duct epithelium and myoepithelium in myxochondroid and hyaline matrix. *(H&E ×162)*

6 A chondroid nodule surrounded by myxoid stroma including dark myoepithelium. *(H&E ×162)*

Behaviour

Slowness of growth is characteristic – a history of 10 to 30 years is commonplace.

Pleomorphic adenoma *(Continued)*

The clinical appearance of these tumours in the parotid is very characteristic. They project laterally displacing the lobule of the ear outwards.

7

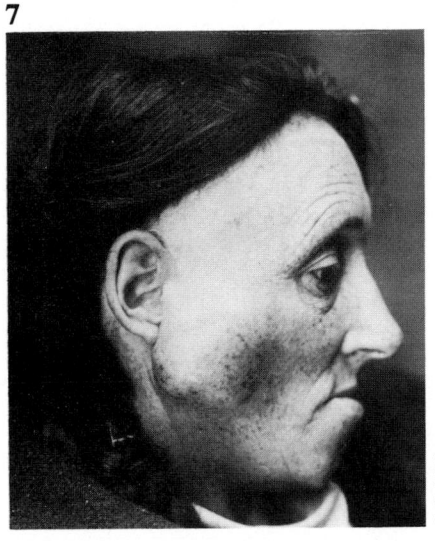

G.C.14270

7 From an elderly female.

Surgical anatomy

These tumours present many difficulties in treatment. Total excision, to avoid leaving satellite nodules, is required.

It has been demonstrated that the parotid gland may be divided into two halves, a superficial and a deep, and in the plane between these lie the facial nerves and a rich venous plexus. Most tumours are found in the superficial segment and surgical removal is facilitated by careful dissection in the plane between the halves. It is also easier to avoid damage to the facial nerve by identifying this plane.

8

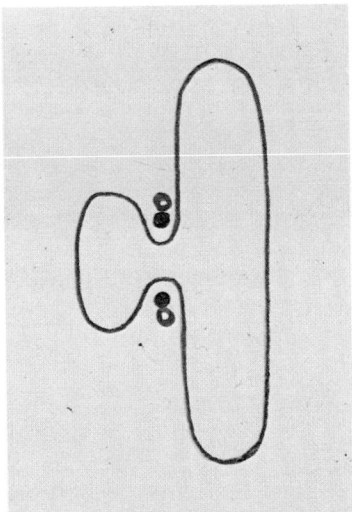

8 Diagrammatic representation of the superficial and deep lobes and the intervening veins and nerves. After Bailey.

9

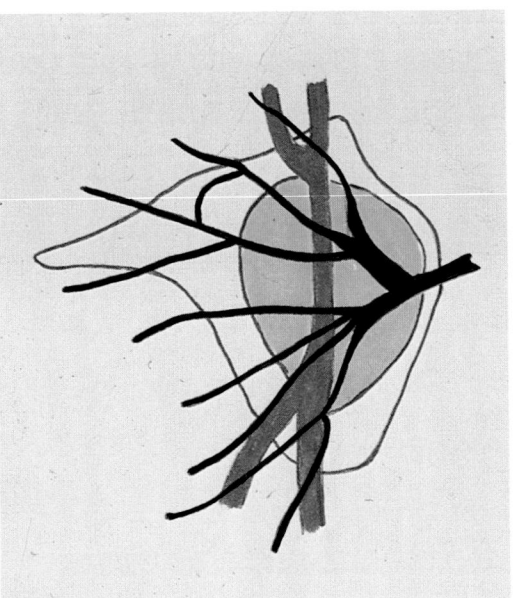

9 Diagrammatic representation of the faciovenous plane showing above the temporal veins, retromandibular and below the drainage to the common facial and the external jugular. After Patey.

Pleomorphic adenoma – Carcinomatous change

Malignant change in a previously simple tumour of long standing occurs in 2 to 4% of cases, is twice as common in female patients and usually becomes obvious during the 6th decade. The clinical features are increasing rapidity of growth of the tumour, increasing fixation and evident nerve involvement.

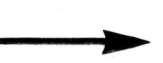

The tumour shows evidence of greater infiltration at its periphery and disruption of its capsule. On histological examination evidence of the pre-existing pleomorphic adenoma persists but there are areas of malignancy indicated by the epithelial elements which show greater pleomorphism. The malignant change is evident in the epithelial cells only and lymph node metastases show only the presence of carcinoma.

10a

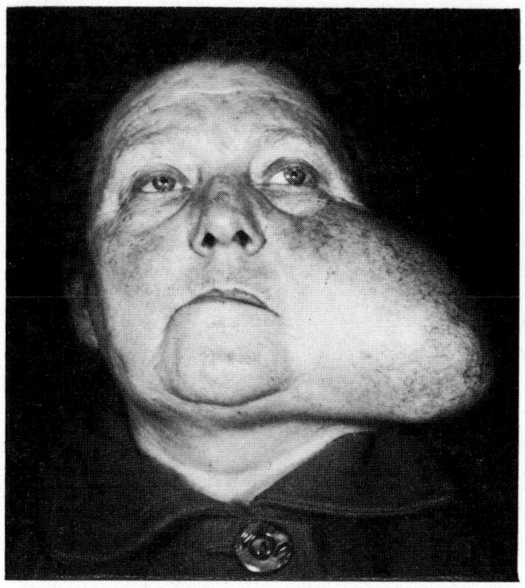

10b

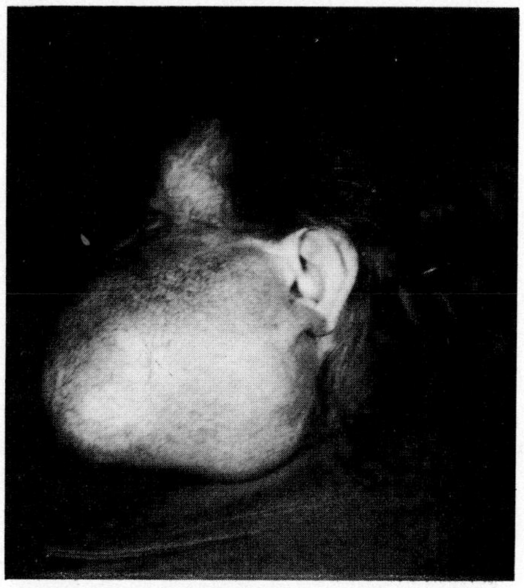

G.C.10443

10a and **10b** From a female aged 65 years. Swelling had been present for 19 years. During the latter 9 years growth was more rapid and at times painful. No facial palsy. Histology demonstrated malignant change in the epithelial element.

11

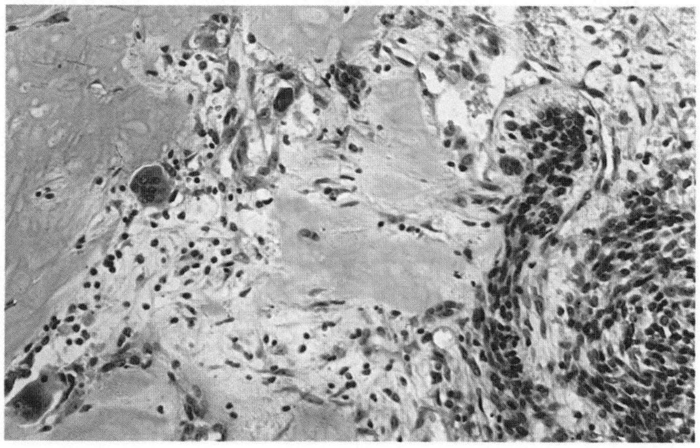

12

11 Portion of the pre-existing adenoma showing osteoid and osteoclast-like cells. *(H&E ×200)*

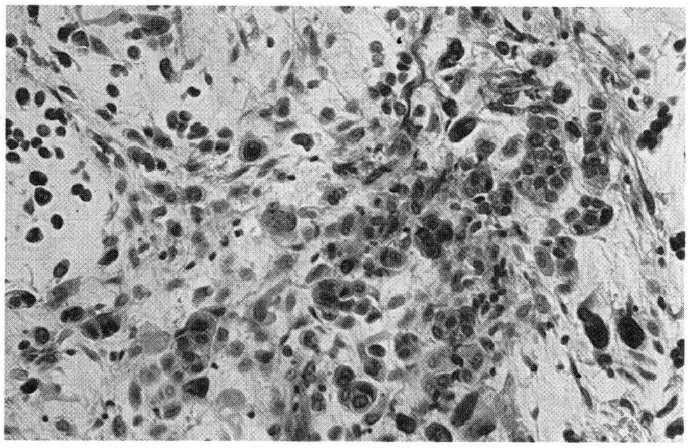

12 Malignant area. Undifferentiated carcinoma with many large hyperchromatic nuclei. *(H&E ×200)*

Monomorphic adenomas

This group includes those benign tumours which show none of the chondro-myxoid tissue found in pleomorphic adenomas. The epithelium is well differentiated and its arrangement tends to be uniform throughout and is often glandular.

Adenolymphoma (Warthin's tumour)

First description – Warthin (1929). This benign tumour is believed to arise from heterotopic gland tissue which has become enclosed developmentally in a lymph node. It constitutes 5 to 6% of salivary gland tumours. It occurs most frequently in males (sex ratio M:F – 5:1) and is usually found over the age of 40 years. An alternative hypothesis is that adenolymphomas represent local areas of immunological over-activity and are not true tumours.

There is a constant relationship to the parotid gland and the tumour presents as a swelling beneath and commonly posterior to the lower pole of the gland. It may lie within the substance of the parotid but more commonly is superficial to it. Multiple tumours, sometimes bilateral, may occur. It is very rare in the minor salivary glands.

13 Tall epithelium is arranged with great regularity around large, irregular glandular spaces which may contain papillae. The cells are non-ciliated, columnar and distinctly eosinophilic. The glands contain eosinophilic secretion. Both the eosinophilic cells and the secretion contain immunoglobulin A in high concentration. The lymphoid tissue is regarded as being part of a normal lymph node and is not an active component of the tumour. *(H&E ×95)*

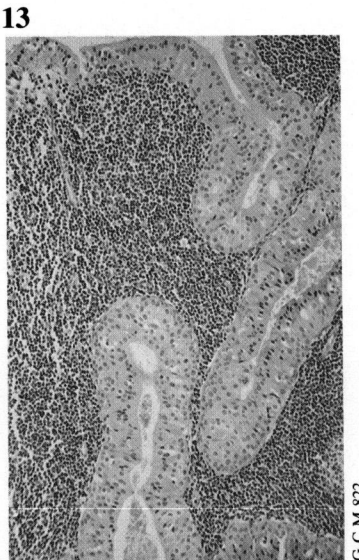

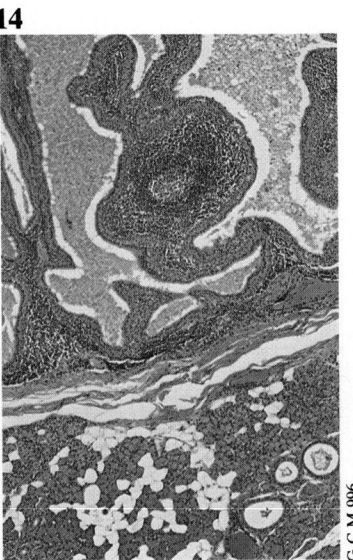

14 The tumour is separated by a thin fibrous capsule from parotid gland. *(H&E ×40)*

Pathology

Is seen as a rounded or slightly lobulated painless mass completely encapsulated. It is soft and cystic. The cysts may contain papillae and also a murky mucinous substance – the appearance can simulate tuberculous adenitis. Growth is slow.

Basal cell adenoma

A very rare tumour usually found in the superficial part of the parotid and of slow growth. Age incidence – over 60 years.

These tumours are encapsulated and rarely wholly solid. The constituent cells have round nuclei, are isomorphic and are arranged in bands forming an interlacing network or as sheets. The picture is very similar to that found in basal cell carcinoma arising from stratified epithelium.

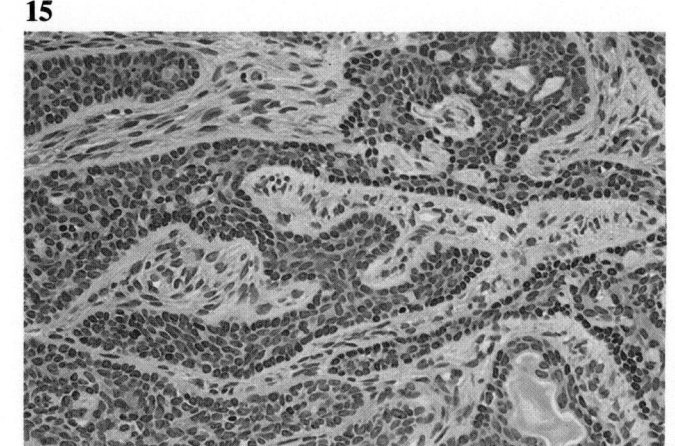

15 Trabeculae of well differentiated basal cells are supported by moderately cellular fibrous stroma. *(H&E ×250)*

Malignancy

Very rare

Oxyphil adenoma (oncocytoma)

These tumours are round or ovoid, encapsulated and solid and occur usually in a higher age group. They are very uncommon and of slow growth. Microscopically the cells are rather large and intensely eosinophilic. The cells are rich in oxidising enzymes and have a large mitochondrial content.

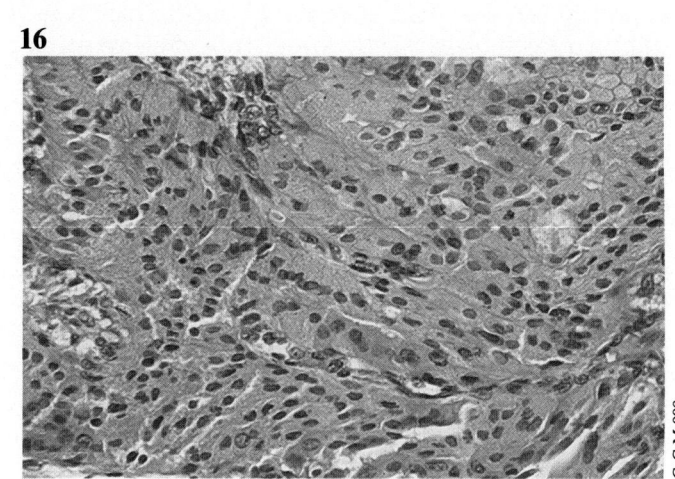

16 Closely packed eosinophilic cells with very regular nuclei. *(H&E ×312)*

Malignancy

Extremely rare

Other rarely encountered monomorphic adenomas with differing histological patterns have also been described – tubular, clear cell, trabecular and sebaceous.

Mucoepidermoid tumour

Forms 2 to 5% of all salivary gland tumours. The majority arise in the superficial lobe of the parotid gland. The minor salivary glands are also a recognised site for this tumour.

Sex incidence – probably equal. Age incidence range 10 to 70 years. Commonest 3rd to 5th decade. Growth very slow.

Pathology

Forms an ovoid and fairly well circumscribed but not encapsulated tumour. Infiltration may be evident with ulceration of the overlying surface. When the tumour occurs in palatal salivary glands, bone destruction is common. These tumours always show an attachment to fascia. The cut surface shows both solid elements and cysts filled with a viscid mucin.

Both epidermoid and mucous elements can be seen. The proportion of these varies. In some instances the dominant feature is the presence of keratinised epidermoid tissue with only small foci of mucoid change in the epidermoid masses. Alternatively, ducts, mucous glands and mucoid cysts form the main elements of the tumour. There is no myxochondroid matrix. The mucin liberated by rupture of small cysts may cause inflammation in the surrounding tissues. The duct epithelium adjacent to the tumour often shows mucoepidermoid metaplasia and the appearances sometimes suggest that the tumour has originated from ducts.

17

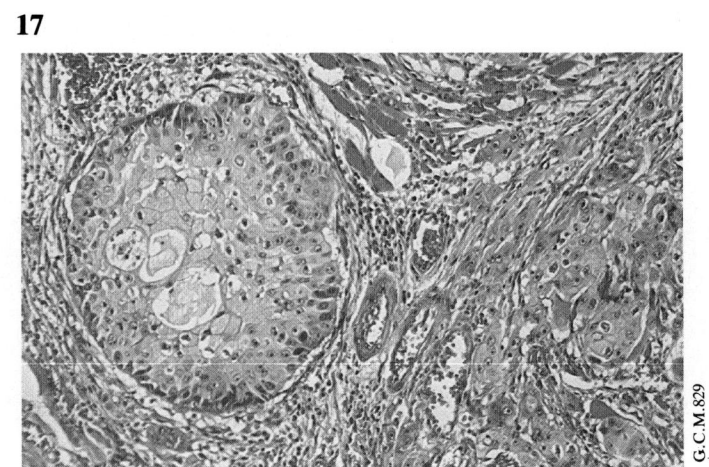

17 In the fibrous stroma of the tumour a mass of epidermoid cells shows mucous change centrally. Other parts of the tumour were mainly mucoid. (*H&E ×125*)

Malignancy

Local infiltration only. Metastases exceedingly rare.

Acinic cell tumour

Forms 1% of all salivary gland tumours. Is usually found in the superficial lobe of the parotid.

Sex ratio F:M – 2:1. Cases have been reported in an age range of 11 to 78 years.

These are solitary lesions, compact, hard, knobbly and mobile. They are apparently encapsulated and present a moist, grey – white cut surface flecked with brown areas. Small cysts containing serous or blood-stained fluid may also be found.

Uniformly round or polygonal cells with abundant basophilic cytoplasm are commonly arranged in solid or mosaic fashion. Large clear cell variants may be present and these often simulate the appearance of renal carcinoma and are described as 'hypernephroid'. The tumour is believed to arise from the serous secreting cells.

18

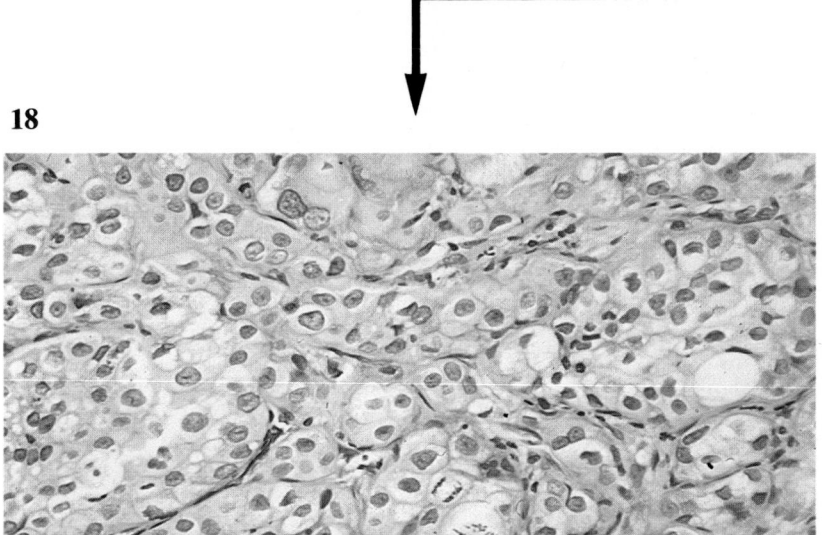

18 A malignant example. Clear cells and granular cells are arranged in solid masses. Two of the cells show mitotic divisions – one abnormal. *(H&E ×300)*

Malignancy

Both benign and malignant variants have been described. After removal of the malignant variety late recurrence with distant metastases has been reported.

Primary carcinoma

The term 'primary carcinoma' of the salivary gland refers to those malignant tumours which do not arise in pre-existent pleomorphic adenomas. They constitute 12 to 15% of all salivary gland neoplasms and half of them occur in the parotid.

Carcinoma

Primary carcinoma arising from the parenchymal cells of the salivary glands is a relatively uncommon tumour affecting the sexes equally with a peak age incidence of 50 to 60 years.

Three varieties have been described

19 A solid undifferentiated highly malignant carcinoma. *(H&E ×320)*

21 An adenocarcinoma – some of the cells producing mucin. *(H&E ×120)*

19

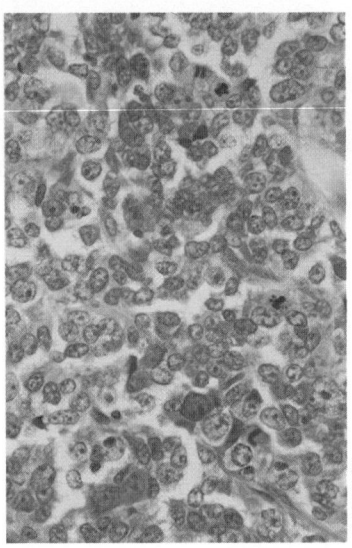

20 A squamous carcinoma. This is most frequently found in the submandibular gland. *(H&E ×100)*

20

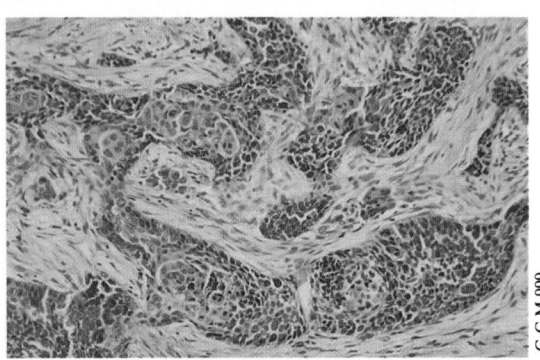

21

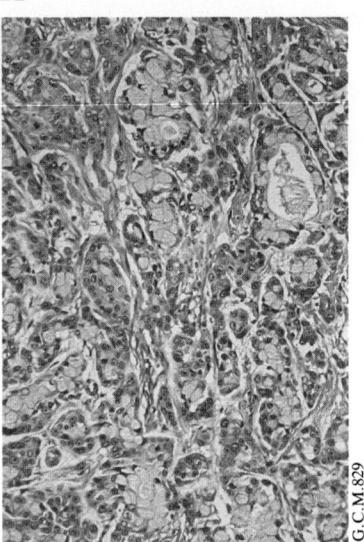

Adenocystic carcinoma

This is a distinctive variety of carcinoma. It usually presents as a firm tumour composed of pink–grey tissue with a moist cut surface. It infiltrates slowly so that its margins are often ill-defined and its limits difficult to identify at operation.

This is the most common malignant tumour of the submandibular and minor salivary glands. Sex ratio equal. Age incidence range 20 to 80 years. Usually found in the 4th to 5th decade.

Pathology

The tumours are composed of basal-type epithelial cells and of a stroma which is variably hyaline. These elements are constantly present and are always sharply demarcated from one another. Within this basic morphology a great variety of histological patterns is found. The epithelial cells may be arranged in solid, glandular, cribriform or cystic masses. The stroma may show marked hyalinisation so that trabeculae or 'cylinders' of hyaline material may separate or infiltrate the epithelial masses. The epithelial cells are small with scanty cytoplasm and dark regular nuclei. Mitotic figures are seldom seen. Neural invasion is often observed.

22
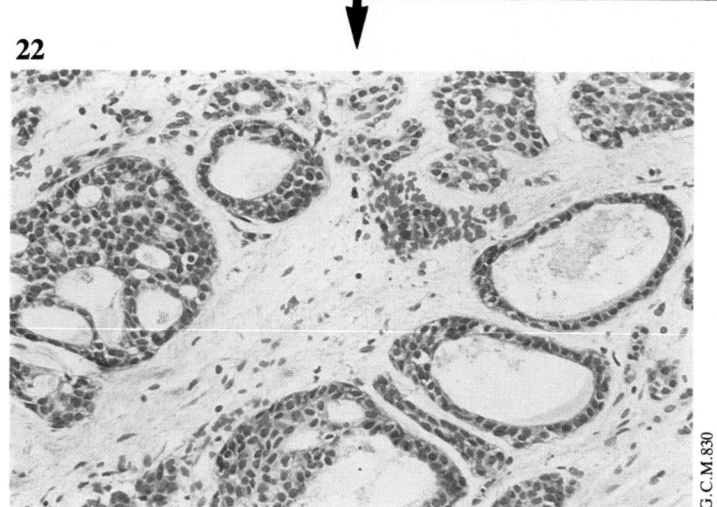

23
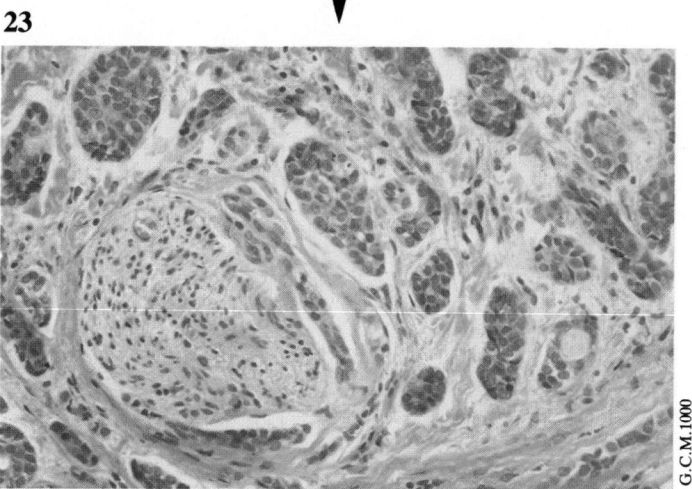

22 Small cells with uniform nuclei are arranged in solid or cystic groups in abundant, often hyaline, stroma. *(H&E ×250)*

23 Solid masses of tumour cells invading a nerve and the perineural spaces. *(H&E ×250)*

Progress

Invasion is slow but unremitting and recurrences after excision are frequent. Metastasis to lymph nodes and other organs is usually late.

N.Maclean

Traumatic perforation

Perforation of the oesophagus may result from direct injury caused by instrumentation, foreign bodies, caustic fluids and acids, or continuous intubation. (Non-traumatic perforation may result from inflammatory lesions – penetrating ulceration, or carcinoma.) Spontaneous rupture is also described.

Oesophagoscopy is a skilled procedure and especially when older patterns of rigid instruments are employed there is a definite risk of injury to the organ. The modern flexible oesophagoscope is much less dangerous. Perforation is liable to occur at two sites:
(a) Post-cricoid perforation. The beak of the instrument catches on the unrelaxed cricopharyngeal sphincter and tears the mucosa in the piriform recess.
(b) Above the diaphragm. The oesophagus here deviates from a straight line, forward and to the left and the tip of the instrument may therefore impinge and perforate the wall.
Perforation at the site of the lesion can also occur due to the fragility of the tissues or due to stretching of a stenosed area.

1

Either by immediate penetration or infection spreading after mucosal injury, the following complications result:

1 Surgical emphysema
2 Pleural infection
3 Mediastinitis
4 Fistula formation to bronchus or aorta

1 From a female aged 80 years with a carcinoma of the lower end of the oesophagus. Oesophagoscopy was carried out and the instrument passed beyond the lesion. The perforation of the oesophageal wall was not detected at this time. Chest pain suggested the need for immediate further investigation and the perforation was demonstrated radiologically. Resection of the lower oesophagus with gastric replacement was successful.

G.C.14272

Spontaneous rupture

H. Boerhaave (1724) described the first classical case.

This form of rupture of the oesophagus most commonly occurs during a bout of vomiting especially after the patient has had an excess of food and/or drink, when the pressure within the lower oesophagus rises sharply. Typically the tear occurs just above the diaphragm, most commonly on the left side. The tear is usually 2 to 3 cm in length. Unless treatment is undertaken death ensues invariably within a few hours or days.

Such cases have been reported in infants and adolescents but the majority of patients are males aged between 50 and 60 years.

Radiology

The signs of rupture of the oesophagus irrespective of the cause include the escape of gas into the mediastinum, the development of pleural effusion and by the use of contrast medium, the escape of oesophageal content into the adjacent tissues or spaces. These features are demonstrated in this X-ray. The rupture in this case was in the mid oesophagus.

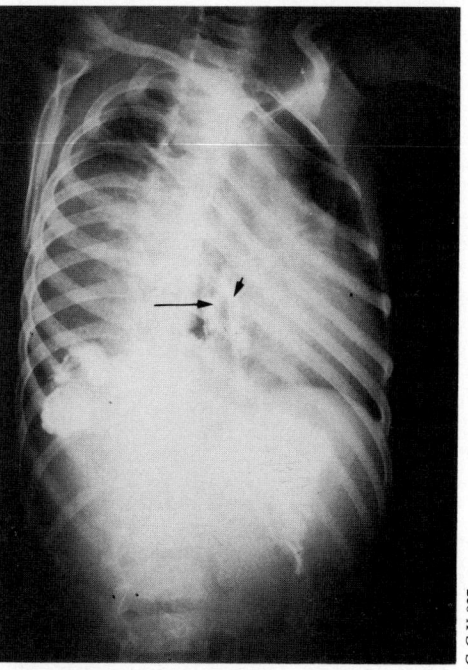

2

G.C.X.927

2 Rupture of the mid oesophagus.

Corrosive oesophagitis

Stricture of the oesophagus may result from swallowing by accident or in attempted suicide corrosives, of which the commonest is caustic soda (Lye). This is frequently observed in the orient. Less commonly sulphuric acid, carbolic or lysol are swallowed.

Acid produces a superficial necrosis. Caustic soda causes a liquefying necrosis with penetration and the subsequent inflammatory reaction can extend to the mediastinum and other adjacent structures. The whole length of the oesophagus may be affected but maximum damage occurs usually at the level of the bifurcation of the trachea.

The acute phase lasts 2 weeks during which there is intense inflammation and oedema. Subsequently, after separation of sloughs, healing is by granulation tissue and fibrosis.

During the acute phase there is initially intense shock followed by general toxaemia and prostration. A fatal outcome is common.

Lye

1

Lysol

2

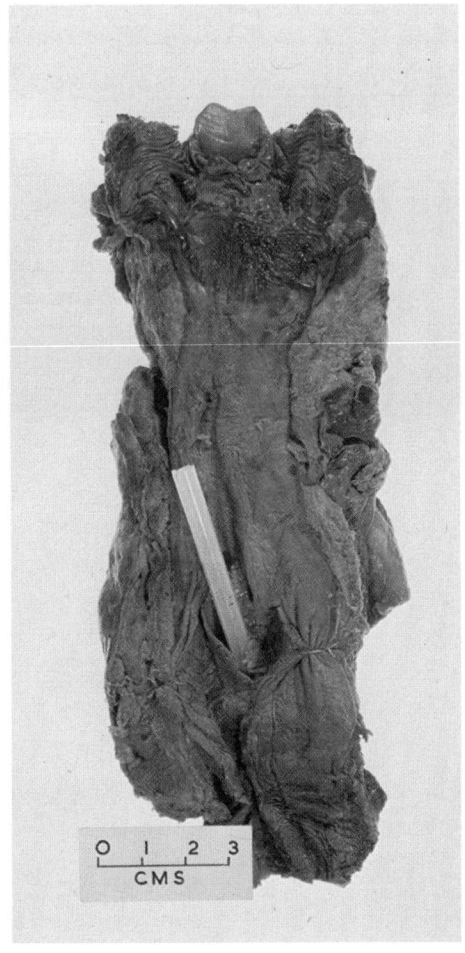

1 From a female aged 33 years who had swallowed caustic soda 5 years previously. She developed complete dysphagia and 1 week later gastrostomy was performed. Later the stricture was repeatedly dilated. Oesophago-jejunostomy was performed but mediastinitis supervened with fatal result.

This specimen shows a stricture affecting the whole length of the oesophagus and is associated with fibrosis of the wall and peri-oesophageal tissues.

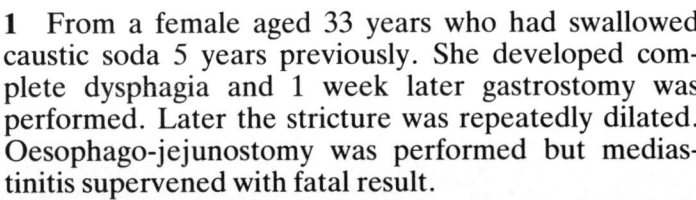

2 From a female aged 16 years who suffered from a stricture following attempted suicide by lysol. The stricture could not be dilated by bougies. Following oesophagoscopy she developed mediastinitis and death occurred 42 hours later.

G.C.10616

G.C.8863

peri-oesophageal tissues. This feature renders attempts at operative removal of the stricture difficult and hazardous.

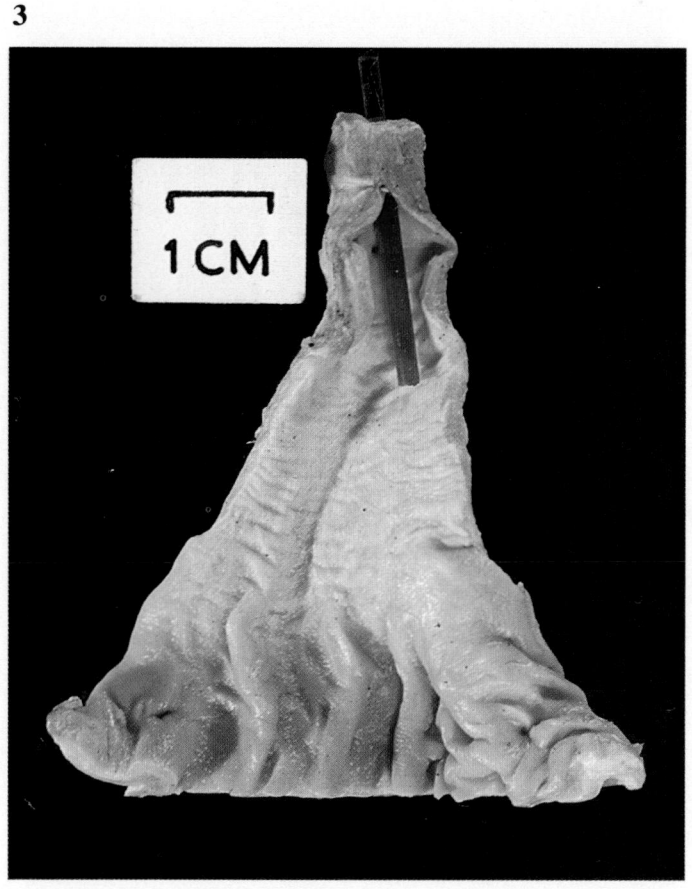

3 From a female child who died following the accidental ingestion of lye (caustic potash). This is a localised stricture of the oesophagus but with marked narrowing.

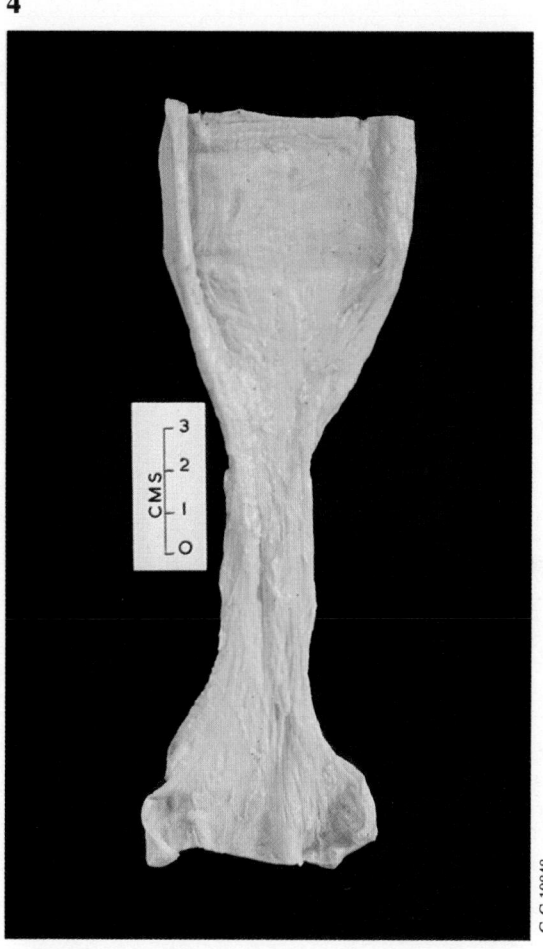

4 From a female who died 20 years after the accidental ingestion of lye. This is an old specimen dating from 1816. It is a tubular form of stricture of the lower part of the oesophagus. There is dilatation above the level of the stricture but the specimen shows little or no peri-oesophageal fibrosis.

Complications

1. Local – perforation, mediastinitis, broncho-oesophageal fistula.
2. Corrosion of gastric and pyloric mucosa is not uncommon leading to ulceration and subsequent stenosis (approximately 5%).

Embryology

Separation of the respiratory and upper alimentary tract in the foetus commences about the 4th week of life. The generally accepted concept is that a longitudinal laryngo-tracheal groove develops in the foregut caudal to the pharyngeal pouches. From this groove is formed the larynx and trachea; the distal end lengthening to give rise to the lung buds.

The tubular structure so formed is flattened laterally and divides in a caudo-cephalic direction to create two separate tubes, the oesophagus dorsally and the trachea ventrally.

The primitive oesophagus is formed by a core of multi-layered epithelium. By vacuolation a lumen develops. The lining cells are initially both columnar and ciliated but after the 5th month the primitive mucosa is formed by squamoid cells. The mesodermal tissues surrounding this primitive epithelial core undergo transition into muscle tissue which at the cephalic end of the primitive oesophagus is striated and in the lower part plain muscle.

Incomplete separation will result in a fistula without atresia. Imperfect development of the lateral oesophageal groove may result in a separation of the upper and lower oesophagus and may leave a communication between lower oesophagus and trachea producing the common type of atresia.

Other embryological abnormalities of the oesophagus include duplications (enterogenous cysts) and posterior enteric remnants. Both are thought to arise when buds of epithelium protrude into the subepithelial tissues to form diverticula which may or may not remain in communication with the oesophagus. An enterogenous cyst lies in close proximity to the oesophagus and may share a common blood supply and muscle coat. A posterior enteric remnant may be associated with splitting the primitive notochord and may result in either a cystic lesion or a fistula which involves vertebrae, spinal cord and overlying skin. The cysts may have gastric mucosa in the lining causing ulceration and even perforation.

Tracheo-oesophageal fistula and atresia

The incidence of tracheo-oesophageal fistula and atresia is 1:1000 to 1:4000 live births. There is no sex difference or familial incidence. The birth weight of the baby with oesophageal atresia tends to be lower than average, and pregnancy resulting in a baby with oesophageal atresia is often complicated by hydramnios from a failure of absorption of amniotic fluid during intra-uterine life.

Tracheo-oesophageal fistula is associated with congenital heart disease in 20% of patients. Other co-existing congenital anomalies which have been reported include imperforate anus and hydrocephalus.

The condition presents as an inability to swallow after birth, with secondary inflammatory changes in the lung as a result of aspiration.

A variety of anomalies occurs depending upon:
(a) the nature, character and site of the communication between the oesophagus and the trachea.
(b) the nature and degree of the oesophageal atresia.
The most common of these anomalies are illustrated below.

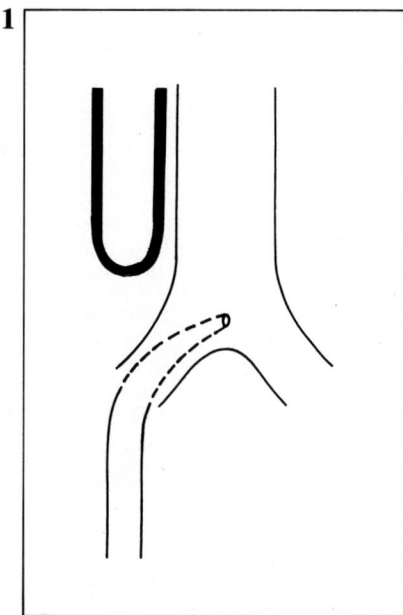

1 Complete occlusion of the oesophagus. The lower segment of the oesophagus communicates with the trachea. This is the most common lesion and found in approximately 90% of cases.

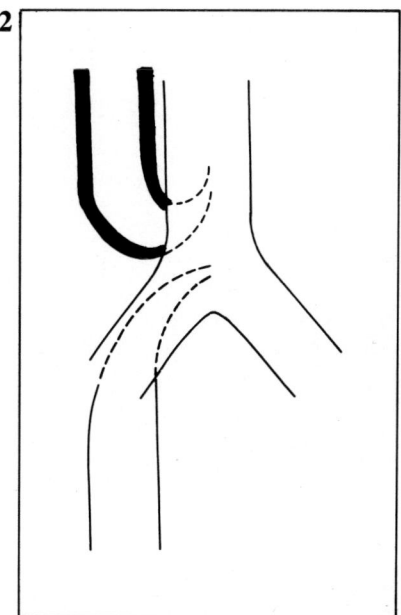

2 Complete occlusion of the oesophagus but both the lower and upper segments have a fistulous communication with the trachea (double fistula). This is found in 1% of cases.

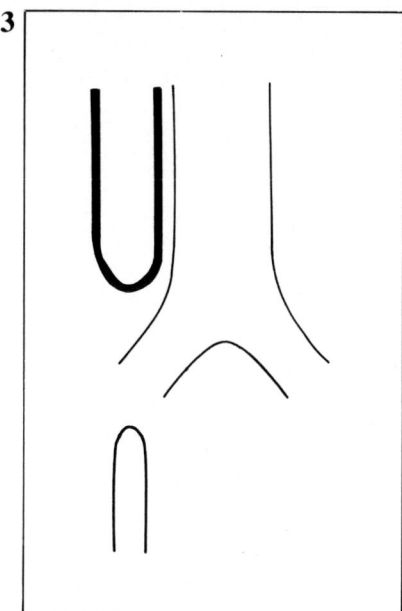

3 Complete occlusion of the oesophagus with wide separation of the two segments. No fistula formation. This lesion is found in approximately 9% of cases.

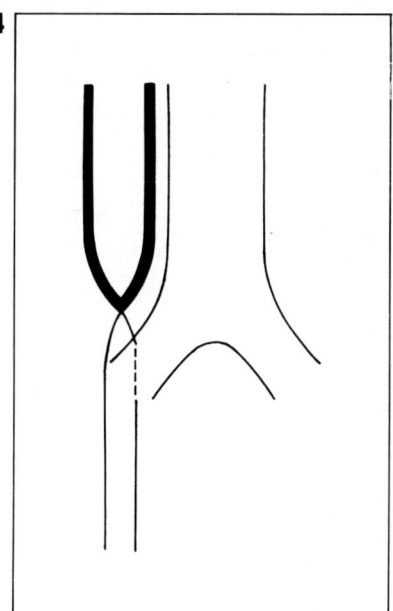

4 Occlusion of the oesophagus partial or complete and representing a narrow ring of stenosis. This is a rare lesion.

Tracheo-oesophageal fistula and atresia *(Continued)*

5

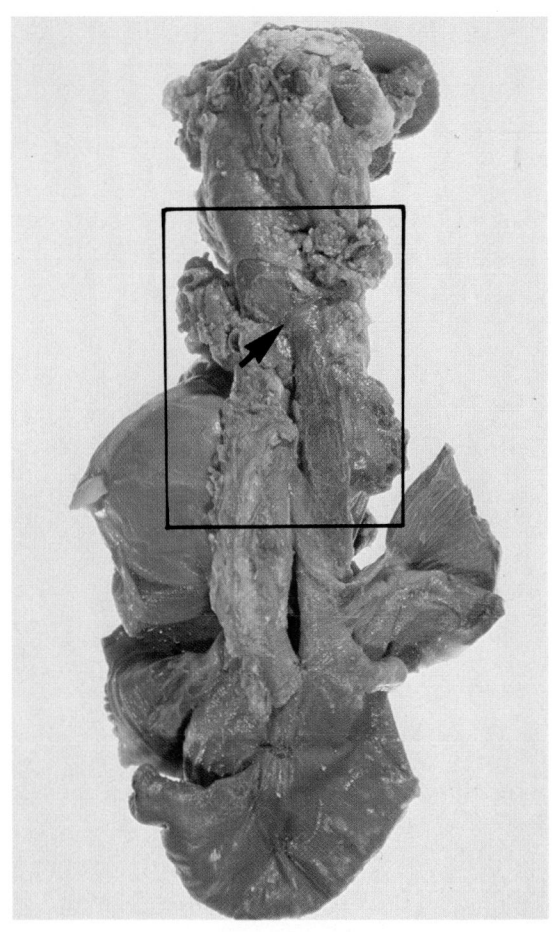

5 A full term female child who survived for 4 days. After feeding, the milk taken was regurgitated. The cephalad 30mm of the oesophagus forms an elongated sac terminating distally in a smooth, rounded extremity. The lower oesophageal segment communicated with the right main bronchus rather than the trachea in this specimen which illustrates the blind upper pouch overlapping the lower segment (arrow).

5a Enlargement of the area of atresia.

5a

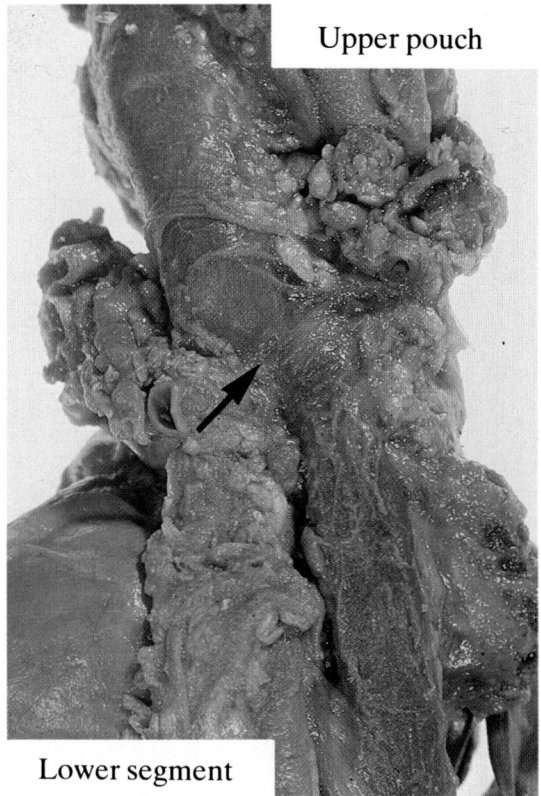

Upper pouch

Lower segment

A further variety of fistula is the 'H type' which occurs in 3 to 4% of all anomalies of the upper oesophagus. This isolated fistula is at a higher level than that seen in association with atresia of the oesophagus and the diagnosis is made by ciné radiography using aqueous barium with the patient in a prone position. It may be diagnosed in adult patients.

6

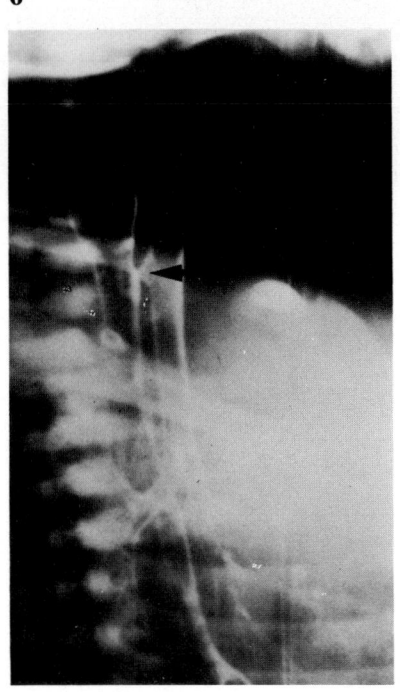

6 Ciné barium swallow taken in the prone position to show an isolated cervical 'H type' fistula.

7 Post mortem specimen showing an isolated tracheo-oesophageal fistula near the carina.

7

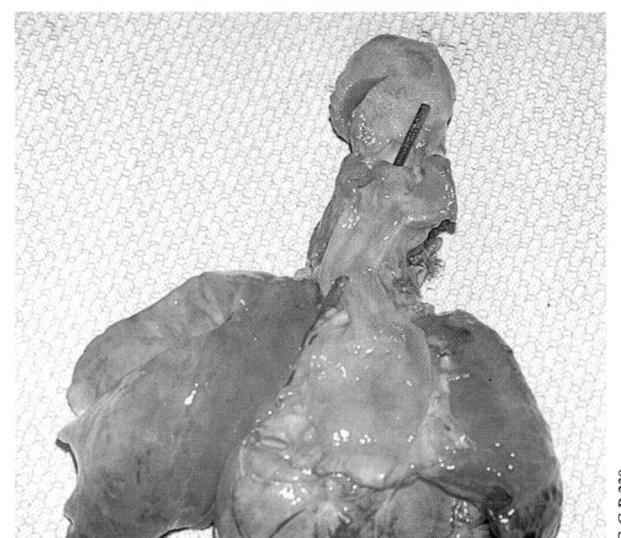

8

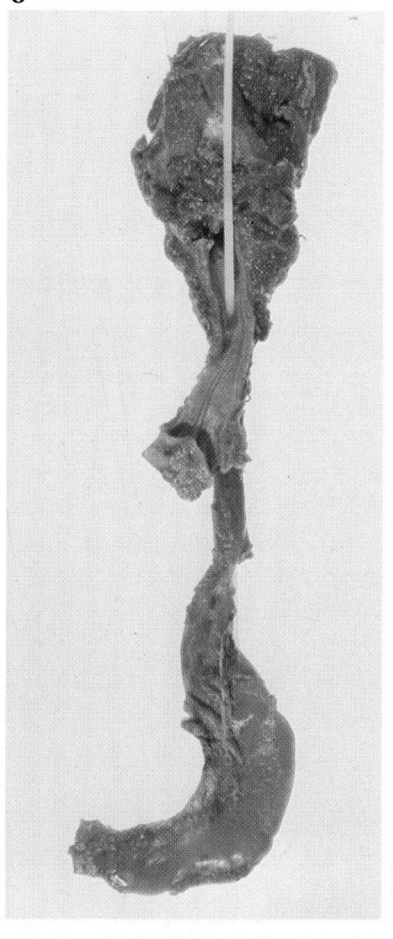

G.C.14335

8 Anterior aspect.

A specimen illustrating an uncommon type of oesophageal atresia. There is a high tracheo-oesophageal fistula shown by the white rod (anterior aspect) and a repaired oesophageal atresia shown by a second white rod (posterior aspect).

8b

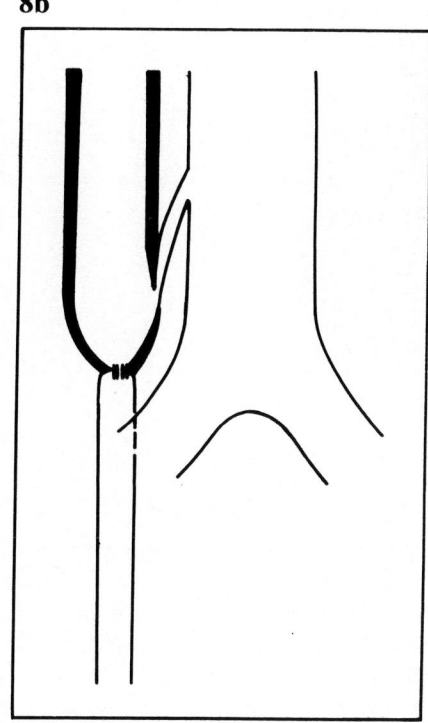

8a

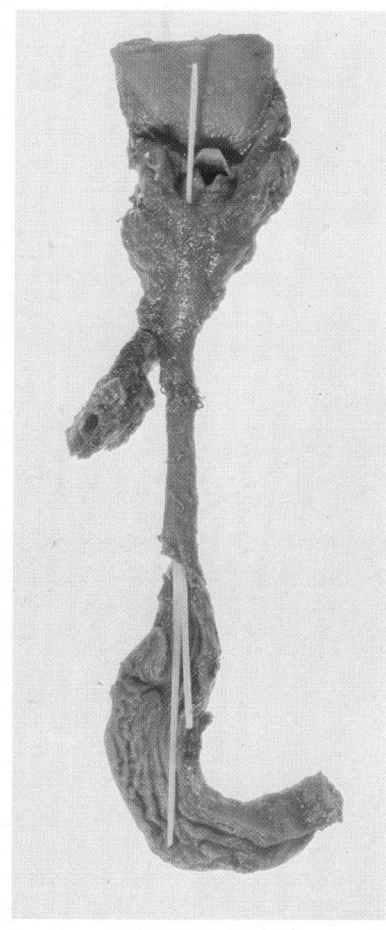

8a Posterior aspect

Diagnosis

9 The diagnosis of oesophageal atresia is confirmed by the passage of a stiff radio opaque catheter which will be held up approximately 10 cm from the mouth. Opaque medium may outline the upper oesophageal pouch.

An X-ray will indicate the level of the obstruction and gas filled bowel distally indicates the presence of a fistula. This X-ray shows the blind upper pouch and associated duodenal atresia (see Section 15B).

9

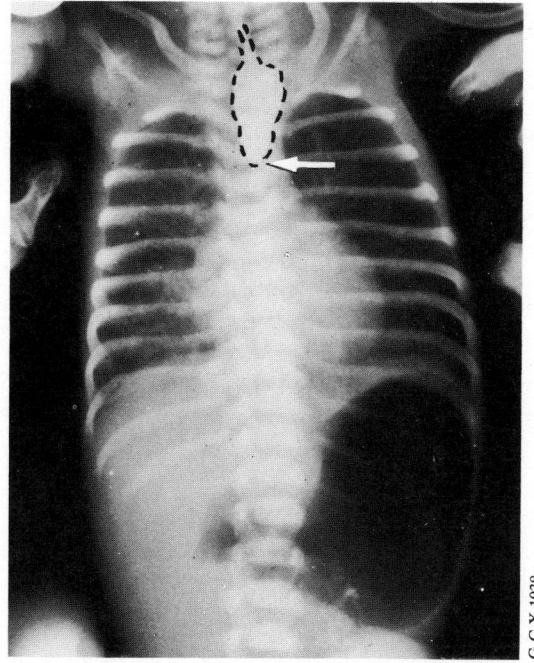

G.C.X.1038

Enterogenous cyst

Enterogenous cyst in association with oesophageal atresia without fistula.

10

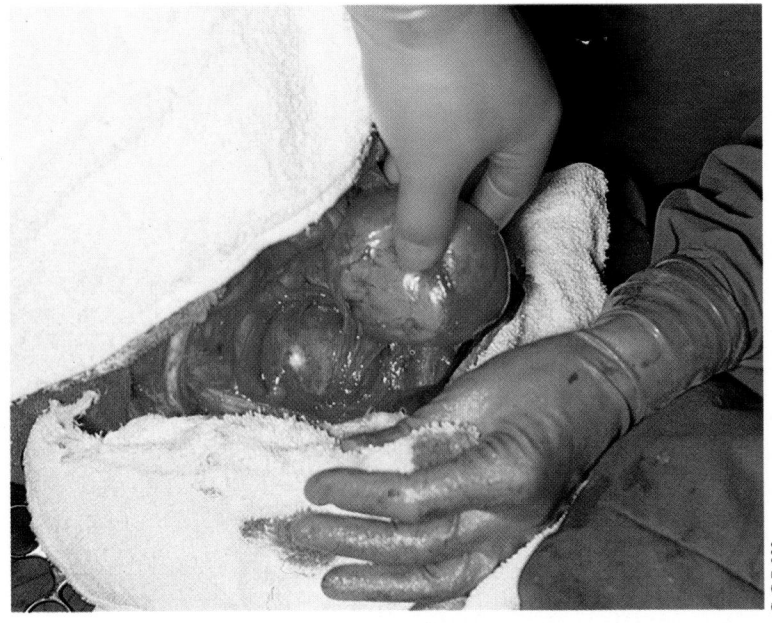

10a

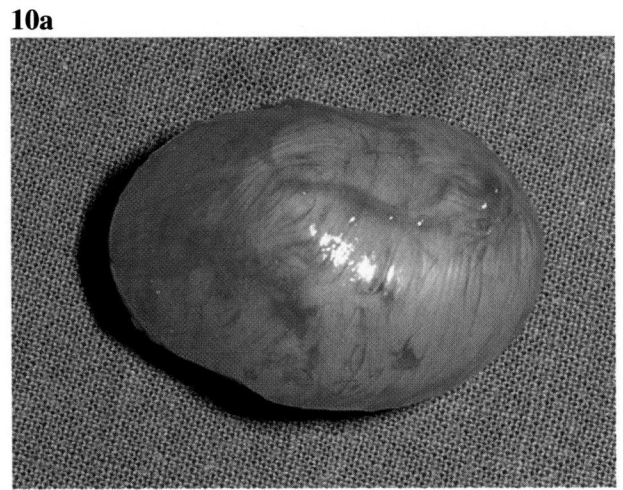

10 and **10a**   This was an incidental finding in a male aged 1 year undergoing colonic replacement of the oesophagus for oesophageal atresia. The cystic swelling was located in the posterior mediastinum just above the apex of the left lung when a tunnel was being made from the chest into the neck. The cyst was not attached to the oesophagus which had been brought out in the neck as an oesophagostomy at a previous operation. There was an associated thoracic hemivertebra.

Typically the cyst wall consists of rather flattened stratified squamous epithelium, with small foci of ciliated cells. Below is a scanty submucosa and two distinct layers of smooth muscle with fibres orientated in different directions. Between the muscle layers are small blood vessels, nerve fibres and a few ganglion cells. An alternative name for this lesion is an oesophageal sequestration cyst.

11

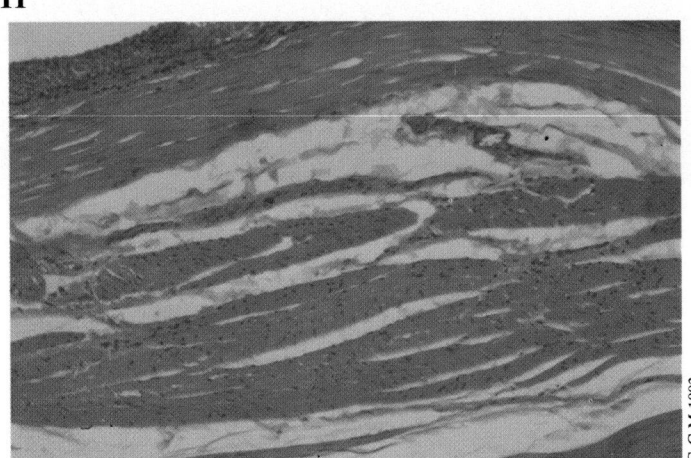

11   Part of the wall of an oesophageal enterogenous cyst. Fibrous tissue separates the epithelial lining (top left) from the underlying muscle. *(H&E)*

Anomalies of the oesophagus are not infrequently associated with abnormalities of the notochord and thoracic vertebrae.

Split notochord syndrome

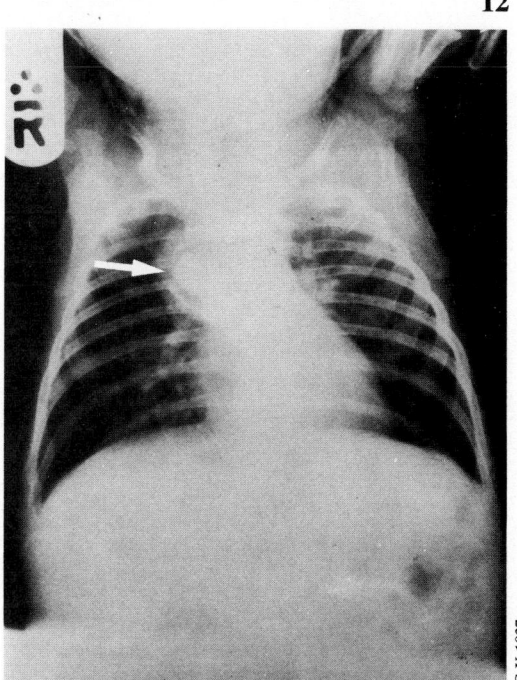

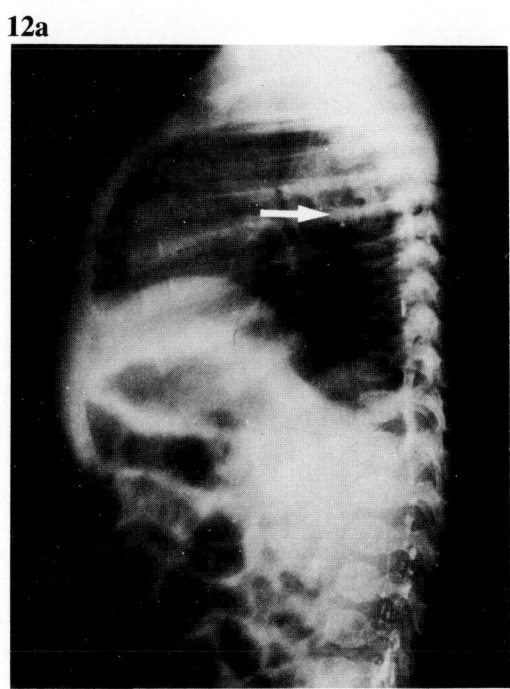

12 and **12a** X-rays of a female aged 7 years who presented with recurring attacks of aseptic meningitis. A myelogram shows contrast in a cyst in the posterior mediastinum which communicates with the subarachnoid space through a split in the 4th thoracic vertebra. Vertebrae above and below this level were also split.

A thoracotomy was performed to remove the major part of the cyst which was 10 cm in diameter and had gastric mucosa in the lining. The remainder of the cyst was removed by laminectomy.

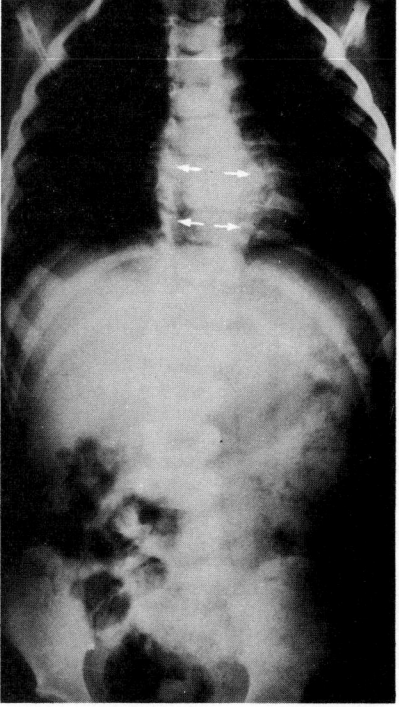

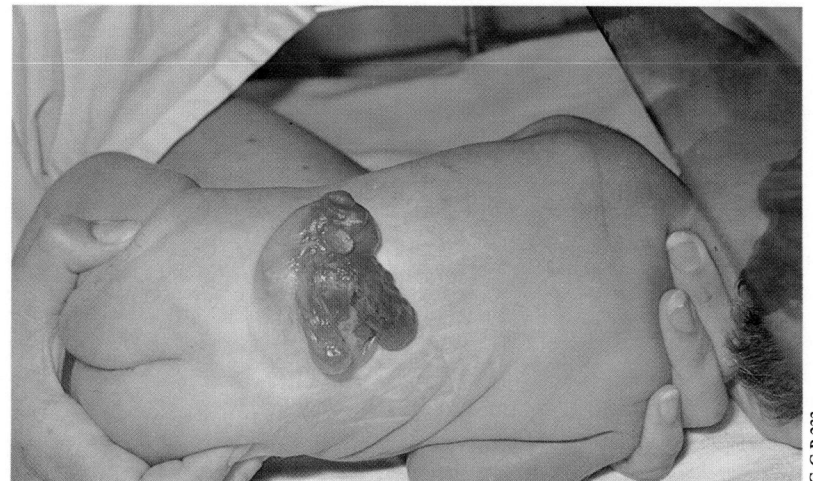

14 A lumbar myelomeningocele with ectopic mucosa. The defect communicated directly with the pelvic colon through a split lumbar vertebra and split cord.

13 Abnormal thoracic vertebrae showing widening of the interpeduncular distance from T7 to T10.

W.G. Scobie

Achalasia

Achalasia of the gastro-oesophageal junction (cardiospasm) has been long recognised and was first described in 1674.

    It occurs in patients of all ages, but mainly in patients aged between 40 and 50 years. Both sexes are equally affected.

This is a complex disorder of motility the cause of which is failure of relaxation of the 'cardiac' or gastro-oesophageal sphincter and is attributed to disturbance of neural control. Histological studies demonstrate degeneration of Auerbach's plexus with absence of ganglion cells. Some authorities believe this to be secondary to more central disturbance of vagal control.

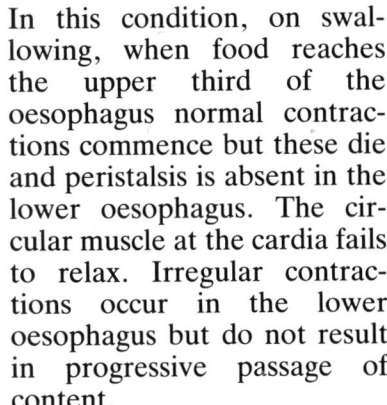

In this condition, on swallowing, when food reaches the upper third of the oesophagus normal contractions commence but these die and peristalsis is absent in the lower oesophagus. The circular muscle at the cardia fails to relax. Irregular contractions occur in the lower oesophagus but do not result in progressive passage of content.

The oesophagus shows gross dilatation with retention of contents and elongation resulting in a sigmoid conformation. The muscle wall is hypertrophied. The mucosa shows inflammatory change due to decomposing contents and superficial ulceration occurs. In very long-standing cases a degree of fibrosis occurs with true stricture formation at the lower end.

Radiology

The recognition of achalasia is established by radiological examination. The following features are diagnostic:
1. Dilatation of the oesophagus as shown either by the wide 'air space' seen in the central mediastinum indicating the lumen of the oesophagus, or by the breadth of the shadow of a barium swallow.
2. The elongation of the oesophagus and the sigmoid formation at the lower end.
3. The coniform termination with the narrow gastro-oesophageal junction.

Carcinoma

Malignancy occurs in approximately 10% of cases of achalasia. It is typically located in the dilated lower oesophagus and in 90% of cases is a squamous carcinoma.

Post mortem specimen of achalasia of the oesophagus. Note the elongation with an S-curvature in outline. The specimen has been opened throughout its whole length and displays the thickened mucosa with, in areas, a few longitudinal rugae but in its upper and lower parts the mucosa is flattened and stretched.

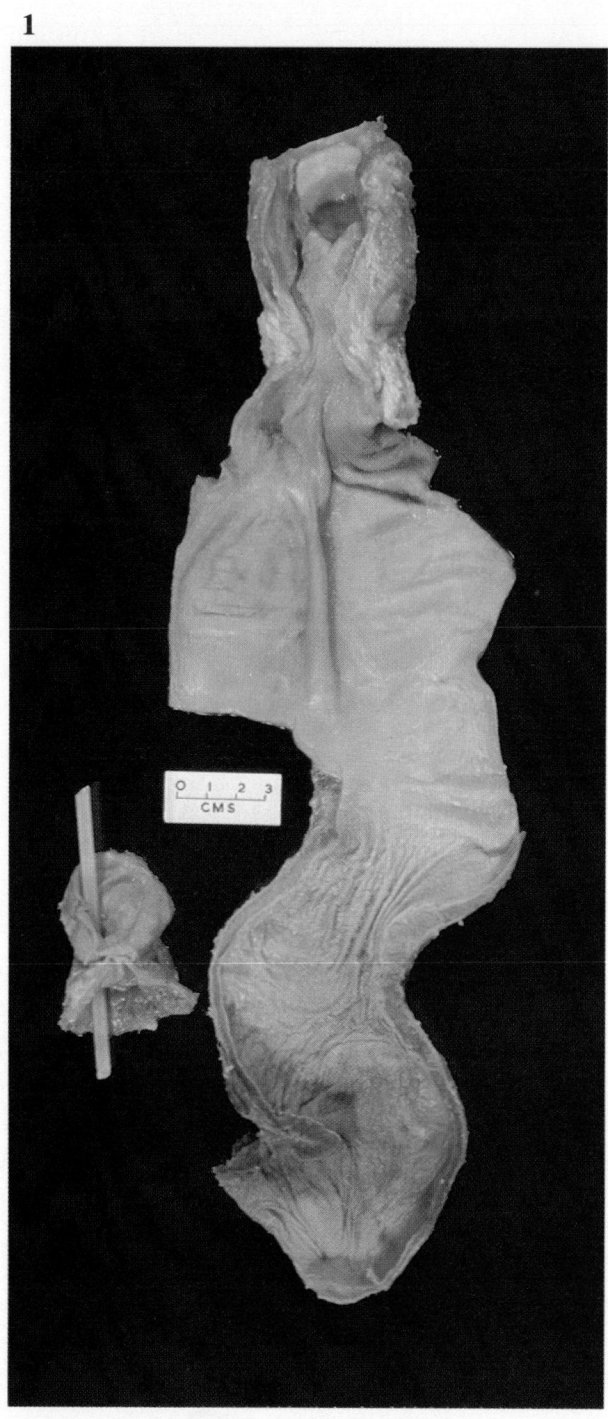

1

Note the flattened mucosa indicative of a chronic inflammatory reaction caused by the fermentation of food within the viscus.

Note the hypertrophied muscular coat which is especially marked in the lower third of the oesophagus and is attributable to the persistent irregular muscular contractions.

Gastro-oesophageal junction. The glass rod has been inserted through the narrow aperture. Note how the circular muscle is hypertrophied and narrowing of the canal is occasioned by failure of this muscle to relax.

G.C.14625

1 From a male aged 66 years. Recurrent dysphagia for many months. A Heller's operation had been performed some years previously and had been partially successful.

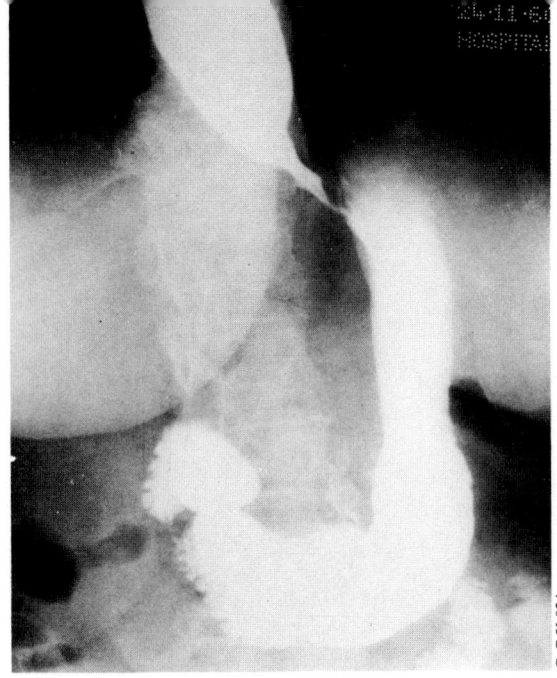

2 From a female aged 55 years. The oesophagus shows gross dilatation with coning at the entrance to the stomach and failure of relaxation of the high pressure zone.

←

G.C.X.924

3 From a male aged 60 years. Dilatation of the oesophagus with lengthening and sigmoid angulation. Coning at the entrance to the stomach.

→

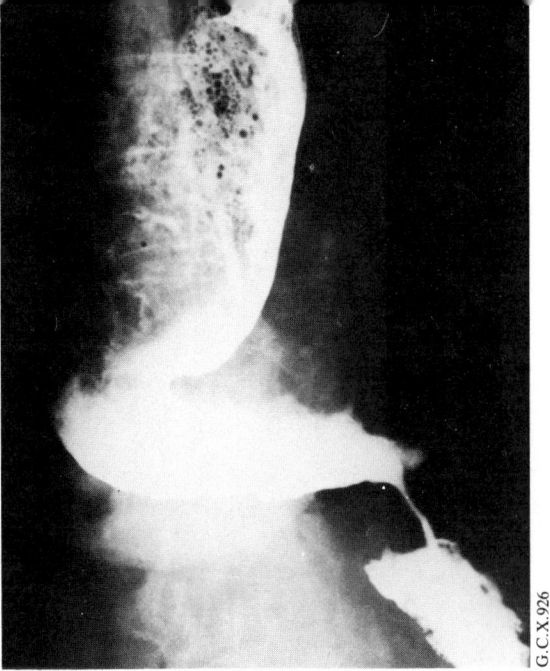

G.C.X.926

With carcinoma

4

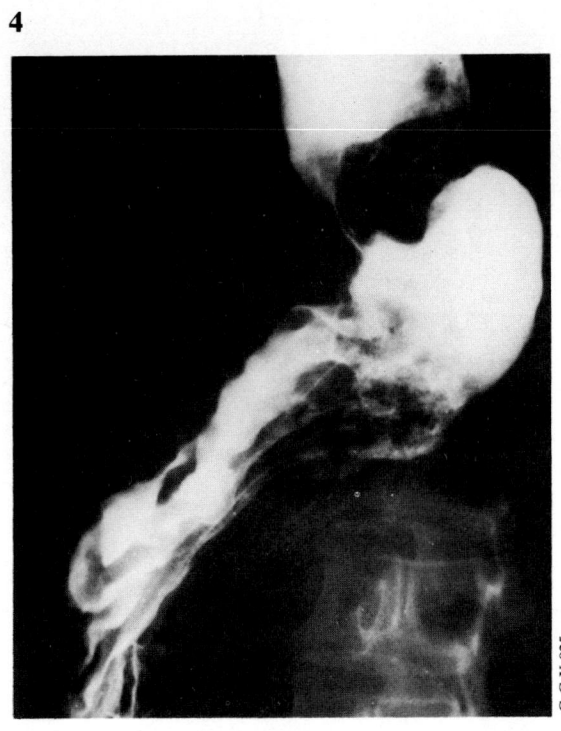

4 From a male aged 47 years. Dilatation of the oesophagus. In addition there is shouldering at the lower end of the distended gullet due to the development of a carcinoma.

←

G.C.X.925

Idiopathic muscular hypertrophy

This condition is attributed to long-standing irregular spasmodic contractions of the muscular coat in the lower two-thirds of the oesophagus. It is chiefly seen in the elderly and is associated with dysphagia and pain. It differs from achalasia in that there is no abnormal contraction of the cardiac sphincter and food passes into the stomach adequately. The muscle becomes hypertrophied. The condition has been ascribed to vagal hyperactivity.

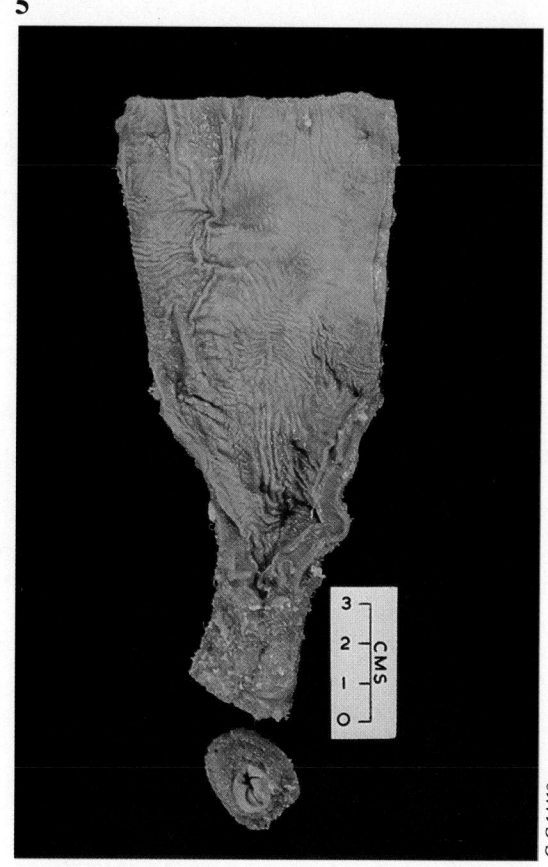

5 From a male aged 76 years who was admitted to hospital with an acute coronary thrombosis from which he died. There was no history of previous dysphagia. The abnormality was found at post mortem examination.

Corkscrew oesophagus

Irregular spasmodic churning contractions also due to vagal hyperactivity are sometimes recognised radiologically. The picture is bizarre and the term 'corkscrew' oesophagus has been applied. Only the lower two-thirds of the oesophagus are affected. The condition occurs in elderly patients. The oesophagus nevertheless empties adequately into the stomach and in contrast to achalasia no residue remains.

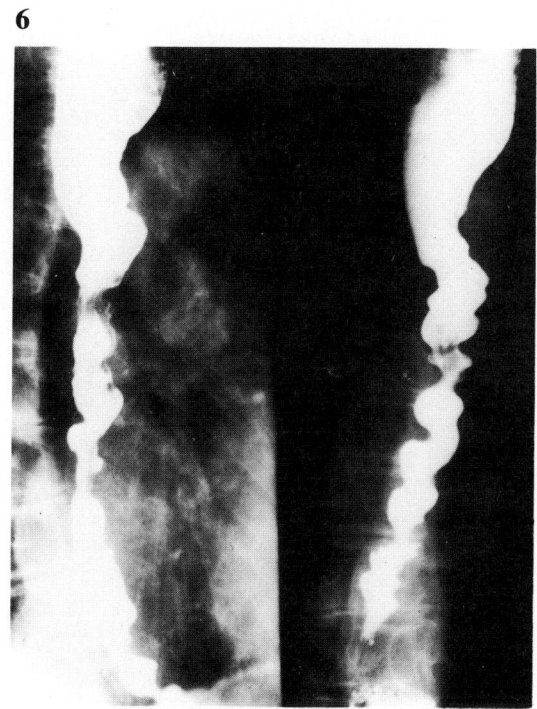

6 From a female aged 77 years who suffered from dysphagia and regurgitation of food.

Oesophagitis

A complex of lesions is found at the lower end of the oesophagus. These lesions are respectively reflux oesophagitis, oesophageal stenosis and hiatus hernia. While these conditions can be present and described individually they frequently occur in combination.

Reflux oesophagitis

Gastro-oesophageal sphincter

The oesophageal content is relatively bland and alkaline in reaction but the oesophageal mucosa is susceptible to injury from acid-pepsin digestion and bile salts. There is therefore an elaborate mechanism to prevent the reflux of acid gastric content into the oesophagus.

1 Factors involved in the prevention of gastro-oesophageal reflux.

1

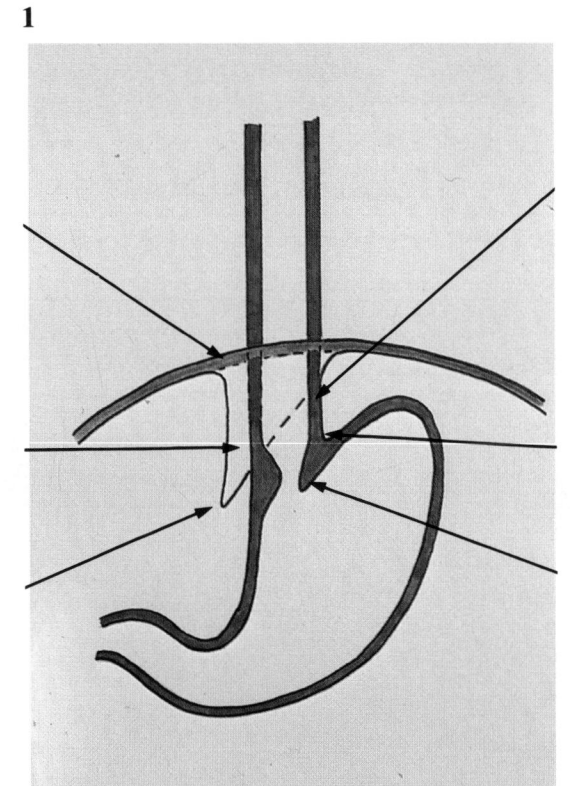

Phreno-oesophageal ligament.

Physiological sphincter or high pressure zone (H.P.Z.).

Pinchcock effect of the diaphragmatic crura.

Segment of oesophagus subjected to intra-abdominal pressure.

Fundo-oesophageal angle (of His).

Gastro-oesophageal mucosal rosette or flap valve.

The most important factor in the prevention of gastro-oesophageal reflux is the presence of a high pressure zone (H.P.Z.) which is under hormonal control (chiefly gastrin which increases sphincter pressure) and intrinsic neural control. Acid (gastric) or alkaline (biliary) agents may be implicated.

Aetiology

Reflux oesophagitis is due to abnormal regurgitation of gastric juice into the lower oesophagus. The squamous epithelium of the lower oesophagus does not possess an inherent protection against the chemical and enzymatic action of gastric juice and is therefore subject to damage. It may be recurrent or persistent. The reflux is facilitated or caused by:

1 H.P.Z. malfunction associated with congenital or acquired factors (scleroderma)
2 Increased intra-abdominal pressure – pregnancy
3 Hiatus hernia (sliding)
4 Vomiting
5 Obesity with local fatty infiltration leading to loss of fundo-oesophageal angle

Pathology

Reflux oesophagitis may be superficial but if prolonged, ulceration occurs and extends into the muscular coat and peri-oesophageal tissues. Superficial lesions heal completely. Deeper lesions are associated with fibrosis which may be followed by stenosis or contracture. Permanent mucosal changes also occur. Reflux oesophagitis commences at the gastro-oesophageal junction and extends upwards (2).

Colour code

Blue = Squamous epithelium
Red   = Area of oesophagitis
Green = Gastric mucosa

2

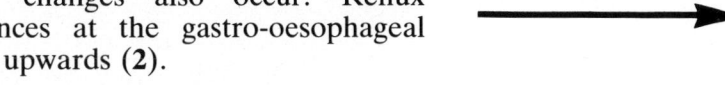

2 Reflux oesophagitis.

Mucosal changes

Changes in the character of the lower oesophageal mucosa have been described as apparently a sequel to reflux oesophagitis. These merit special consideration.

The gastro-oesophageal junction is a developmental site at which two types of mucosa meet; stratified squamous epithelium of the oesophagus and the columnar mucosa of the stomach. At such a site congenital variation is commonly found and at the gastro-oesophageal junction the anomaly seen is a replacement of stratified epithelium in the oesophagus by columnar epithelium. This may be circumferential or patchy and it extends upwards for a variable distance in the oesophagus. Following inflammation in which squamous epithelium has been destroyed, when healing occurs areas of apparent replacement of the lost stratified epithelium by columnar epithelium may be observed. The significance of this finding is controversial. It has been held that:

1 There has been metaplasia of the stratified epithelium into columnar epithelium.
2 Islets of columnar cells have been present prior to the inflammation. These were not destroyed during the inflammatory process and are able during the period of recovery to proliferate.
3 There has been an upward extension of columnar mucosa over the ulcerated lower oesophageal surface as a replacement lining.

The present view is that the latter two mechanisms are the most prominent.

Reflux oesophagitis *(Continued)*

3a

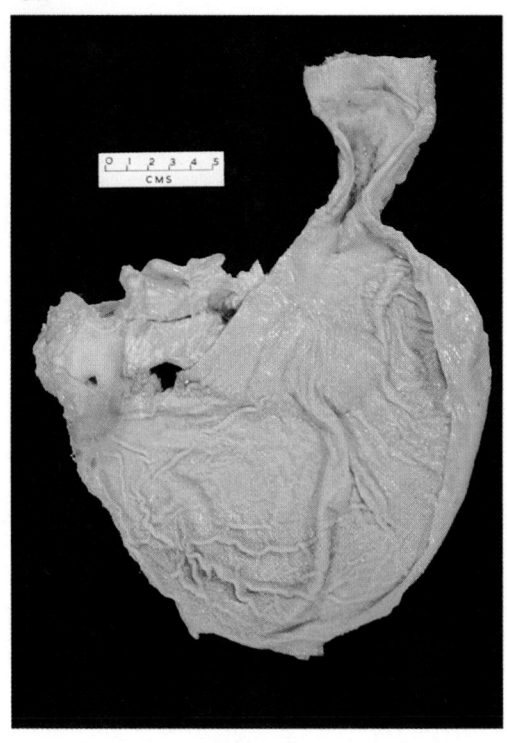

G.C.14635

3a and **3b** This is a specimen which demonstrates reflux oesophagitis associated with a perforated duodenal ulcer. It can be presumed that in this patient hyperchlorhydria was probably present.

3b Is an enlarged photograph of the gastro-oesophageal junction demonstrating an area of congestion and ulceration in the lower oesophagus associated with stenosis.

3b

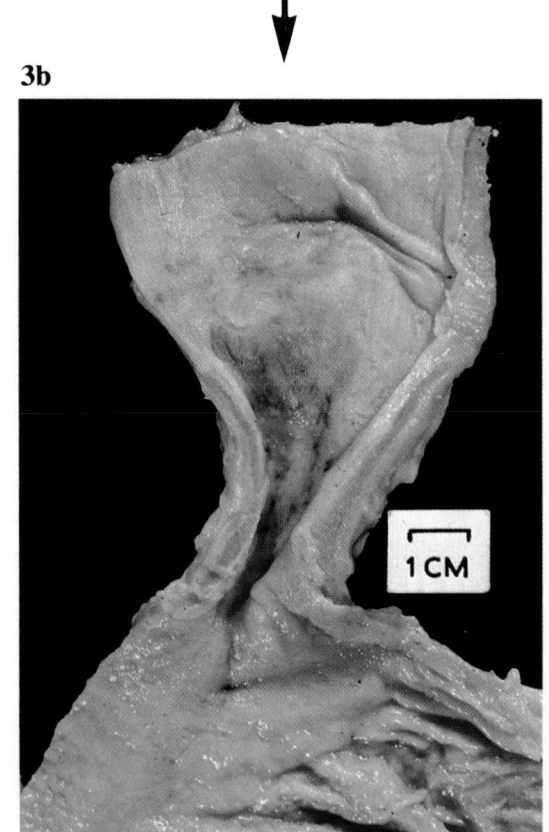

1CM

G.C.14635

4

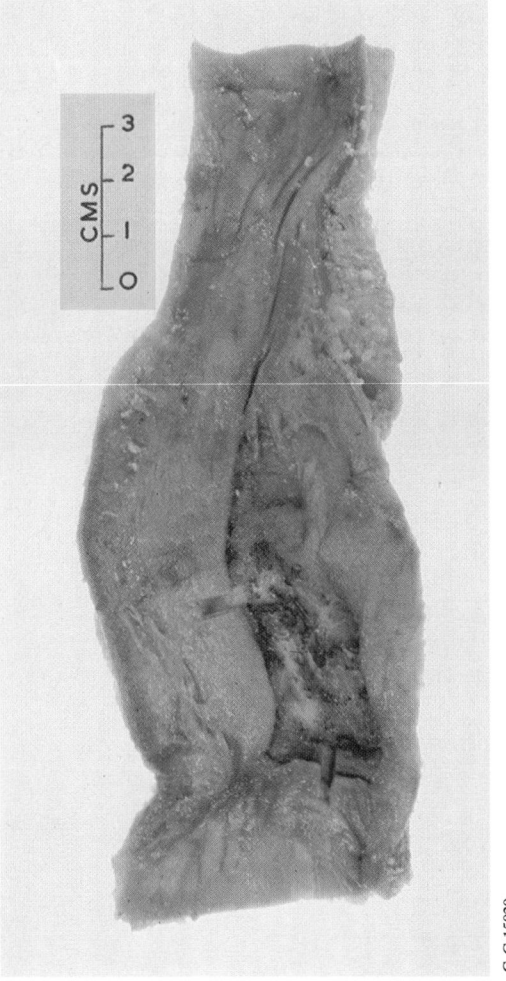

G.C.15029

4 Post mortem specimen of a patient who died from an unrelated condition. The man was 82 years of age and had a 10-year history of dyspepsia attributed to a hiatus hernia.

The specimen shows an ulceration 5 cm in length associated with fibrosis. Haemorrhage had occurred before death. The stomach was found to be full of clot.

From the naked eye appearances it would be difficult to state whether the ulcer is of a simple or malignant type.

Oesophageal peptic ulceration

A specific form of ulceration ccurs in the oesophagus arising in areas where gastric type mucosa exists. This form of ulceration is commoner in the lower part of the oesophagus although it has been reported at higher levels. The ulcer has the characteristics of a peptic ulcer and may lead to haemorrhage, perforation or stenosis. First described by Barrett, it is commonly known as a 'Barrett ulcer'.

5

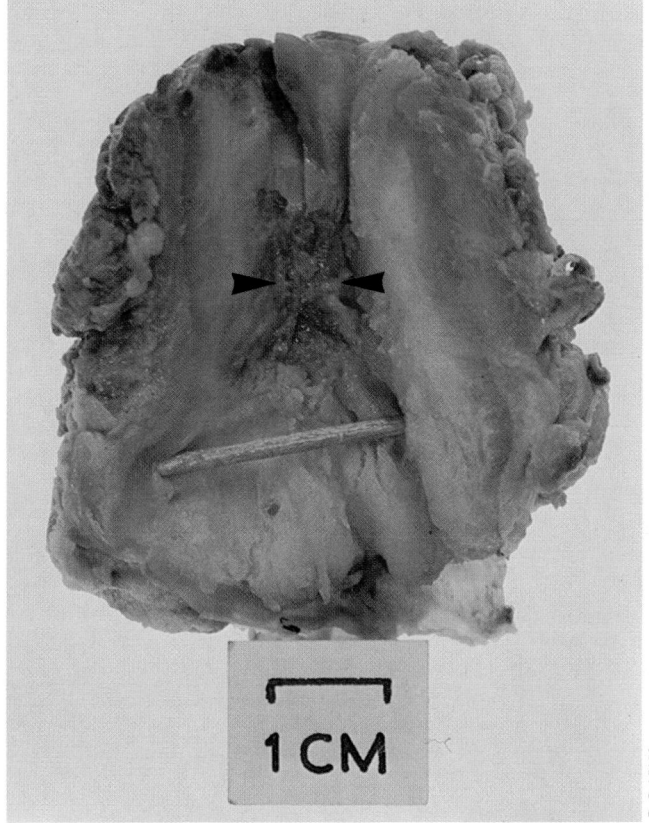

1 CM

G.C.15183

5 From a female patient with a 6-year history of epigastric pain, dysphagia and loss of weight. X-ray examination demonstrated the presence of a sliding hiatus hernia with peptic stricture and the appearances of a gastric ulcer at the gastro-oesophageal orifice. At operation a large ulcer of the lower oesophagus was found eroding into the sheath of the thoracic aorta. Oesophago-gastrectomy was performed successfully.

Stenosis

When the inflammatory process spreads more deeply affecting the muscle and outer coats of the oesophagus a degree of transient stenosis resulting from the oedema and inflammatory reaction occurs. If the condition continues, fibrosis develops leading to the formation of an oesophageal stricture.

Short oesophagus

The term 'congenital short oesophagus' has been applied where on radiological or operative evidence the gastro-oesophageal junction appears to be above the diaphragm or where the lower part of the oesophagus is lined by columnar epithelium without evidence of a preceding oesophagitis. These observations have been most fequently made in the presence of a sliding hernia in childhood. This developmental anomaly has to be differentiated from the upward displacement of the gastro-oesophageal junction which results from fibrosis consequent upon a reflux oesophagitis.

Stenosis *(Continued)*

Post inflammatory stricture

Stricture of the lower end of the oesophagus resulting from oesophagitis whether recurrent, chronic or with ulceration, is well recognised. The stricture may be limited to the point of junction of squamous and columnar epithelium where the normal squamous epithelium has been replaced by mucosa of a gastric type. It may involve a segment of the oesophagus extending to as much as 2 to 3cm. The fibrosis may pull the gastro-oesophageal junction upwards – acquired short oesophagus.

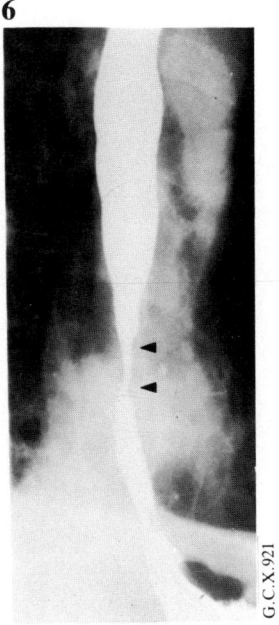

6 Barium swallow showing benign oesophageal stricture.

Endoscopic appearances

Endoscopic examination will establish the diagnosis. In reflux oesophagitis it will demonstrate the nature of the reaction and the presence of ulceration or stenosis. It is emphasised that the procedure can be dangerous owing to the friability of the oesophageal wall but this risk is somewhat reduced with modern flexible instruments.

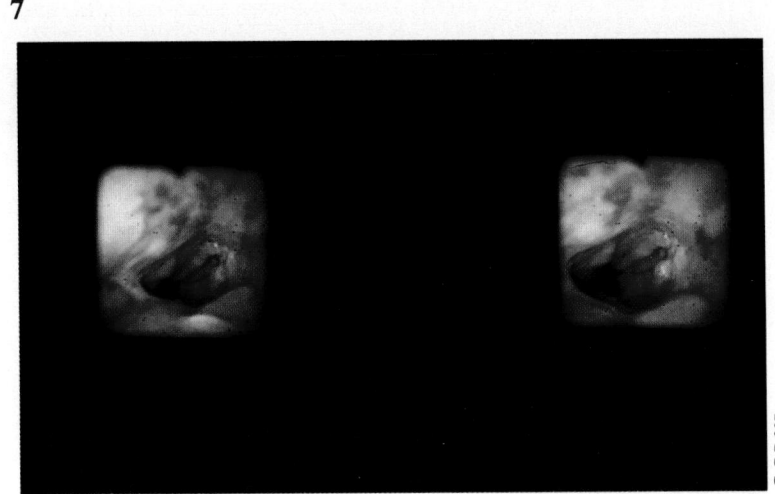

7 Endoscopic picture illustrating florid oesophagitis with superficial ulceration.

Reflux oesophagitis is not infrequently associated with hiatus hernia and it is appropriate, therefore, to link the study of the two conditions.

Hiatus hernia

The majority of herniae which pass through the diaphragm do so at the oesophageal orifice. Three types are recognised: Para-oesophageal, Sliding and Mixed.

Para-oesophageal hernia

This is a true hernia of a portion of the fundus of the stomach through the hiatus close to the oesophagus but possessing a separate sac in which the herniated portion of stomach lies. The gastro-oesophageal junction is normally sited.

Gastro-oesophageal sphincter function is normal and therefore reflux and consequent oesophagitis does not occur.

Complications are generally serious and include:
1 Incarceration and obstruction.
2 Gastric ulceration with bleeding or perforation.
3 Volvulus and strangulation.

8

9

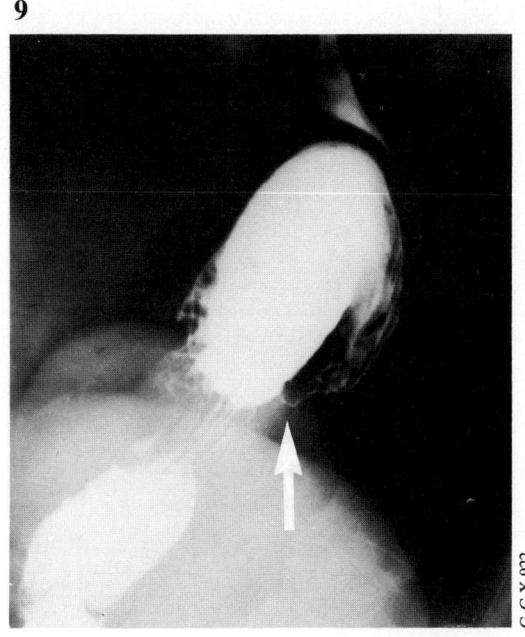

G.C.X.922

8 Diagram of a para-oesophageal hernia. Note that the gastro-oesophageal junction is normal in position and the hernia rises above this level in a separate sac passing through the hiatus.

9 Female aged 52 years. Radiograph shows a large para-oesophageal hernia which caused marked dysphagia. The gastro-oesophageal junction is normal in position.

Hiatus hernia *(Continued)*

Sliding hernia

This is the most common form of hiatus hernia.

(a) Congenital – found in the neonate and may be associated with failure to thrive.
(b) Acquired – a lesion of later life (40 to 70 years). Three times as common in females. Associated with a rise in intra-abdominal pressure and laxity of the oesophageal hiatus. Obesity is a common associated feature.

Surgical anatomy

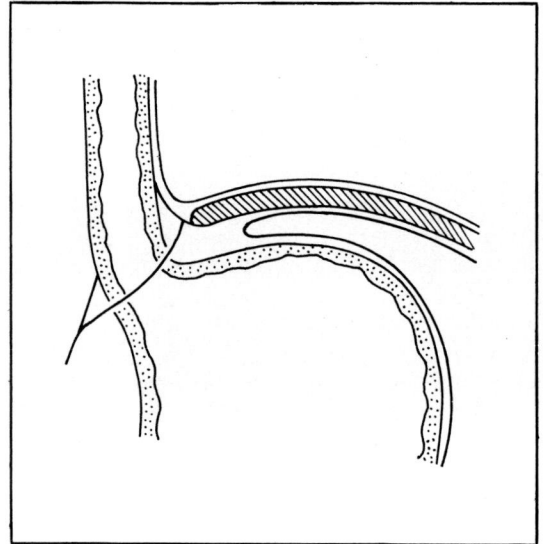

10 Normal.

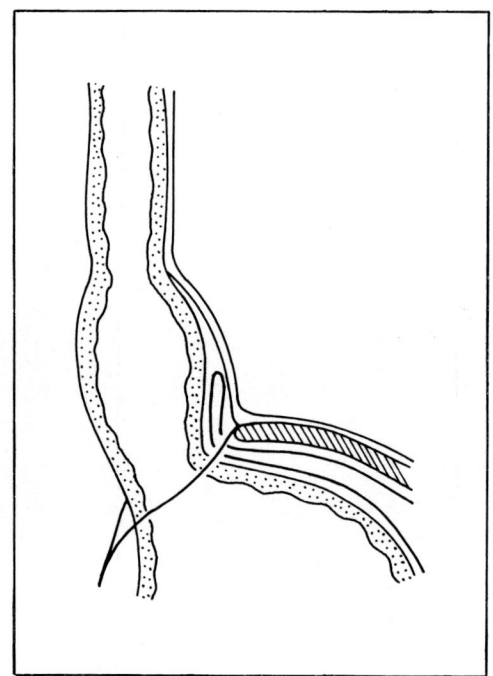

11 Small hernia. Sac anterior to the hernia.

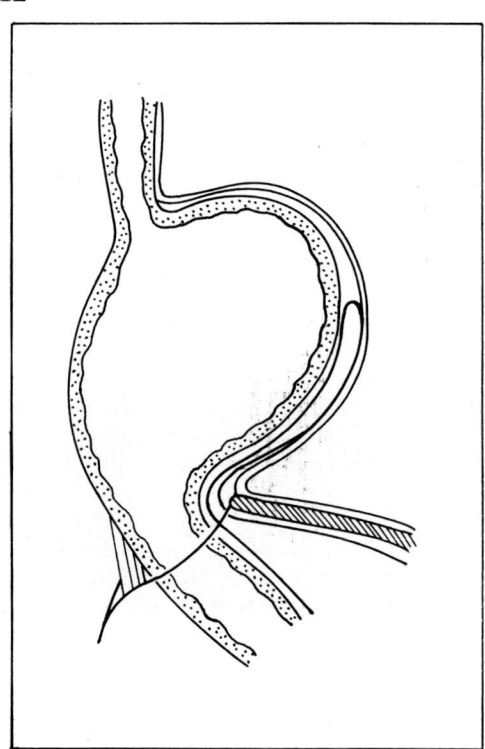

12 Large hernia. Peritoneal sac constitutes only a partial covering.

The diaphragmatic orifice is enlarged and the gastro-oesophageal junction, together with a portion of the fundus of the stomach, passes upwards into the thorax. In front of the stomach and oesophageal junction is a pouch (sac) of peritoneum.

The displacement may or may not be associated with dysfunction of the gastro-oesophageal sphincter. If the function is disturbed reflux oesophagitis, in one of its several forms, occurs, with or without complications.

13

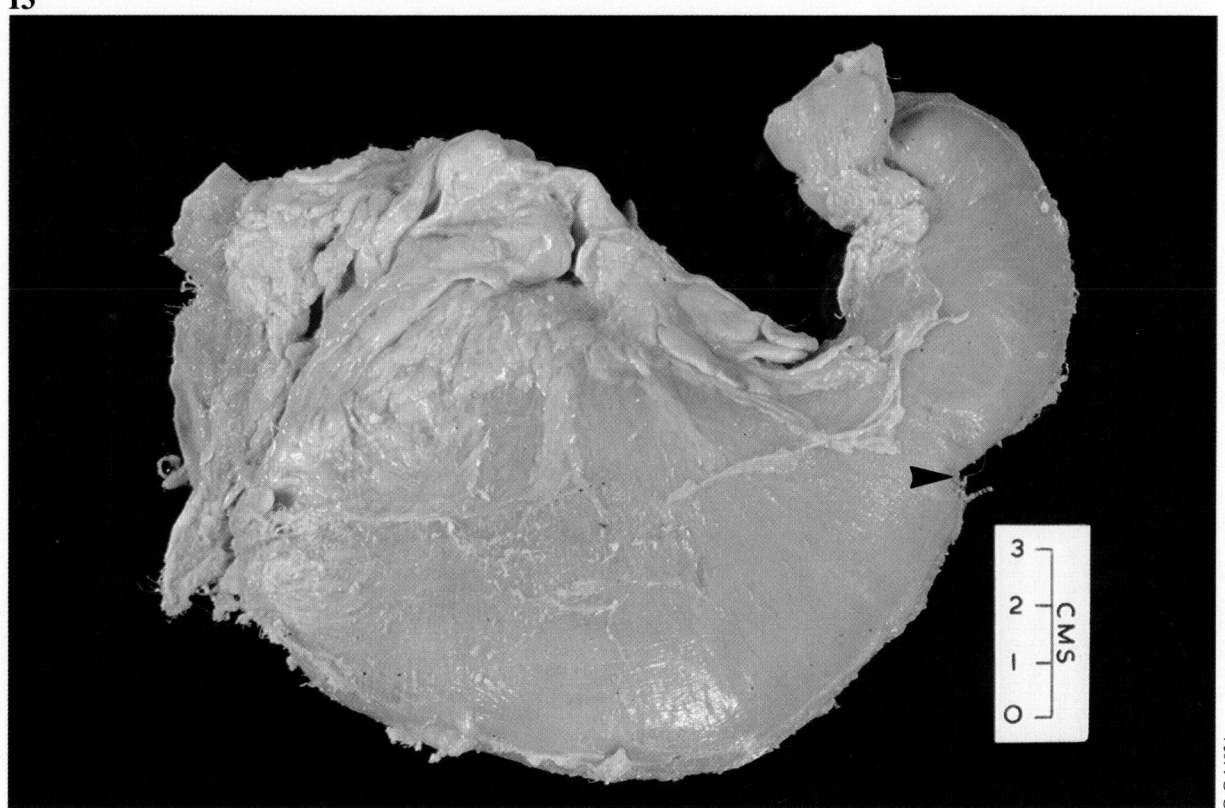

13 Post mortem specimen illustrating a sliding hiatus hernia. The arrow indicates the position of the hiatus above which will be seen the herniated portion of the fundus of the stomach and the gastro-oesophageal junction.

14

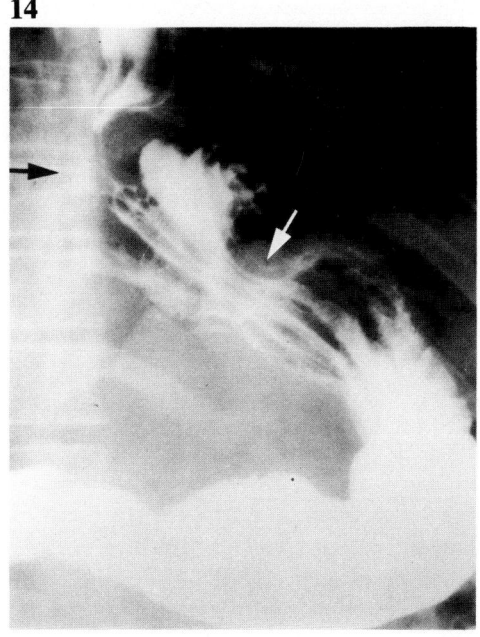

14 Radiograph showing the typical appearances of a sliding hiatus hernia in a female aged 40 years with symptoms of reflux.

The arrows indicate the position of the gastro-oesophageal junction high above the diaphragm (black arrow) and the level of the hiatus through which the herniated segment of stomach has passed (white arrow).

A. H. McLean Ross

Carcinoma

Incidence

Cancer of the oesophagus is common and in England and Wales accounts for 5% of all deaths from cancer. In the USA it is the third most frequent form of malignancy in the alimentary canal. Squamous carcinoma is an occasional late complication of achalasia (see Section 13 C).

There is a high incidence of the disease in Japan and China. It is also very prevalent amongst the Bantu in Africa in whom a nutritional deficiency is held to be of aetiological significance, especially when associated with alcoholism.

Age and sex incidence

Rare in young people, the peak incidence is in the 6th and 7th decades. There is a marked male preponderance (sex ratio M:F – 5:1).

Pathology

The majority of malignant neoplasms fall into two groups: the squamous carcinomas (squamous epitheliomas) – 90%, and the adenocarcinomas – 10%. The squamous carcinomas are found throughout the whole length of the oesophagus possibly most frequently at the points of physiological narrowing:

  at its upper limit (upper third)
  at the arch of the aorta (middle third)
  at the level of transit of the left bronchus (middle third)
  at the diaphragm (lower third)

The adenocarcinomas are chiefly found in the lower third of the oesophagus.

Squamous carcinoma

Histology

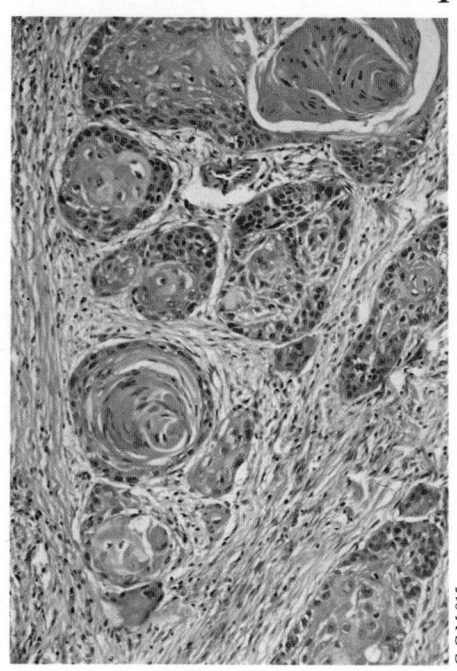

G.C.M.915

Squamous carcinomas of the oesophagus vary in their degree of differentiation. Most are well differentiated and in them prickle-cells and cell nests may be seen. At the other extreme solid masses of cells or spindle cells streaming into the stroma may predominate. Both can be associated with a variable amount of fibrous stroma.

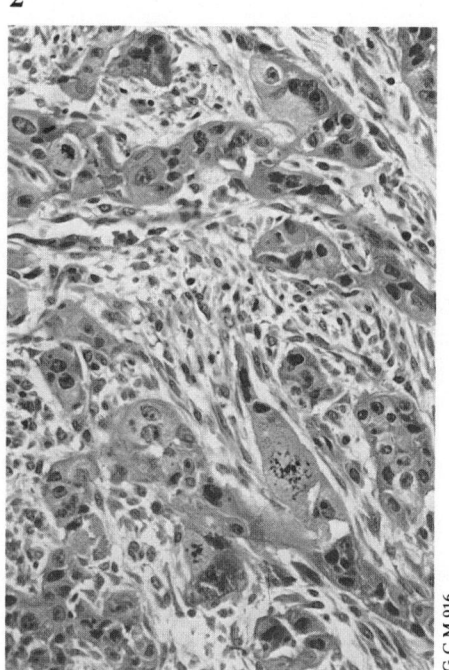

G.C.M.916

1 Well differentiated squamous carcinoma with cell nests. (*H&E ×125*)

2 Poorly differentiated squamous carcinoma with numerous mitotic divisions. (*H&E ×250*)

Macroscopic types

Ulcerative type

The ulcerative lesion is most frequently found in the lower oesophagus. The margins of the ulcer may project into the lumen and be associated either with deep excavation or have a polypoid appearance. The ulcer gradually spreads around the whole circumference.

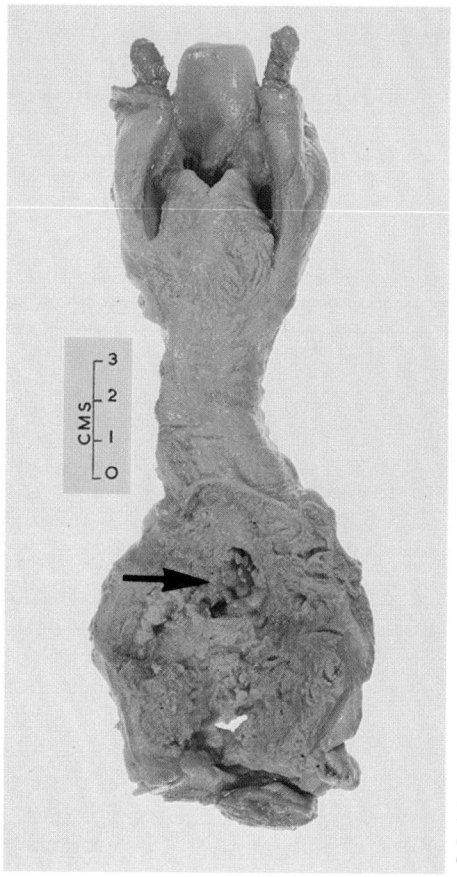

G.C.10854

3 The oesophagus at the level of the bifurcation of the trachea is extensively ulcerated. The edges of the ulcer are well-defined and the floor is irregular and shreddy. In the depth of the ulcer a communication with the trachea has formed just above the commencement of the left bronchus. Microscopically the ulceration is of a squamous-cell carcinoma with much round-cell infiltration.

Squamous carcinoma *(Continued)*

4

Tubular or stenosing type

Annular lesions are typically seen in the upper two-thirds of the oesophagus. Such tumours cause early obstruction and consequent starvation. The early lesion may be limited locally but rapid and extensive spread in the submucosa leads to involvement of a considerable length of the oesophagus producing a more 'tubular' form of tumour.

4 From a male aged 86 years. Squamous carcinoma of the oesophagus. Treated by routine course of irradiation but died 3 months later. The specimen illustrates a neoplasm in which there has been narrowing of the lumen but the tumour is still limited to the oesophageal wall. The main tumour is ovoid and 5cm in length (bracket). It has spread distally in the submucosa and there is ulceration both at this site (arrow) and in the main tumour.

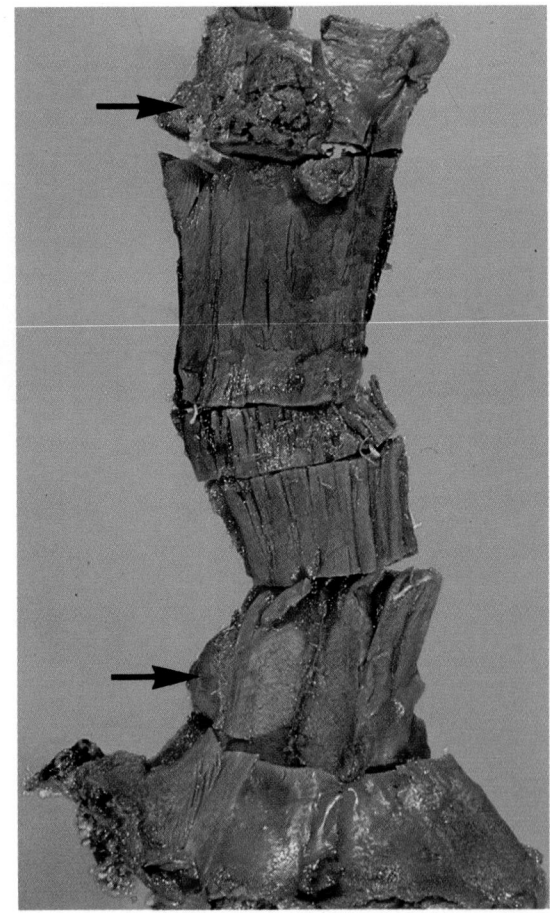

5

Submucous spread

In the submucosa of the oesophagus there is a rich lymphatic plexus in which the early spread of the neoplasm occurs. This is both upwards and downwards: as much as 10cm beyond the macroscopic edge of the tumour. The overlying mucosa may remain intact or ulcerate in places giving the appearance of multiple primary tumours.

5 The submucous spread has been held on occasion to be responsible for the appearance of two or more apparently separate naked eye tumours. In the specimen illustrated, which was from a male aged 66 years, two tumours of the oesophagus were found but repeated sections taken at intervals (note how the specimen has been reconstructed) failed to demonstrate any malignant cells apparently passing from one site to the other. This, therefore, would appear to be a true example of multiple carcinoma but even in this case the evidence is not conclusive.

Lymphatic spread

Lymphatic dissemination outwith the wall of the oesophagus is common. From lesions in the upper third, lymphatic spread is generally to the lower cervical nodes. From the lower two-thirds spread is to the mediastinum, to the nodes along the lesser curvature of the stomach, and to the nodes about the coeliac axis.

Even in lesions of the middle third which appear to be resectable, it is common to find lymphatic metastasis below the diaphragm around the gastro-oesophageal junction (30%).

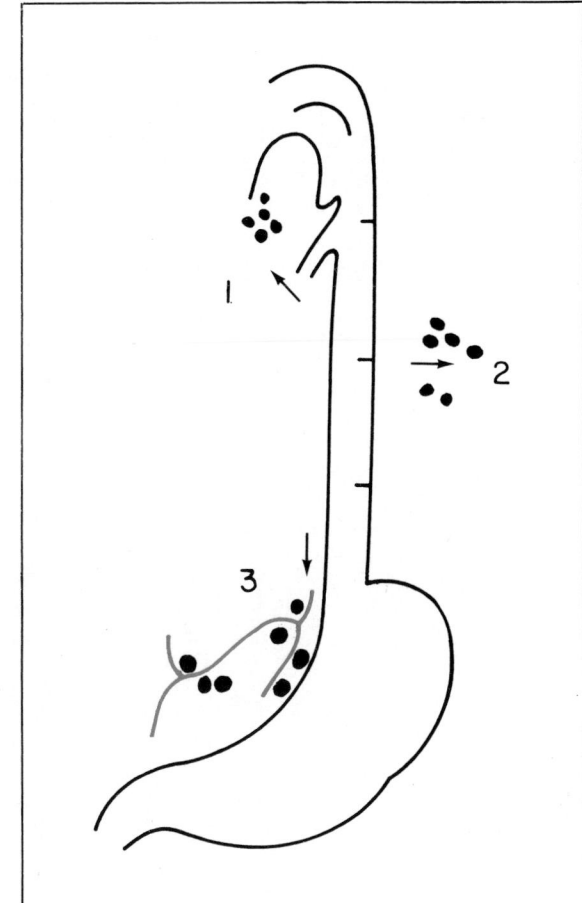

6

1 Lower cervical
2 Mediastinal
3 Coeliac axis and left gastric artery

Involvement of adjacent tissues

Direct spread with involvement of adjacent tissues and organs is common. In tumours of the upper third, involvement of the trachea may lead to tracheo-oesophageal fistula formation. Involvement of the left recurrent laryngeal nerve is, however, very rare. In lesions of the middle third the trachea or bronchi again may be involved as in upper third lesions.

7

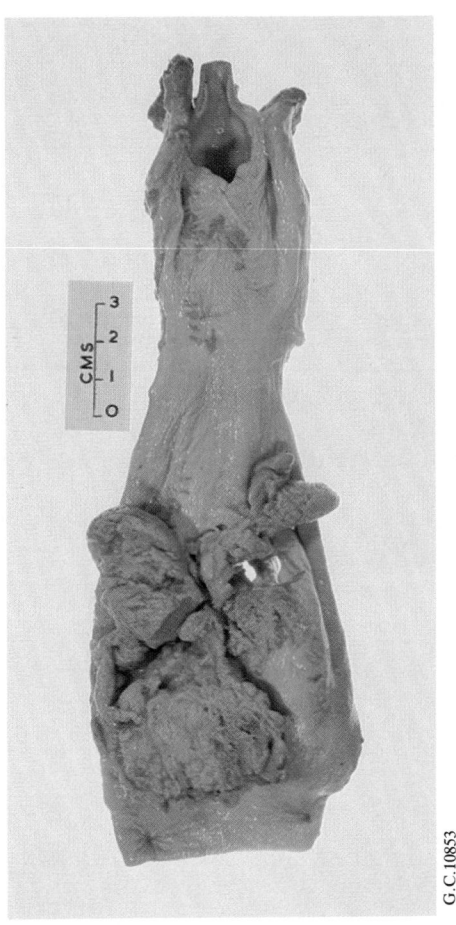

7 From a male aged 70 years. A historical specimen originally described by Sir Charles Bell in 1816. This is a large ulcerating carcinoma with polypoidal masses which has perforated the wall of the oesophagus leading to a para-oesophageal abscess which eventually tracked to the left axilla where a large abscess was present.

Squamous carcinoma *(Continued)*

Involvement of aorta

Extensive spread into the mediastinal tissues occurs and the aorta may be invaded with fistula formation and fatal haemorrhage. In the lower third invasion of the aorta also occurs.

8a

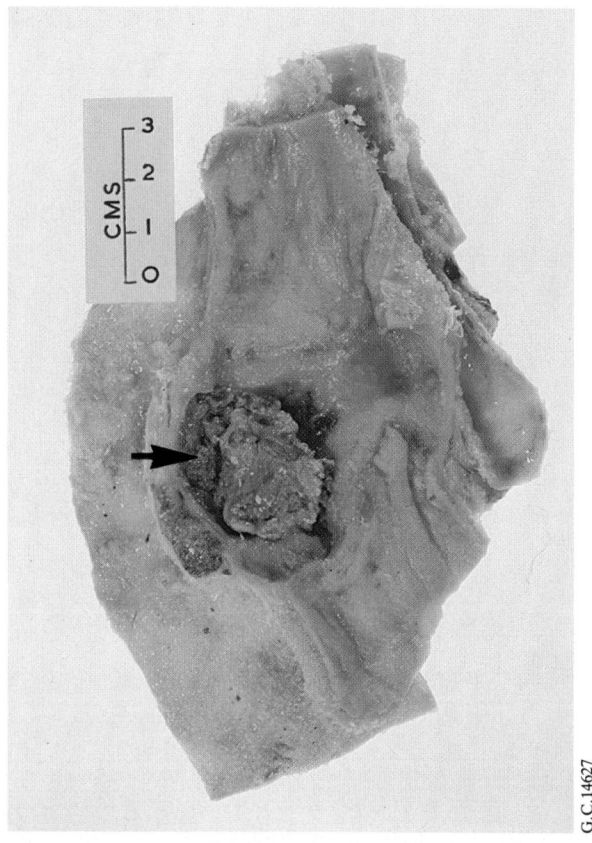

8b

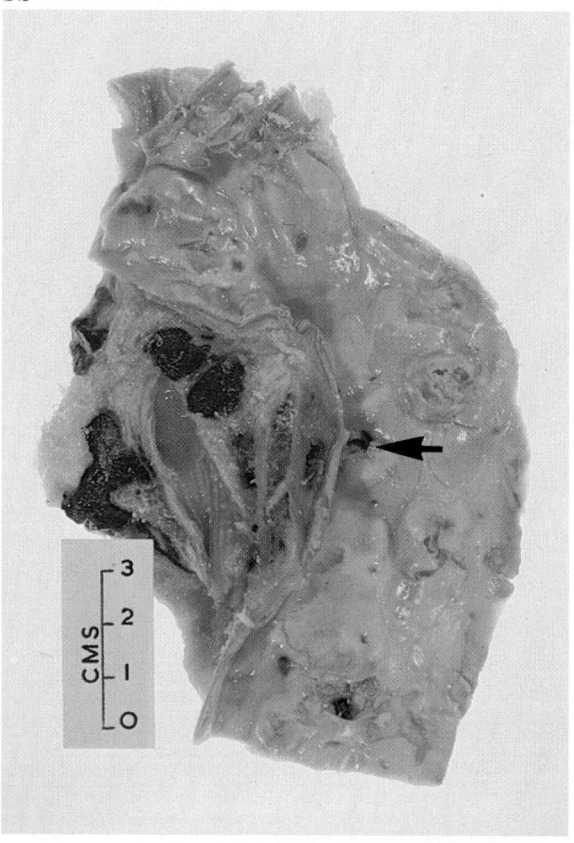

8a and **8b**   From a female aged 71 years. Dysphagia 8 months. Received radiation treatment followed temporary improvement. Later severe fatal haemorrhage.
(a) A large carcinomatous ulcer at the level of the bifurcation of the trachea. At the base of the ulcer v a narrow aperture communicating with the aorta at the site of an atheromatous plaque.
(b) Shows the atheromatous aorta. The fistulous opening lies near the origin of one of the right intercos arteries and there is a haematoma in the para-aortic tissues.
The fistula formation may be partially attributable to radiation necrosis.

Haematogenous spread is usually late but is seen in 33% of post mortem studies.

Respiratory complications are common. While some may be the sequel to fistula formation, many occur as the result of regurgitation of oesophageal contents into the trachea. This leads to a bronchopneumonia which frequently is terminal.

Radiology

9

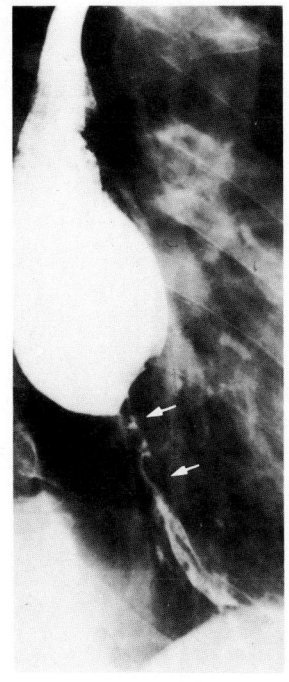

The radiograph will show either the 'rat tail' narrowing at the level of a stenosing carcinoma or the irregular surface of an ulcerative carcinoma. The oesophagus proximal to the lesion will show dilatation but never of gross degree.

9 Male aged 50 years. Irregular stricture: carcinoma with proximal dilatation.

G.C.X.105

10

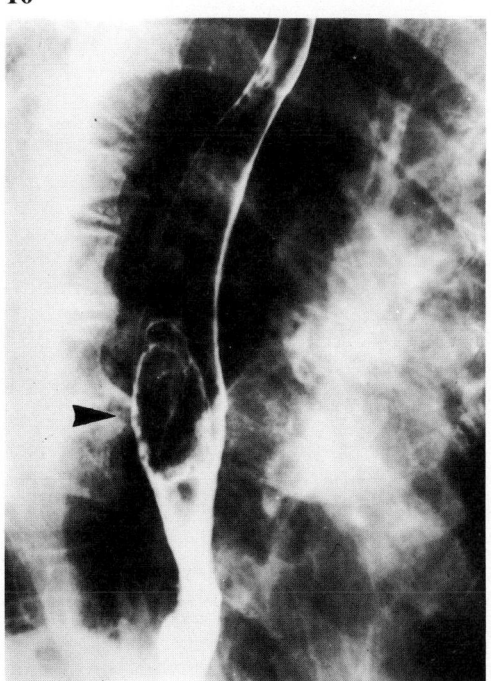

10 Polypoid type of tumour.

G.C.X.126

Carcinoma (upper third)

Squamous carcinoma of the upper part of the oesophagus is frequently comparable to carcinoma of the hypopharynx in that there is a high female incidence and the age of onset is early. Other features of the Plummer – Vinson syndrome may be present such as dysphagia, hypochlorhydria, hypochromic anaemia or Vitamin B deficiency.

11

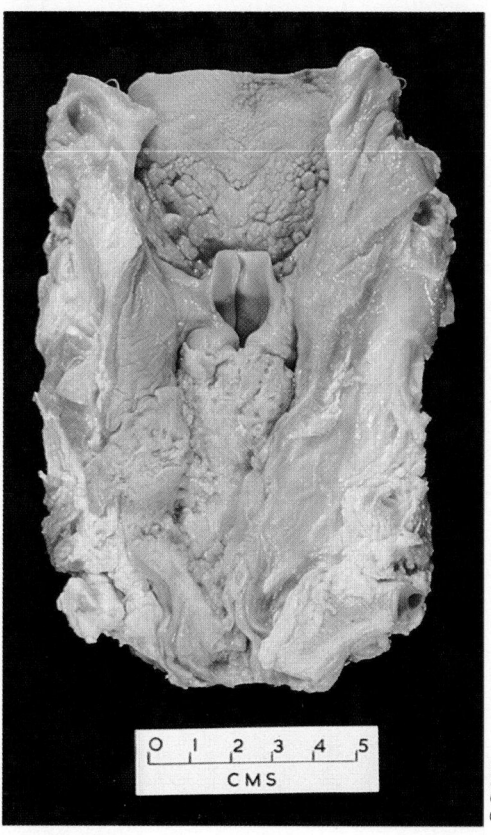

11 From a female aged 46 years. History of painful dysphagia for many months and oesophageal haemorrhage. Evident upper cervical lymphatic metastasis.

A tumour of the upper 4cm of the oesophagus is present especially involving the anterior wall. The surface shows a warty ulceration.

G.C.8520

53

Adenocarcinoma

Adenocarcinoma is most frequently found in the lower third of the oesophagus. The tumour is held to originate in three possible ways.

12

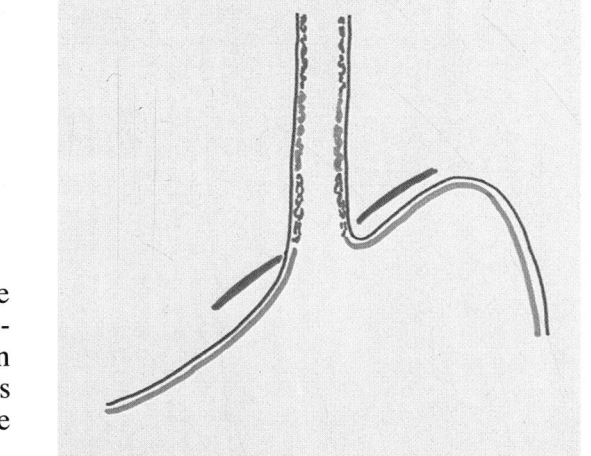

12 The relatively rare 'true' adenocarcinoma of the oesophagus arises from submucous glands or heterotopic gastric mucosa. These tumours may be found in any part of the oesophagus. The adenocarcinoma is surrounded by squamous epithelium and this is the criterion of diagnosis.

13

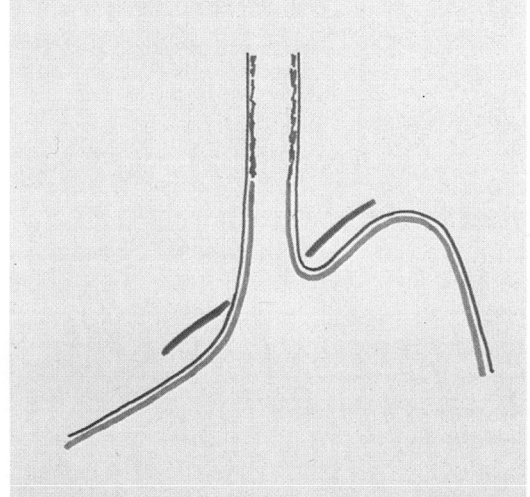

13 The adenocarcinoma arises from glandular epithelium which has replaced squamous epithelium eroded by reflux oesophagitis. It is not surrounded by squamous epithelium but is in a mucous membrane which passes downwards to be continuous with the gastric mucosa.

Colour code

Blue = Stratified epithelium
Green = Columnar mucosa
Brown = Diaphragm
Black = Carcinoma

14

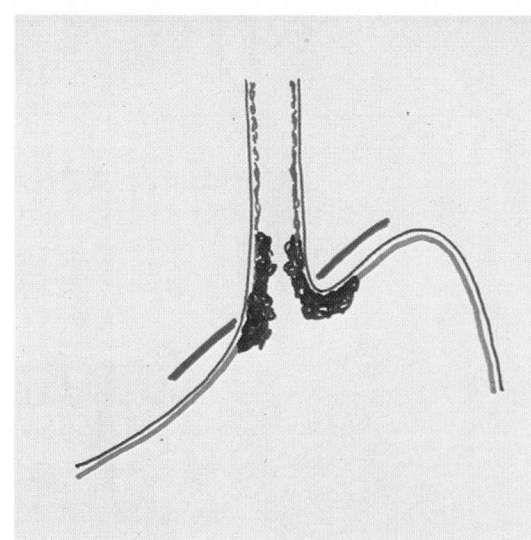

14 The adenocarcinoma represents invasion of the lower end of the oesophagus by a carcinoma of the cardia. There is difficulty in many instances in ascertaining whether an adenocarcinoma at the lower end of the oesophagus is a true oesophageal tumour or whether it represents the upward extension of an adenocarcinoma of the stomach.

These tumours are often polypoid with extensive ulceration. The oesophagus is expanded and the tumour infiltrates into surrounding tissues. Lymphatic spread is early and is both upwards and downwards into the lymph nodes about the left gastric artery and coeliac axis.

15

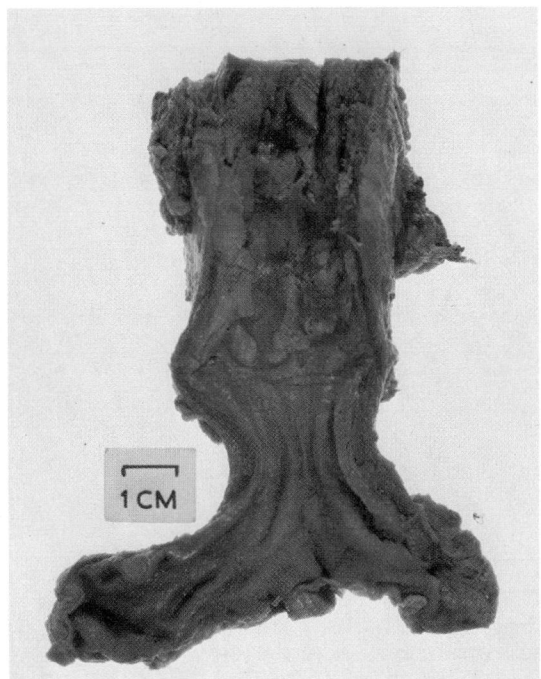

G.C.10978

15 From a female aged 65 years. Dysphagia for 5 years which suggests a preceding reflux oesophagitis. The diagnosis was established by radiology and oesophagoscopy. Ulceration is present in the lower part of the oesophagus and completely encircles the lumen. The surface is ulcerated and haemorrhagic. The edges of the ulceration are raised and irregular and the appearance is typical of a carcinomatous ulceration. The tumour appears to have arisen in the oesophagus approximately 2.5 cm above the cardiac orifice. Histologically the tumour is a well differentiated papillary adenocarcinoma.

This specimen illustrates the difficulty of determining the precise site of origin of the neoplastic change and the histological examination does not determine whether stratified epithelium is present distal to the tumour and accordingly whether the tumour is of type 1 or 2.

16 From a female aged 76 years. Dysphagia 3 weeks. Jejunostomy performed. The patient died of cardiac failure.

The oesophageal wall at the gastro-oesophageal junction is infiltrated and the lumen encroached upon by tumour which does not appear to have ulcerated. The primary tumour lies in the cardia as a projecting mass close to the oesophageal orifice. Several small shallow ulcers can be seen above the obstructing tumour – erosive oesophagitis.

Histologically the tumour is an adenocarcinoma which can be seen to originate in the mucosa of the cardia from which it extends deeply into the muscle layer of the stomach and upwards into the oesophageal wall in the submucosa and muscle layer.

This is an example of type 3.

16

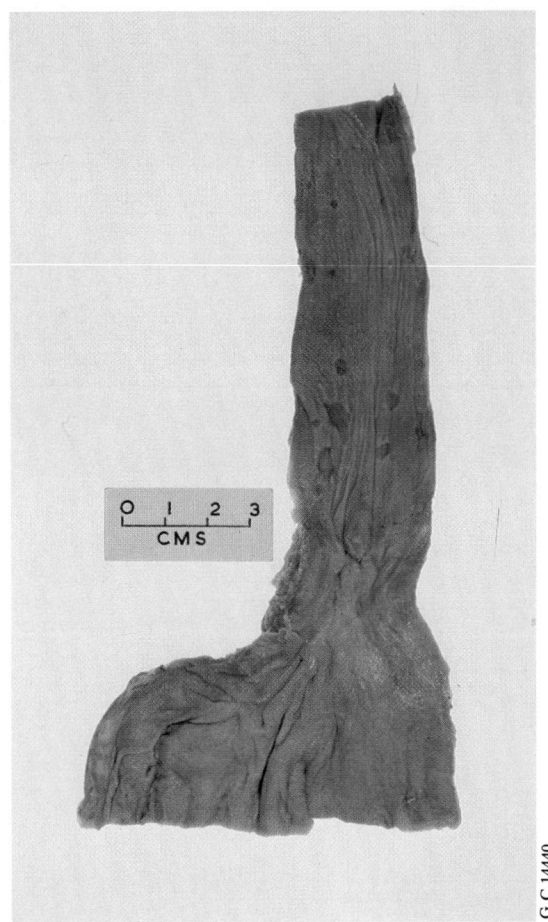

G.C.14440

Adenocarcinoma *(Continued)*

Adenocarcinoma of the oesophagus may occasionally be diffuse, extending over a long segment of the viscus. Like squamous carcinoma it may perforate into the aorta.

17

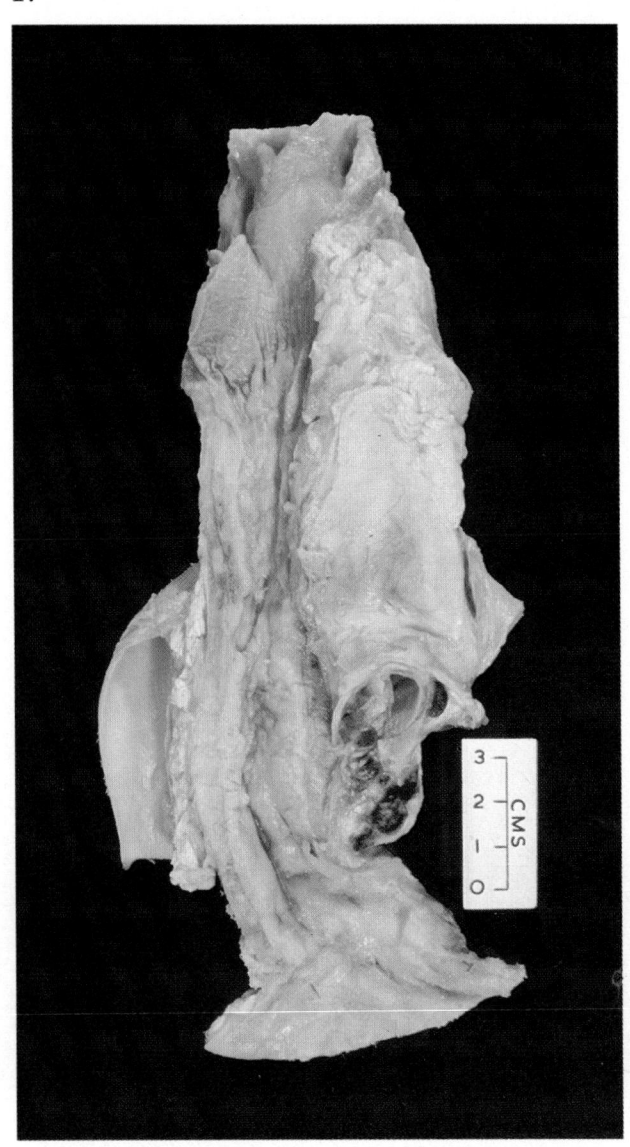

17 A diffuse carcinoma extending along almost the whole length of the oesophagus. The walls of the oesophagus are thickened throughout with ulceration of the mucosa and the tumour has extended beyond the wall of the oesophagus to become adherent to and involve the aorta. As the result of perforation of the aorta haemorrhage has occurred into the mediastinum. The cardiac portion of the stomach shows no abnormality and this would appear to be a 'true' adenocarcinoma of the oesophagus.

18

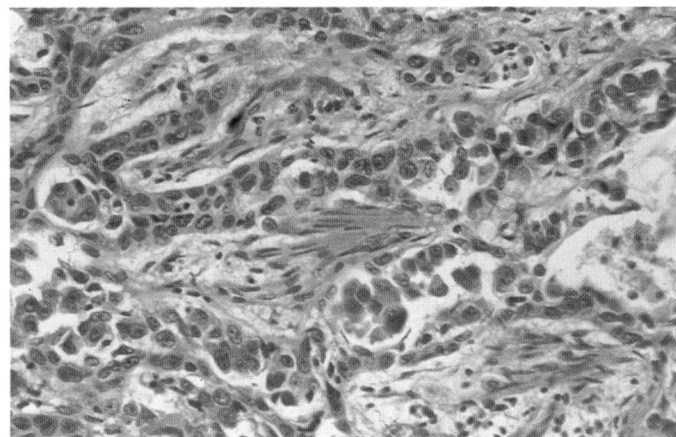

18 This illustrates the typical appearances of a rather poorly differentiated adenocarcinoma. *(H&E ×250)*

Carcinoma associated with hiatus hernia

Occasional difficulty in diagnosis occurs where there has been a sliding hernia with an upward displacement of a gastric pouch through the hiatus and an adenocarcinoma develops in this pouch.

19

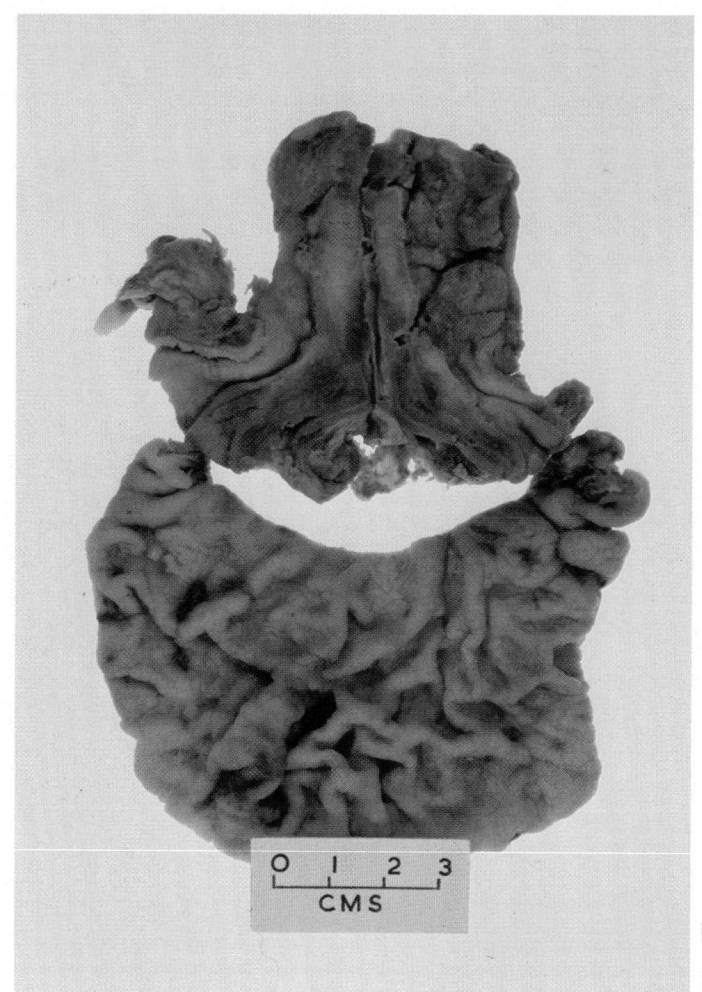

19 From a female aged 60 years. 12 year history of dysphagia, vomiting and nausea. Hiatus hernia demonstrated radiologically. Oesophagoscopy disclosed a stricture of the oesophagus at 30 cm, leucoplakia and peptic ulceration distal to the stricture. During examination the oesophagus was perforated and immediate resection undertaken. The specimen shows a carcinoma of the oesophagus with a gross perforation. Note the involvement of the wall with homogenous malignant tissue. Histologically the tumour is a mucoid adenocarcinoma. Mucoid change is an occasional finding which this case illustrates as well as the occurrence of the tumour in association with hiatus hernia.

20

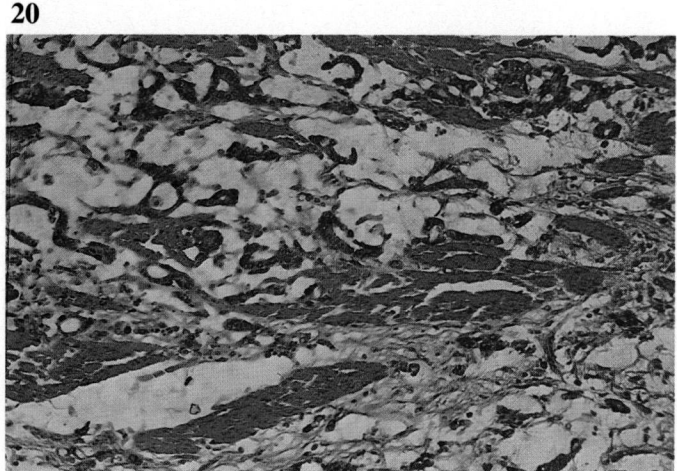

20 Mucoid carcinoma invading the oesophagus. Extracellular mucin separates the muscle fibres. *(H&E ×125)*

Miscellaneous tumours

Benign tumours of the oesophagus are rare and are most commonly found in the middle aged. There is a male preponderance. Of the benign tumours the leiomyoma is the most frequent. Fibromas and lipomas have also been reported.

Leiomyoma

Leiomyomas of small size are most frequently found at post mortem examination. Larger examples causing clinical features are rare. The tumours may be solitary or multiple and arise in the muscular coat of the oesophagus especially in the lower third. They may project into the lumen and therefore cause dysphagia or be disclosed on radiological examination. The overlying mucosa shows no ulceration. The cut surface of the tumour is greyish in colour, clearly circumscribed and has typical fasciculation. Malignant change is rare.

21

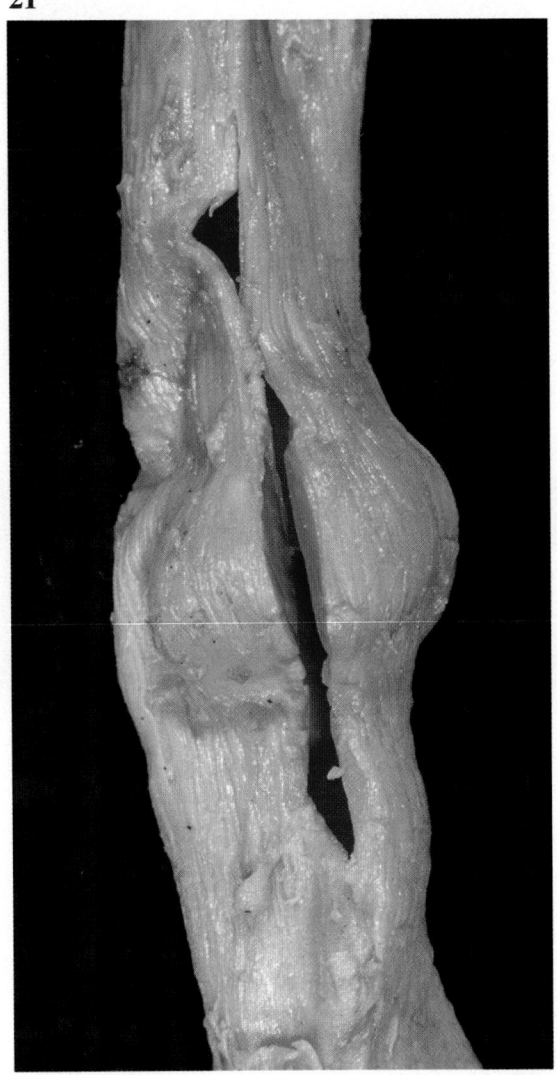

21a

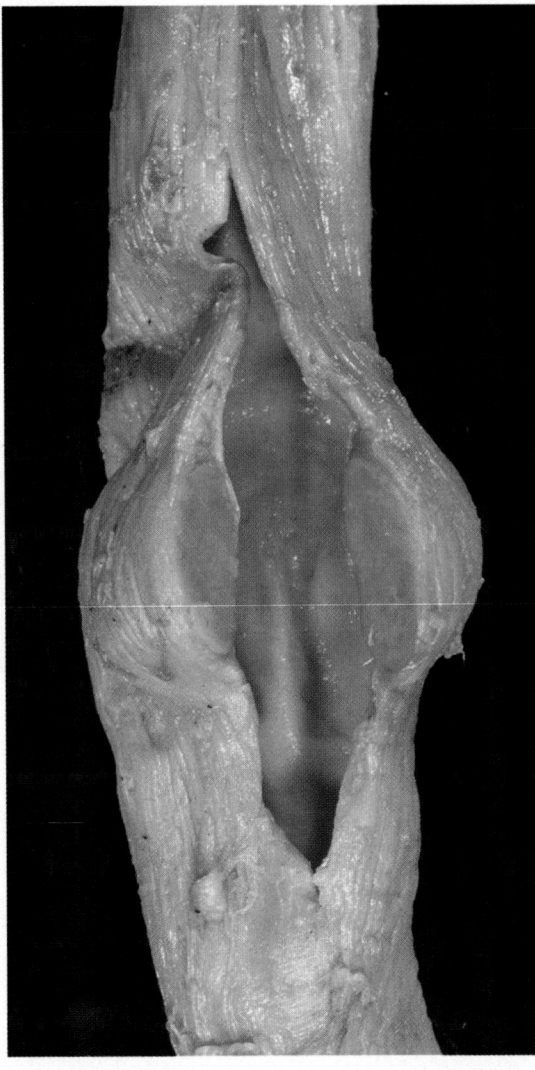

G.C.1547

21 and **21a**   An incidental post mortem finding from a female aged 45 years. The tumour is well defined, moderate size measuring 15 mm at its maximum diameter and localised in the posterior wall of the oesophagus. Microscopically the structure is that of a leiomyoma.

Polyp

Submucous tumours of the hypopharynx and the oesophagus whether leiomyomatous, fibromatous or lipomatous, which project into the lumen may become pedunculated and without treatment the pedicle may be of considerable length. They may extend downwards along the oesophagus or frequently upwards into the pharynx and mouth.

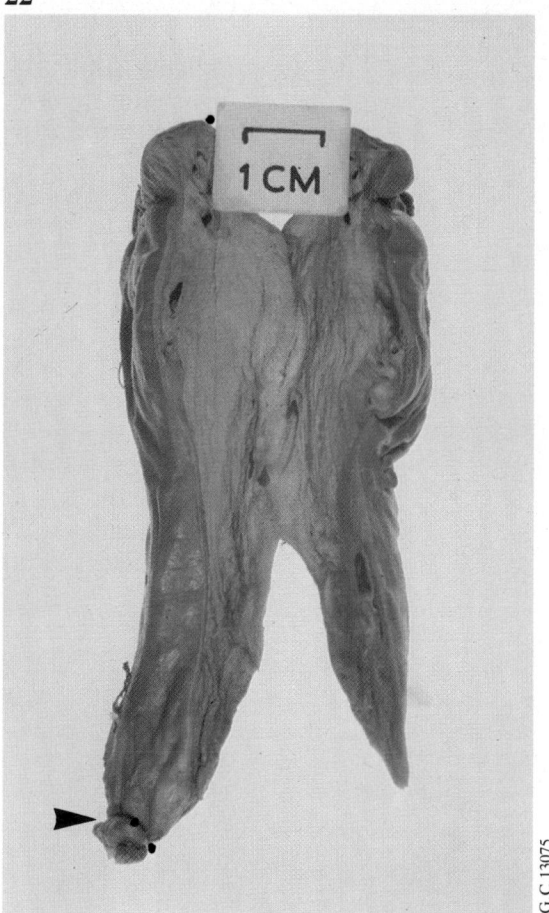

22

22 Polyp of the pharynx. When the patient vomited the polyp was forced up to the back of the mouth and was removed after ligature of its pedicle. The polyp is an elongated cylindrical mass with bulbous tip measuring some 10cm in length and approximately 2.5cm in transverse section in its proximal part. The specimen after removal has been split along one side in order to demonstrate the character of the interior of the mass. The outer cover of the polyp is a smooth mucosa while the cut surface demonstrates a loose fibrous texture possibly inflammatory. Note the ligature at the base of the polyp.

Melanoma

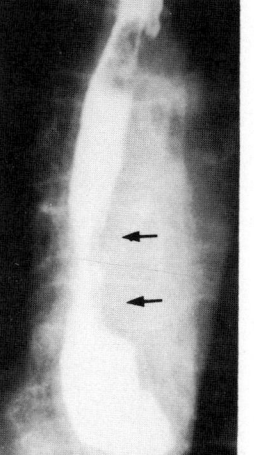

23

Primary melanoma of the oesophagus has been reported and has on occasion been associated with diffuse melanomatosis.

This tumour is very rare and is only accepted if no other melanomatous lesions are present and if histological examination shows the lesion arising from junctional epithelium. Both pigmented and non-pigmented varieties have been described. The occurrence of melanoblasts in normal oesophageal mucosa has been rarely shown. These lesions are malignant and usually pedunculated.

23 From a female aged 84 years.

A case of dysphagia investigated radiologically disclosed a filling defect of the lower mid oesophagus. Biopsy disclosed that the tumour was a lobulated melanoma. No other melanomatous lesions were found on clinical examination.

R.J.M. McCormack

First described by Maier in 1885. In 1912 Rammstedt introduced myotomy as a curative method of treatment. The same operation was independently devised by Harold Stiles in Edinburgh some months prior to the publication of Rammstedt but the child died following the operation and the case was not reported.

Modern management with earlier operation and the correction of preoperative biochemical disturbances has reduced the mortality almost to nil.

1   There is both hyperplasia and hypertrophy of the circular muscle coat of the pylorus which forms a firm ovoid mass approximately 2 to 3cm in length and which ends abruptly at the commencement of the duodenum. Structurally this represents the point at which gastric and duodenal musculature meet. The overlying peritoneum is smooth. When sectioned, the thickened muscle mass is seen to end distally, projecting knob-like into the duodenum. This projecting mass is surrounded by a duodenal mucosal sulcus. This last point is of great significance in the operation of myotomy.

1

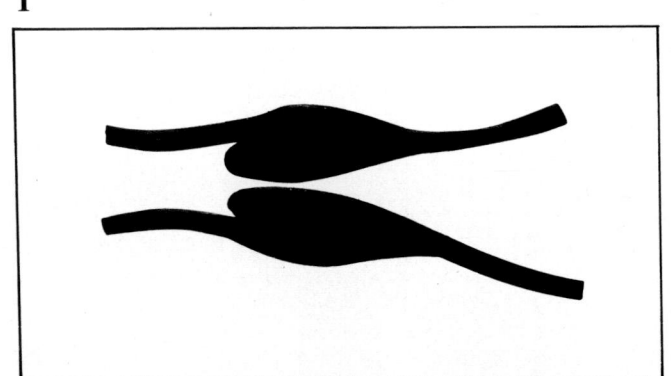

There is no evidence of neurological abnormality and no underlying cause for the obstruction has been found.

The mucosa of the pyloric canal if examined immediately after birth, is normal but later becomes oedematous and shows inflammatory change. The pyloric canal therefore becomes increasingly diminished in calibre. The stomach is enlarged and shows hypertrophy of all layers of its wall.

If patients who have had a myotomy for pyloric stenosis in infancy are examined in adult life it will be found that all evidence of muscular hypertrophy will have disappeared.

Pyloric stenosis in later life rarely may be attributable to a persisting congenital lesion in which the degree of narrowing of the lumen has been slight and health has been maintained by careful diet.

2

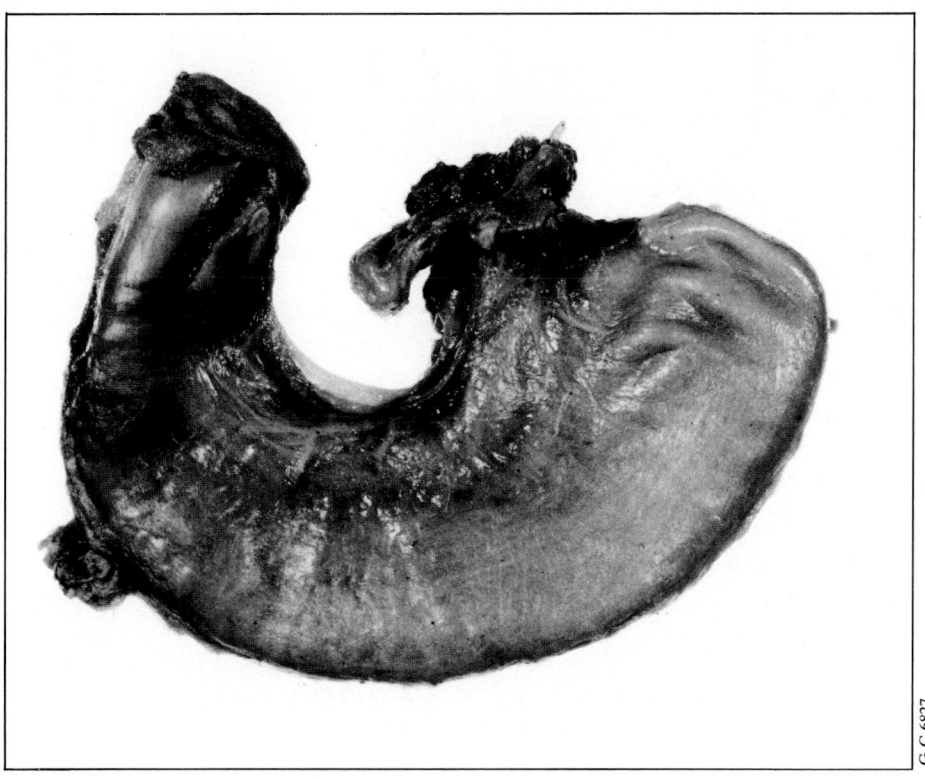

G.C.6827

2 From a male hydrocephalic aged 12 weeks. Symptoms commenced 7 weeks after birth. The child did not respond to initial conservative methods and death occurred suddenly 9 days after emergency operation.

Note the prominence of the pyloric bulb in which the incision (Rammstedt) has been made to relieve the obstruction.

3

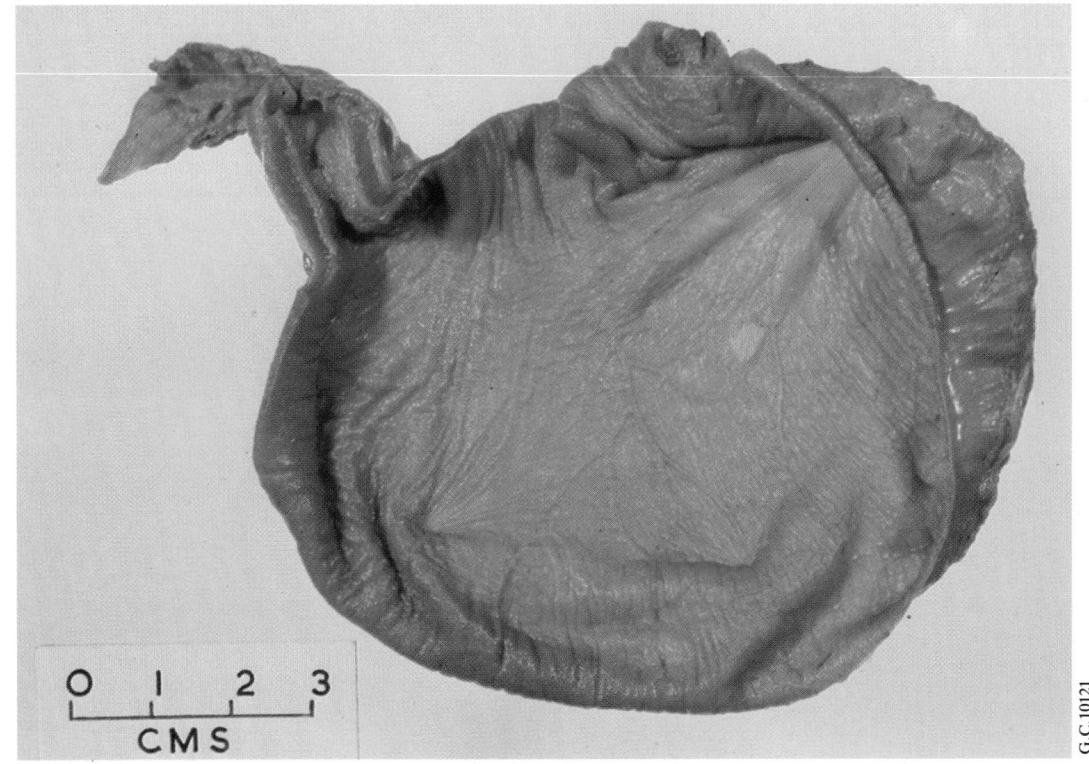

G.C.10121

3 From a male child aged 2 months. Death occurred shortly after admission to hospital.

The pyloric canal has been sectioned and demonstrates the hypertrophy of the muscular tissue at the pylorus. Note how this mass projects into the duodenum.

Ian S. Kirkland

The function of the stomach is to secure the admixture of the swallowed food with gastric secretion of acid and pepsin and to retain the gastric chyme for a sufficiently long period to permit the phase of gastric digestion to be completed. This complex activity is secured by the specialised secretions of the gastric mucosa and the regulated activity of the muscle wall and sphincters. These secretory and muscular activities are controlled by complex neurohormonal mechanisms.

A knowledge of the relevant specialised anatomy and physiology is essential for an understanding of the aetiology and pathology of peptic ulceration. For clarity these elements are described separately.

The stomach may be divided into two functionally distinct parts. These differ both in regards to their secretory and motor function and the line of separation of these two zones varies considerably in its level.

Secretory function

1 The fundus and body are primarily concerned with the secretion of hydrochloric acid and pepsin (red).

The antrum is chiefly concerned with the secretion of gastrin (brown).

Motor function

2 The body and fundus is the capacitance area (red) and holds and mixes the contents during digestion. The antrum is the gastric pump area (green) which ensures orderly gastric emptying. Following the ingestion of a meal regular gastric contractions commence sweeping downwards from the fundus to the pylorus. These occur in response to increased intragastric tension, direct stimulus of the gastric mucosa and changes in the pH of the gastric content.

In the antrum the contractions rhythmically project (2 to 5 ml) into the duodenum through the relatively narrow pyloric canal.

1

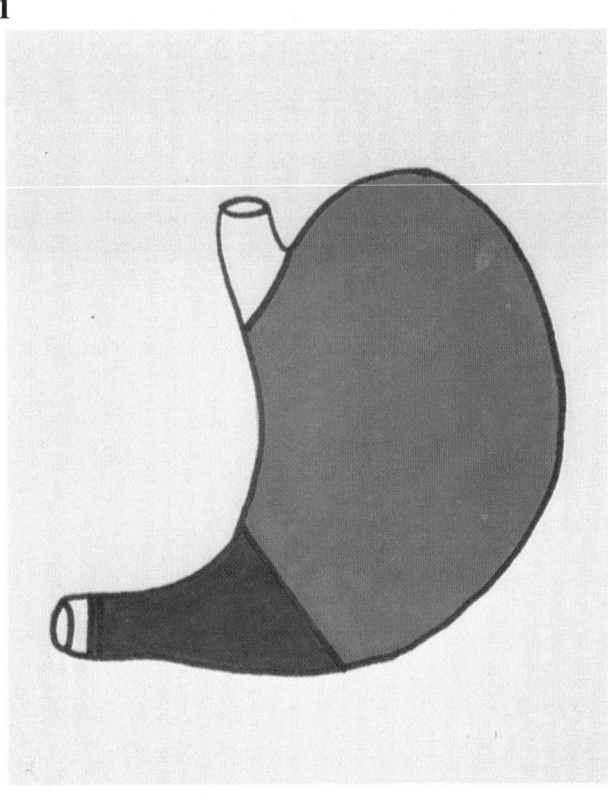

2

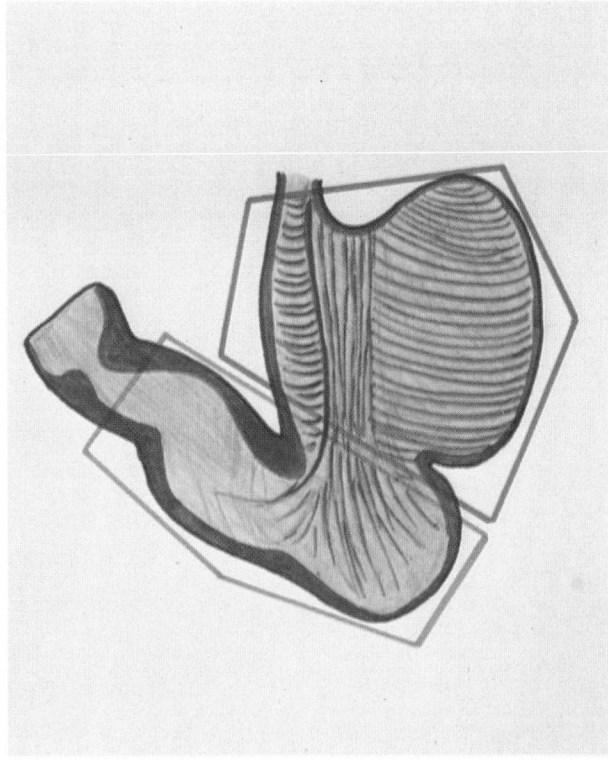

Parietal cell mass

The volume of acid secreted is proportional to the cell mass. The ability to produce increased amounts of acid results from the presence of increased numbers of parietal cells within the gastric corpus, an increased parietal cell mass. Whether parietal cell mass variations are congenital or result from chronic hormonal or neural stimulation is debated. Both factors are probably implicated.

3

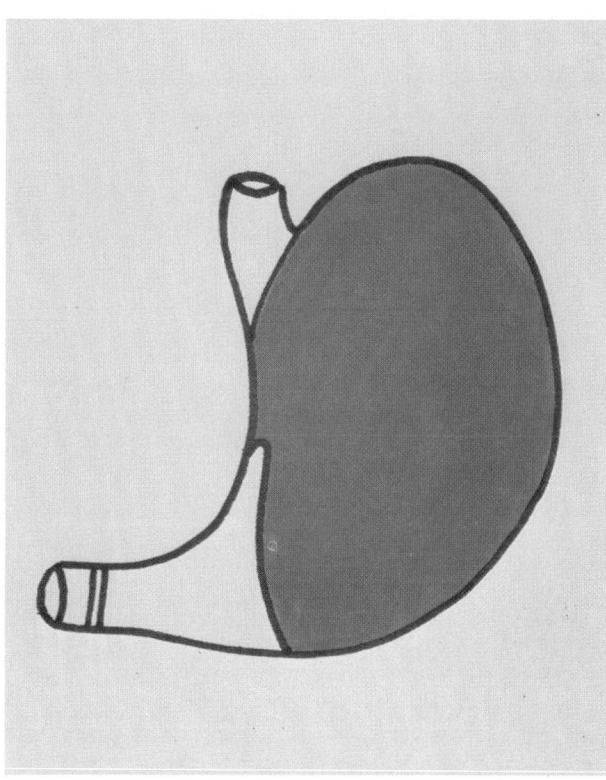

3 Normal distribution of cell mass.

4

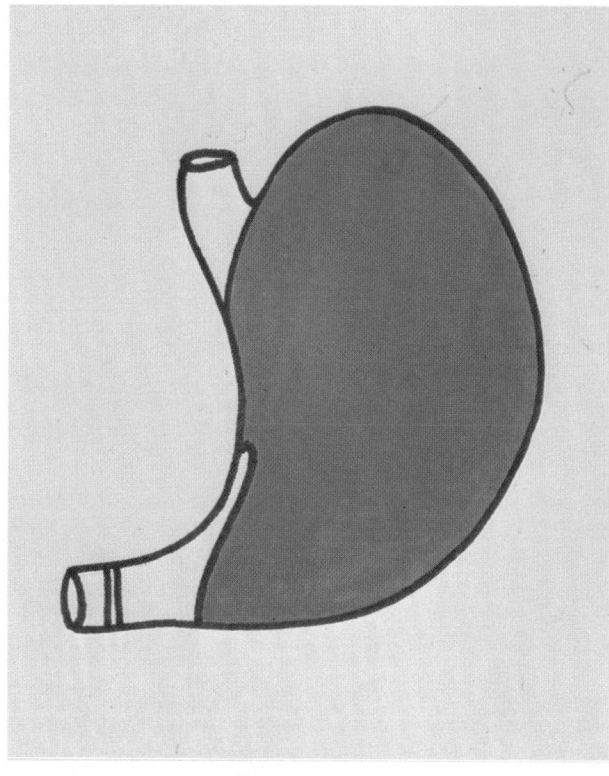

4 Distribution of increased cell mass.

5

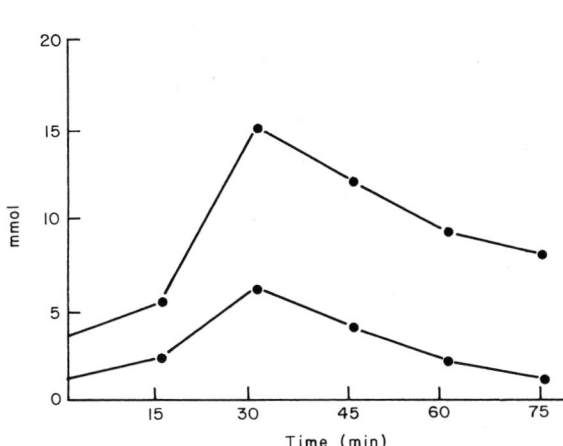

5 The response in mmol/15 minutes to intramuscular injection of pentagastrin at zero time in two subjects.

The adjacent graph indicates the acid secretory response of two subjects following the intra-muscular injection of the synthetic peptide pentagastrin. At a dose of between 1 and 6μg/kg body weight this produces maximal HCl secretion from the parietal cell mass.

The upper curve demonstrates the curve obtained in a patient with acid hypersecretion as a result of an increased parietal cell mass and the lower curve that obtained in a patient with a normal parietal cell mass.

Two values are commonly quoted in tests of secretion:
1 Basal acid output (B.A.O.) = the total amount of acid secreted by the stomach for one hour prior to pentagastrin stimulation after an overnight fast (Normal < 5 mmol).
2 Maximal acid output (M.A.O.) = the sum of four 15-minute samples taken in the hour following pentagastrin stimulation. Upper limit of normal 35 mmol/hour.

Gastric mucosa – Structure

An authoritative account of the intimate structure, microscopic and ultramicroscopic, was published by Ito and Winchester in 1963 in the *Journal of Cell Biology*, Volume 16 p.541. The material was obtained from the bat.

6

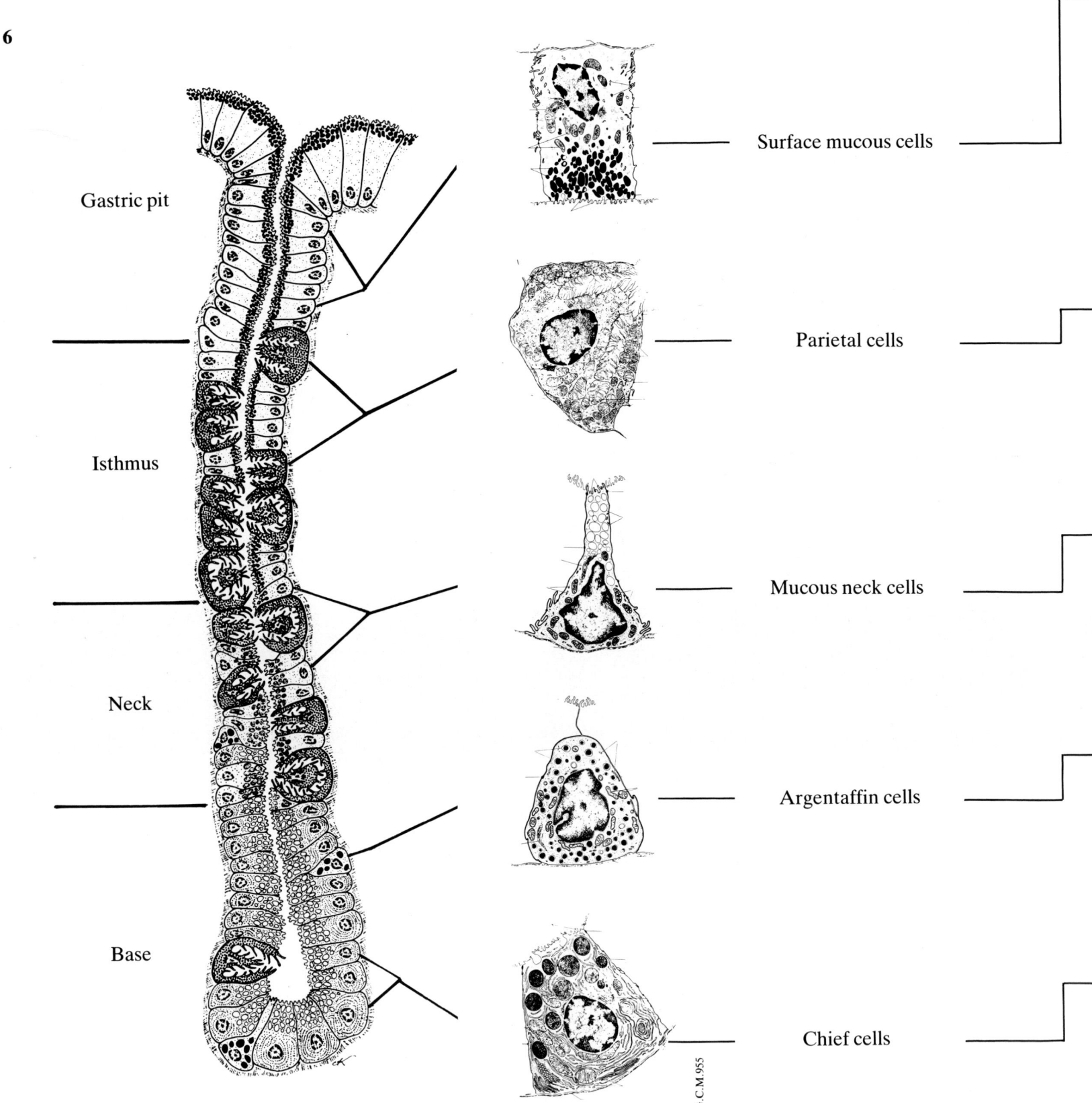

Gastric pit

Isthmus

Neck

Base

Surface mucous cells

Parietal cells

Mucous neck cells

Argentaffin cells

Chief cells

G.C.M.955

Structure	**Function**
These cells form a single layer of columnar cells lining the surface of the lumen of the viscus and extend into the gastric pits. These cells show projecting filaments and microvilli on their surface margin as far as the isthmus. The cells also extend into the isthmus of the gastric gland. The nuclei are basal, have a well developed envelope and a centrally sited dense nucleolus. Mucous droplets are found in the cytoplasm and are more numerous after a period of fasting. These droplets are aggregated close to the surface of the cell. Mitosis is rare and seen most frequently in the cells in the isthmus and neck regions.	The mucin in these cells, when discharged, forms a lubricant and protective layer against the acid peptic activity of the stomach secretions. In addition to mucus, glyco-protein blood group specific substances are also secreted.
Parietal cells are found in the main glands of the fundus and body of the stomach. They occur mainly in the mid part of the gastric glands lying between the surface mucus cells above and the peptic cells below. They are large pyramidal cells, eosinophilic because of the many mitochondria in the cytoplasm. Intracellular canaliculi surround the nuclei, channelling the cell secretions into the lumen.	These cells secrete HCl and are the site of production of the mucoprotein, Intrinsic Factor.
These cells are recognised by their position in the neck of the gland and by the specific nature of their PAS positive granules located between the nucleus and luminal surface. The cells are isolated or in small groups. They may simulate chief cells but can be differentiated by specific staining methods. The cells are generally columnar but show variation. The surface microvilli of these cells are sparse. The mitochondria are less marked than in the surface cells.	These cells serve as the source of replenishing cells for the rapid turnover surface epithelium and for the slow turnover parietal and chief cells. They are believed to secrete blood group antigens A and B.
This is an enterochromaffin cell found throughout the whole length of the alimentary canal but relatively uncommon in the stomach. They occur as isolated cells which are identified by their specific affinity for silver stains. The cytoplasm may or may not contain granules. They appear as pyramidal cells with a broad base resting on the basement membrane but do not reach the lumen of the gland.	These cells are a part of the hormonal system and are the site of endocrine synthesis (5 H-T).
The chief (peptic or zymogenic) cells are also found mainly in the fundus and body of the stomach occupying the deep portion of the glands. The cells are basophilic having a rich content of endoplasmic reticulin and ribosomes. Microvilli are present on the surface and zymogen granules are present in the cytoplasm near the apex of the cell.	These cells contain large numbers of zymogen granules which are released following neural or hormonal stimulation. Pepsinogens are liberated.

65

Gastric mucosa – Human

Fundus

The main gastric glands are tubular and lie perpendicular to the surface in their upper two-thirds and coiled in their deepest one-third. The parietal cells are found in the upper two-thirds and in the middle and deep thirds are the chief cells. Mucous neck cells and argentaffin cells are also present, the latter being rare.

A variation in the number of cells (cell mass) may be observed. Increase in the number of parietal cells (parietal cell mass) is associated with hyperacidity.

7

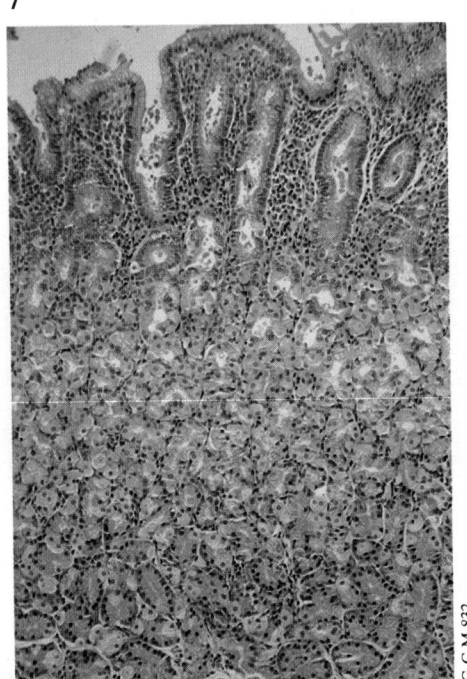

8

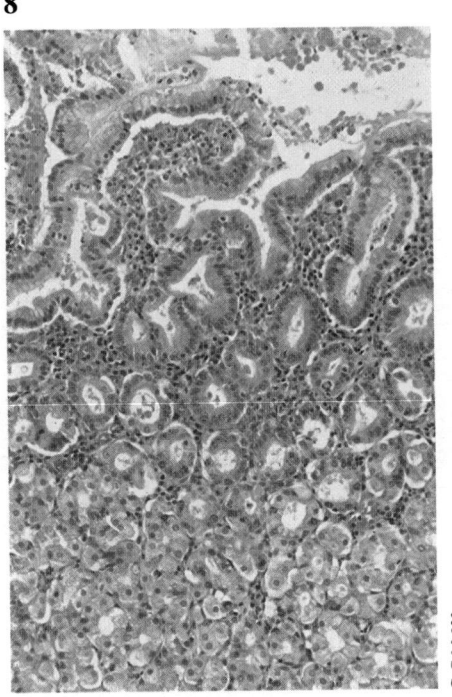

9

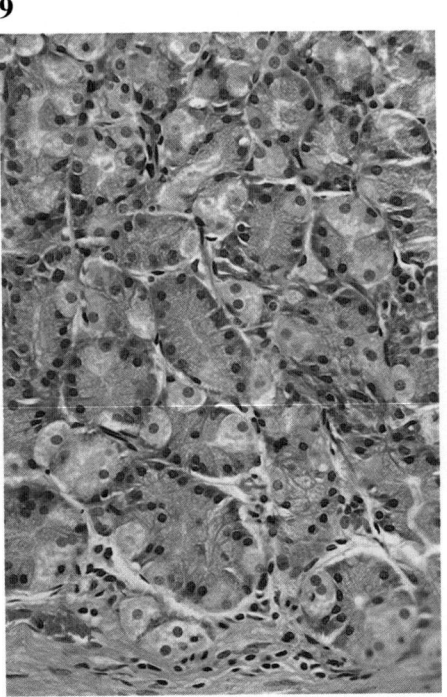

7 Human fundic mucosa showing gastric pits and full depth of main glands. Parietal cells red, chief cells blue. *(H&E ×100)*

8 Upper layer of fundic mucosa showing surface mucous and parietal cells of upper part of main glands. *(H&E ×150)*

9 Bases of main glands resting upon muscularis mucosae. Chief cells predominate but parietal cells can also be seen. *(H&E ×250)*

Antrum

The gastric pits are deeper than in the fundus and body and the glands are extensively coiled and branching. The lining cells are similar to mucous neck cells. Argentaffin cells and gastrin containing cells may also be demonstrated by special techniques including immunofluorescence.

G cells

First described in 1967, gastrin cells (G cells), identified by immunofluorescent techniques, lie between the bases of the mucous cells in deep portions of the glands.

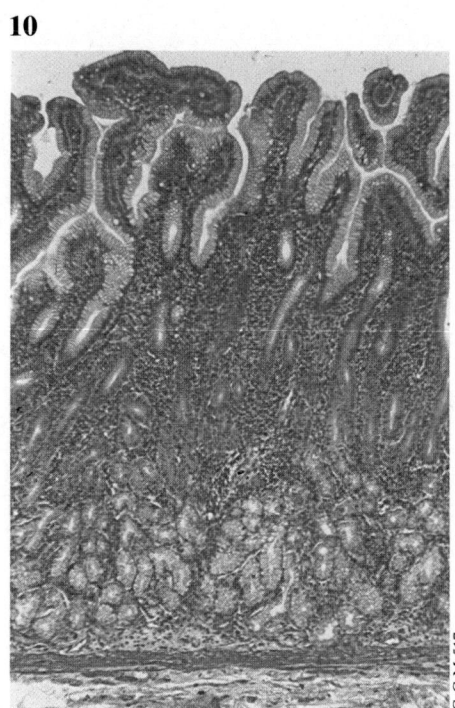

10 Antral or pyloric mucosa showing branching glands and deep gastric pits. The upper two-thirds of the mucosa is heavily infiltrated by plasma cells and lymphocytes. *(H&E ×70)*

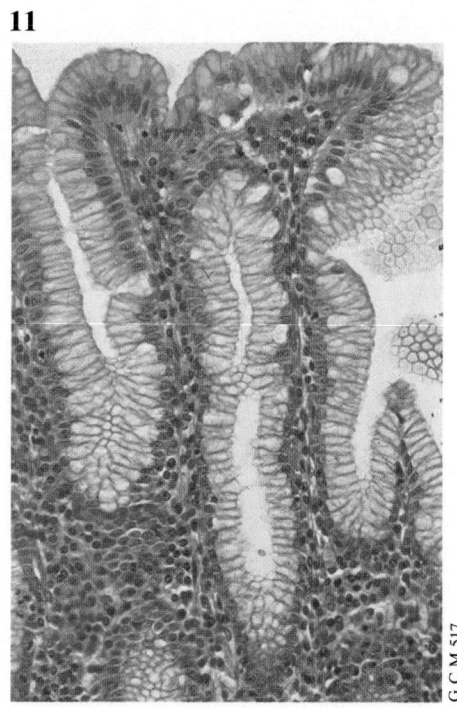

11 Antral mucosa. Mucous cells in gastric pits. *(H&E ×250)*

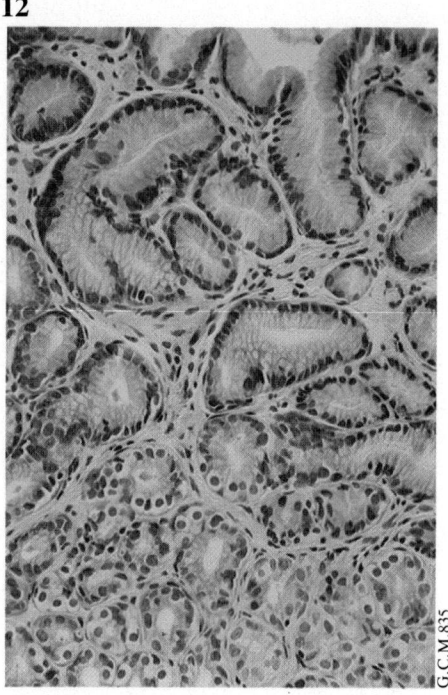

12 Antral mucosa. Round cells with central nucleus and clear cytoplasm, G cells, lie on the basement membrane between mucous cells. *(H&E ×250)*

Physiology

Gastric secretory and motor activity are both under neural and hormonal control the main components of which are stimuli transmitted through the vagus nerves, and the action of the hormone gastrin.

Vagus nerves

The abdominal vagi enter through the oesophageal hiatus as two main trunks – anterior and posterior.

Anterior trunk

This is commonly present as two or more separate divisions from which a number of nerves or groups of branches arise:
1   On entering the abdomen hepatic branches pass from the main trunks through the lesser omentum to the porta hepatis
2   Vagal fibres pass to the cardia and fundus
3   Further elements pass down the lesser curve within the lesser omentum as the nerve of Latarjet from which nerve fibres pass obliquely to the body of the stomach. This nerve terminates by dividing to form the 'crow's foot' which supplies the gastric antrum

13

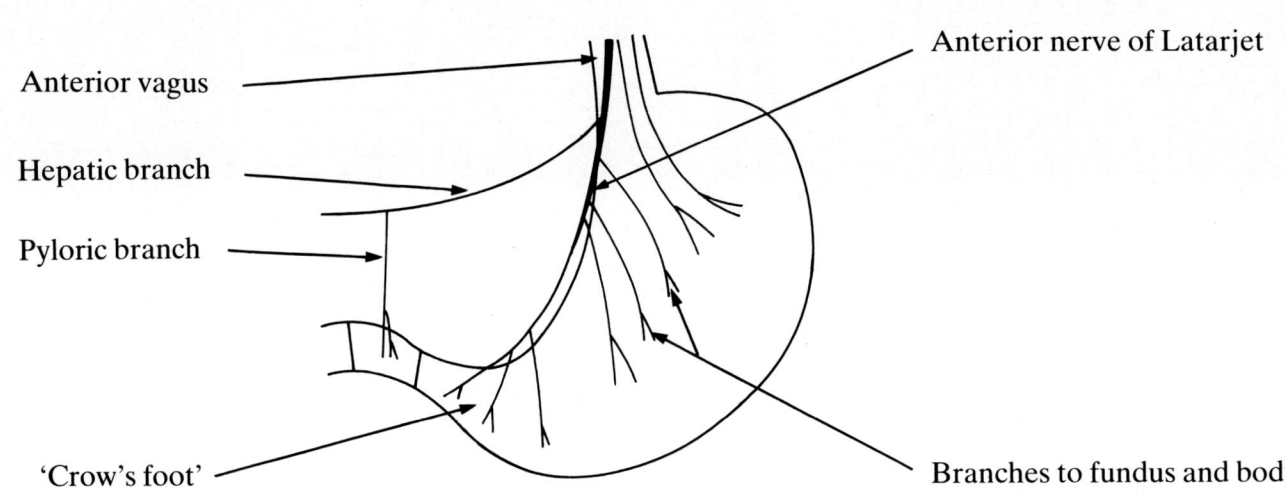

Posterior trunk

This enters the abdomen as a single large trunk in most cases. Vagal branches are given off to the coeliac ganglion, as are branches to the stomach from the posterior nerve of Latarjet which runs within the lesser omentum terminating with the anterior nerve in the antral 'crow's foot'.

14

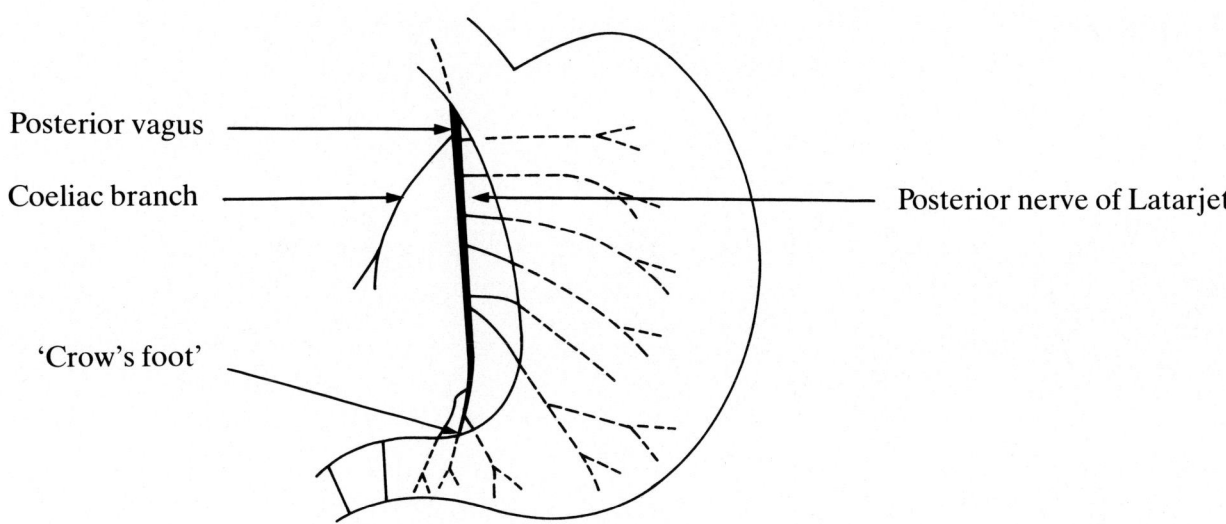

Posterior vagus

Coeliac branch

Posterior nerve of Latarjet

'Crow's foot'

Gastrin

The hormone gastrin consists of a number of peptides of similar structure but differing in size. The most physiologically important of these contains 17 amino acids and is a potent stimulator of the gastric secretion of HCl produced by the parietal cells. Gastrin is found in greatest concentration in the antral mucosa. It may also be found in much lower concentrations within the duodenal and to a still lesser extent the upper small bowel mucosa. In addition cells within the pancreatic islets can be shown to contain gastrin-like substances.

Additional physiological activities of gastrin are:
(a) Increase in the tone of the lower oesophageal sphincter (cardia)
(b) Stimulation of pepsin secretion
(c) Stimulation of intrinsic factor release

Gastric secretion

Gastric acid secretion can be broadly divided into two phases:
1 The inter-prandial phase which relates to the previously mentioned basal acid output.
2 The post-prandial phase.

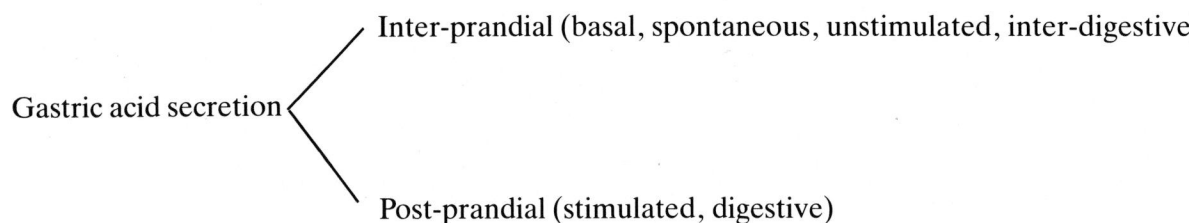

Gastric acid secretion
- Inter-prandial (basal, spontaneous, unstimulated, inter-digestive)
- Post-prandial (stimulated, digestive)

There are three mechanisms of control of the post-prandial gastric secretion:
1 Cephalic
2 Gastric
3 Intestinal

Cephalic

Cortical and hypothalamic connections to the dorsal motor nuclei allow gustatory, olfactory and visual stimuli to alter gastric secretion in both stimulatory and inhibitory ways. The vagus nerve must be intact for such stimulation or inhibition.

Vagal stimulation of the stomach excites acid secretion by three mechanisms:
1 Direct cholinergic stimulation of the parietal cells. Pre-ganglionic vagal fibres synapse within the sub-mucous plexus of the stomach wall and post-ganglionic fibres pass to the parietal cells.
2 Cholinergic stimulation of release of the hormone gastrin from the G cells of the pyloric antrum.
   Pre-ganglionic vagal fibres synapse in the sub-mucous plexus in the wall of the pyloric antrum and post-ganglionic fibres innervate the antral G cells.
   Gastrin on release passes via the blood stream to stimulate the parietal cells to secrete acid (possibly via histamine and cAMP).
3 Sensitisation of the parietal cells to stimulation by gastrin, histamine or other stimulants.

A.H. McLean Ross

Gastric

There are two components:

1   Direct cholinergic stimulation of the parietal cells by ⟨ local reflexes / vago-vagal reflexes

Distension of the parietal gland area leads to stimulation of receptors whose afferent fibres synapse in the submucous plexus. Efferent fibres pass to the parietal cells to cause acid secretion. This local reflex is reinforced by a long vago-vagal reflex. Afferent fibres from the distension receptors pass upwards in the vagus to the dorsal nucleus, and fibres from this centre pass down the vagus to the submucous plexus and thence post-ganglionic fibres innervate the parietal cells.

2   Cholinergic release of gastrin from the antral G cells by the mechanical stimulus of distension of the pyloric antrum.
    Chemical stimuli: extracts of meat, liver, amino acids, and alcohol.
    As in 1, there are local reflexes, impulses passing from the receptors to the submucous plexus and thence to the G cells, and also vago-vagal reflexes which potentiate the local response.

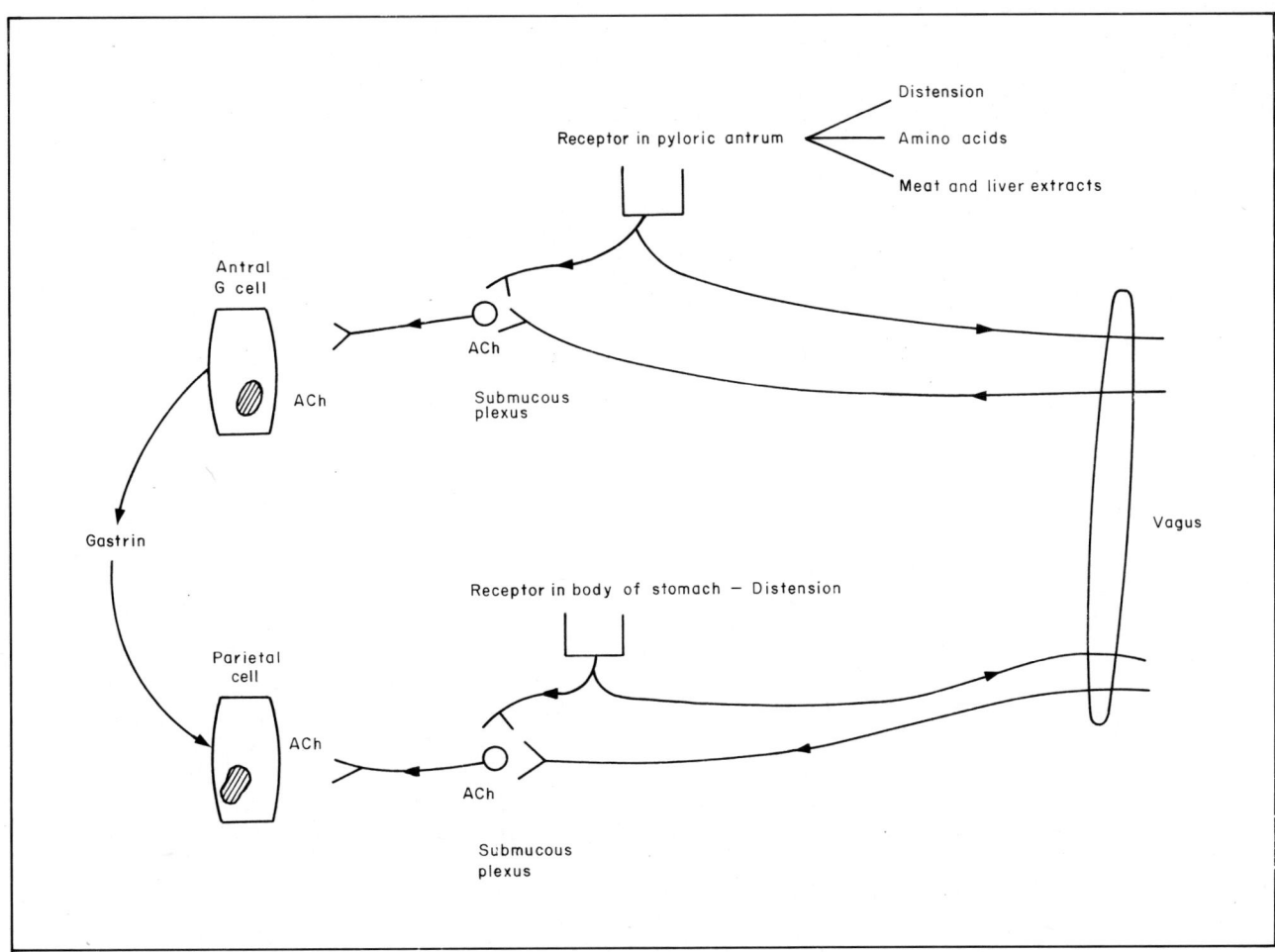

Possible interactions at the parietal cell membrane

Histamine is known to be a potent stimulus of gastric acid secretion. Drugs have been synthesised which block the action of histamine on acid secretion by causing blockade of Histamine 2 receptors (H_2 receptors). H_2 receptor antagonists not only inhibit acid secretion induced by histamine, but also that induced by pentagastrin, feeding, urecholine and insulin. This suggests a dominant role for histamine as a common final stimulator of the parietal cells. Evidence suggests that the H_2 receptor is an adenyl cyclase, stimulation of which causes the formation of cAMP within the cell, and this leads to acid secretion.

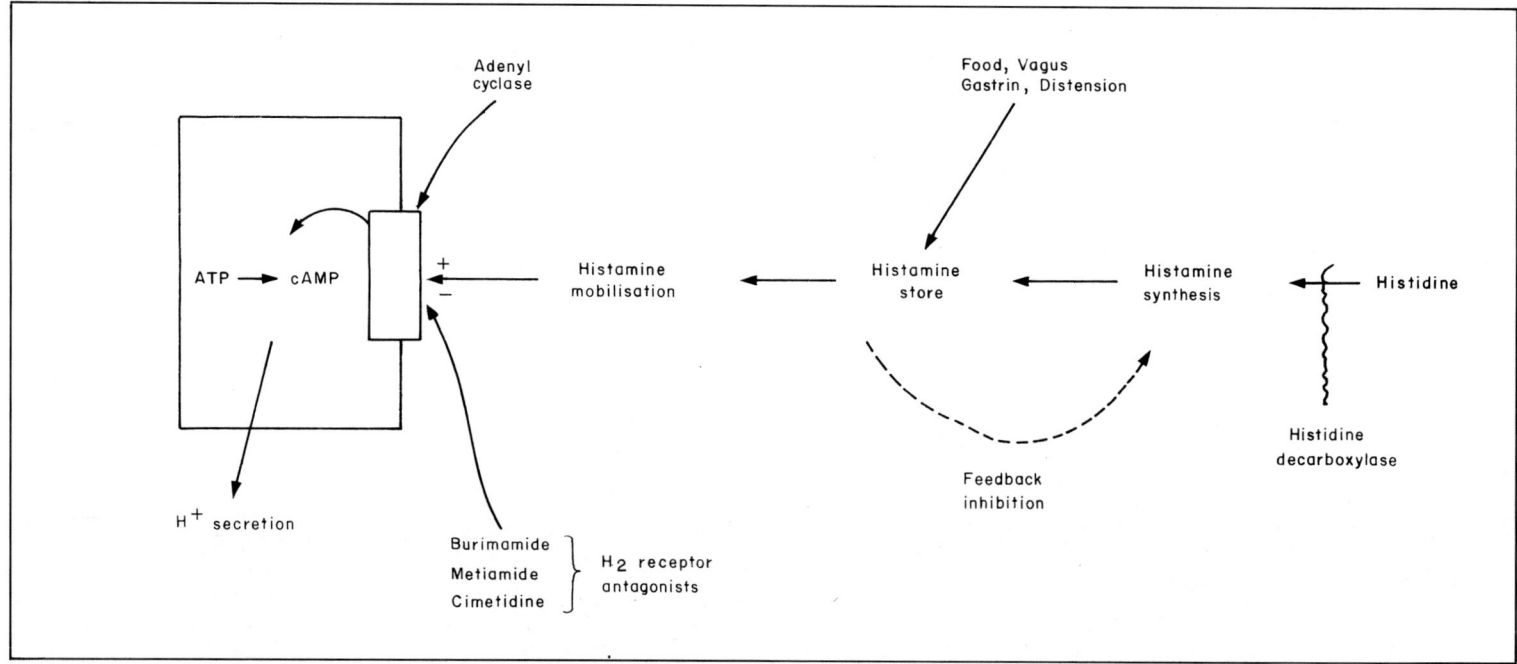

Intestinal

Following the ingestion of a meal gastric secretion continues weakly, for a period of up to 6 hours. This phase has both gastric stimulation and inhibitory mechanisms. Food in the duodenum can cause secretion of acid from the parietal cell area of the stomach, which is mediated by at least two mechanisms:

1   via the release of gastrin present in cells of the upper duodenal mucosa
2   via the release of the peptide, Bombesin, which in turn causes the release of gastrin from the antral G cells

M.O. Wright

Mechanism of control

Inhibitions of gastric secretion

Under physiological circumstances a number of factors combine to reduce or abolish the gastric secretory response:

1. Unpleasant cortical stimuli, unpleasant surroundings or fear will, through central pathways, inhibit gastric secretion via the vagi.
2. pH. The release of gastrin from the antral mucosa is modified by the pH of gastric content. Increasing acidity decreases gastrin release which ceases below a pH of 1.
3. Intestinal factors. The entry of acid solutions into the duodenum and proximal small bowel results in inhibition of acid production.

   Secretin (released from the duodenal mucosa) in addition to its effects on the pancreas blocks both the release of gastrin from the antral mucosa and the action of gastrin on the parietal cell.

Enterogastrone (Bulbogastrone). This as yet uncharacterised hormone inhibits gastric secretion after it is released by acid solutions or fat suspensions bathing the duodenal mucosa. Whether enterogastrone is a distinct entity or actually represents one or a number of the intestinal A.P.U.D. cell peptides is presently debated.

Other substances produced by the small intestine are known to have inhibitory effects on gastric secretion. Among these are: gastric inhibitory peptide (GIP), vaso-active inhibitory peptide (VIP), glucagon, somatostatin and neurotensin. Their exact role is uncertain but it seems likely that multiple hormonal factors are involved in the inhibition of gastric secretion.

Gastroduodenal motility

Continuous peristaltic waves pass from the cardia to the antrum mixing gastric content and moving it towards the antrum. Periodically a stronger peristaltic wave passes along the length of the antrum forcing about 5 ml of gastric chyme through the pylorus which has relaxed prior to the arrival of the peristaltic wave.

Vagal stimuli increase the frequency and amplitude of gastric peristalsis as does gastric distension. Total gastric vagotomy abolishes forceful co-ordinated peristalsis for a variable period of time. Retention of those vagal fibres supplying the antrum will retain normal gastric emptying.

Other factors that slow the rate of gastric emptying are:

1. Acid duodenal content.
2. Fat in the duodenum.
3. Hyperosmolar duodenal content.
4. Noxious small bowel stimuli, e.g. distension or stretching.

Aetiology

Gastric mucosal barrier

The mucous cells of the stomach are protected from the corrosive action of hydrochloric acid by a barrier consisting of a film of mucus. This mucous barrier overlies the gastric and duodenal mucosa.

Peptic ulceration results from an imbalance between the corrosive action of gastric content and the protective mechanisms of the mucosa.

This mucus is secreted by the mucous cells and contains complex mucoproteins resistant to acid hydrolysis and prevents access of acid peptic gastric content to the mucosa.

15

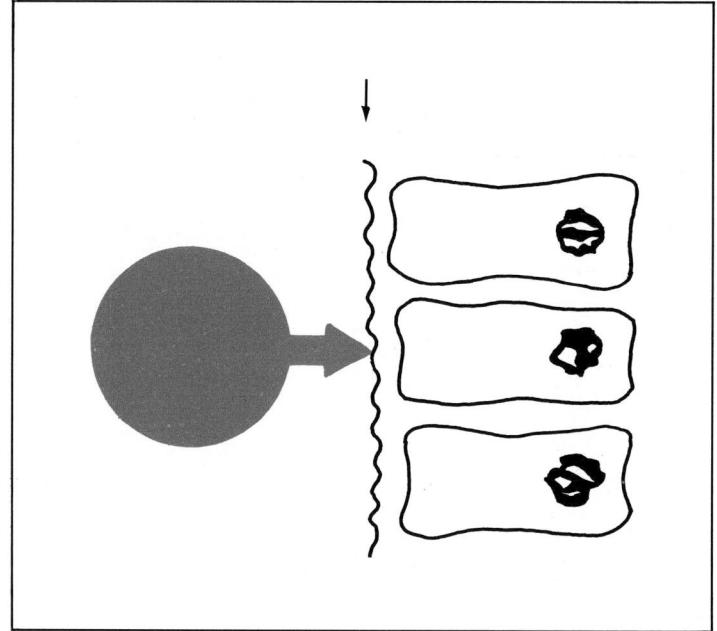

15 Normal protective mechanism of gastric mucosa by mucous film (indicated by arrow). Acid gastric content represented by red circle.

The alkaline nature of the mucus may inactivate acid-activated pepsin before it reaches the mucosa. It is postulated that defects in the efficacy and nature of this secreted mucus may be of significance in the aetiology of both duodenal and gastric ulceration although the precise nature of any such defect has not been identified.

Alteration in the nature of lining mucus by agents such as steroids may be the basis for certain drug induced ulcers.

16

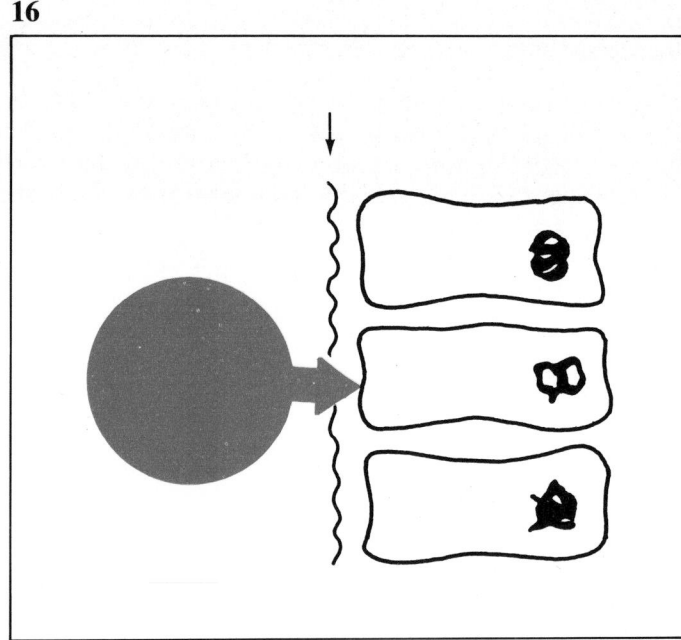

16 Defective mucous film. HCl penetrating mucous cells.

Ulceration will result if this barrier is defective since the acid will reach unprotected cells and tissues lying below the mucosa. The mucosae of other parts of the alimentary canal do not possess this protective mechanism and if acid reaches these parts e.g. oesophagus or intestine, ulceration may result.

The effects of hydrochloric acid on the mucosa may be deleterious (*per se*) when (a) there is delayed gastric emptying and (b) there is disturbance of the regulation of gastric secretion by neural and hormonal feedback resulting in hypersecretion.

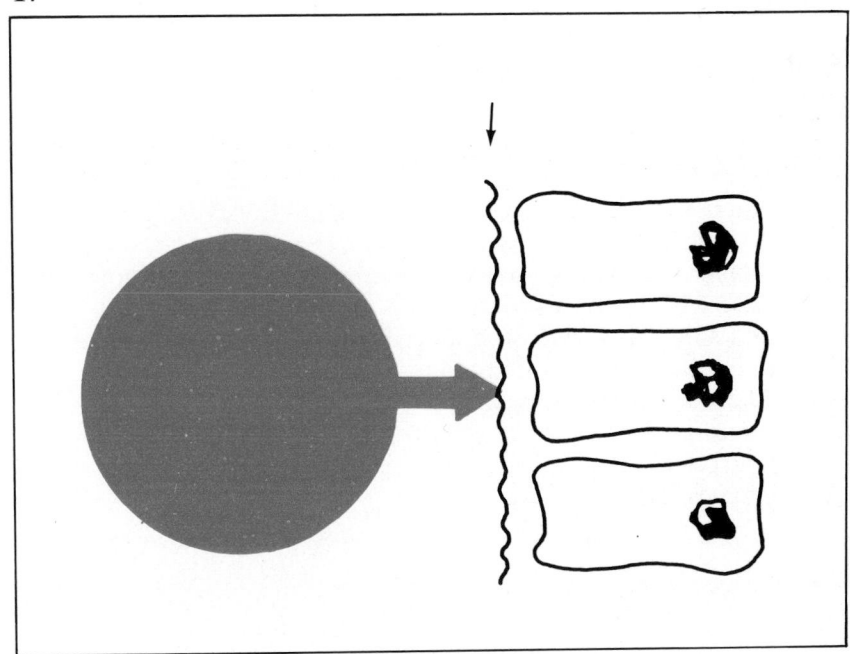

17 The mucous film continues its protective role even in the presence of hyperacidity.

Variations of acidity

Achlorhydria: Peptic ulceration cannot occur where there is achlorhydria.
Normal secretion: Ulceration can occur in individuals whose output of hydrochloric acid is normal.
Hyperchlorhydria: Increased secretion of hydrochloric acid is associated with an increased parietal cell mass.
Patients with prepyloric, pyloric ('channel') or duodenal ulceration typically have higher capacities to produce acid due to an increased cell mass than do individuals without ulcers. The range of acid producing capacity in patients with duodenal ulcer overlaps with that of the normal population.

Two other factors contribute toward the hyperchlorhydria:
1 Increased sensitivity of the parietal cells to a given acid producing stimulus.
2 An inherently high parietal cell drive by either hormonal or neural mechanisms.

Acid production in gastric ulceration is generally low or within the limits for a normal population. Correspondingly the parietal cell mass is low. As with duodenal ulceration the congenital or acquired nature of the parietal cell mass is disputed.

Hydrogen ion diffusion

In normal circumstances the permeability of the mucosa to hydrogen ions is slight. However, under circumstances such as extreme stress, after application of bile salts to the mucosa, or the corrosive action of drugs such as salicylates, this permeability increases and acid 'back diffusion' occurs into the mucosa which may then result in mucosal damage and ulceration. There is presently no evidence to support the view that there is a breach in the gastric mucosal barrier to hydrogen ions as the initial event in gastric ulcerogenesis.

Acetylsalicylic acid

Salicylates taken for therapeutic purposes especially when a coarse granule preparation is given are known to cause gastric mucosal erosions associated with haemorrhage. It would appear that if the drug is administered for short periods as an analgesic the hazard, although present, is seldom serious but where employed for long-term treatment as in rheumatoid arthritis a significant percentage of patients will develop gastric ulcers.

The role of bile salts

Bile and pancreatic fluid neutralise gastric content as it enters the duodenum and this provides a measure of duodenal protection. Biliary reflux into the stomach may cause damage to:
1 The mucous film lining the gastric mucosa.
2 The underlying mucous cells.
   These two factors together lead to a breach in the 'mucosal barrier' to acid.
   Biliary reflux may thus be an aetiological factor in the origin of gastric ulceration. In established gastric ulcer biliary reflux is commonly observed.

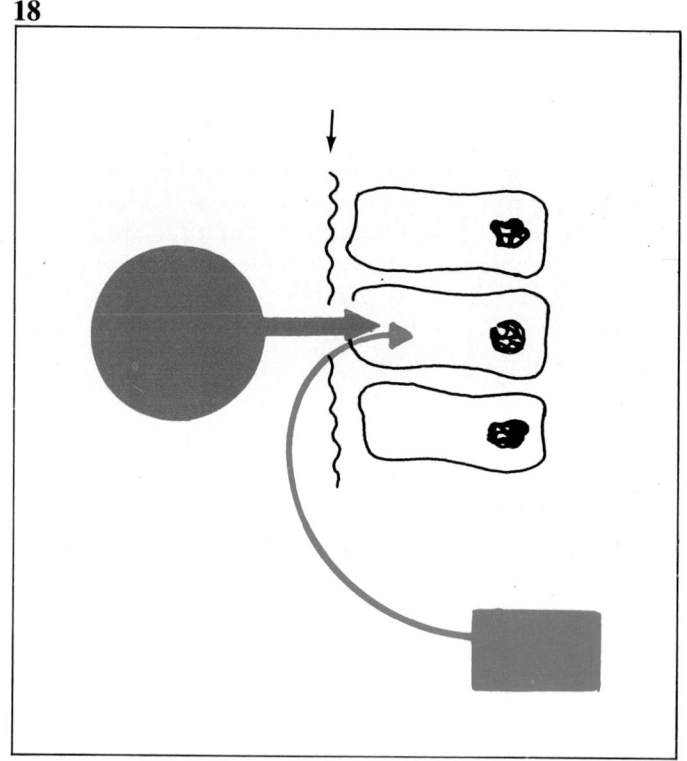

18

18   Damage to mucous film by biliary reflux (green).

Vascularity

A system of functional end arteries supplies the mucosa of the lesser curve in distinction to the rich submucosal anastomoses, including arterio-venous shunts, found in the remaining areas of the stomach. The lesser curve is thought to be more prone to mucosal ischaemia which as a result renders the mucosa more susceptible to ulceration. The predominance of gastric ulcers on the lesser curve may be a reflection of this. Ischaemia is not considered an aetiological feature of duodenal ulceration.

19

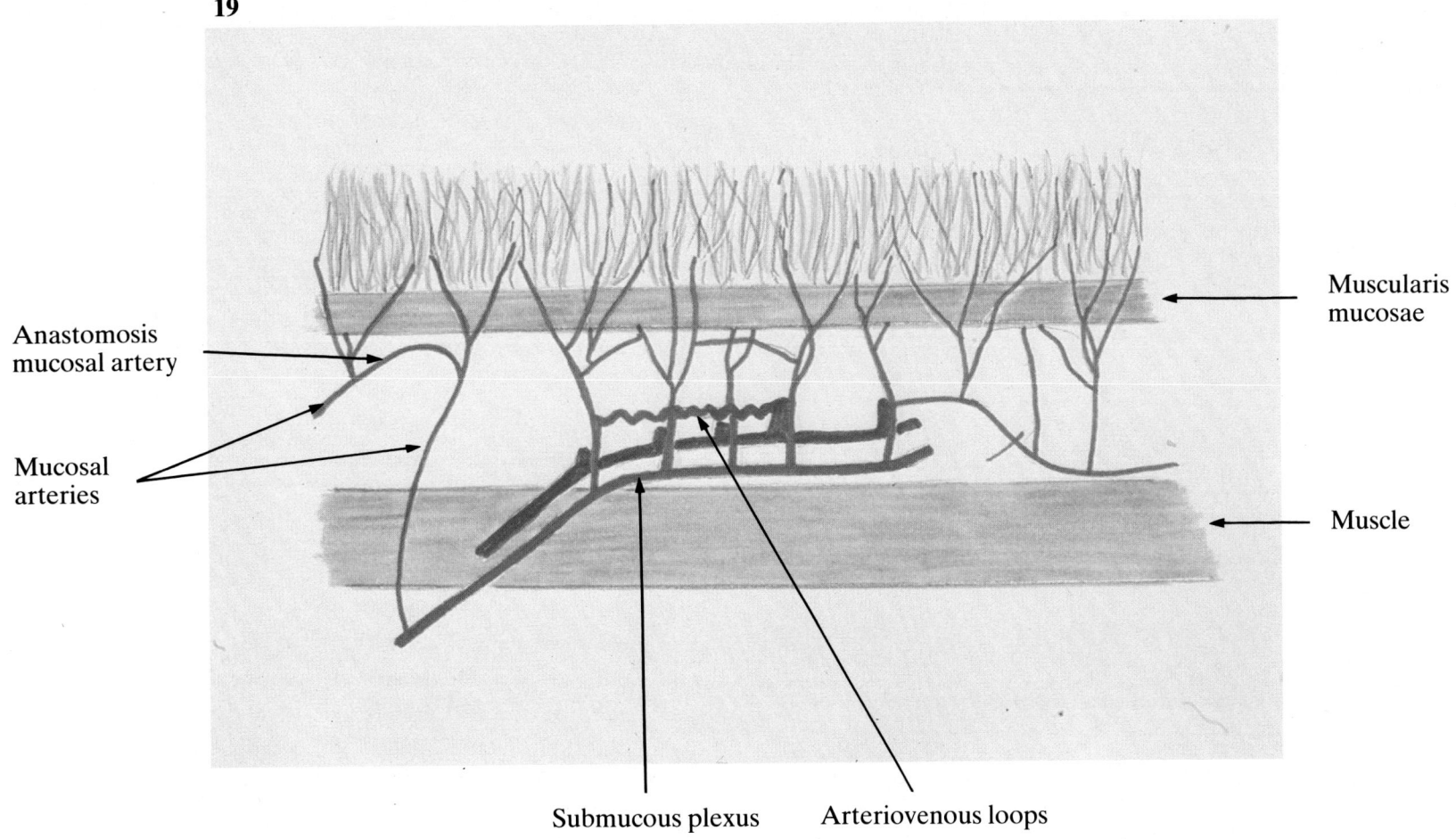

Anastomosis mucosal artery

Mucosal arteries

Muscularis mucosae

Muscle

Submucous plexus   Arteriovenous loops

Aetiology – Additional factors

A number of other factors which are known to be related to the incidence, location, course and nature of peptic ulceration have been described but their precise role has not been determined.

Incidence

Peptic ulceration of the duodenum is commoner than gastric ulceration. The ratio between the two ulcers has been reported and the figures vary between 2:1 and 3:1. These figures show variation according to diet and geographical distribution.

Sex and age incidence

Peptic ulcers are more common in men than women.

The sex ratio between men and women differs from duodenal ulcer (D.U.) (M:F – 7:1) to gastric ulcer (G.U.) (M.F. – 2:1).

Approximately 10% of males and 4% of females will have developed duodenal ulceration at some time before 50 years of age. After this age there is little increase in prevalence. The peak incidence for gastric ulceration occurs at 50 years and for duodenal ulcer at 40 years of age. These are based on the United Kingdom figures.

Social status

Gastric ulcer predominates in the lower socio-economic groups whereas duodenal ulcer is more common in the higher groups.

The ratio of the incidence of duodenal to gastric ulceration has changed over the century.

Heredity

It is established that there is a strong familial tendency to peptic ulceration. This tendency is the result of environmental and genetic influences. The genetic influence is specific for gastric or duodenal ulceration.

Hormones

Gastric ulcer may occur in association with primary hyperparathyroidism. Ulceration also occurs in relation to a complex disorder of the endocrine glands known as the multiple adenoma syndrome in which there may be a pituitary adenoma associated with adrenal hyperplasia, hyperparathyroidism and hypergastrinaemia due to pancreatic islet hyperplasia or adenoma. There is a relationship between peptic ulcer and the female sex hormones. During pregnancy patients with peptic ulceration usually experience a remission of ulcer symptoms. After the menopause the sex ratio differences in both forms of ulceration become less distinct. The precise mechanism of such hormonal effects remains uncertain. Adrenocortical imbalance is not a factor in chronic peptic ulceration although it probably has a role in stress induced acute ulceration.

Blood groups

There is an association between peptic ulceration and blood groups. Duodenal ulceration is more commonly associated with Group 0 and gastric ulcers with blood Group A. In addition patients who secrete Lewis antigen into their peptic juice ['non (ABO) secretors'] instead of ABO groups are at increased risk of peptic ulceration.

Smoking etc.

Cigarette smoking delays the healing of gastric ulcers and is likely to be a contributory factor in the aetiology of both duodenal and gastric ulcers. Excessive alcohol consumption is not an aetiological factor. Certain diseases are associated with an increased incidence of duodenal and gastric ulcer. These include hepatic cirrhosis, rheumatoid arthritis, chronic obstructive airway disease and hyperparathyroidism.

Superficial erosions

There is destruction of the mucosal layer only. The muscularis mucosae is not involved. Surrounding inflammation is not prominent and fibrosis does not occur. These lesions are self limiting and are not regarded as a precursor of chronic ulceration. Superficial erosions may be found in association with both acute and chronic ulceration.

Superficial erosions may result from:
1 Abnormal cephalic stimuli as seen in periods of marked stress or due to cerebral disturbance, e.g. trauma.
2 In toxic states as occur in burns and severe infection.
3 In severe shock.
4 Following drug therapy (steroids, salicylates).

In the latter three circumstances the mode of action is debatable.

Acute ulcers have a similar aetiology.

5 Following gastric surgery reflux of bile into the stomach may result in severe gastritis and erosions.

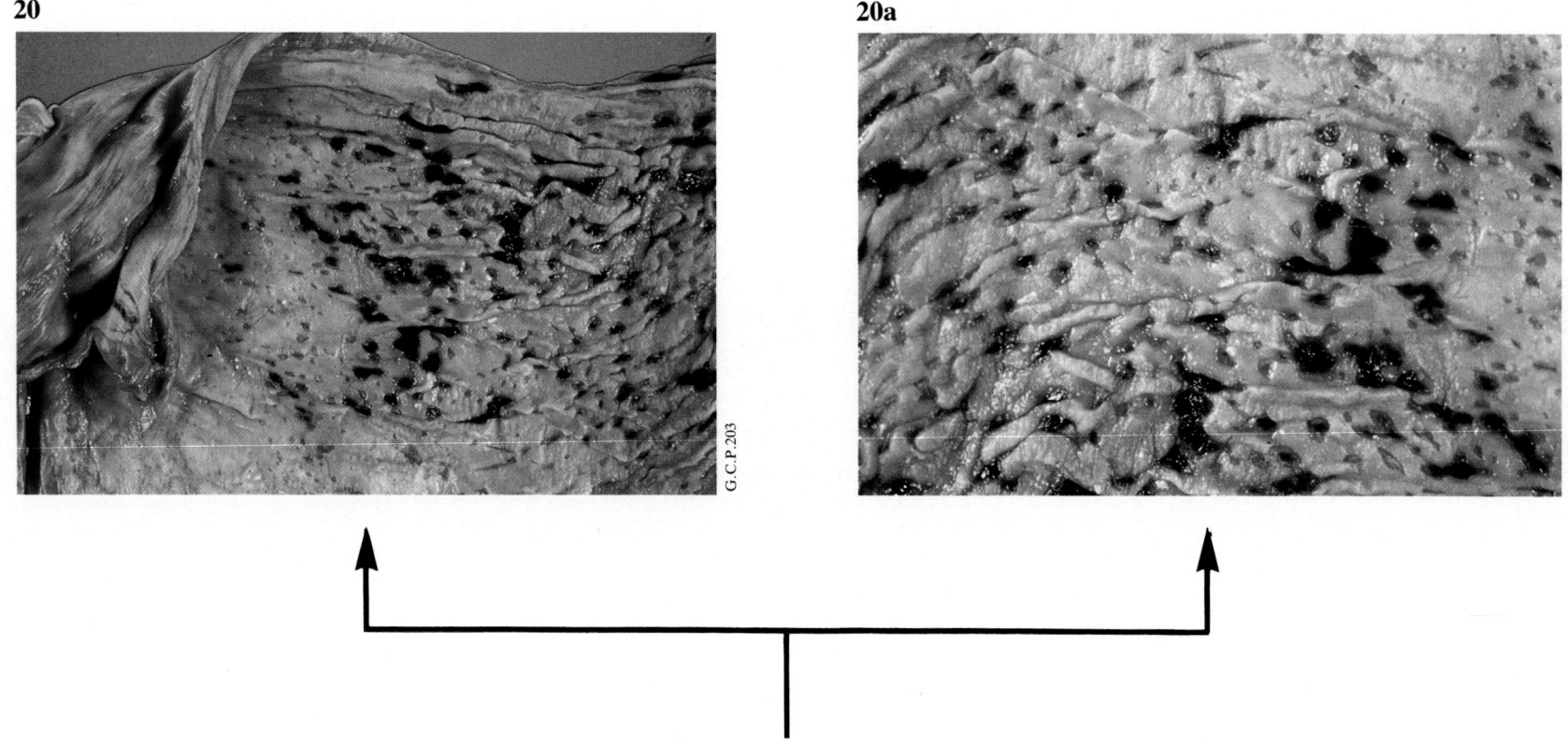

20 and **20a** Superficial erosions present in the stomach of a woman aged 56 years who died following massive haemorrhage. She suffered from severe rheumatoid arthritis which had been treated by cortisone. The illustrations show the numerous erosions with foci of swollen necrotic mucosa blackened by altered blood.

21

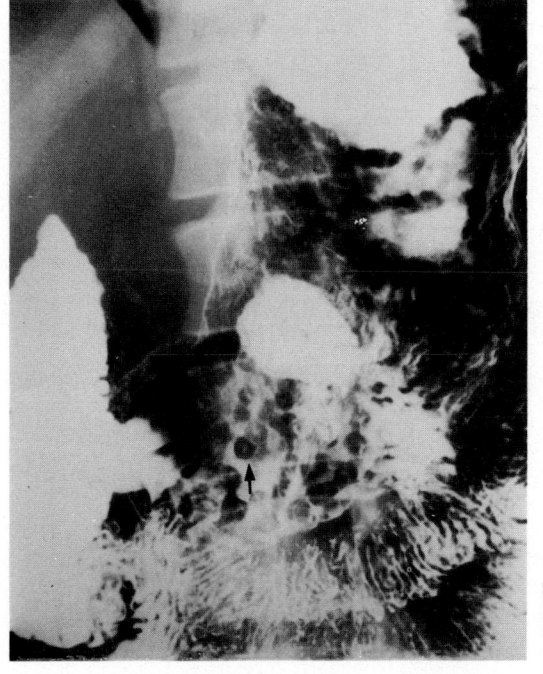

21a

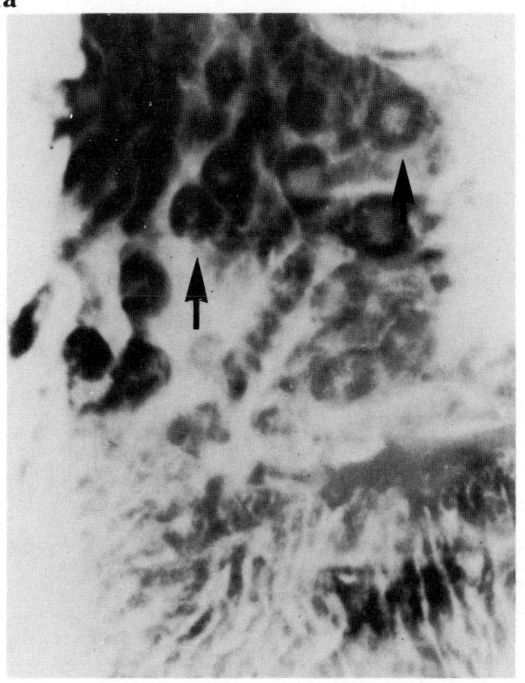

21 Superficial erosions may be demonstrated radiologically. This double contrast barium meal demonstrates severe acute gastric erosions in a male aged 23 years with a 7-year history of dyspepsia. The central mucosal erosion is filled with a spot of barium while the surrounding oedematous mucosa, uncoated by barium, produces the characteristic dot and circle appearance.

21a Close up view of the affected mucosa.

Acute peptic ulceration

Mucosal destruction is accompanied by extension of tissue necrosis deep into the wall and may penetrate all layers leading to perforation and escape of contents into the peritoneal cavity (*vide infra*). Inflammation, though present around the ulcer, is minimal and fibrosis is absent. Peritoneal reaction is also minimal. The consistency of the affected part on palpation is relatively soft in comparison with the firm thickening associated with chronic ulcer. Haemorrhage is a hazard. The great majority of these ulcers heal without scarring. In a minority the ulceration continues and the features of chronic ulceration become superimposed.

22

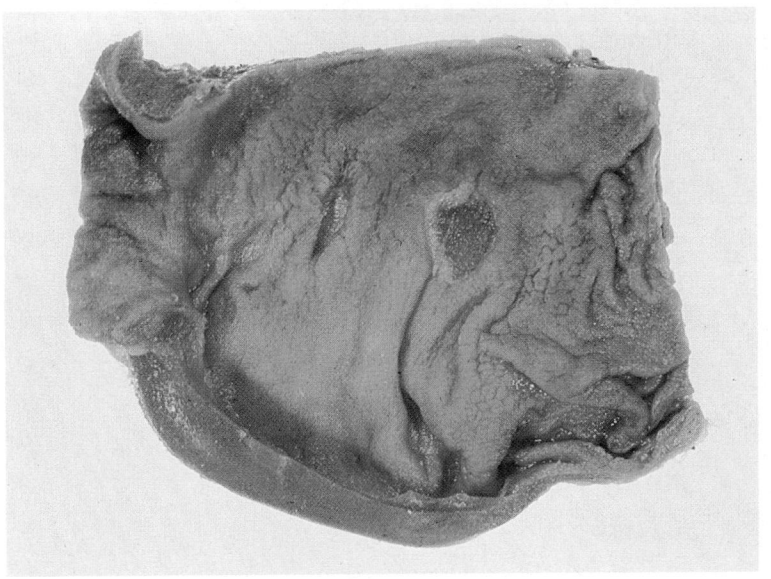

22 This example of acute peptic ulceration was discovered at post mortem examination of a patient who died from pulmonary embolism. Two ulcers are obvious in the pyloric antrum. The larger proximal ulcer measuring approximately 1 × 1.5cm is shallow and its floor is partly covered by blood clot. The distal ulcer is deeper and appears older. In the fresh specimen numerous acute erosions involving only the surface mucosa could be seen and varied from pin-point size to a few millimetres in diameter.

Chronic ulceration

Geographical variation

Peptic ulceration occurring in the stomach and duodenum occurs throughout the world. The incidence of the disease, its course, complications and mortality, however, show variation. These differences have been demonstrated by the statistical studies which have been undertaken universally but the standard of the material on which the statistics have been compiled is not always comparable. It is difficult, therefore, to collate the figures given.

The incidence in Western Europe and North America is high and approximates to that of the United Kingdom as already quoted (10%).

In South Africa it is known that the incidence of peptic ulcer amongst the Bantu is one seventh that of Europeans but that when the native population moves into the towns and adopts a more European mode of life and diet the divergence of incidence becomes less.

In Asia several reports indicate the varying incidence of peptic ulceration. In India the disease is less common in the north than in the south and it has been reported from Travancore that gastric ulceration is common in the lower social classes and is of a chronic character. In Java it has been shown that as between Indonesian and Chinese of the lower social classes the incidence amongst the Chinese is ten times more common.

In reports from Singapore and Hong Kong the high incidence of gastric ulcer as opposed to duodenal ulcer has been recorded.

Observers in India have related their findings to diet and malnutrition and the incidence especially amongst the lower social classes seems to play a prominent part. There is evidence throughout the world that the incidence of gastric and duodenal ulcer is changing possibly in relation to alteration in economic and social conditions. This is another factor to be taken into consideration in the comparison of different statistical studies.

Chronic peptic ulceration is a widespread disease and occurs in those parts of the alimentary canal exposed to hydrochloric acid and pepsin. Such ulcers irrespective of site exhibit a uniform pathology.

23a

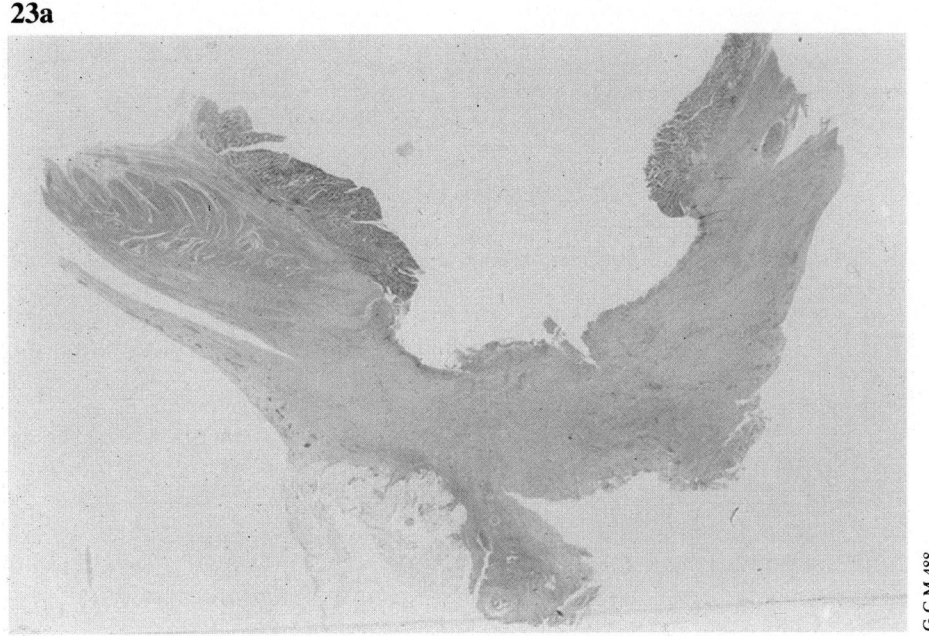

23b

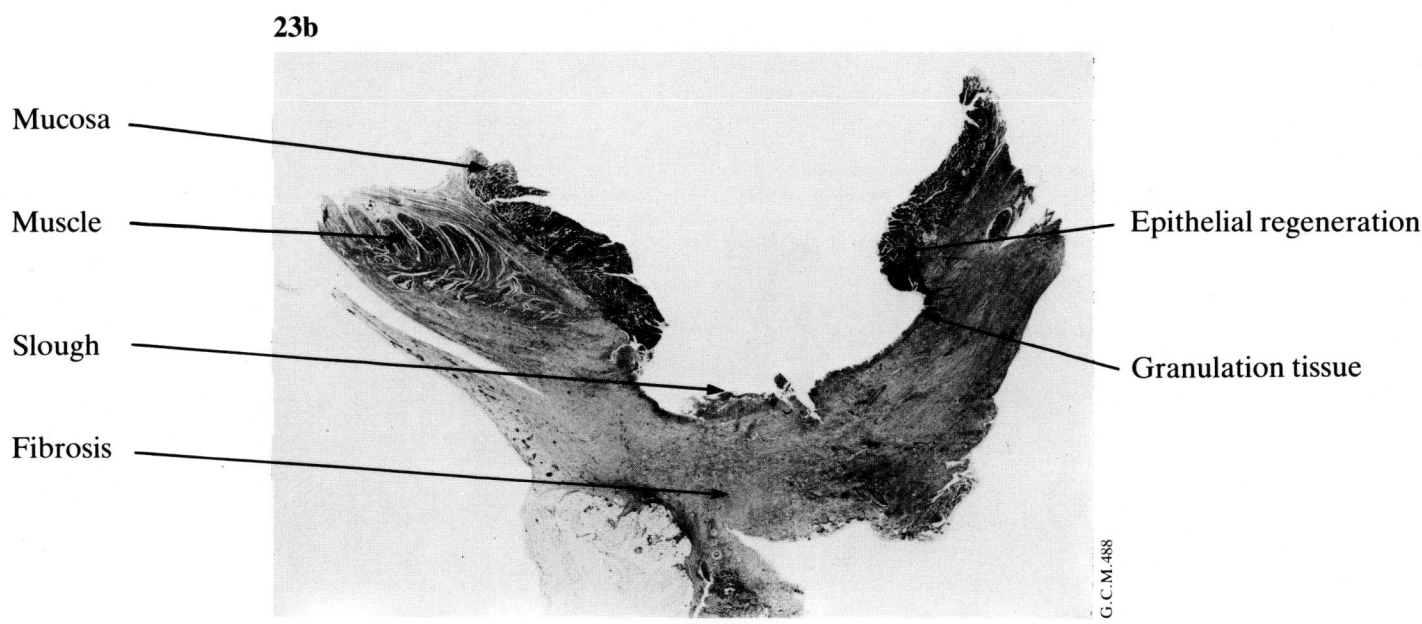

Mucosa

Muscle   Epithelial regeneration

Slough

                                     Granulation tissue

Fibrosis

23b Diagrammatic representation of the pathological layers of a chronic ulcer.

Chronic ulceration *(Continued)*

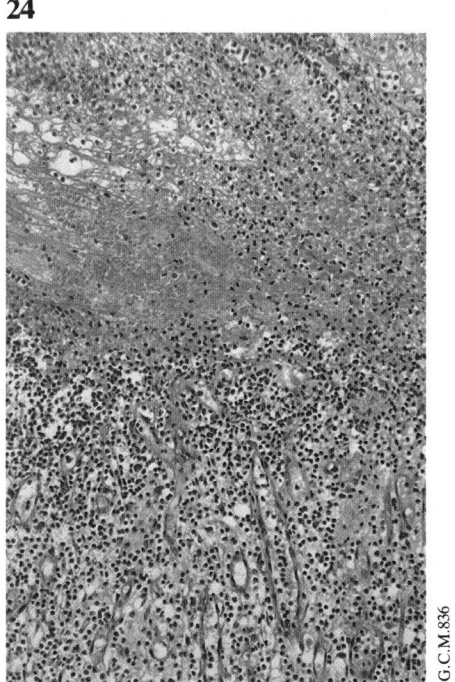

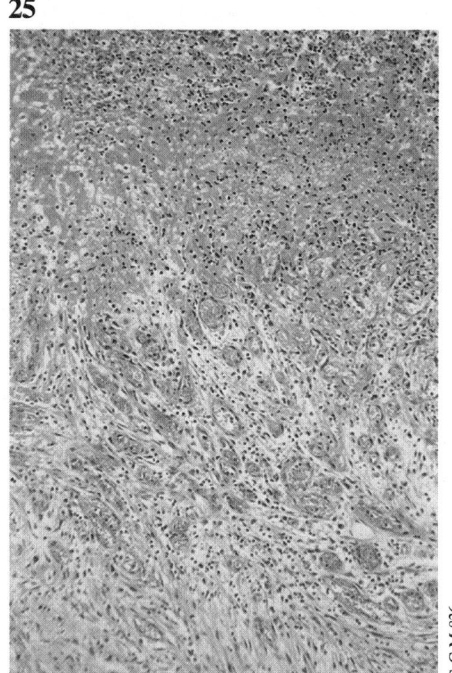

24 The ulcer base is covered by necrotic debris, inflammatory exudate, fibrin and blood. The underlying granulation tissue is infiltrated by acute and chronic inflammatory cells. *(H&E ×125)*

25 Lying below the slough a zone of granulation tissue exists which is being transformed into young fibrous tissue. *(H&E ×100)*

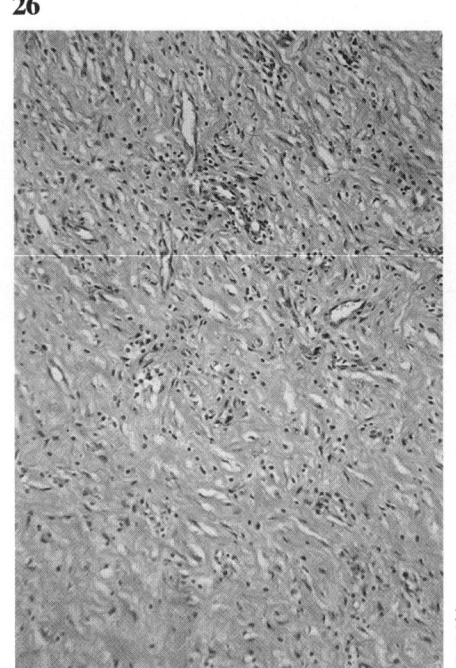

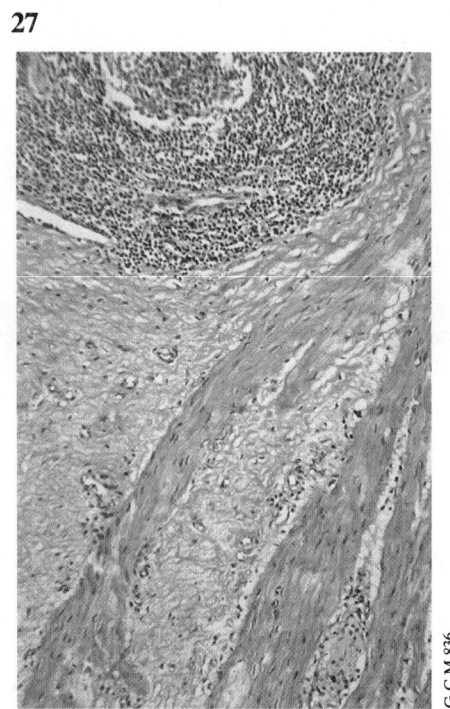

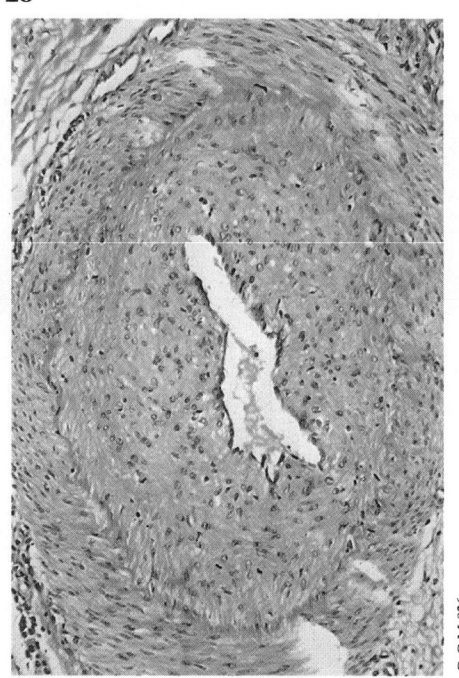

26 Transition of granulation tissue to mature fibrous tissue. *(H&E ×100)*

27 Ulcer base showing fibrosis of muscularis. The lymphoid follicle is hyperplastic. *(H&E ×100)*

28 The lumen of an artery near the base of the ulcer is narrowed by fibrosis – endarteritis obliterans. *(H&E ×125)*

29

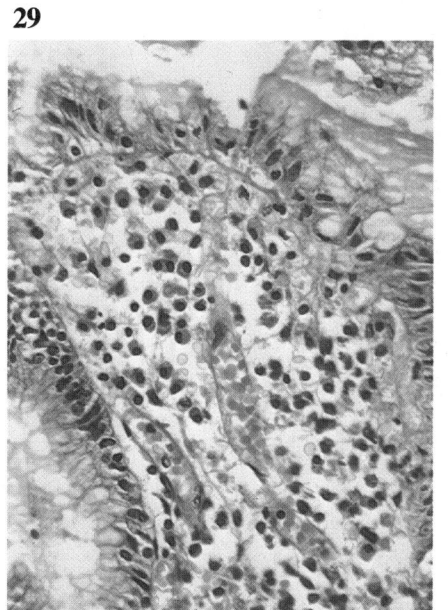

G.C.M.836

29 Plasma cells infiltrate the mucosa around the ulcer. *(H&E ×310)*

30

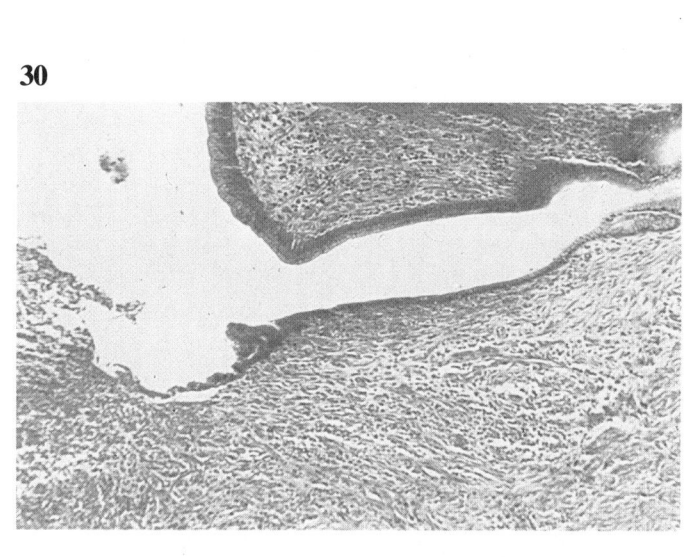

G.C.M.837

30 The mucosa overhangs the margin of the ulcer. A single layer of hyperchromatic regenerative epithelium covers the periphery of the ulcer in an attempt at healing. *(H&E ×100)*

31

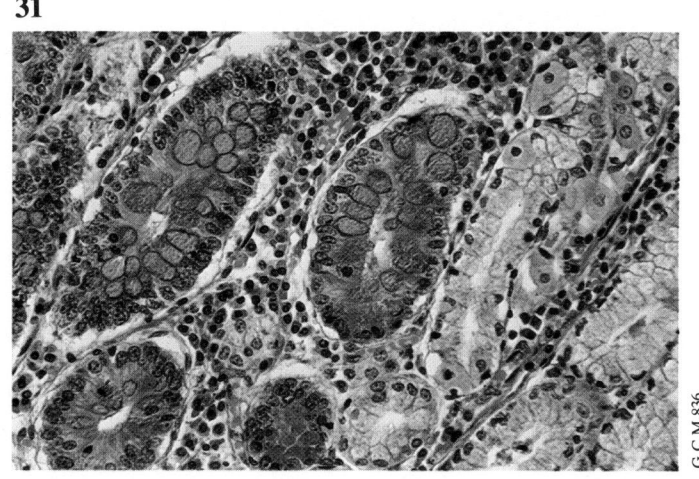

G.C.M.836

31 Intestinal metaplasia near a chronic gastric ulcer. The main glands have been replaced by intestinal-type epithelium. Paneth cells have formed at the base of the crypts. The mucin is strongly stained by alcian green indicating that it is of intestinal type. *(Alcian green, phloxine, tartrazine ×250)*

Chronic ulceration *(Continued)*

Chronic ulceration characteristically runs an episodic course. Periods of greater activity associated with expansion of the ulcer and increased destruction of tissue alternate with periods of healing when the ulcer contracts. In the expanding phase there is evidence of greater inflammatory cell infiltration, congestion and oedema and mucosal destruction is evident.

In the healing phase congestion and oedema subside, cellular infiltration is decreased, increasing fibrosis at the base is evident and at the edges of the ulcer regeneration of the mucosa is present but may show disturbed arrangement.

Chronic peptic ulceration may occur at five sites: oesophagus, stomach, duodenum, at the stoma between stomach and small intestine following partial gastrectomy or gastroenterostomy, and in relation to Meckel's diverticulum. The characteristics of ulceration in each of these sites is described separately.

Gastric ulcer

In the stomach ulceration occurs in non acid secreting areas and accordingly most commonly appears on the lesser curve, in the antrum distal to the junction of antral and body mucosa and in the pyloric canal. A tendency to mucosal ischaemia (*vide supra*) and maximal exposure to refluxed duodenal content, particularly bile, are implicated in these locations.

Gastritis usually surrounds chronic gastric ulceration and whether this is caused by bile reflux and then proceeds to ulceration or whether gastritis and reflux are secondary to duodenal ulceration is debated.

Intestinal metaplasia is frequently found in association with gastritis and forms an area unduly susceptible to the action of acid. Occasionally an ulcer is found very high on the lesser curvature close to the hiatus and may be associated with the presence of a hiatus hernia.

Acid production in gastric ulceration is generally low or within the limits for a normal population. Correspondingly the parietal cell mass is small.

It is noted, however, that distal ulceration involving the pre-pyloric region or the pyloric canal is commonly associated with a relatively high acid level thus bearing a close relationship to the high acid associated with duodenal ulcer.

Chronic gastric ulcers are usually solitary. They present as punched out areas in the gastric mucosa, usually circular in outline but as they become larger they assume an oval shape. The edges of the ulcer are overhanging and are relatively steep on the proximal edge and more shelving at the pyloric edge. The floor of the ulcer is covered by slough overlying the fibrotic base of the ulcer. Characteristically the mucosa of the stomach is arranged in folds which appear to radiate from the ulcer and the mucosa may show a variable degree of oedema and congestion depending on the state of activity of the ulcer. On the peritoneal aspect there may be an area of subserosal fibrosis which causes the area to be pale and firm on touch in comparison with adjacent parts. Peritoneal reaction and the formation of adhesions and fixation of the stomach especially to the liver or pancreas may be present. If the ulcer is in an acute phase some stippling may be observed. When healing occurs contraction takes place and leaves a puckered scar on the serosal surface.

32

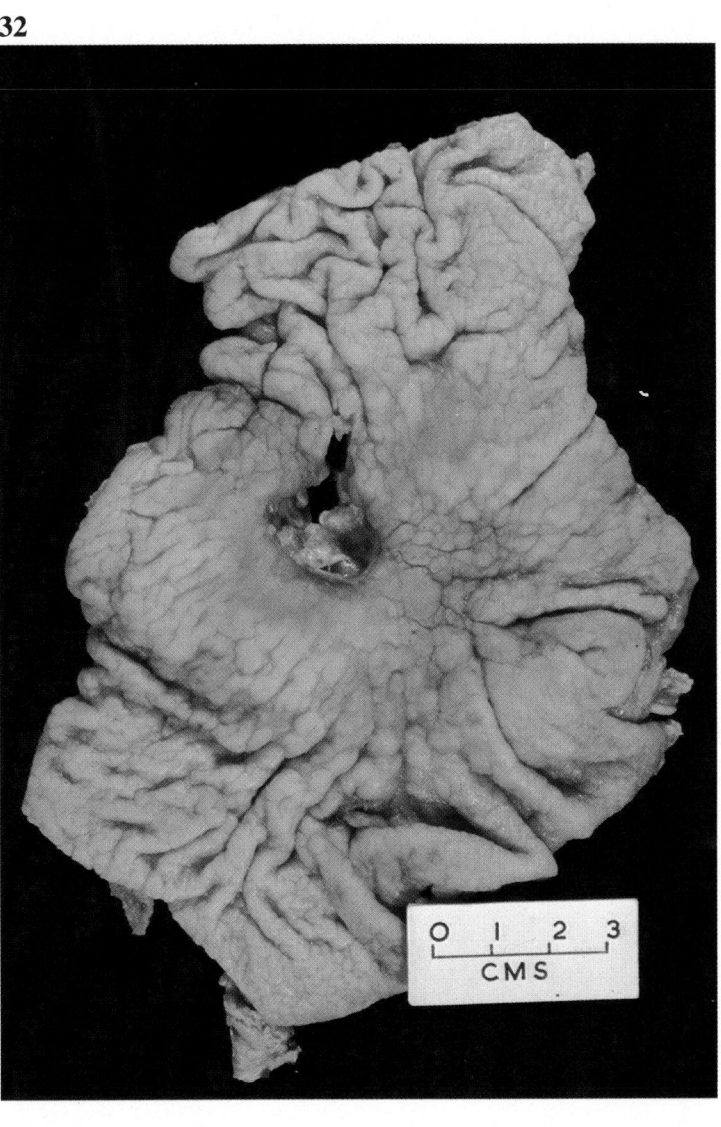

32 From an adult female who gave a 10-year history of dyspepsia, pain in the epigastrium and vomiting. An X-ray taken at the commencement of her illness demonstrated a peptic ulcer. When admitted to hospital the pain had increased and was radiating into her chest. This was associated with considerable vomiting. The specimen shows a large ulcer on the lesser curvature which at operation was located midway between the cardiac and pyloric sphincters. It is deeply penetrating with a sloughy base. Note the sharp outline and the radiation of the mucosal folds about the ulcer. The mucosa in the vicinity of the ulcer appears to be oedematous. The ulcer at operation was adherent to the pancreas.

Chronic ulceration *(Continued)*

Gastric ulcer *(Continued)*

33

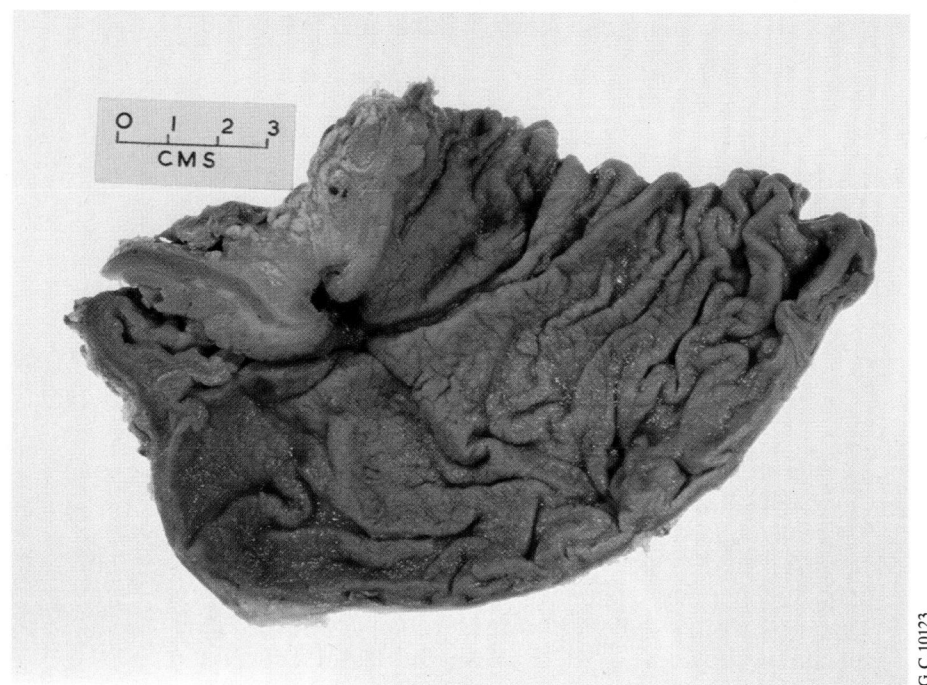

33 From a male aged 40 years. History of dyspepsia for 'many years'. Pain in the epigastrium, left hypochondrium and through to the back. Pain occurred 1 hour after food. Two years prior to admission to hospital the ulcer perforated and simple closure was carried out. Eight months later admitted for definitive treatment. Partial gastrectomy was performed.

The stomach presents a chronic ulcer situated on the lesser curvature. The ulcer is 15 mm in its long axis, is saddle-shaped and has transgressed the whole thickness of the stomach wall. It has a deep crater with typical overhanging margins. The stomach wall in the vicinity and the connective tissues of the lesser omentum adjacent are thickened and fibrous as a result of the chronic inflammation. The mucous membrane adjacent to the crater is drawn into radiating folds as a result of the fibrosis.

34

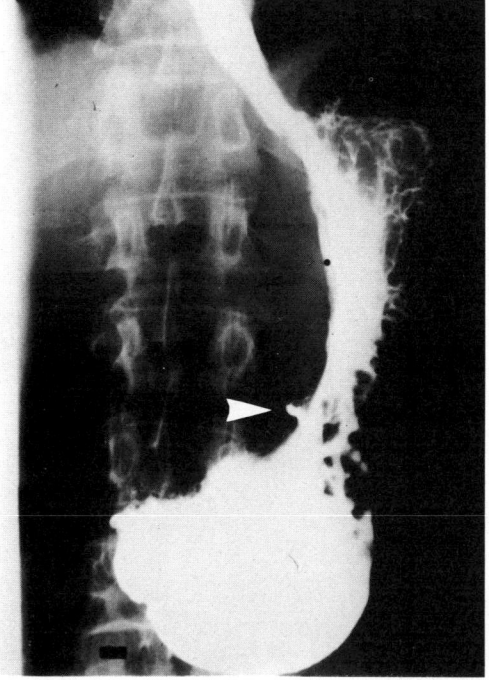

34 From a male aged 55 years. Typical picture of a penetrating ulcer on the lesser curvature of the stomach demonstrated by a barium meal. Note that the outline of the mucosa of the stomach remains normal and that the defect is penetrating into the wall and not protruding in any way into the lumen of the viscus; 'an ulcer niche'.

On the greater curvature there is evidence of irregular hyperactive muscular contraction.

After the barium in the stomach has passed on into the intestine it is frequently found that a residual flake of barium remains in the base of the crater of the ulcer.

Gastric ulceration may present less commonly in an atypical manner:
1 'Kissing' ulcers
2 Giant ulcers
3 Ulcers of the greater curvature

Kissing ulcers

Where two ulcers occur (one on either side of the lesser curvature) but are in contact with each other when the stomach is empty, the term 'kissing' ulcer is applied.

If by extension the two ulcers coalesce they form an ulcer which is described as a saddle ulcer. The saddle shaped ulcer may also arise when a single lesion of the lesser curvature has extended on to both the anterior and posterior walls.

35

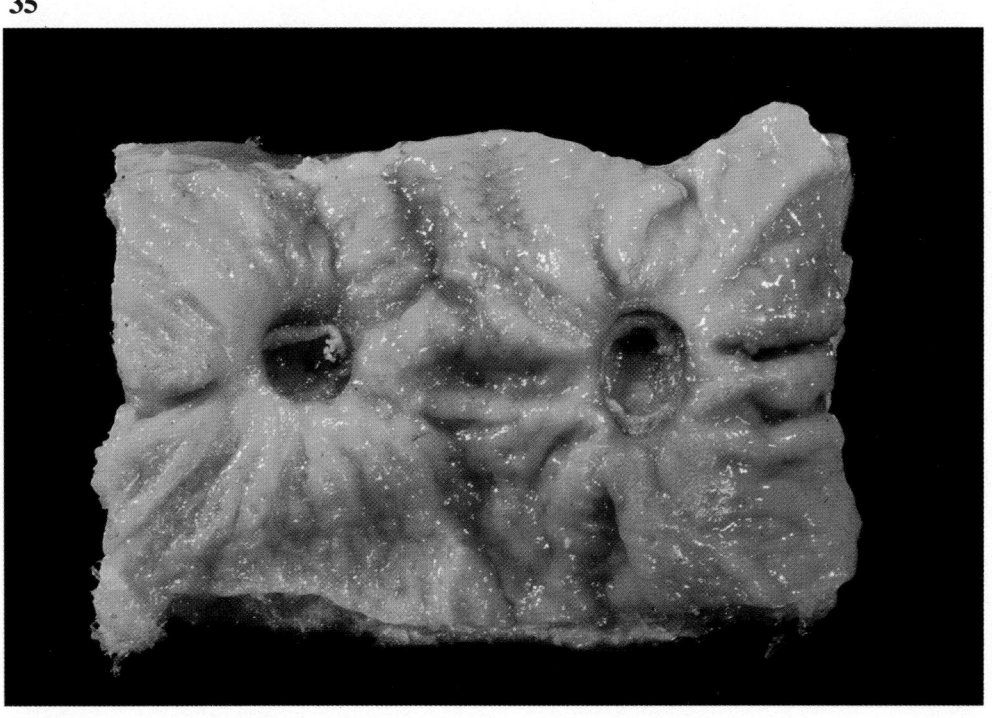

G.C.14645

35 From a male aged 51 years. History of pain characteristic of peptic ulcer. The presence of an ulcer was confirmed by radiological examination. At operation a resection of the ulcer bearing area was carried out.

The specimen shows two chronic peptic ulcers arranged like a pair of spectacles on the lesser curvature of the stomach. The proximal and distal ulcers are rounded and measure roughly 1 cm in diameter. Each of the ulcers is covered by inflammatory exudate and their margins are rather puckered, but the ulcers are themselves sharply punched out. The distal ulcer lay approximately 2 cm proximal to the pylorus.

Chronic ulceration (*Continued*)

Giant ulcer

Examples of atypical ulceration are giant ulcer and lesions occurring in the fundus or greater curvature. It is not improbable that these ulcers are preceded by a gastric mucosal metaplasia leading to the cell formation of intestinal type which has been caused by an earlier gastritis.

36

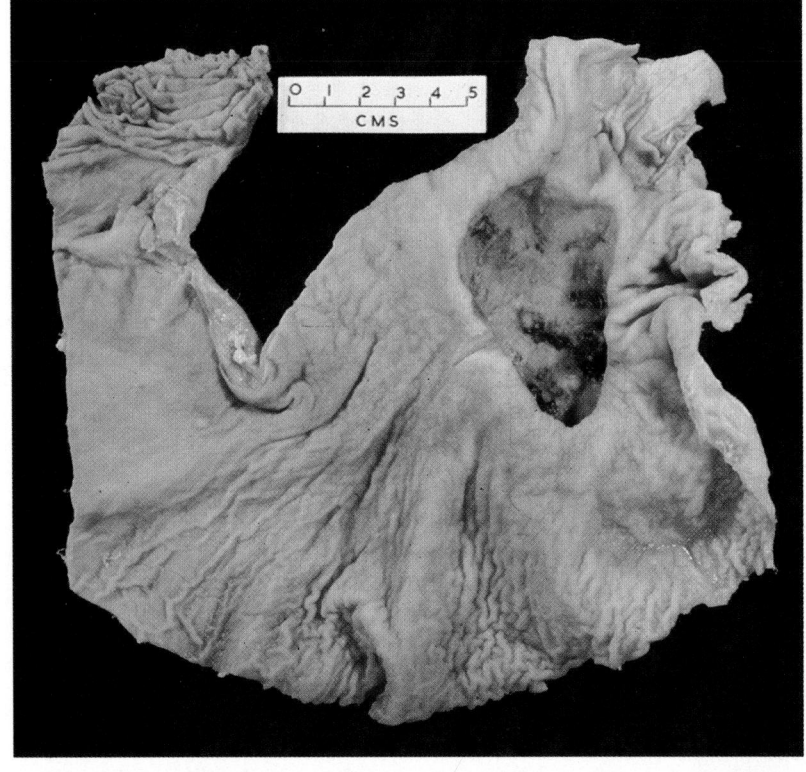

36a

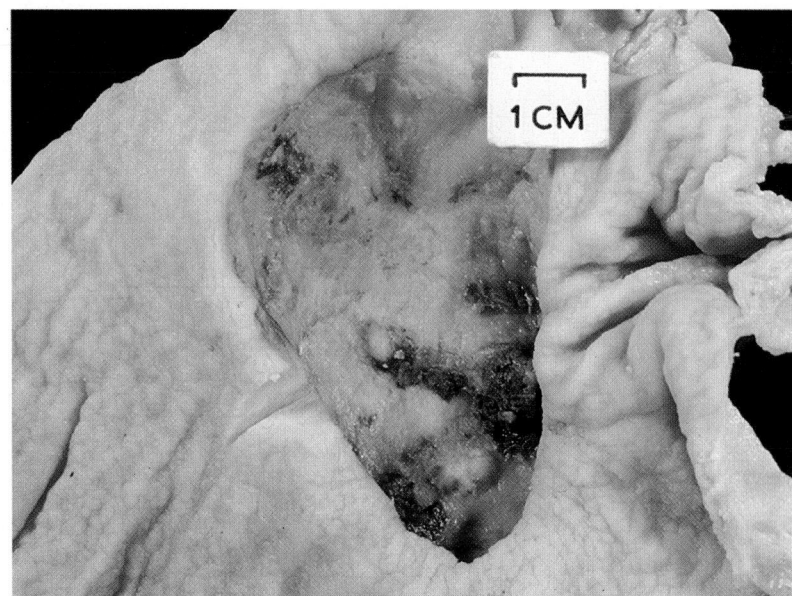

36a   Enlarged view of the ulcer.

36   From a male aged 61 years. This patient ran a relatively asymptomatic course with minimal dyspepsia but was admitted because of 'fainting'. The patient died as the result of an acute massive haematemesis. A very large ovoid ulcer covers the posterior wall of the pyloric antrum. The edges are sharp and clear cut, the wall steep and the floor smooth except for a few nodular elevations one of which, covered with blood clot, represents the site of bleeding from an eroded blood vessel. Histological examination showed chronic simple ulceration.

Ulcers of the greater curvature

Ulcers of the fundus and greater curvature are rare and frequently of giant type. These ulcers commonly have an atypical clinical history of long duration and the diagnosis is initially made by radiological examination.

37

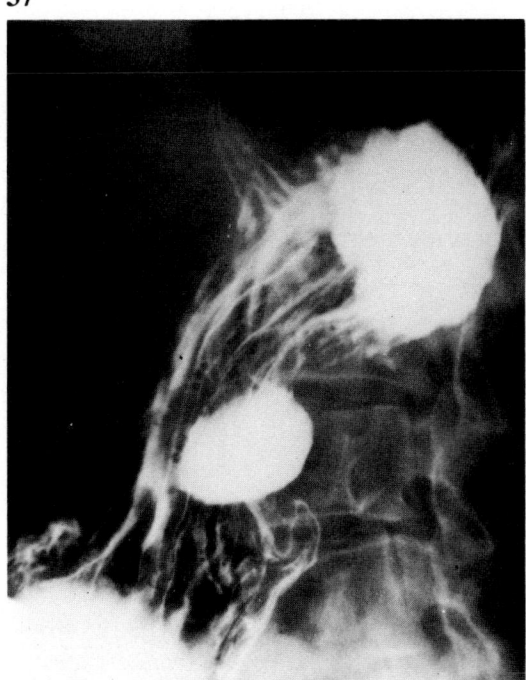

G.C.X.953

37 From a female aged 61 years with a long history of dyspepsia. The barium meal shows a giant ulcer measuring 3 × 5 cm on the greater curvature with considerable surrounding oedema.

Biopsy

Gastric ulcers and in particular giant ulcers and those located on the greater curvature have to be differentiated from carcinoma. This differentation is achieved by histological studies obtained by endoscopic biopsy. Similarly, ulcers especially on the lesser curvature which are suspected of being carcinomatous can be examined. Such examinations are particularly appropriate in older patients in whom a decision to carry out major operative intervention is difficult in view of the increased operative risk. Four quadrant examination of the margin of the ulcer with special attention to any areas which may suggest proliferative activity is undertaken and material from the floor of the ulcer (brushings) is also taken for cytological examination (see Section 14 U).

Chronic ulceration *(Continued)*

Duodenal ulcer

Duodenal ulceration most commonly occurs in the first part of the duodenum and less commonly in the first segment of the second part proximal to the ampulla of Vater. This part of the duodenum receives the acidic gastric content prior to neutralisation and thus bears the brunt of its corrosive action. Earlier studies were more familiar with a relatively acute ulcer on the anterior wall in which the complication of early perforation was common. Present experience in the United Kingdom indicates that posterior ulceration is now more frequent and is of a more chronic and penetrating character.

Patients with duodenal ulceration have higher capacities to produce acid than do individuals without ulcers. The range of acid producing capacity overlaps with that of the normal population.

Two other factors contribute toward the hyperchlorhydria of duodenal ulcer patients:
1 Increased sensitivity of the parietal cell to a given acid producing stimulus
2 An inherently high parietal cell drive by either hormonal or neural mechanisms

38

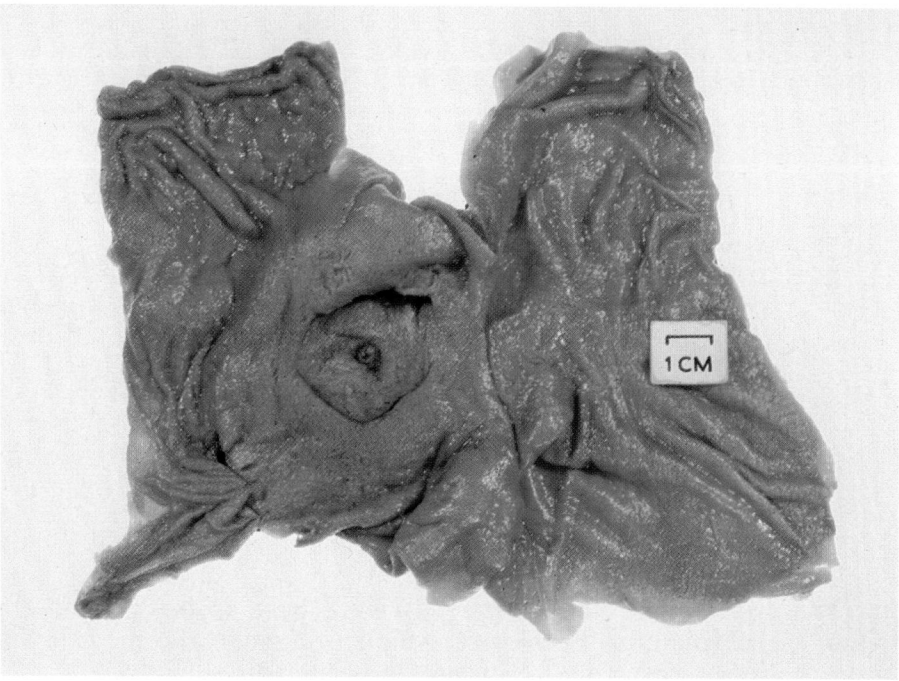

1 CM

G.C.6538

38 From a male aged 75 years who died of an unconnected condition. At post mortem examination ulceration of the first part of the duodenum was disclosed.

On the posterior wall of the duodenum some 10 mm distal to the pylorus commences a quadrilateral ulcer measuring some 33 mm in its long axis with a well defined, smooth but deeply undermined margin and a slightly irregular floor in the centre of which a raised blood-stained papilla indicates the site of haemorrhage from the gastroduodenal artery which was shown on the posterior surface in immediate proximity to part of the head of the pancreas.

Chronic ulcers are usually solitary and if on the anterior wall are small. Kissing or opposing ulcers occurring simultaneously on the anterior and posterior wall are not infrequent. When healing occurs, especially when the ulcer is on the anterior wall, scarring can be observed with puckering of the peritoneal coat. Coexisting gastric ulcers are not infrequently encountered. This may relate to acid hypersecretion or to gastric stasis induced by pyloric spasm or stenosis.

39

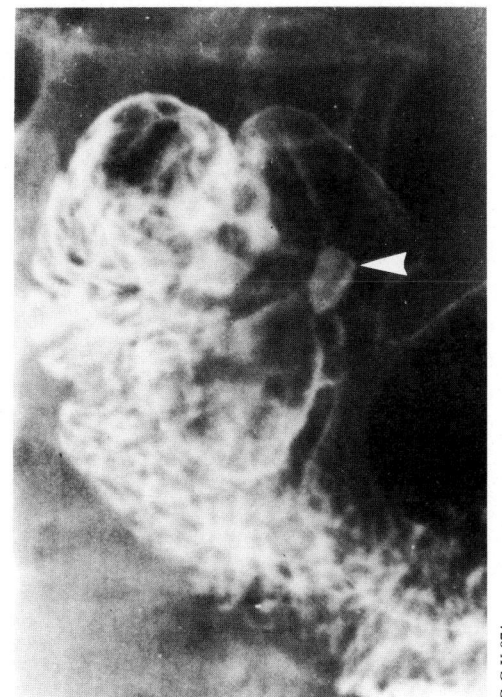

G.C.X.974

39 From a male aged 37 years with a long history of dyspepsia and one previous haematemesis.

Double contrast barium meal shows deformity of the duodenal cap with a large ulcer crater from which radiate folds of duodenal mucosa.

40

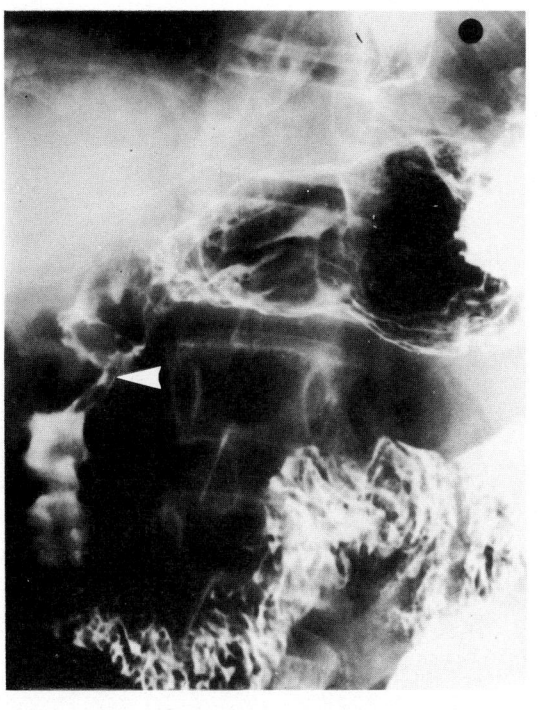

G.C.X.332

40 From a male aged 62 years who suffered from longstanding dyspepsia.

The ulcer lies in the second part of the duodenum and is associated with a degree of retention of barium. Ulcers in this region may cause a deformity which suggests carcinoma by reason of an apparent filling defect.

Peptic ulceration occurring in the distal part of the duodenum is usually the result of the endocrine disturbance known as the Zollinger–Ellison syndrome. Such ulcers may be single or multiple. The Zollinger–Ellison syndrome is associated with the presence of non-beta adenoma(s) of the pancreas which cause a marked rise of acid secretion and there is inability of the biliary and pancreatic fluids to neutralise the overproduction of acid (see Section 17U).

Chronic ulceration *(Continued)*

Gastro-jejunal (stomal) ulcer

Following gastrojejunostomy even if combined with vagotomy or partial gastrectomy, ulceration at, or close to the site of the anastomosis, may occur. The incidence of stomal ulcer is difficult to assess with accuracy as many reports are based on comparatively short (5 to 10 years) studies and has been variously estimated between 2 and 20%, but the long-term studies have revealed that the true incidence of stomal ulceration steadily increases with the passage of time and figures of 30% have been recorded. Stomal ulcer is five times more common following simple gastrojejunostomy than after partial gastrectomy and the majority develop within 3 years but the late development of ulcers up to 30 years after an operation is well recognised.

The great majority of stomal ulcers occur in young males who have been operated on for duodenal ulcer associated with hyperchlorhydria.

41 From a male aged 43 years with a 6-year history of dyspepsia complicated by a duodenal perforation. This was treated by simple closure but within 2 years he developed evidence of duodenal stenosis. A posterior gastrojejunostomy was performed. One year later he developed evidence of a stomal ulcer and a partial gastrectomy was performed.

The illustration is that of the posterior wall of the stomach and the stoma. Note how the gastric mucosa of the stomach is congested and markedly rugose but in the vicinity of the ulcer and pyloric segment is flattened. The stoma is small, approximately 1 cm and showed ulceration on the lower lip.

(a) Commonly the ulcer arises in the jejunum (80%) exposed to the gastric juices against which the jejunal mucosa is poorly protected. The ulcer may arise close to the anastomosis or occur in the efferent loop more distant from the anastomosis.
(b) The stomal ulcer is most commonly caused (90%) by the persistence of hyperchlorhydria and is therefore usually the sequel to operation performed for duodenal ulcer. It may also occur with a low level of acidity.
(c) The ulcer may arise at the line of suture and be attributed to faulty technique, e.g. the use of non-absorbable sutures, haematoma formation, crushing of tissues, etc.

41

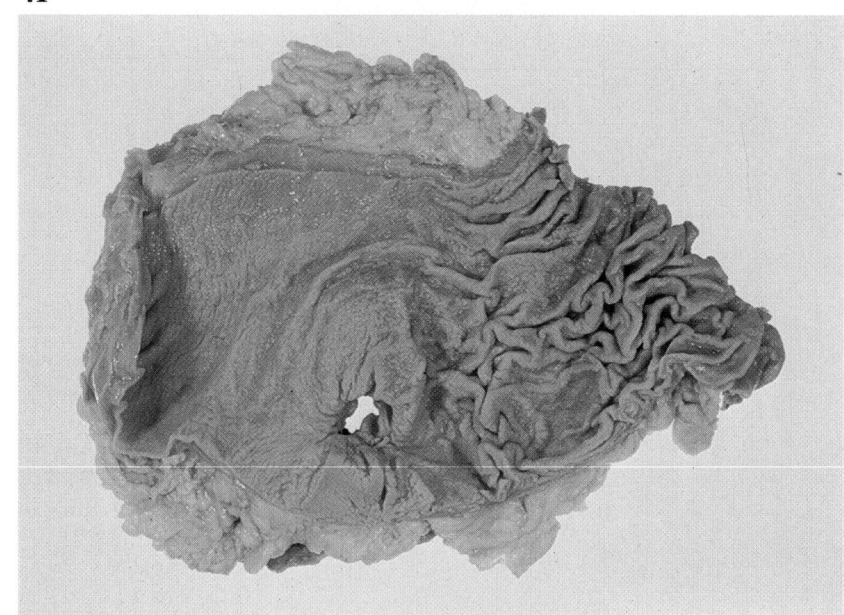

G.C.10213

In common with other peptic ulcers the disease may run an acute or chronic course and may be intermittent. The ulcer crater may be small but is surrounded by much inflammatory reaction and tends to penetrate deeply. There are frequently dense adhesions whereby the stomach becomes fixed to adjacent structures especially the colon. Occasionally in longstanding ulceration contraction of the fibrous tissue leading to occlusion of the stoma occurs. In this event recurrence of an original duodenal ulcer is common even if the stomal ulcer heals. Occult blood in the stools is common and massive haemorrhage can occur.

42

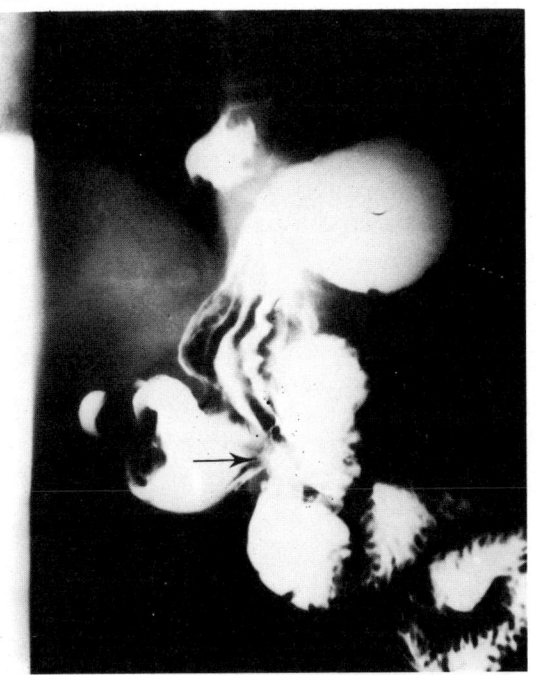

G.C.X.327

42 From a female aged 58 years who had a previous duodenal ulcer for which a gastro-enterostomy was performed. Recurrence of symptoms due to the formation of an anastomotic ulcer.

Note the prominence of the mucosal rugae in the stomach and the ulcer crater at the anastomosis in which an irregular mass of barium is lodged.

43

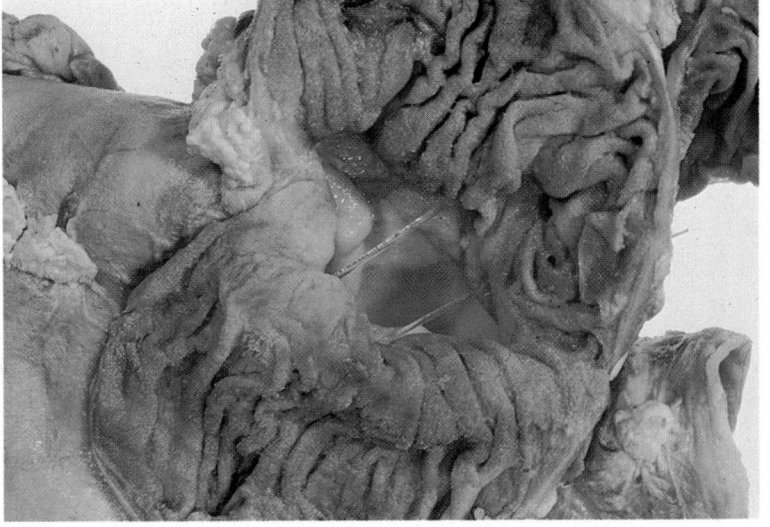

G.C.11808

43 From a male aged 59 years. Illustration of a stomal ulcer of very long duration. Gastrojejunostomy 1931. Operation for stomal ulcer 1958. This is an enlarged picture to show the detailed characteristics of the ulcer.

Complications

The specially important complications of gastro-jejunal ulcer are fistula formation and the development of a carcinoma at the site of the stoma (see Section 14 U).

Complication – Perforation

An ulcer may transgress the wall of the stomach or duodenum:
1　Where the peritoneum is not attached to adjacent structures free perforation into the peritoneal cavity occurs.
2　When the stomach or duodenum becomes adherent to a hollow viscus, e.g. the colon or kidney, a fistula may form.
3　When the stomach or duodenum becomes adherent to an adjacent solid viscus, e.g. the pancreas or liver, the floor of the ulcer is formed by that organ. These are referred to as penetrating ulcers.

The typical perforation is seen as a punched out hole in the wall of the viscus when observed from the peritoneal aspect and frequently occurs during the earlier active phase of ulceration. The most common site is the anterior wall of the duodenum. The edges of the perforation are sharply demarcated with surrounding oedema and thickening of the wall of the duodenum. At operation the escape of contents can be clearly observed. In such cases the wall of the duodenum is firm but is frequently friable making operative closure difficult. Enlargement of the adjacent lymph nodes is sometimes present. These features show variation according to the activity or chronicity of the ulcer.

Perforation of an ulcer results in the escape of liquid and gaseous content from the stomach or duodenum. This results in an initial chemical peritonitis and is followed within 6 to 12 hours by the onset of bacterial peritonitis, primarily streptococcal. The peritoneal reaction and the outpouring of fluid may be localised or become diffuse.

Where perforation occurs in a more gradually penetrating ulcer the final transgression of the serous coat may be minute initially and this may be sealed by an adjacent omental tag or by coagulation of lymph on the surface. To this the term 'sealed perforation' is applied. This sealing may be curative or the process continue with reperforation within a short period of time.

44

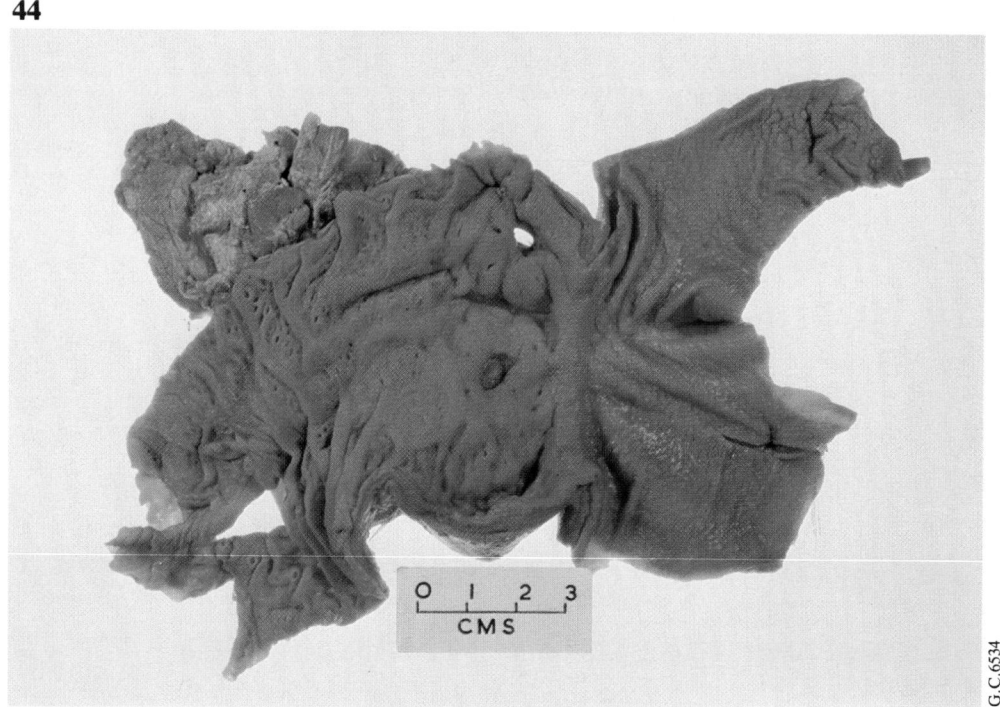

O 1 2 3
CMS

G.C.6534

44　From an adult. Some 15mm distal from the pylorus a small circular ulcer, 6mm in diameter, perforates the thickness of the anterior wall of the duodenum. The edge of the ulcer is smooth and rounded, slightly undermined and about half of the floor is occupied by the perforation. An ulcer of the same size, shape and character is present on the posterior wall (kissing ulcer) at the point of contact with the anterior ulcer when this portion of the duodenum is collapsed. The posterior wall is not completely perforated and to it the pancreas has become adherent.

This second example of perforation illustrates the features from the peritoneal aspect.

45

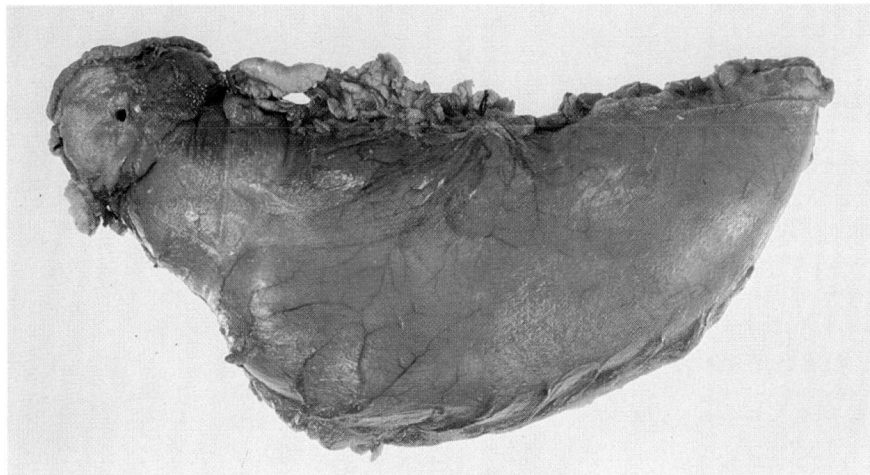

45a

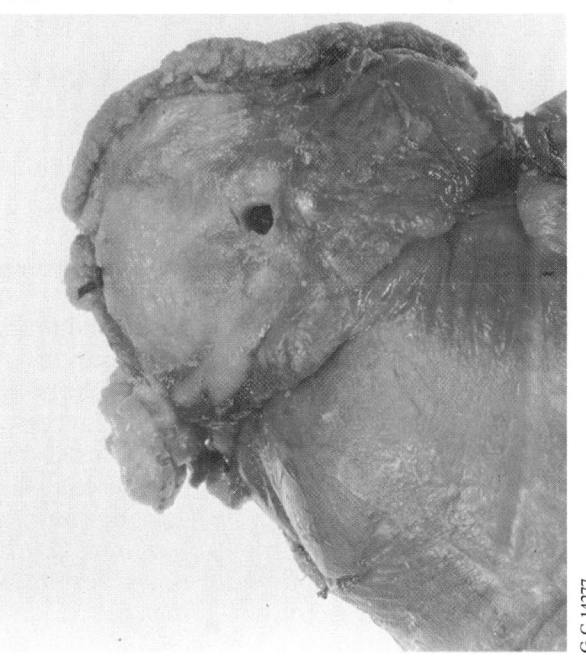

45 and **45a**   From an adult male who had a long history of duodenal ulcer. The ulcer perforated on two occasions. On the first occasion the perforation was treated by simple closure. After a period of time, during which symptoms continued, perforation again occurred and a partial gastrectomy was performed. This case illustrates that perforation may recur after a considerable interval.

The gas which escapes into the peritoneal cavity following perforation rises and accumulates between the diaphragm and the liver (subphrenic space) (**46**), and below the liver in the vicinity of the perforation. This may be demonstrated best on a plain, upright, chest X-ray.

An alternative radiological method of demonstrating a perforation is by the administration (orally or by tube) of a water soluble radio opaque substance e.g. gastrografin (**47**) which escapes from the duodenum and tracks downwards along the right para colic gutter.

47

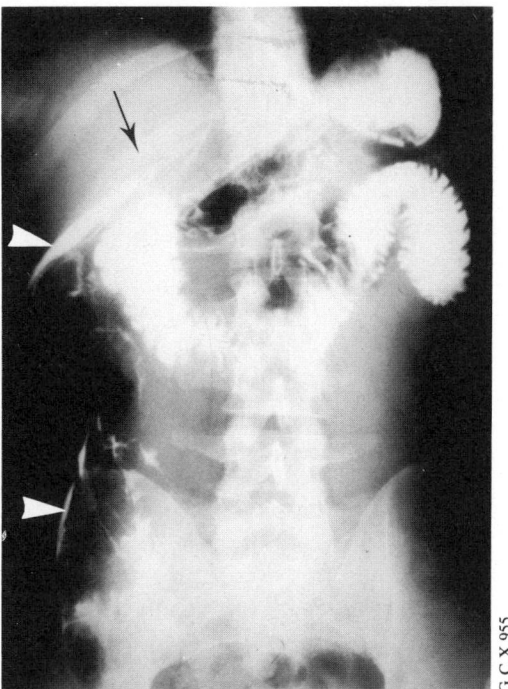

46

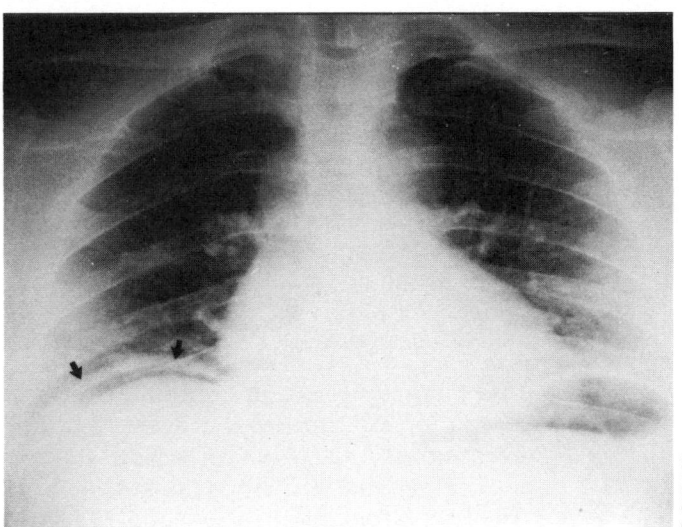

46   Male aged 47 years.

47   Male aged 35 years.

97

Perforation *(Continued)*

Gastro-jejuno-colic fistula

Because of the dense adhesions and fibrous tissue reaction about a stomal ulcer, frank perforation into the free peritoneal cavity is uncommon. A localised peritonitis or abscess formation can occur. Deep penetration through a mass of adhesions into the colon causes a fistula (gastro-jejuno-colic fistula). This occurs in 5 to 8% of gastrojejunal ulcers. The colon lies as an immediate relation to the line of anastomosis to which it has become firmly bound by adhesions. In the presence of ulceration a fistulous tract, which may be either short and direct or long and tortuous, forms between the stomach, jejunum and colon. The fistula formation may be a speedy (months) or delayed (years) complication.

Faecal material may regurgitate into the stomach causing faecal vomiting. The faecal material which enters the jejunum induces a severe jejunitis which leads to diarrhoea. At the same time gastric content and jejunal secretions enter the colon and this too causes diarrhoea. The result of the diarrhoea is malabsorption and debility.

Gastro-colic fistula

48 and **48a** From a male aged 54 years. History of vomiting offensive material and diarrhoea with passage of porridge-like stools in the morning.

48

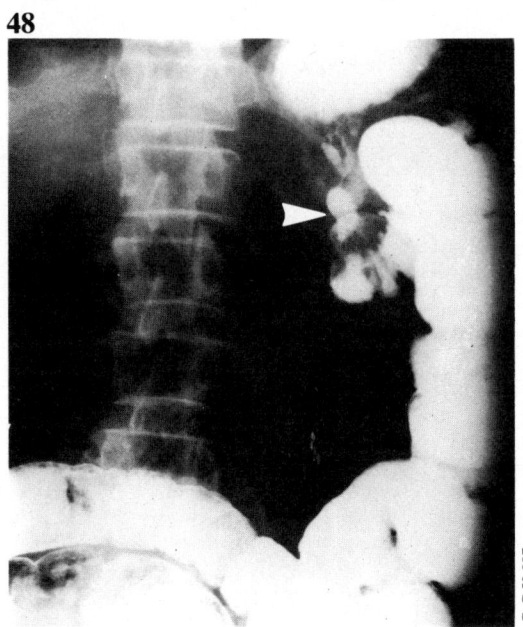

G.C.X.887

48a

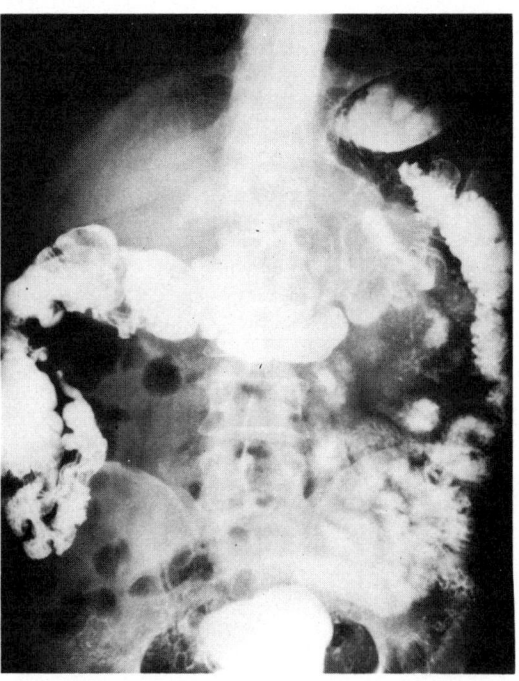

48 Barium enema reveals a gastro-jejuno-colic fistula due to a benign peptic ulcer of the stomach eroding the splenic flexure of the colon.

48a Post-evacuation film showing emptying of the distal colon, retained barium in the colon proximal to the fistula and barium from the stomach in the small intestine.

Pyeloduodenal fistula

49 and **49a**   This is an unusual specimen in which a communication has been established between the renal pelvis and the second part of the duodenum. No clinical notes are available.

The specimen is a right kidney on the anterior surface of which, at the lower pole is attached a small portion of duodenal wall apparently the site of an ulcer the base of which communicates with the lower calyx of the kidney. There is a degree of hydronephrosis. The mucous membrane of the pelvis is oedematous and congested, indicative of an inflammatory reaction.

The most probable explanation is that a duodenal ulcer has become adherent to the anterior surface of the underlying kidney and slow penetration (perforation) has occurred, the renal infection being secondary to the entry of duodenal contents into the renal pelvis.

49

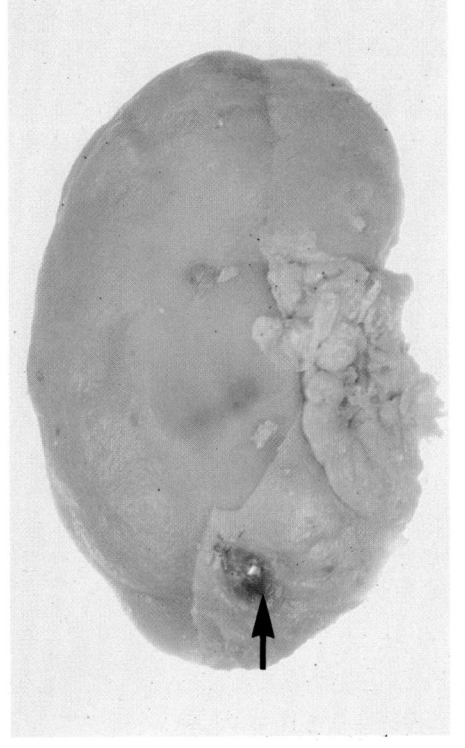

G.C.14746

49a

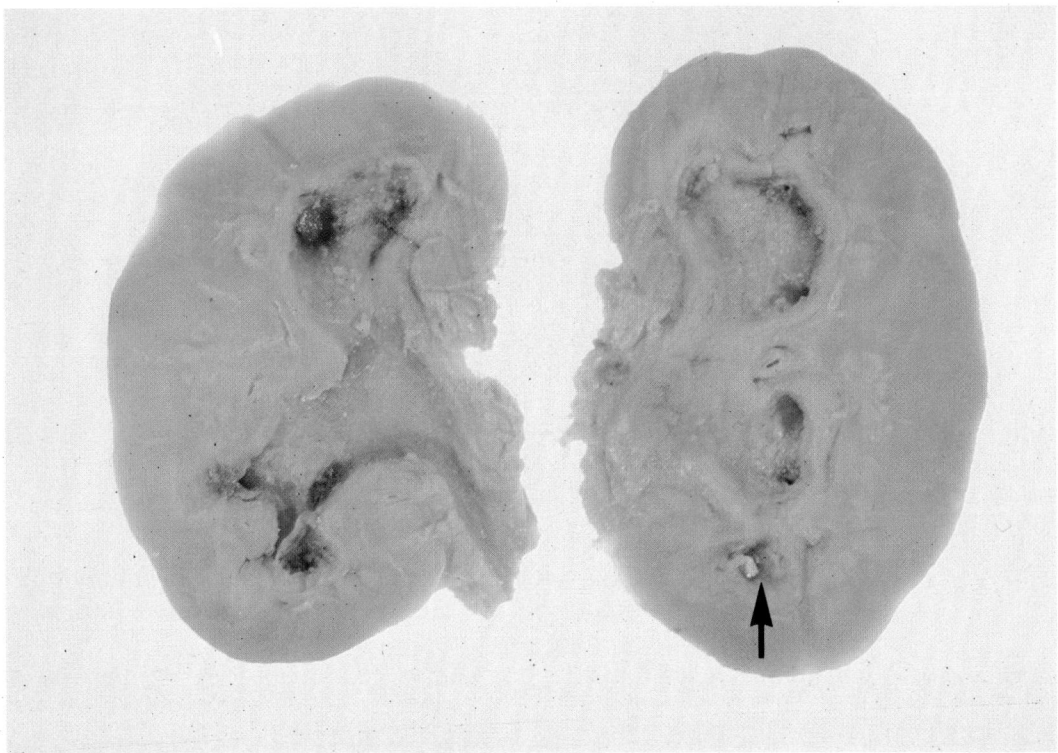

This ulcer must have arisen in the second part of the duodenum and therefore may be an example of the Zollinger–Ellison syndrome.

Ulcers of the second part of the duodenum may present great difficulty in radiological diagnosis and technical difficulties at operation.

Perforation *(Continued)*

Fistula formation

50 and **50a**   From a female aged 45 years. Ten-year history of periodic suprapubic pain associated with dysuria and the passage of malodorous urine. There was a short history of epigastric pain occurring before meals and relieved by the ingestion of food. This pain was especially severe at night. Some vomiting. The left kidney was palpable and presented as a hard mass. Barium meal was normal (**50**). Pyelography showed a normal right kidney and a non functioning left kidney. On retrograde pyelogram the left renal pelvis showed hydronephrosis and distortion of the pelvis. The contrast medium was seen to enter the duodenum (**50a**). Left nephrectomy and repair of the fistula was carried out.

50

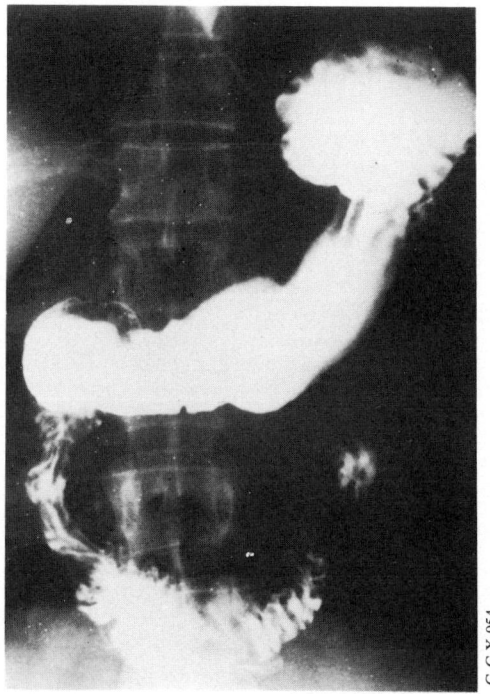

50a

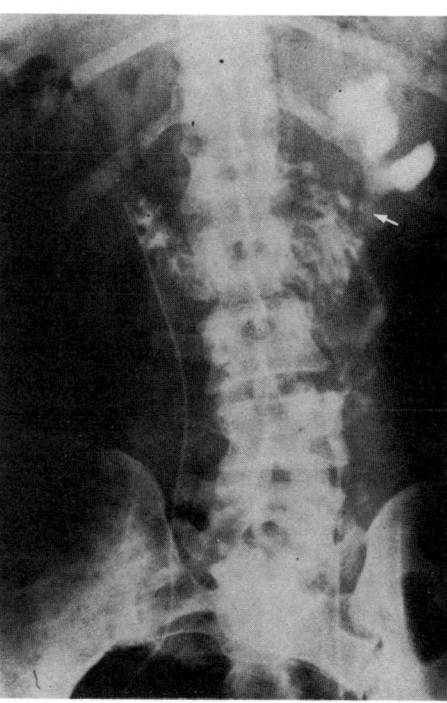

Pyeloduodenal fistula on the left side is extremely rare. Probably this fistula was the sequel to a primary renal lesion. It could well be that an acute pyonephrosis complicated by a perinephric abscess which ruptured into the duodenum was the cause of the fistula.

Penetrating ulcer

The danger of a deeply penetrating ulcer is not damage to the viscus itself but the grave risk of massive haemorrhage which is described later.

Complication – Haemorrhage

Haemorrhage is a common complication of ulceration but the amount is usually small and detected only by examination of the stools. Overt, often massive haemorrhage leading to haematemesis or evident melaena is less frequent but is serious and may be fatal.

Sites of haemorrhage

Haemorrhage may arise from congested mucosa with or without superficial erosions. The haemorrhage may be slight or massive but at operation in such cases or at post mortem examination the source of the bleeding may not be evident.

In acute ulceration haemorrhage may occur but is not common and usually there is spontaneous arrest. The haemorrhage may be minimal or considerable and arises from the congested mucosa or erosion of small vessels in the wall of the viscus. In chronic ulceration haemorrhage is also usually slight though massive bleeding is a serious and often fatal complication.

The haemorrhage may arise from surrounding congested mucosa or from granulation tissue at the base of the ulcer. It may arise from a smaller vessel in the wall of the stomach close to the ulcer which has probably become the site of endarteritis. This interferes with spontaneous arrest. Where the ulcer has penetrated more deeply a large vessel (extragastric) adjacent to the base of the ulcer e.g. the left gastric, the splenic or the gastroduodenal is eroded and haemorrhage is massive. It is not uncommon for small initial (warning) haemorrhages to precede the erosion of a major vessel.

51

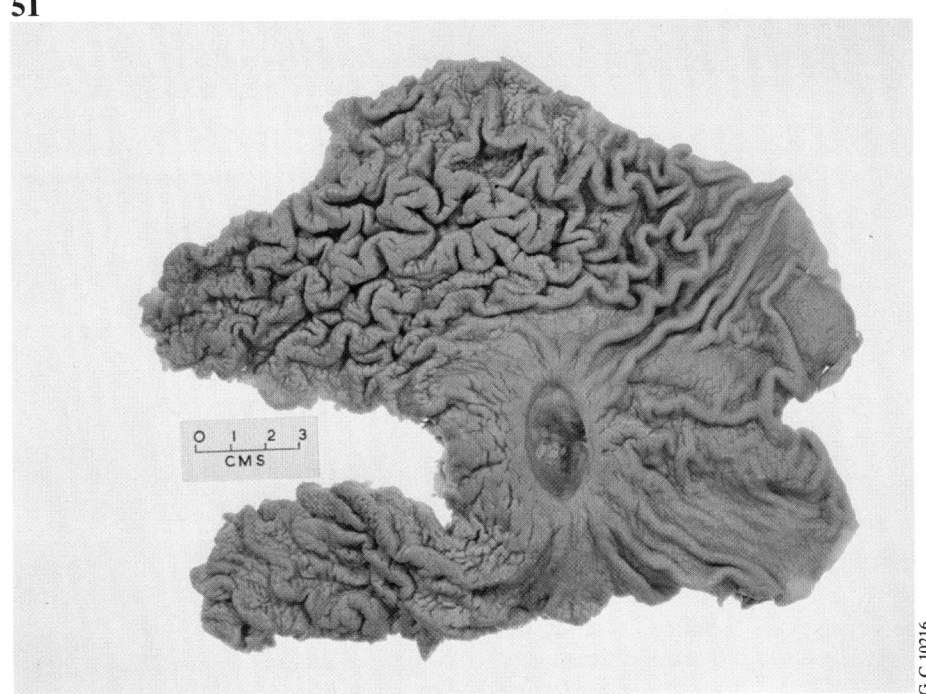

G.C. 10216

51 From a male aged 40 years. Ten-year history of ulcer. A severe haematemesis occurred 11 days after the ulcer had perforated and been repaired. A partial gastrectomy was performed.

A typical gastric ulcer is located on the lesser curvature. The feature of note in this instance is the presence of blood clot in the base of the ulcer but no single bleeding point is identified.

101

Haemorrhage *(Continued)*

52

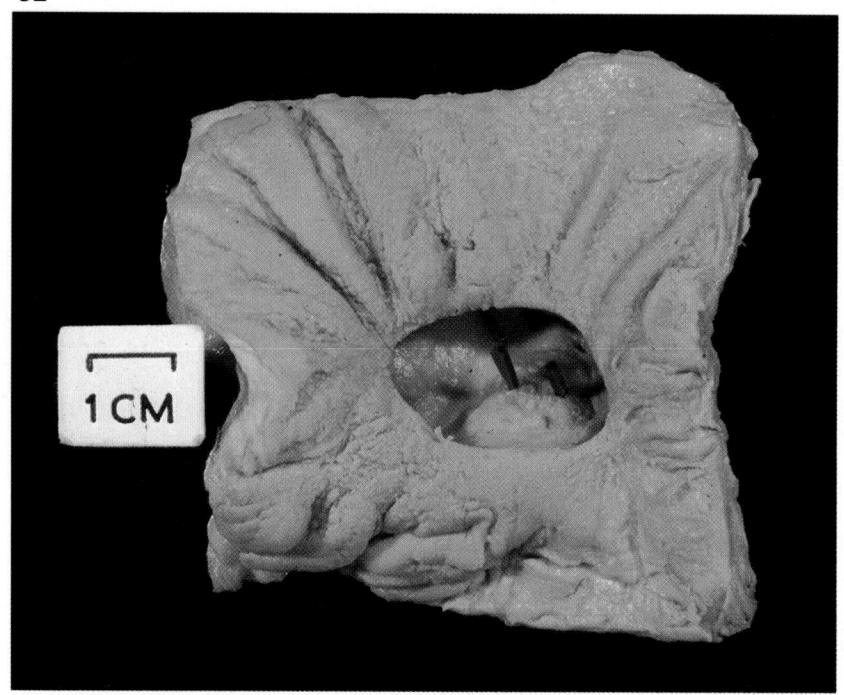

G.C.12078

52 Post mortem specimen. From an adult who died following a massive haematemesis. A large ulcer on the posterior wall of the stomach close to the lesser curvature adherent to the pancreas. Two arteries in the substance of the pancreas and in the floor of the ulcer have been eroded.

53

53 From a male aged 72 years who suffered from indigestion for 'several years'. Admitted with a severe haematemesis.

At operation the stomach was opened and a shallow ulcer was seen on the posterior wall of the antrum with, protruding from its base, a large rounded hollow mass partly open and with blood welling up from its base. This simulated an aneurysm and a polya partial gastrectomy was performed. The patient made a satisfactory recovery. When the specimen was examined it was observed that haemorrhage had occurred from a branch of the gastro-duodenal artery.

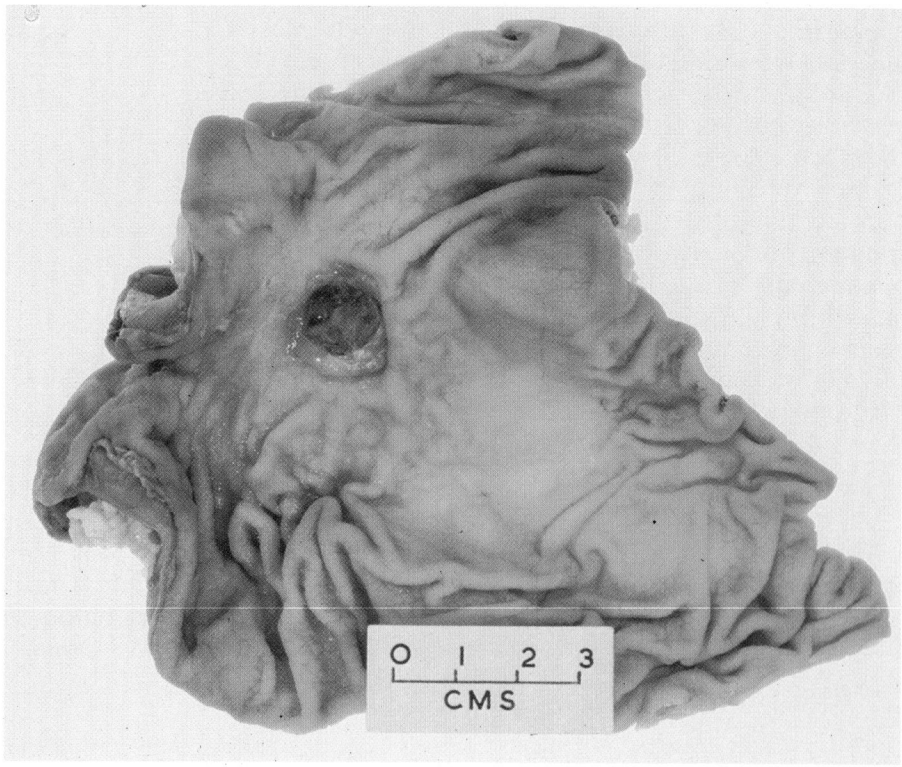

G.C.14021

54

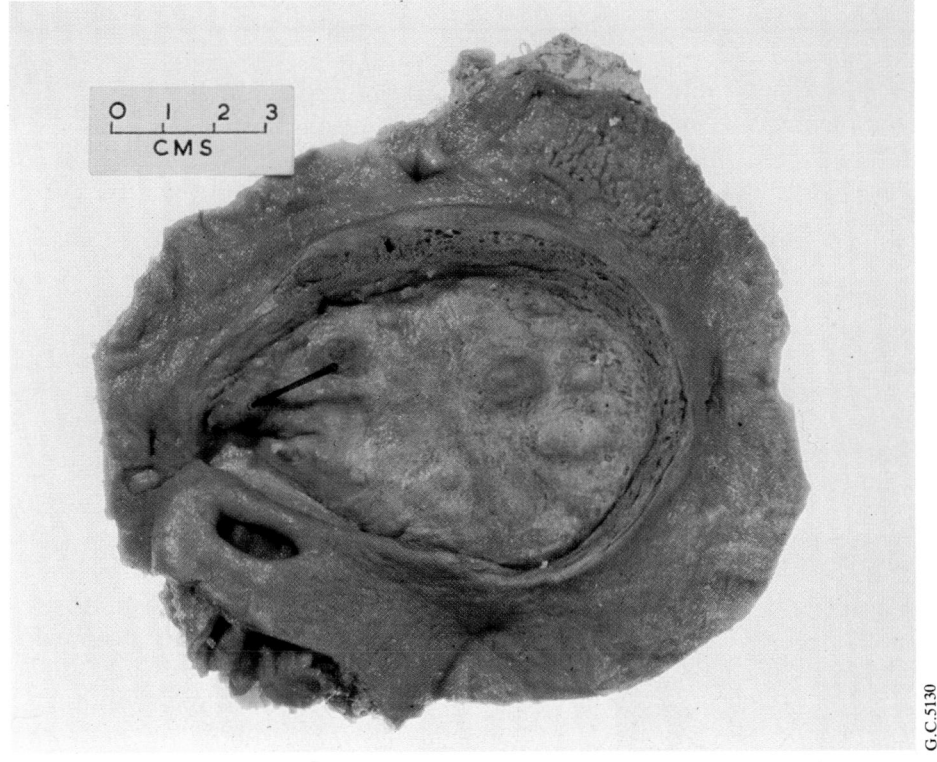

G.C.5130

54 From an adult who died of massive haematemesis. A large chronic gastric ulcer located on the lesser curvature and posterior wall of the antrum. The stomach has been opened along the greater curvature exhibiting the piriform shape of the ulcer the maximal diameters of which measure 95 × 65 mm. The margin of the ulcer is raised, smooth and is composed of mucosa and the whole thickness of the muscular coat. The floor of the ulcer is nodular and is formed by the pancreas covered with newly formed fibrous tissue. Towards the apex of the ulcer a glass rod indicates an opening into an artery, probably the gastroduodenal. Not far from the apex of the large ulcer is a small triangular ulceration of the mucosa and the pylorus forms an oval opening into the duodenum.

The opening into the artery appears to be oblique suggesting that it has been eroded laterally and therefore retraction of the artery does not occur and the haemorrhage is in consequence massive.

Other causes

Other causes of bleeding into the stomach include:
1. Rupture or erosions of oesophageal varices
2. Mallory Weiss syndrome – haemorrhage, occasionally severe, resulting from a tear in the oesophageal mucosa immediately cephalad to the hiatus, brought about by minor trauma, vomiting or retching
3. Gastric carcinoma
4. Acute erosions or gastritis (alcohol or drug induced)
5. Disorders of blood coagulation

Complication – Stenosis

Pyloric stenosis

Gastric outlet obstruction of benign causation most commonly results from pyloroduodenal fibrosis related to, or consequent upon, chronic duodenal, prepyloric or pyloric 'channel' ulceration. Duodenal ulceration is the most common cause (80%).

Non-fibrotic obstruction in the presence of an active ulcer may be caused by oedema of the wall or spasm of the encircling muscle particularly in children.

55

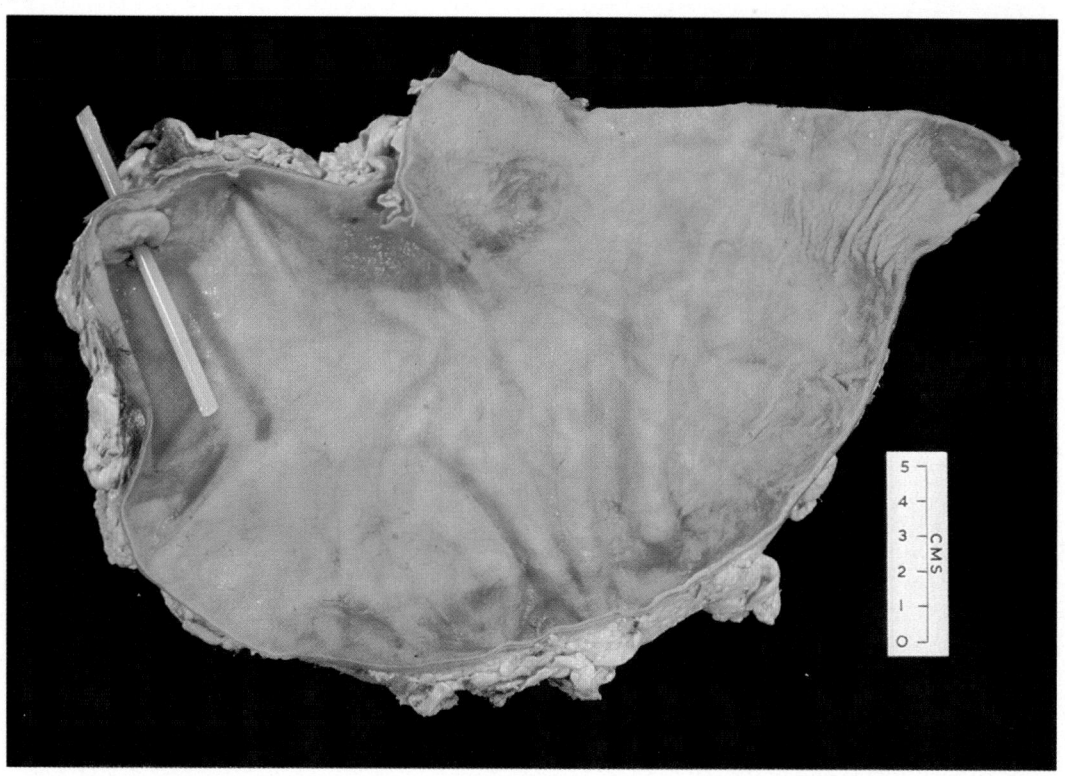

G.C. 10730

55 From a male aged 42 years. Fourteen-year history indicating presence of a duodenal ulcer with two episodes of haematemesis. Seven months prior to operation he complained of severe flatulence, a sense of fullness and vomiting on one occasion. Gastric succussion was present on examination. The specimen (the distal 3/4 of the stomach) shows gross distension.

The wall is thin and the pyloric canal shows marked stenosis and permits only the passage of a 3mm rod. The mucosa on the gastric side of the canal is roughened and scarred as the result of previous ulceration. Only a very small portion of normal duodenal mucosa is visible but at operation two ulcers were present in the first part of the duodenum but beyond the line of section. The gastric mucosa is stretched and all the rugae have been lost. The mucosa is atrophic and congested throughout.

Histological examination showed the mucosa flattened and the muscle atrophied.

Gastric outlet obstruction causes chronic retention of gastric contents and results initially in hypertrophy of the muscular coats and dilatation of the stomach if the obstruction is not relieved. Its capacity may reach 2 to 3 litres.

56

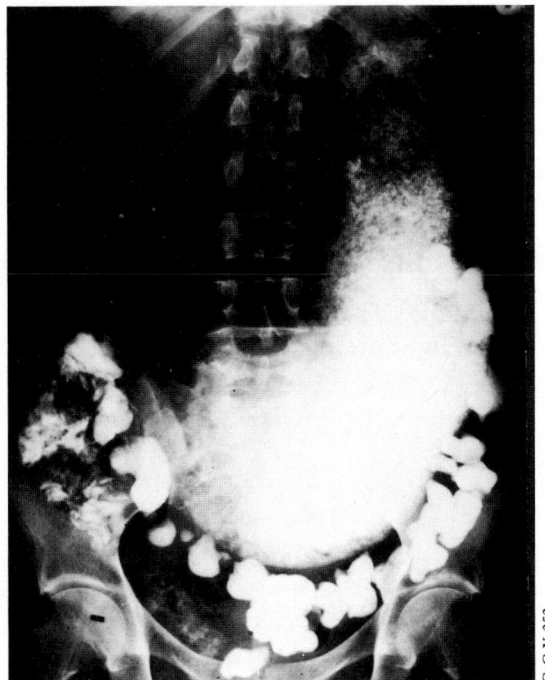

G.C.X.353

56 From a female aged 75 years. The radiograph shows gross retention of stomach content with the greater curvature lying in the pelvis. This degree of stenosis and distension may occur following simple ulceration.

Vomiting is a feature of 90% of cases of pyloric stenosis and this produces characteristic biochemical features of hypochloraemic alkalosis.

Stasis results in multiple gastric erosions and in the proliferation of anaerobic and coliform bacteria within the stomach content.

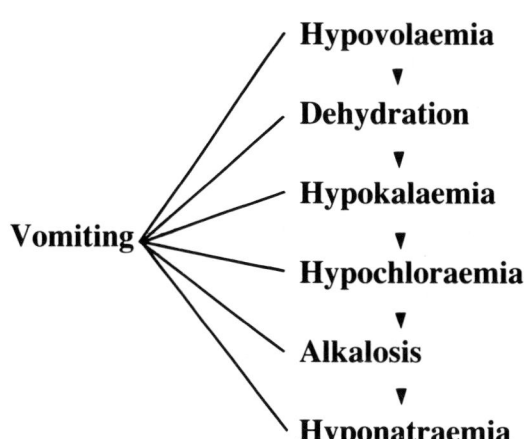

Pyloric stenosis is occasionally a late manifestation of congenital stenosis and is also a feature of pyloric carcinoma. These two conditions must be differentiated from that consequent upon ulcer.

Stenosis *(Continued)*

Hour-glass contracture

An uncommon but recognised complication of ulcer located high on the lesser curvature but the incidence appears to be lessening. Co-existent pyloric stenosis is common. Usually occurs in elderly female patients.

57

The lesion on the lesser curvature initially is a large ulcer of the saddle type but when the contracture occurs this ulcer may be active or have healed. Fibrosis in the submucous and subserous coats extend towards the greater curvature and on shortening this causes a deep indentation (hour-glass deformity). The stomach forms two pouches and the opening between these may be small (mid gastric stenosis).

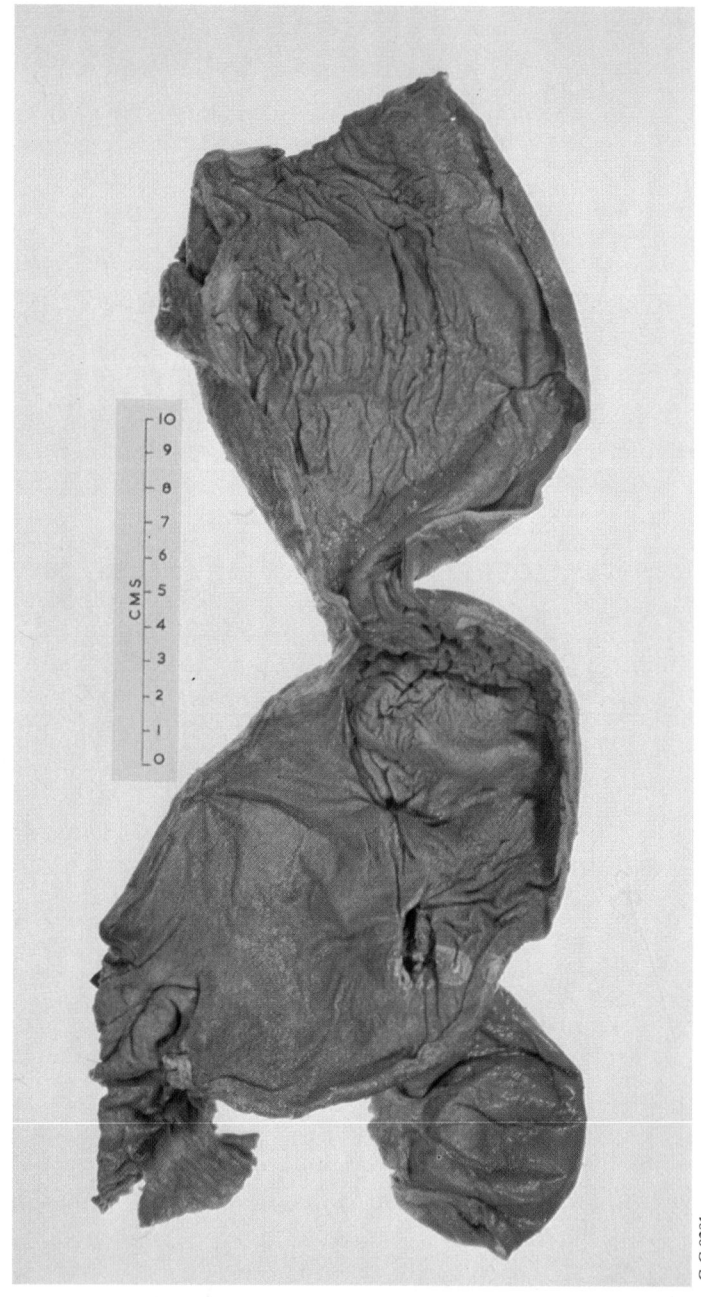

57 This is a classical example of an hour-glass contracture. It is an older specimen (1906) and for the relief of vomiting a gastrojejunostomy was performed. This was clearly an inadequate measure and the patient died shortly after operation. The stomach is divided into two equal sacs each of considerable size. The saccular cavities communicate through a narrow isthmus some 15 mm in diameter and 30 mm in length. This portion of the stomach is soft and pliant and has no evidence of cicatrix. The gastrojejunostomy opening is on the posterior wall about the middle of the distal sac, the union has been effected by sutures and in the neighbourhood there is on the serous coat of the stomach, a slight recent deposit of fibrin.

G.C.9281

Spasm of the circular muscle fibres in acute ulcer but without fibrosis of the stomach wall may lead to a similar appearance.

This is more common in males than in females. Radiologically volvulus and hiatus hernia require to be differentiated.

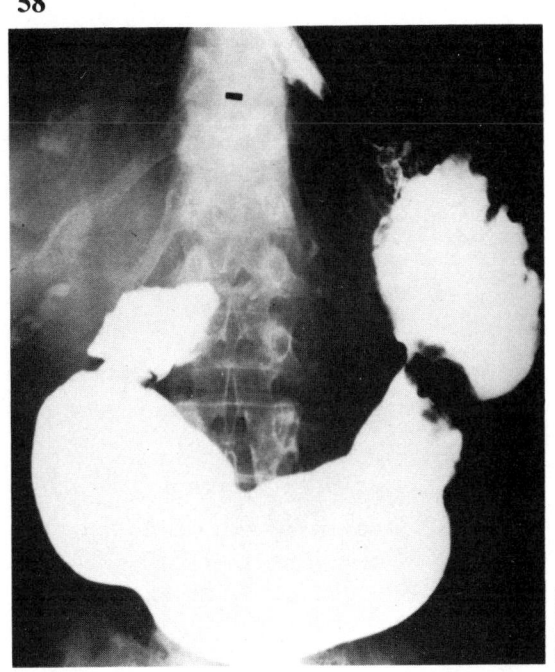

58 From a male aged 81 years. The stomach is divided into two segments. At the junction of the upper and middle thirds of the organ a circumferential band of tissue has encircled the stomach and by counter action drawn upwards the greater curvature. A narrow channel exists between the two segments.

Vomiting, especially if repeated, may result in aspiration of stomach content into the respiratory tract. It results in a chemical and infective pneumonitis which progresses to pneumonia if untreated.

59

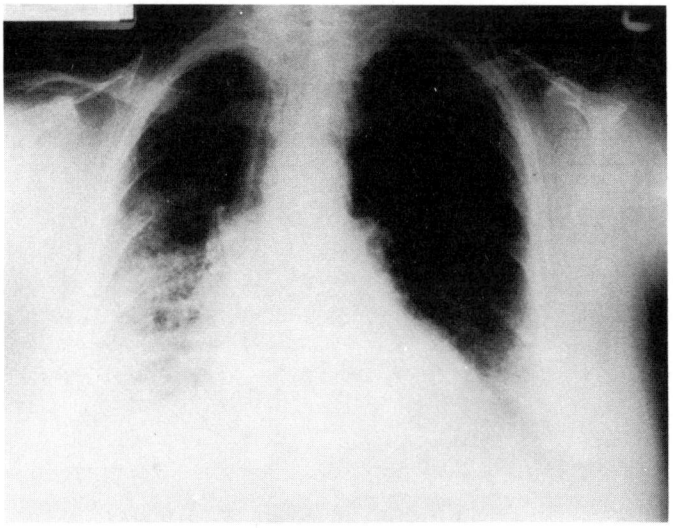

59 From a female aged 81 years suffering from a hiatus hernia with reflux. The radiograph of the chest shows marked loss of translucency in the right lung field due to aspiration of gastric content during vomiting.

Other causes

Hour-glass deformity of the stomach may be congenital (very rare), be due to a stenosing carcinoma, stricture following corrosive poisoning, gastro-jejunal ulcer, or perigastric adhesions.

Complication – Malignancy

The occurrence of malignant change in peptic ulcers has long been a subject of controversy and only occurs in relation to gastric ulcers. Malignant change in duodenal ulcers is unknown. Earlier writers considered that the frequency of malignant change was high, in some cases figures of 50% being quoted.

The naked eye appearance of a chronic ulcer and an ulcerating carcinoma may be similar. The history of the patient may indicate that the development of a carcinoma was preceded by a dyspepsia which could be attributed to simple ulceration. Such evidence is not conclusive.

The present assessment of the risk of malignant change in a gastric ulcer is as low as 1% to 2%. This view is based on the following considerations:

1 In longstanding simple ulceration epithelial changes about the margins of the ulcer seldom show evidence of malignant change.

   Long term follow-up of patients with gastric ulcers treated medically has not revealed a substantially increased incidence of carcinoma as compared with a non-ulcer population.

2 Evidence of marginal malignancy in longstanding ulcers with a fibrous base indicative of a longstanding chronic ulcer is rare.

3 Having regard to the frequency of peptic ulcer only a disproportionately small number of gastric carcinomas show clear evidence of preceding chronic ulceration.

4 Gastric ulceration reflects an unstable gastric epithelium with evidence of intestinal metaplasia, a known precursor of malignancy in the surrounding mucosa.

   Benign ulceration may therefore coexist with gastric carcinoma.

The final diagnosis depends on histological studies. To be certain that the malignancy has arisen in a pre-existing ulcer the pathologist accepts only those cases which satisfy Newcomb's criteria as modified by Nakamura [Nakamura K. *et al.* (1967) Gann 58. p.377]:

1 Destruction of the muscularis mucosae in the ulcer bed.

2 Fusion of the muscularis mucosae with the muscularis propria at the margin of the ulcer.

3 Dense fibrosis involving all layers of the gastric wall.

4 Cancer at a relatively early stage of development and limited to one side of the ulcer margin.

If the carcinoma is in a more advanced state absolute proof is difficult to establish.

Carcinomatous change at the site of a gastro-enteric anastomosis is a well recognised entity of considerable frequency. The interval may be prolonged between the time of operation and the onset of neoplastic change and statistically the risk appears to become greater after an interval of 15 to 20 years. Further evidence of the linkage of the carcinoma to the previous operation is the fact that the tumour is frequently located close to the greater curvature of the stomach, a most unusual site for malignant change in otherwise normal stomachs.

It would appear that following anastomotic operations the risk of malignancy is increased six-fold.

Oesophagus – Peptic ulcer

Peptic ulcer may occur when islets of ectopic gastric mucosa are present in the oesophageal wall. The condition is most commonly found in the lower oesophagus. These ulcers may penetrate deeply, perforate or be the site of severe haemorrhage especially in the acute phase. This condition is described in Section 13.

Meckel's diverticulum – Peptic ulcer

The mucosa of the diverticulum may contain cell elements of gastric type including both fundic and pyloric glands (12%). Secretion of HCl by these cells leads to ulceration either in the neck of the diverticulum or in the adjacent ileum. Haemorrhage and perforation are recognised complications. Clinical features may become manifest at any age but are most common in infants and young children, the majority presenting with haemorrhage before the age of 5 years. Approximately half the cases are diagnosed after perforation.

60

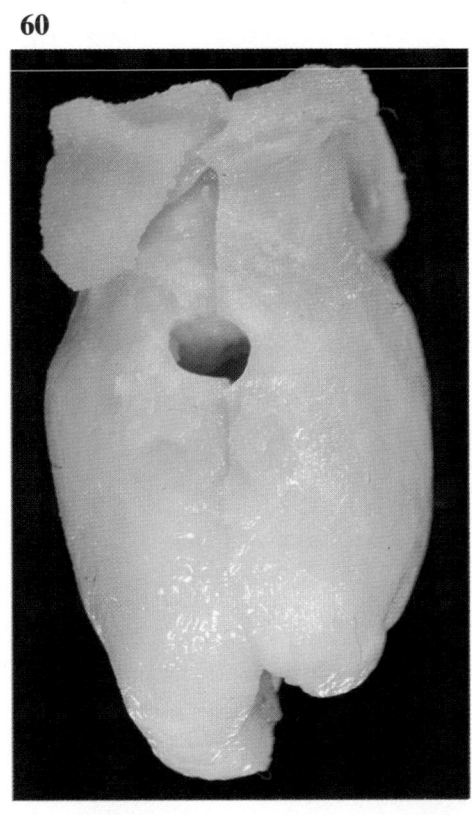

60a

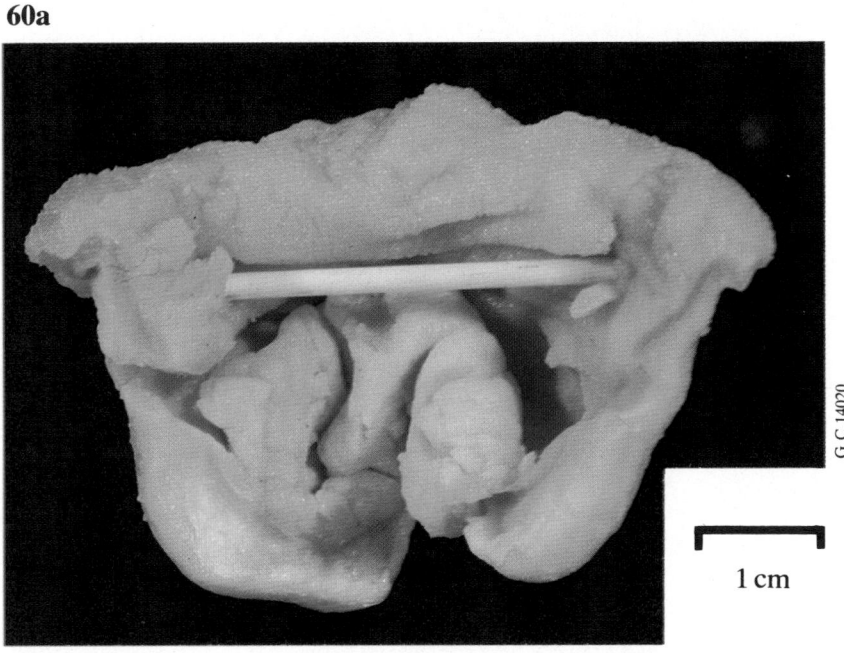

1 cm

60 and **60a**   From a male child. There was a history of blood in the stools and episodes of central abdominal pain. After admission to hospital, on investigation, the pain became acute and operative intervention was immediately undertaken.

The specimen shows an acute perforation. Note how the edges are sharply demarcated. In the sectioned specimen note how the ulcer has penetrated and how the wall of the diverticulum has thickened (see Section 15 B 1).

Endoscopy

Modern endoscopy employs the principle of light conduction along glass fibre bundles. These are bound together in a sheath which helps to minimise loss of visual acuity by ensuring the maximum transmission from the intracavitary source along the conduction bundles. The instruments used may be forward or side viewing and are highly flexible but may be steered towards the lesion or made to pass natural obstacles such as the pylorus. It was the development of the modern flexible instrument which allowed panendoscopy of the oesophagus, stomach and duodenum or colonoscopy as far as the ileo-caecal valve. Most instruments have channels mounted in them for washing the inspected mucosal surface and for biopsy or brushing lesions for cytology, and there are channels for inflation or collection of secretion. The modern endoscopist only sees the living pathology of lesions in the upper and lower gastrointestinal tract but can biopsy tissue or remove cell brushings and aspirate secretions. He can further cannulate important secretory channels such as the main biliary and pancreatic ducts and can perform therapeutic manoeuvres such as dilatation of strictures or the removal of polyps.

Four examples of endoscopic appearances of peptic ulceration in the upper gastrointestinal tract are shown:

61

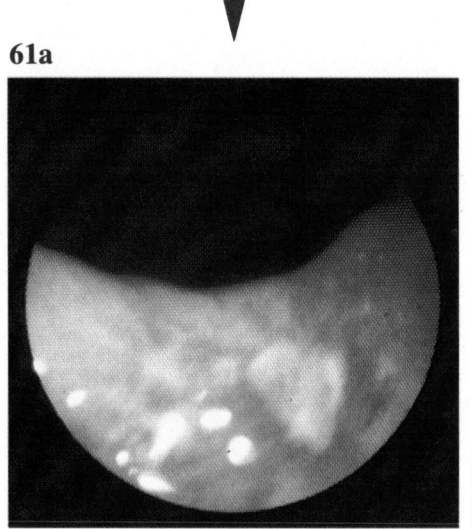

61 A superficial gastric ulcer lying on the mucosa.

61a

61a A second view of the above.

62

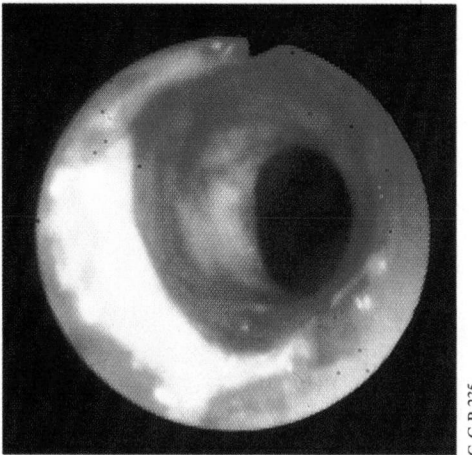

62 Severe oesophagitis with granular friable mucosa and membrane formation.

63

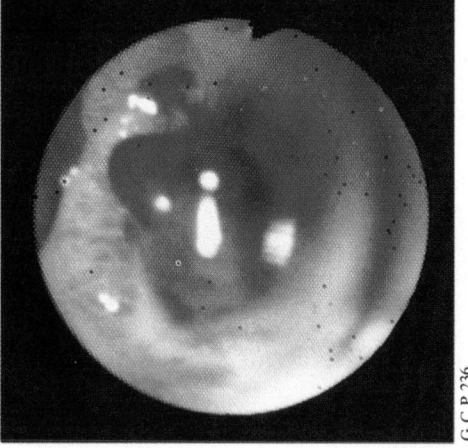

63 A large chronic duodenal ulcer the edge of which is well seen. In the centre of the ulcer is a large blood clot lying on a blood vessel. The ulcer is surrounded by severe duodenitis.

A.H. McLean Ross

110

Epithelial metaplasia

A change in the nature of the lining epithelium may occur in many parts of the alimentary tract and is seen most often in the presence of inflammation or ulceration. Thus the squamous epithelium of the lower end of the oesophagus may be replaced by mucin-secreting epithelium, whilst less commonly the columnar epithelium of the rectum may be replaced by transitional or squamous epithelium. Both changes occur as a concomitant of ulceration and could therefore result from migration from gastric or anal epithelium respectively.

The term epithelial metaplasia is usually reserved for those examples of epithelial change where there is no possibility of migration of the atypical epithelium from an adjacent site. All forms tend to be promoted by the destabilising influence of inflammation. Thus metaplasia to colonic-type epithelium may occur in the stomach in chronic gastritis, and metaplasia to pyloric-type epithelium in the ileum in Crohn's disease. The most striking metaplasia, however, is seen where the gastric mucosa shows a transition to small intestinal epithelium. Intestinal crypts formed by cells with brush borders and secreting intestinal-type mucin develop, and Paneth cell and argentaffin cell differentation may be present. This change is common in the stomach but is also met with in the colon in ulcerative colitis.

Some metaplastic epithelium shows a tendency to become dysplastic, a factor probably concerned in the increased incidence of malignancy in cases of chronic gastritis and ulcerative colitis.

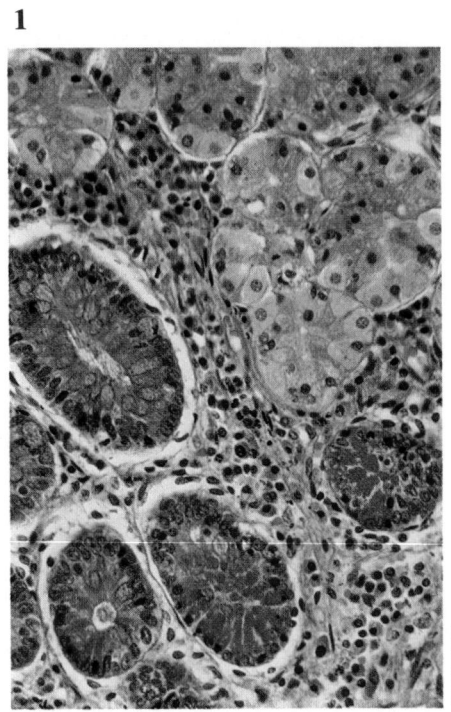

1

1 Intestinal metaplasia in the stomach. The main gastric glands (top right) have partly been replaced by crypts secreting intestinal mucin (bright green) and containing cells with red Paneth granules. (*Alcian green, phloxin, tartrazine ×250*)

G.C.M.836

Gastritis – Specific types

Classification

Acute	Chronic	
	A Affecting body and fundus	**B** Affecting antrum
Corrosive		
Phlegmonous	(i) Superficial (ii) Atrophic	Chronic antral gastritis
Focal erosive (Haemorrhagic)	(iii) Gastric atrophy (iv) Giant hypertrophic (Ménétrier)	

This classification is not fully comprehensive since other rarer forms of gastritis have been described. A and B forms of chronic gastritis can co-exist. On the other hand in many cases of duodenal ulceration antral gastritis may be well marked whilst the body mucosa shows no inflammation. By contrast in pernicious anaemia the antral mucosa is relatively well preserved although that of the body shows advanced atrophy

Corrosive gastritis

Corrosive gastritis results from accidental or suicidal ingestion of corrosive fluids such as strong acids and alkalis, mercuric chloride, or phenol. Contact of the corrosive with the mucosa causes reflex contraction of the muscularis so that the mucosa deep in the folds is protected. By contrast the mucosa on the convexities of the folds and on the lesser curvature becomes necrotic, the colour varying according to the corrosive involved. Recovery may be complicated by chronic ulceration or pyloric stenosis. There is invariably a concomitant comparable oesophageal lesion.

Phlegmonous gastritis

May complicate chronic gastric ulceration but is usually part of a septicaemic process most commonly bacterial and predominantly streptococcal. It may also occur in severe viral infections.

Pathology. The wall of the stomach is swollen by inflammatory oedema and its serosa may be covered by a layer of fibrin. The severe acute inflammation which affects all layers of the stomach can result in necrosis and hence perforation.

113

Focal erosive (haemorrhagic) gastritis

A condition of varying aetiology including severe toxaemia, shock, burns, and ingestion of aspirin. The combination of hyperchlorhydria, aspirin and alcohol is particularly damaging. Substantial haemorrhage may result.

Pathology. Small haemorrhagic spots, usually multiple, are distributed over the gastric mucosa. Microscopic examination reveals that they may be associated with focal mucosal erosion of varying depth.

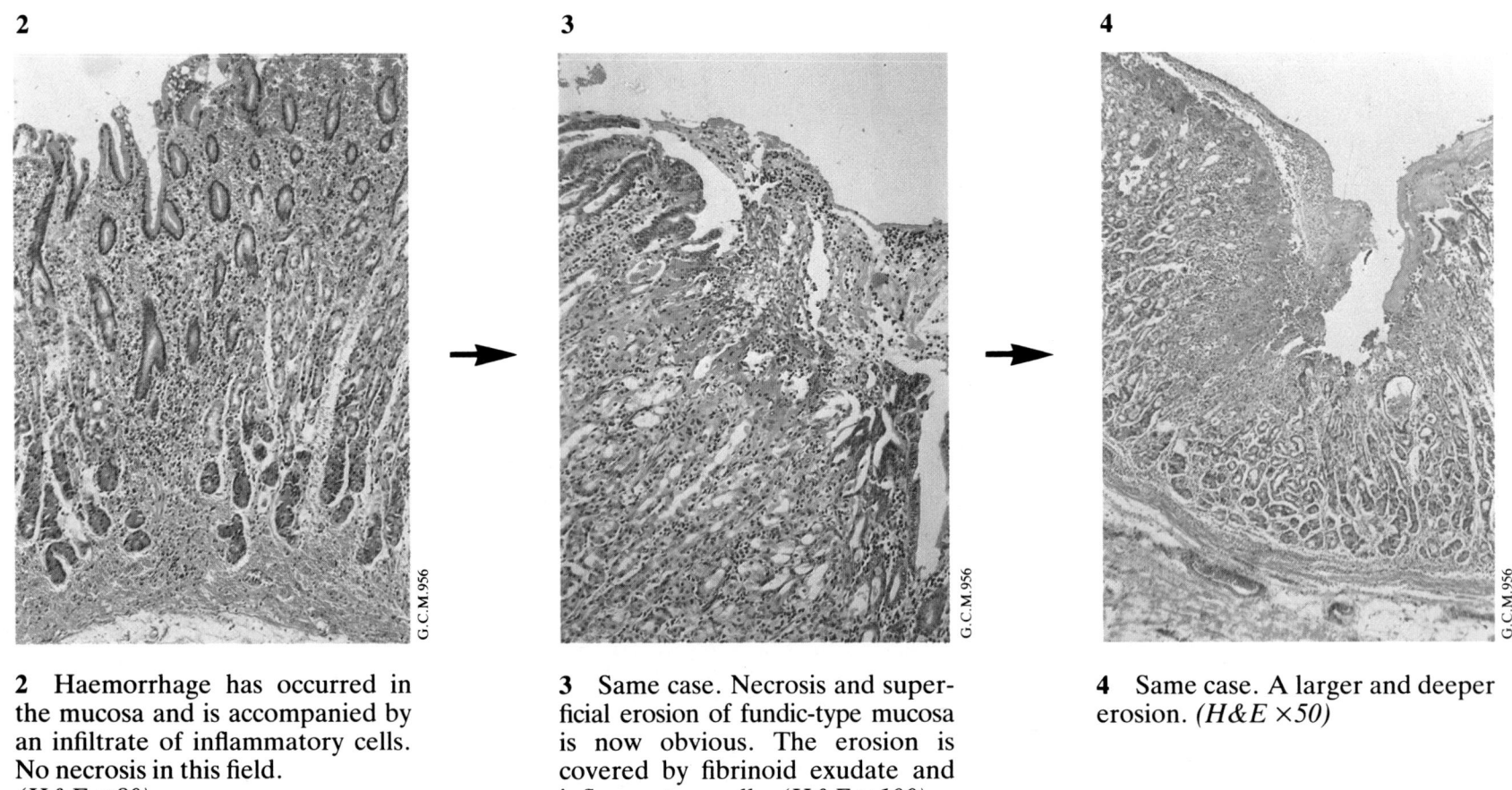

2 Haemorrhage has occurred in the mucosa and is accompanied by an infiltrate of inflammatory cells. No necrosis in this field. *(H&E ×80)*

3 Same case. Necrosis and super-ficial erosion of fundic-type mucosa is now obvious. The erosion is covered by fibrinoid exudate and inflammatory cells. *(H&E ×100)*

4 Same case. A larger and deeper erosion. *(H&E ×50)*

Chronic gastritis of the fundus and body

Definition. Chronic inflammation of varying severity involving the normally acid-secreting portions of the gastric mucosa.

Incidence. A not uncommon finding in adults of all ages. Its incidence and severity tend to increase with age so that in the 7th decade only one-fifth of stomachs appear entirely normal.

Pathogenesis. Many factors, both genetic and dietetic, may be involved. For example, it is more prevalent in those with blue eyes and in relatives of patients with pernicious anaemia and gastric mucosal antibodies may be present in the serum. Two-thirds of all who drink and smoke to excess develop chronic gastritis.

Pathology. The appearances vary from those of mild superficial gastritis to those of the advanced stages of mucosal atrophy.

Superficial gastritis

5

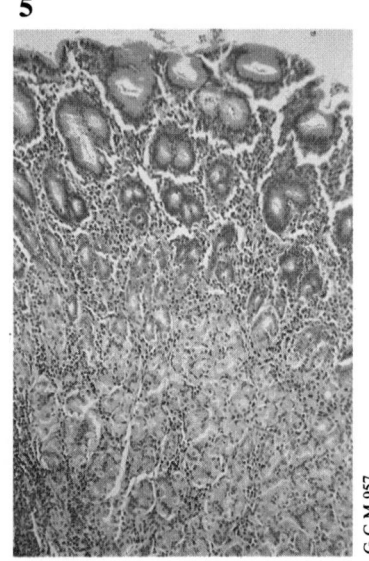

5 Superficial gastritis – A histological finding without consistent symptomatology. At most only the upper third of the mucosa is abnormal. The affected zone is infiltrated by excessive numbers of cells, mainly plasma cells and lymphocytes. There may also be mild epithelial changes such as slight distortion and hyperchromasia. The main glands are normal. *(H&E ×80)*

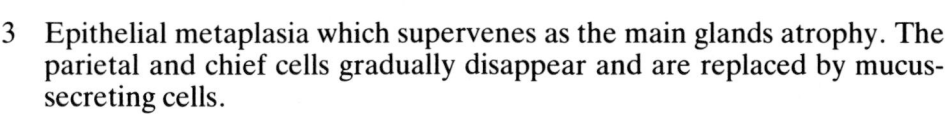

Atrophic gastritis

Only the mucosa is affected. At first the condition is patchy and may not affect the full depth of the mucosa. It tends to be more marked distally but any part of the body and fundus may be affected. The disease is usually progressive and as it becomes confluent it spreads proximally. It has three main histological features.

6

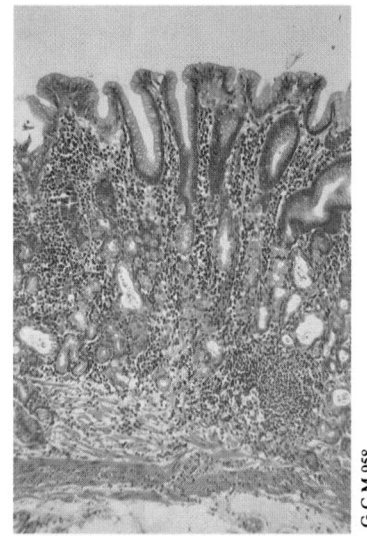

1 Infiltration of the mucosa by chronic inflammatory cells, mainly plasma cells and lymphocytes although eosinophils and other polymorphs are often present. Lymphoid follicles in the deeper layers of the mucosa may be hyperplastic.

2 Atrophy of the main glands which at first tends to be focal and shows in the upper part of the glands. Later it becomes diffuse and affects all or most of the gland. As the glands atrophy the mucosa becomes thinner and less rugose and acid secretion diminishes. *(H&E ×80)*

7

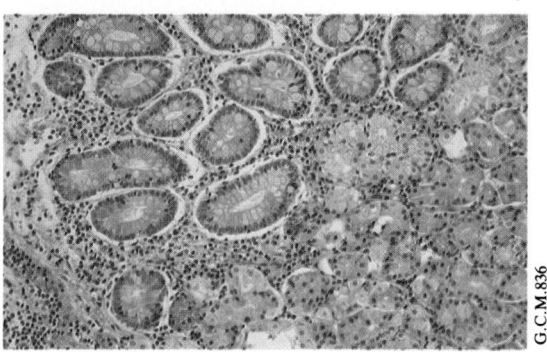

3 Epithelial metaplasia which supervenes as the main glands atrophy. The parietal and chief cells gradually disappear and are replaced by mucus-secreting cells.

In the upper part of the field a few main glands have been replaced by pyloric-type glands with pale mucin-secreting cells. Brightly eosinophilic Paneth granules can be seen in the deeper intestinal glands. *(H&E ×100)*

Gastric atrophy

The end stage of chronic atrophic gastritis is known as gastric atrophy and is the characteristic finding in pernicious anaemia. The inflammatory infiltrate is less than in preceding stages but except in the antrum the mucosa is thin and the main glands have virtually disappeared. Achlorhydria is characteristic and may be accompanied by increased secretion of gastrin and an increased population of G cells in the antral mucosa.

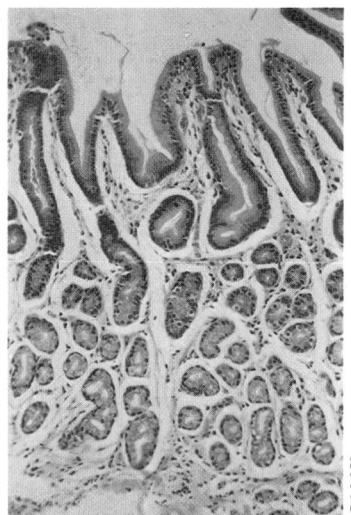

8 Gastric atrophy in a case of pernicious anaemia. The surface epithelium and gastric pits show no atrophy but main glands have disappeared and have been replaced by pyloric-type glands which extend to the muscularis mucosae. In the intermediate zone the pale cells with central nuclei are probably G cells. In this example of gastric atrophy there is virtually no inflammatory infiltrate. *(H&E ×120)*

Pernicious anaemia

The incidence of pernicious anaemia (PA) in persons with blood group A is greater than that in the general population and in PA antibodies to parietal cells and intrinsic factor may be demonstrable in the serum. Utilisation of Vitamin B 12 is impaired and when the liver stock is depleted megaloblastic anaemia develops. In patients with PA the incidence of gastric polyposis and cancer is increased.

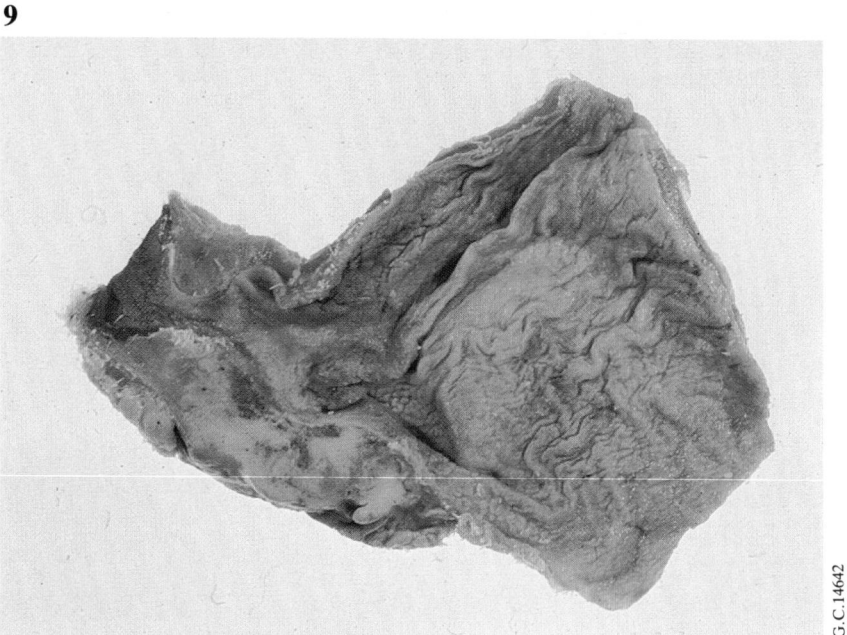

9 From a male aged 81 years who had been treated for pernicious anaemia for 10 years before he died from a carcinoma of the stomach with extensive hepatic metastases.

In the specimen illustrated the gastric mucosa is thin. The carcinoma is situated on the greater curvature of the antrum. It is ulcerated and has infiltrated to the serosa and spread to lymph nodes along the greater curvature. On histological examination the tumour proved to be a well differentiated adenocarcinoma. The mucosa of the body and fundus was atrophic.

Chronic antral gastritis

In duodenal ulceration the fundic mucosa may show no inflammatory changes. By contrast the antrum in most types of peptic ulceration almost invariably shows chronic inflammatory infiltration. It is difficult to establish how much it contributes to the symptomatology.

Pathology

In the early stages the mucosa is thicker than normal due to the heavy inflammatory infiltrate. Infiltration by plasma cells is intense. Lymphocytes and other cells are also increased and large hyperplastic lymphoid follicles may develop in the deeper layers. The upper layers of the epithelium become hyperchromatic due to increased cell turnover and in later stages there is a variable degree of pyloric gland atrophy. Intestinal metaplasia may develop.

10

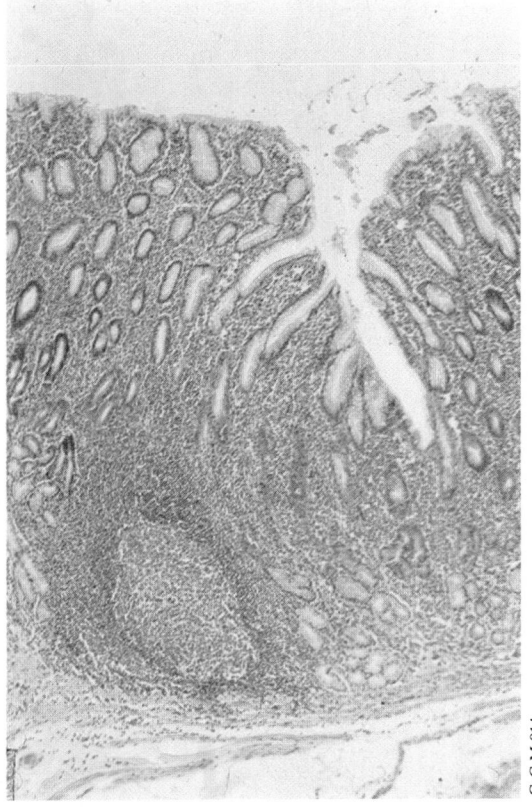

11

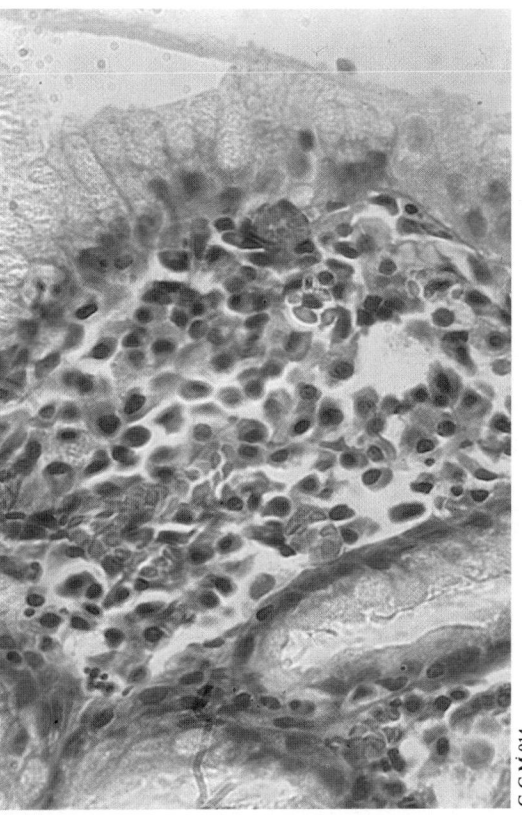

10 The full depth of the mucosa is infiltrated by chronic inflammatory cells. The hyperplastic lymphoid follicle has a large germinal centre. *(H&E ×60)*

11 Plasma cells predominate in the inflammatory infiltrate. *(H&E ×600)*

Ménétrier's disease (Giant hypertrophic gastritis)

A mysterious and uncommon abnormality which shows features both of hyperplasia and inflammation. The pathogenesis is unknown. A few cases have been associated with disturbances of endocrine glands. It may affect either sex at any age but is most often met with in middle-aged men. Loss of blood and protein may lead to anaemia and hypoproteinaemia.

Pathology. The disease affects the mucosa of the body and fundus, and may be diffuse or localised. It tends to affect the greater curvature particularly. The antrum is spared. The mucosal folds are so thickened that they come to resemble cerebral gyri.

12

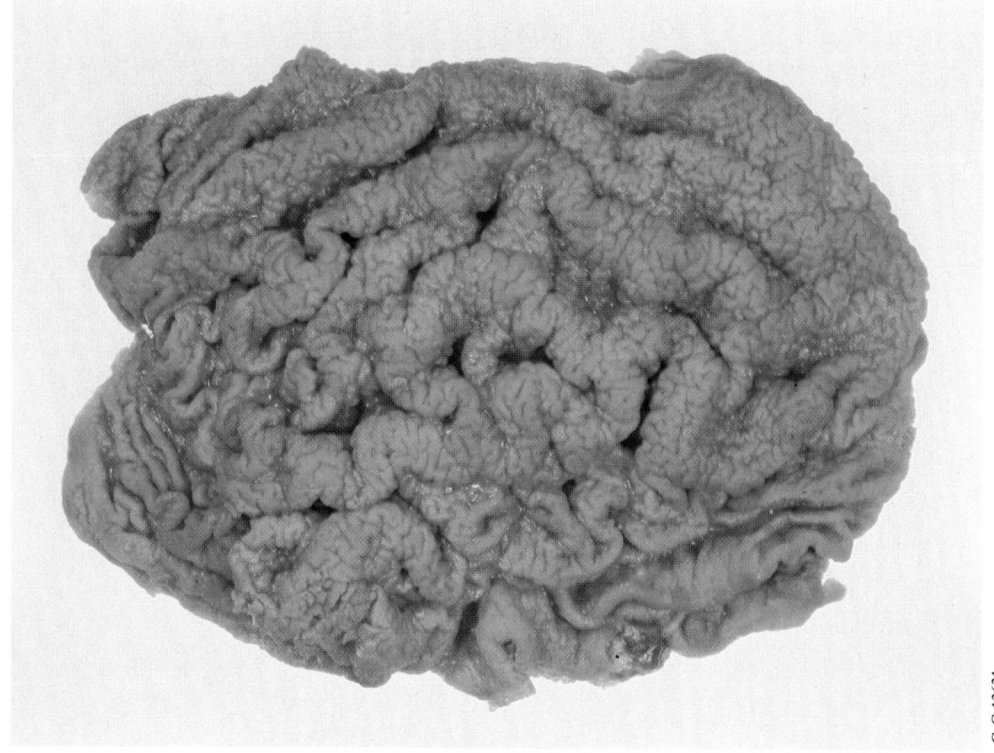

12 The patient was a middle-aged woman who had received treatment for thyrotoxicosis by radio-active iodine. She became euthyroid but later developed anorexia, achlorhydria, and persistent diarrhoea with weight loss and marked hypoproteinaemia. Gastroscopy revealed giant hypertrophic gastritis. Because of the severity of the hypoproteinaemia a partial gastrectomy was performed. The patient recovered well from the operation and her weight and plasma proteins were regained.

G.C.1363I

The mucosa is excessively infiltrated by plasma cells and lymphocytes but the most characteristic abnormalities are epithelial.

13

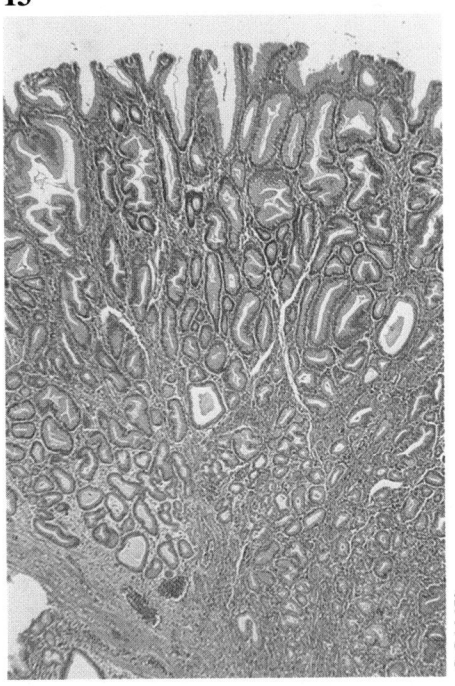

14

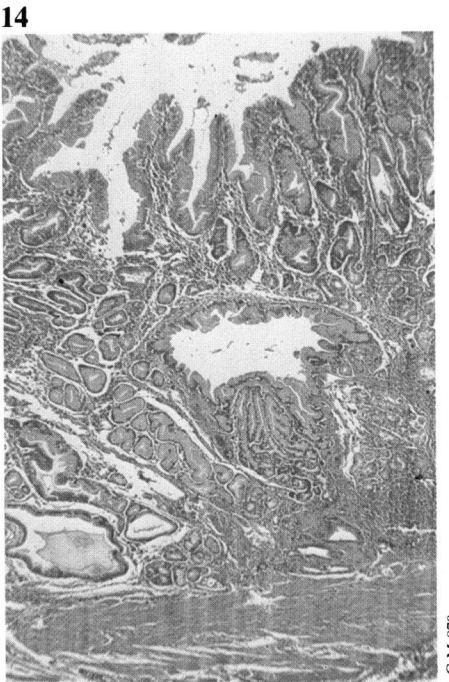

13 The gastric pits and the gastric glands are much enlarged and the parietal and chief cells tend to be replaced by mucin-secreting cells like those of the gastric pits. Pyloric-type metaplasia may be present but intestinal metaplasia is not a feature of the disease. *(H&E ×40)*

14 Small cysts lined by mucin-secreting cells develop in the deeper layers of the mucosa. *(H&E ×40)*

15

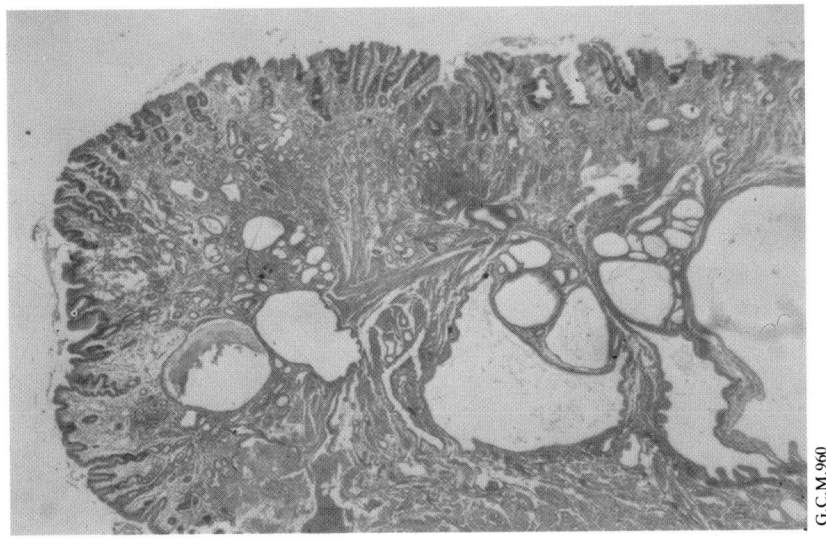

15 As they distend they may cause gross distortion. *(H&E ×17.5)*

N. Maclean

Incidence

In the United Kingdom some 15000 deaths occur annually from carcinoma of the stomach, an incidence of approximately 26 per 100000. This figure is exceeded only by carcinoma of the lung and colon but exceeds that of carcinoma of the breast and uterus. It is a fascinating fact that the incidence of this disease seems at present to be changing.

1 Carcinoma of the stomach is a universal disease but comparative statistical studies demonstrate that there is wide geographical variation.

Age adjusted death rate per 100000 males.

1

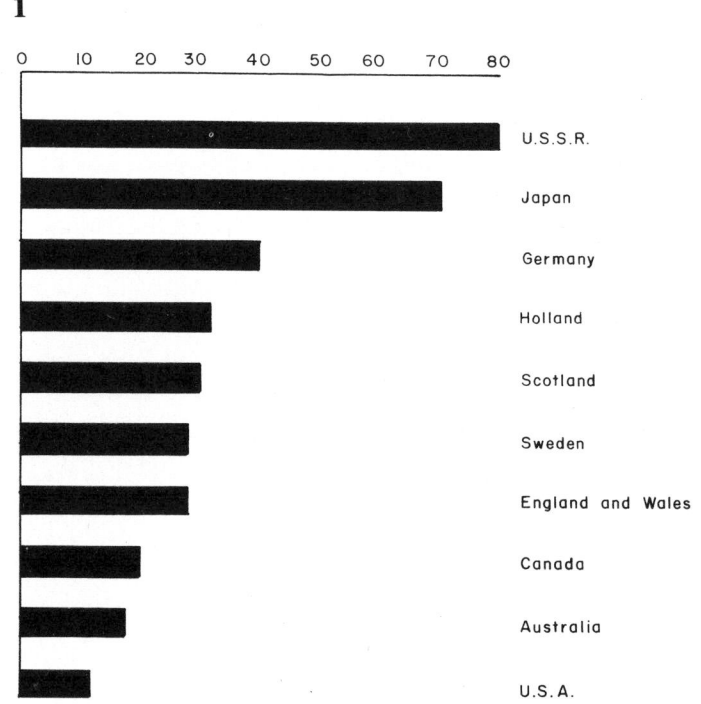

Decline of incidence

It is important in the interpretation of statistics relating to the incidence and course of the disease that the figures quoted refer only to the facts as they existed at the date of the investigation and subsequent study may give a different result. There is evidence that the incidence of carcinoma of the stomach in the U.S.A. and Western Europe is declining but the fall appears presently to have levelled off.

In the United Kingdom the death rate for males per 100000 for the years 1959–1963 was 34.8, a decrease of 1.3 (3½%) when compared with the figures for the 1954–1958 period. G. Melvyn Howe (1970) *National Atlas of Disease Mortality in the United Kingdom.* Thomas Nelson and Sons Ltd. London.

120

The wide variation in the incidence of the disease in different parts of the world suggests two factors are involved:

1 Racial
2 Environmental (including diet)

An interesting observation is made in relation to the Japanese living in the U.S.A. Japanese born immigrants show a high incidence but 2nd and 3rd generation Japanese show a decrease to a figure which approximates to that of the general U.S.A. population. This study strongly supports the view that environmental and dietary factors are more significant than any possible inherent racial trait in determining geographical differences in cancer incidence.

2

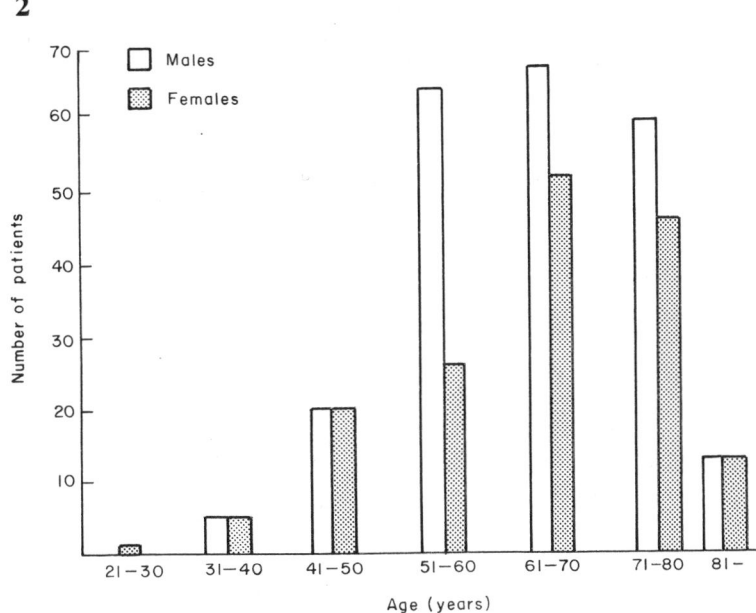

The sex incidence of the tumour is approximately:
2 males/1 female.

2 Sex and age distribution. Edinburgh Royal Infirmary Survey 1959–62.
Female cases shown as stippled column.

Social–economic status (U.K. Social Grade)

There is evidence that carcinoma of the stomach shows an increased incidence in both men and women in the lower social classes.

Willis (1948 *Pathology of Tumours*) quotes the death rate per 100 000 males in the five classes.

I Professional and managerial	59
II Intermediate professions	84
III Skilled occupations (manual and non-manual)	98
IV Partly skilled occupations	108
V Unskilled	124

Conditions associated with a high incidence of gastric cancer

Congenital

(a) An apparent familial factor in the incidence of gastric cancer has been frequently noted. A classical example was the family of Napoleon Bonaparte. Napoleon died of gastric carcinoma as most probably did his father, brother and two sisters. In the United Kingdom 6% of patients give a strong family history of gastric cancer.

(b) Individuals of Blood Group A statistically show a significantly high incidence of gastric carcinoma (Aird). This fact supports the view that a genetic factor is involved.

AIRD, I. (1957) *A Companion in Surgical Studies.* E. & S. Livingstone Ltd. Edinburgh and London.

Acquired

Chronic gastritis

In chronic gastritis studies have shown that the mucosal changes characterised by metaplasia and atrophy (see Section 14 S) frequently precede or are associated with carcinoma. Where atrophic gastritis has existed for a long period and shows areas of metaplasia, malignant change is common. Atrophic gastritis may be a local lesion or associated with a general disease such as pernicious anaemia. This is shown by the fact that 7% of patients with pernicious anaemia die of gastric cancer.

Following gastric surgery reflux of bile into the stomach induces a chronic gastritis with metaplasia.

Peptic ulcer

The relationship of peptic ulcer to carcinoma has been long debated. Earlier observers considered the relationship was close and that carcinoma was a sequel to ulcer in a high percentage of cases (50% or over). The modern view is that the incidence of carcinoma directly attributable to preceding ulceration is relatively uncommon (1 to 2%).

Nevertheless a gastric ulcer reflects a sick gastric epithelium and as such may exhibit the changes of chronic gastritis (see Section 14 EA).

Achlorhydria

Achlorhydria is a common finding in carcinoma of the stomach. The achlorhydria may have resulted from a chronic gastritis preceding the onset of carcinoma and it has been held that it may be a contributory factor to the development of neoplastic change. The achlorhydria, on the other hand, may be a sequel to the carcinomatous change.

When hypochlorhydria arises in association with gastric ulceration or follows the use of agents such as H_2 receptor antagonists to control the acid hypersecretion of duodenal ulcer the nitrosamine content of the stomach increases. This may be a factor in subsequent carcinogenesis. Nitrates whether consumed or secreted endogenously in salivary and gastric secretions are believed to undergo bacterial conversion leading to the subsequent formation of compounds of the nitrosamine class.

Gastric polyps

The relationship between gastric polyps and carcinoma is recognised and discussed overleaf.

Other debated factors

Injury

Physical, caustic or thermal damage to the mucosa of the oesophagus and stomach may result in scarring. If extensive the replacement epithelium may be imperfect in nature. In general direct injury is not a recognised cause of carcinoma.

Alcohol

The higher incidence of carcinoma of the stomach in certain groups, social and occupational, who are believed to be prone to excessive alcohol intake leading to chronic gastritis, has provided some statistical evidence suggestive that alcohol is a causative factor of carcinoma.

Dietary habits

It is difficult to implicate specific dietary habits with cancer of the stomach but a possible linkage exists with a high intake of Vit. A. and methods of cooking at high temperatures resulting in splitting of fats and the possible production of carcinogens. It has also been suggested that certain additives including colouring agents and preservatives may be implicated.

Prognosis

The course of the disease and the final outcome are determined both by the variable rate of the proliferative neoplastic process and the state to which it had advanced when medical aid was first sought. The initial features are often minimal – consequently early diagnosis is rare. When cases reach hospital they are frequently inoperable. The gravity of the disease is reflected in a table by the late Sir Heneage Ogilvie prepared in 1938. There has been little change in these figures since that time in spite of the developments in surgical technique and therapeutic management of malignant disease.

The fate of 200 cases of cancer of the stomach presenting themselves at hospital.

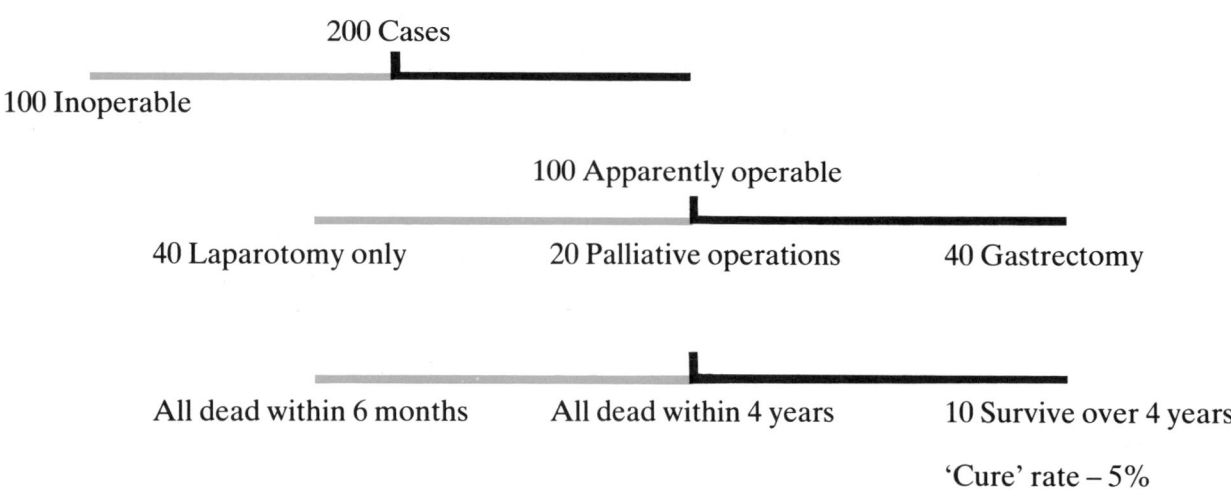

200 Cases

100 Inoperable

100 Apparently operable

40 Laparotomy only   20 Palliative operations   40 Gastrectomy

All dead within 6 months   All dead within 4 years   10 Survive over 4 years

'Cure' rate – 5%

Edinburgh Royal Infirmary Survey

3

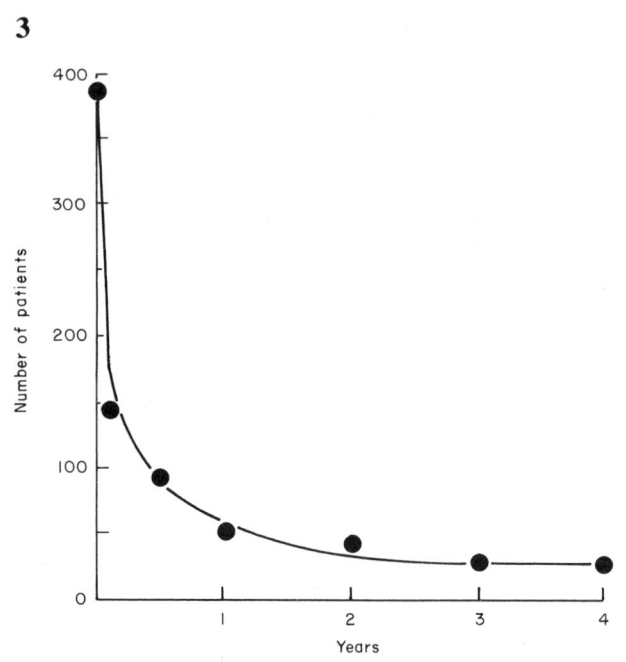

3 Overall survival figures, March 1966 (4-year follow up). Cancer of the Stomach Survey 1959–62. Royal Infirmary of Edinburgh.

Gastric polyps

In addition to metaplasia of the gastric mucosa (see previous section) certain innocent formations have been recognised as capable of undergoing malignant change.

The term 'polyp' is descriptive of appearance and is used frequently without definite pathological meaning and thus includes several pathological entities:

1   The hamartomatous lesions
2   Polypoid remnants of tissue due to the presence of active or past inflammation
3   True adenomatous tumours

Hamartomatous and inflammatory polyps

The polyps may be single or multiple and are found chiefly in the body and antrum. The individual lesions are smooth in contour and may be disparate or forming small confluent masses. Microscopically both mucosal and stromal elements are present. The epithelium is derived from the columnar cells of the gastric mucosa and may form glandular masses which may be solid or papillary and there may be cyst formation. These epithelial masses simulate pyloric glands. Muscle fibres derived from the muscularis mucosae are present and may also form masses of irregularly arranged fibres. Increase in fibrous stroma and inflammatory cell infiltration may be observed. These papillomas are regarded as either hamartomatous formations or may be inflammatory or regenerative in origin. Distinction between the two groups may be difficult. These lesions are usually found in patients in the 6th decade; there is a male preponderance, and an increased incidence in patients with atrophic gastritis. Relationship to carcinoma – 25% of these polyps become malignant. It is also found that where a frank carcinoma of the stomach exists 5% are found to be associated with polyposis.

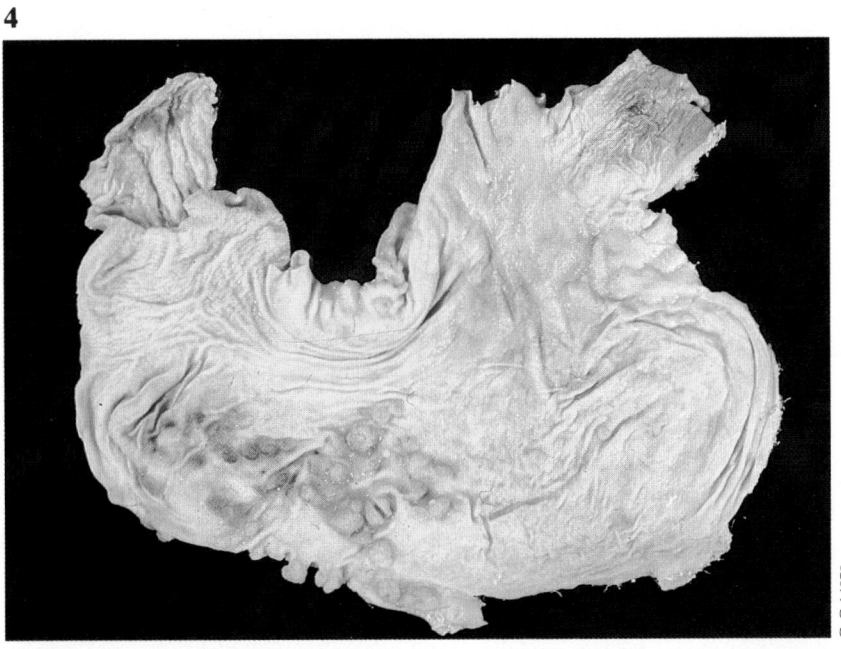
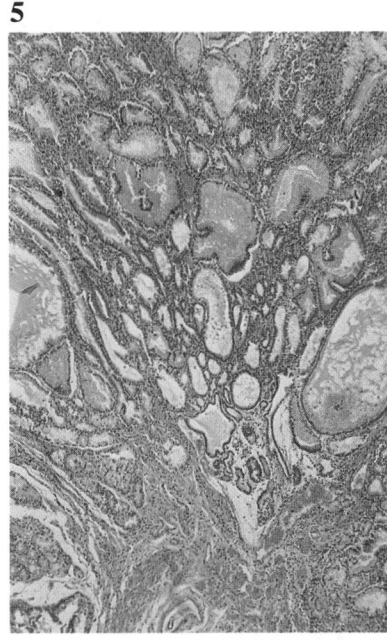

4   From a male aged 64 years. The gastric lesion was a post mortem finding. In the distal half of the stomach the mucosa is studded by rounded polyps with discrete pedicles. At necropsy they were covered by abundant tenacious mucin.

5   Microscopically the polyps are formed by mucus-secreting columnar epithelium of the type normally found in the necks of the gastric glands. The cytoplasm is bloated with mucin and some of the glands are so distended that microcysts have formed. All the tumour is well differentiated and the muscularis mucosae is intact. *(H&E ×40)*

125

Hamartomatous and inflammatory polyps *(Continued)*

6

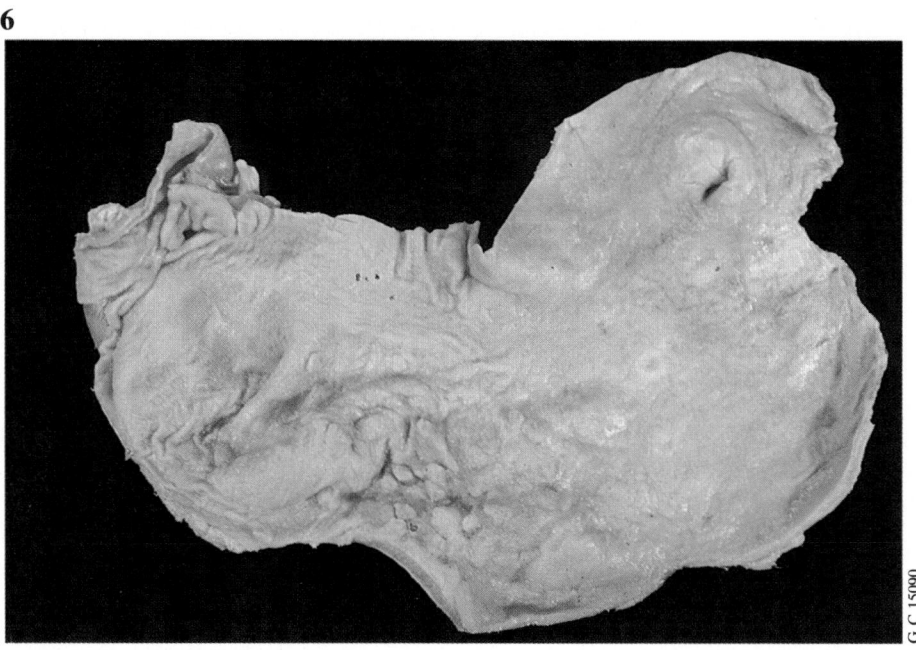

6 From a male aged 76 years. The gastric lesion was a post mortem finding and associated with peritoneal metastases.

In the distal half of the stomach there are multiple mucosal polyps measuring up to 0.5 cm in diameter and from a few millimetres to about 1 cm in length. Where they are most numerous there is an obvious carcinomatous infiltration of the stomach wall and a plaque of tumour on the serous surface. The cut section of stomach wall shows a typical striated marking of the muscle layer where the tumour penetrates between the muscle fibres. Microscopically the infiltrated area of stomach wall and the nodules of tumour in the peritoneal cavity show the presence of well differentiated adenocarcinoma.

7

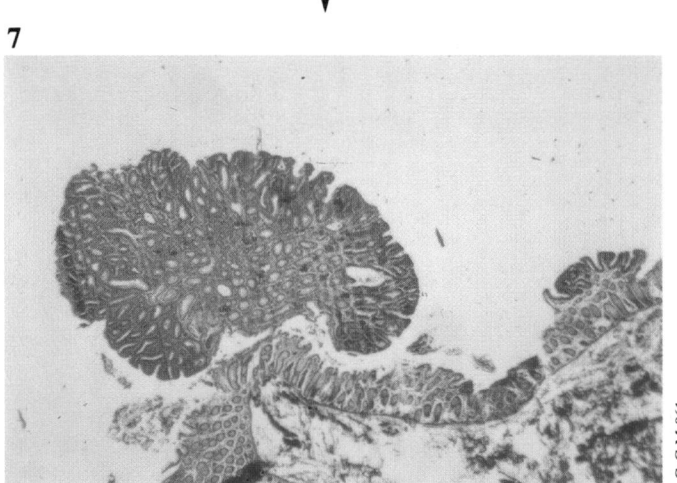

8

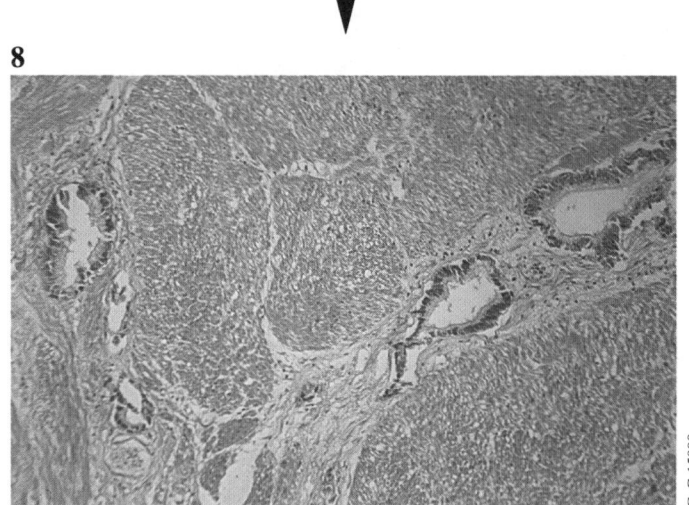

7 Arising from the gastric mucosa there are two adenopapillomas, one fully developed and polypoid and the other a much smaller incipient and sessile tumour. The surface epithelium in both is hyperchromatic but there is no sign of malignancy. *(H&E ×15)*

8 A portion of the stomach wall at the site of invasion showing deep infiltration of muscularis by well differentiated adenocarcinoma. *(H&E ×100)*

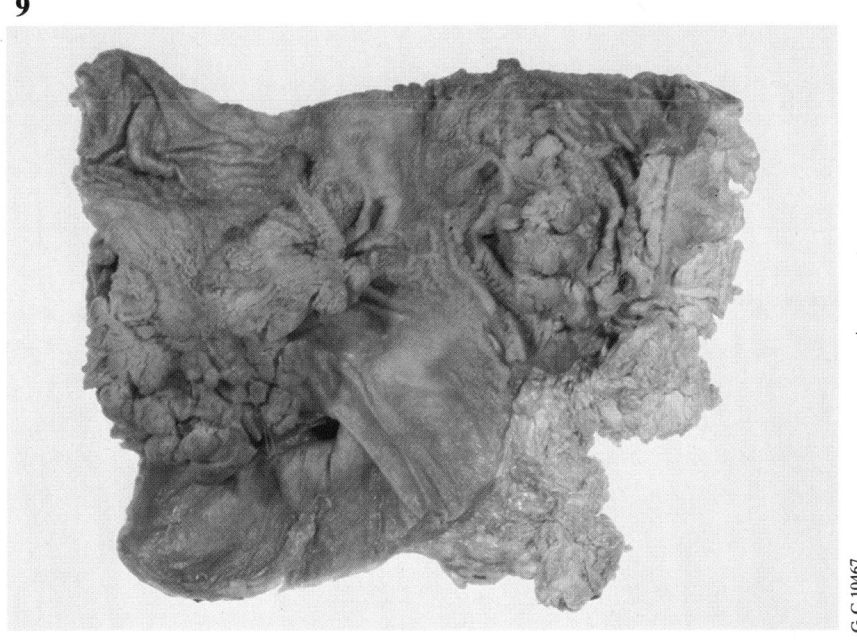

9

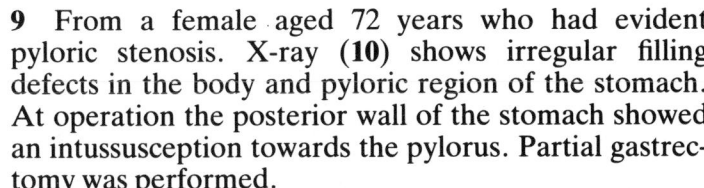

G. C. 10467

9 From a female aged 72 years who had evident pyloric stenosis. X-ray (**10**) shows irregular filling defects in the body and pyloric region of the stomach. At operation the posterior wall of the stomach showed an intussusception towards the pylorus. Partial gastrectomy was performed.

The preparation consists of the distal two thirds of the stomach and the first part of the duodenum. These have been laid open by incising along the lesser curvature. On the posterior wall, the lesser curvature and upper part of the anterior wall of the body of the stomach there are numerous polyps. Some are pedunculated, others sessile and they vary in size, many being about 1.5 cm in diameter. Some of the sessile polyps have fused to form irregular projecting masses. The remainder of the mucosa of the body of the stomach is thickened and the rugae are unduly prominent. The pyloric canal and part of the adjacent antrum are free from polyps. The posterior wall and lesser curvature are invaginated to form an intussusceptum, the apex of which has passed through the pylorus into the duodenum, both being markedly dilated.

11 Microsections show the polyps to consist of closely packed gastric glands. There is no nuclear hyperchromatism or irregularity to suggest malignancy. (*H&E ×40*)

10

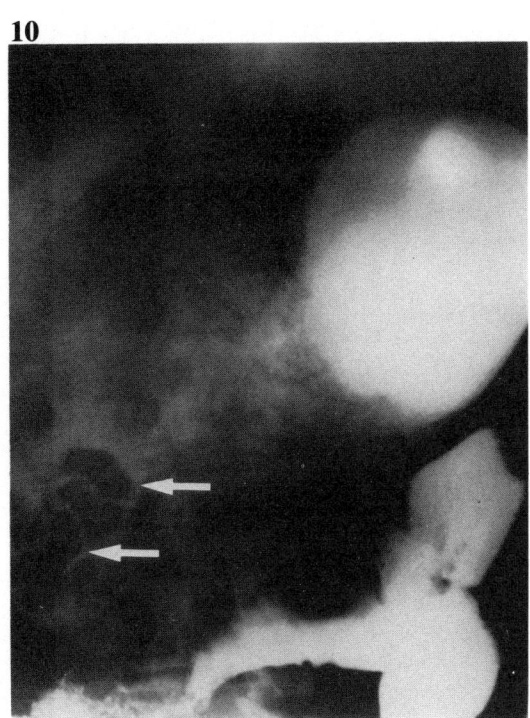

11

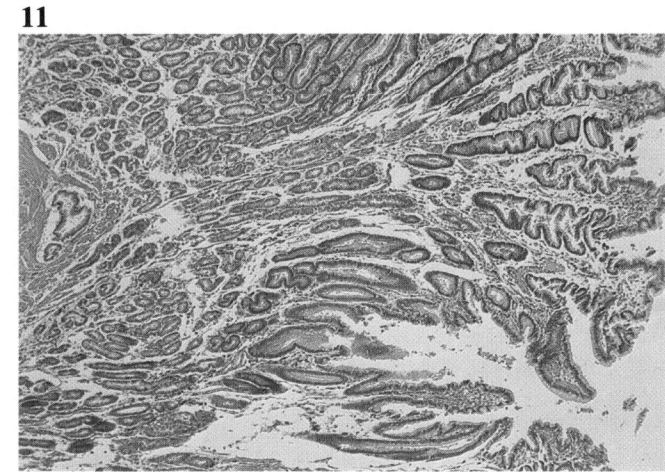

Adenomatous polyps

True adenomatous polyps tend to be larger in size than the so-called 'inflammatory' polyps and resemble similar papillomas arising in the colon. They may be solitary and arise chiefly in the antrum. Occasionally they show surface papillae.

Microscopically the epithelial elements show a glandular structure which is usually orderly in its arrangement. There may be some irregularity of the cells and evidence of mitotic activity. Some polyps are frankly malignant on first recognition.

12

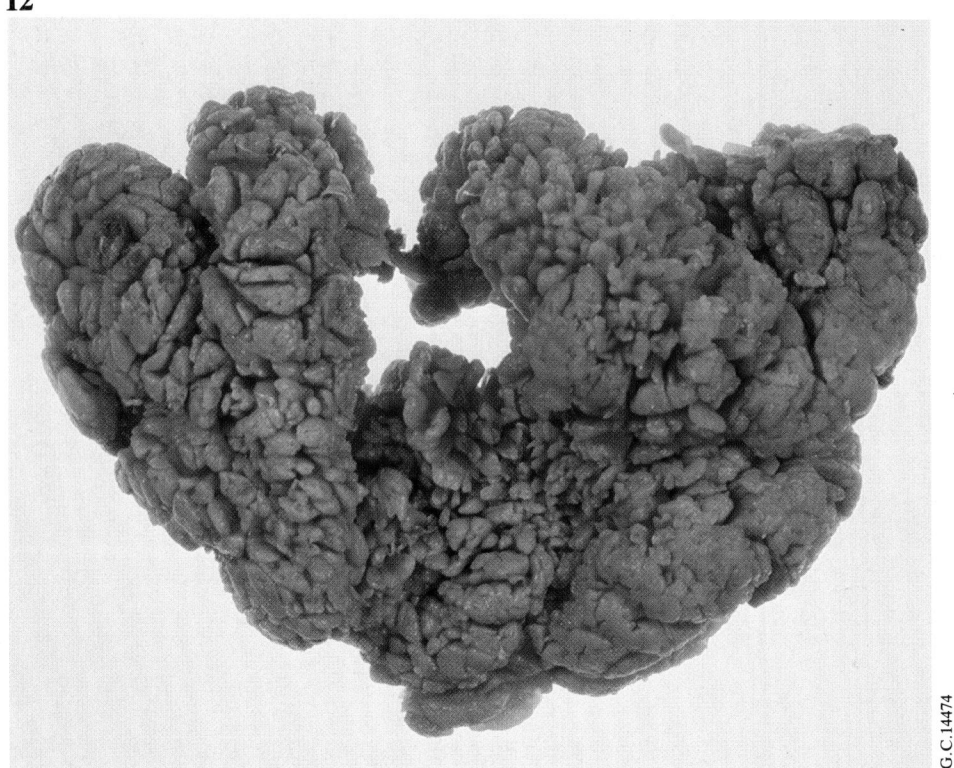

G.C.14474

13

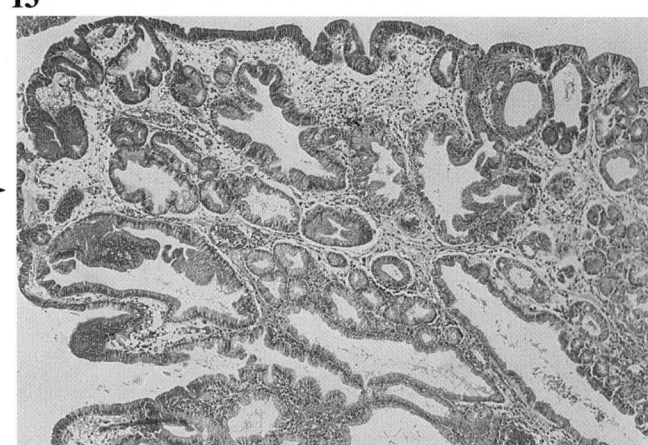

13 A portion of the tumour showing an adeno-papillomatous pattern. The glands vary in size and are formed of well differentiated mucus-secreting cells with low mitotic activity. *(H&E ×48)*

14

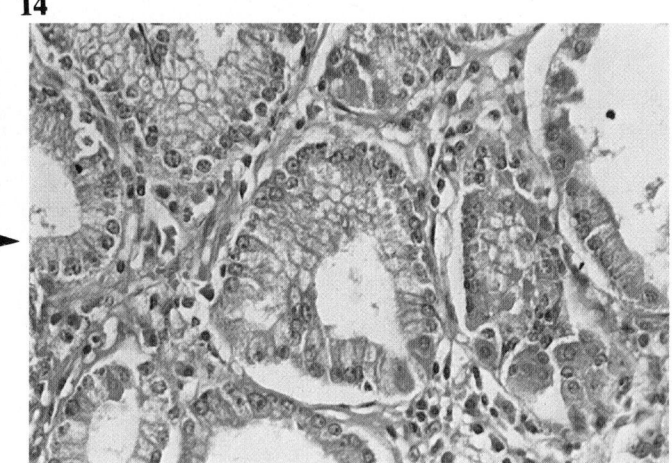

14 A higher power view showing that parietal cells survive in some of the glands. *(H&E ×310)*

12 The specimen is a portion of the stomach in which the whole of the mucosa is covered by a multitude of polyps. In one area they are aggregated to form a larger projecting lobule. Ménétrier used the term *'polyadenome en nappe'* to distinguish this confluent form of gastric polyposis from other forms in which each polyp is discrete and has a well-defined separate pedicle – *'polyadenome polypeaux'*. Numerous portions of the tumour were examined and all appeared well differentiated. Despite this, metastases became obvious a year later suggesting that at least part of the tumour was malignant.

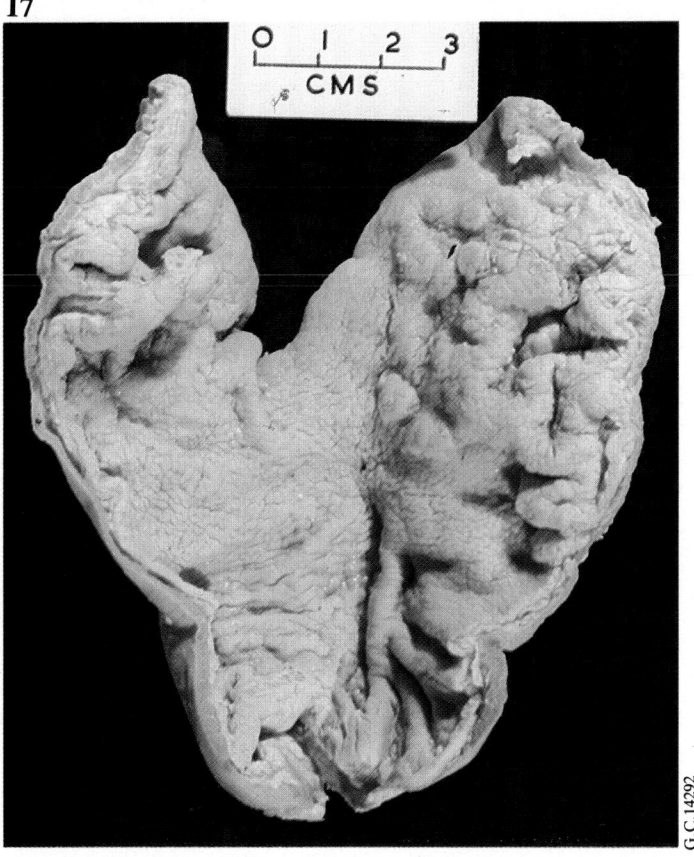

17 From a male aged 70 years admitted to hospital because of haematemesis. Gastroscopy revealed an area of irregular mucosa and several polyps on the greater curvature in the lower part of the body and upper part of the antrum. A partial gastrectomy was performed.

The specimen shows a relatively large polypoid area in the upper part of the antrum which is smooth-surfaced and not ulcerated. More distally there are a few more discrete rounded polyps.

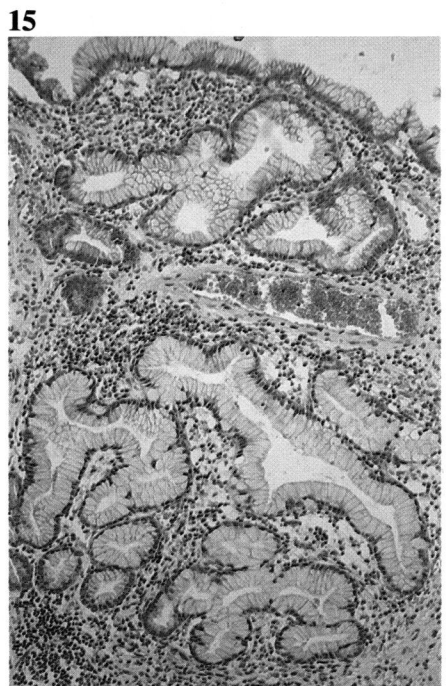

15 Part of a polyp with well differentiated glands formed by tall columnar cells arranged in a single layer. *(H&E ×100)*

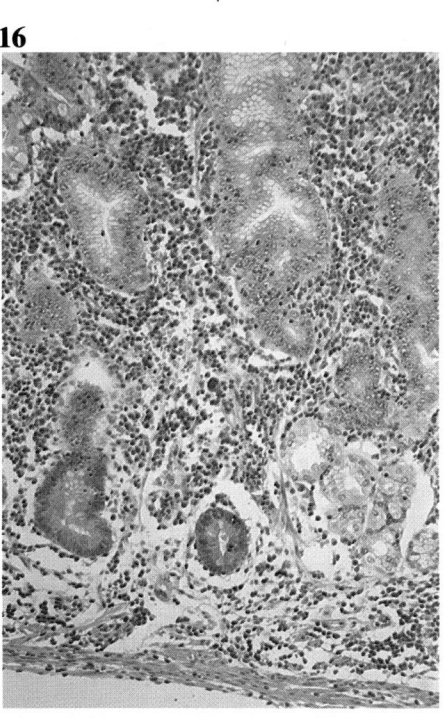

16 The glandular epithelium tends to be heaped up and hyperchromatic. The nuclei are enlarged and show mitotic activity. Foci of intestinal metaplasia can be seen (bottom left). The muscularis mucosae is intact. *(H&E ×125)*

18 Illustration of a small polypoid tumour from another case showing frank malignancy – a 'malignant adenoma'. *(H&E ×100)*

Site incidence

The majority of carcinomas arise in the pyloric antrum and along the lesser curvature. Carcinomas are much less frequent on the greater curvature and in the fundus.

19 Approximate ratio according to site of tumour.

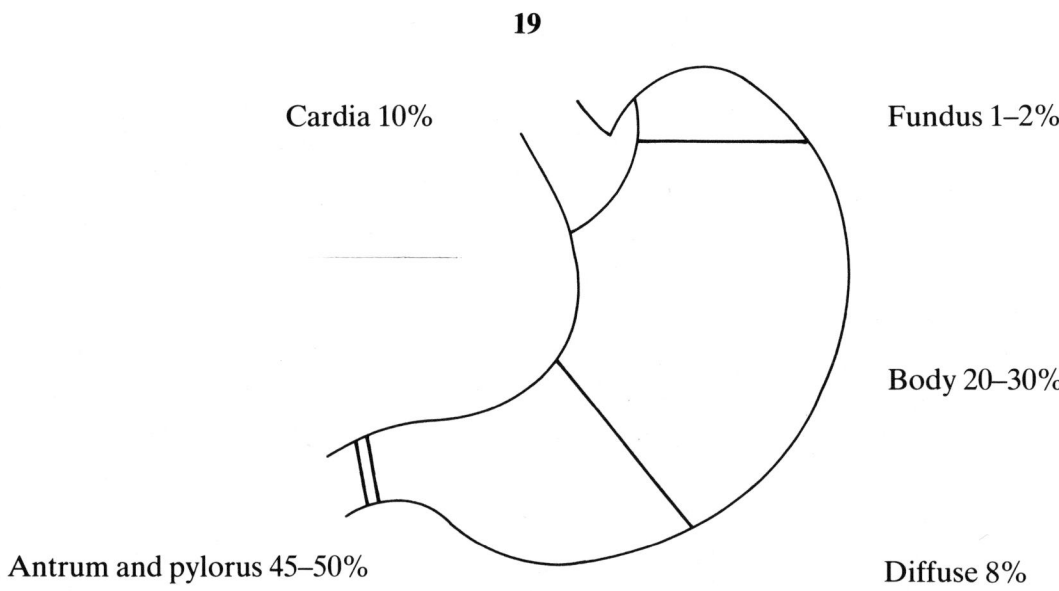

19

Cardia 10%

Fundus 1–2%

Body 20–30%

Antrum and pylorus 45–50%

Diffuse 8%

Carcinoma at the cardio-oesophageal orifice presents the problem of determining whether the neoplasm arose in the oesophageal or gastric mucosa. A glandular carcinoma can occur in the lower end of the oesophagus (see Section 13 U 2).

Lesions in the fundus or on the greater curvature present a difficult differential diagnosis both clinically and radiologically between carcinoma and simple ulceration.

The rule to follow is to regard all these lesions as malignant until proven otherwise by histology. (*Vide infra.*)

Macroscopic features

Since the development of carcinoma of the stomach is insidious and the initial features relatively slight, the diagnosis may be late. When the lesion is exposed at operation the tumour may be found to be extensive. It may present in a variety of macroscopic forms to which descriptive names have been applied. These do not represent different pathological entities since they are of common histological character. The distinction between the varieties is not sharp. Intermediate or combined forms occur. The variation of appearance depends upon the degree of epithelial proliferation, infiltration in the submucous coat and the extent of ulceration. Certain tumours are characterised by excessive production of mucin which is also evident histologically. The term mucoid (or colloid) is applied to this form. The characteristics of these forms of tumour are most readily appreciated by the study of vertical sections through the tumour bearing wall of the stomach.

The different gross forms of carcinoma are illustrated on the following pages

Form	I	(ulcerating)	Figures **20 – 22**
Form	II	(polypoid)	Figures **23 – 25**
Form	III	(obstructing)	Figures **26 – 28**
Form	IV	(diffuse)	Figures **29 – 31**
Form	V	(mucoid)	Figures **32 – 34**
Form	VI	(atypical)	Figures **35 – 37**

Differentiation of carcinoma and benign chronic ulcer

The naked eye appearances of a chronic benign ulcer and a carcinoma are often difficult to differentiate. The terms malignant ulcer or ulcer carcinoma are commonly used but add to the confusion and are applicable both to the innocent ulceration which has become malignant or the carcinoma which ulcerates. These are the lesions which especially require histological verification to establish the true diagnosis.

The differentiation is particularly difficult in relation to saddle ulcers on the lesser curvature – whether simple ulcers or carcinoma. The mass is usually hard, fixed and the edges of the ulcerated mass may be inverted or project.

Early lesion – Endoscopy

Using endoscopic methods attention has been directed to the early lesion which may appear as a small plaque in the mucosa (carcinoma *in situ*), a depressed ulcer or a small papilla which may or may not show ulceration. These are early lesions in which the diagnosis can be established only by biopsy. (*Vide infra.*)

Form I (ulcerating)

20 This is a relatively rapidly growing carcinoma. The mass of proliferating cancer cells into the lumen has become the site of excavating ulceration characterised by raised margins and an irregular penetrating base. The lesion may have originated as a flat plaque and ulceration has commenced at the centre of the cell mass. The muscularis mucosae is breached and invasion of the underlying submucosa and muscularis is evident. Involvement of the peritoneal coat occurs and the tumour may become adherent to and invade an adjacent viscus.

(a) Raised margin of ulcer not over-hanging the floor.

(b) Floor of ulcer with penetration and destruction of muscularis.

20

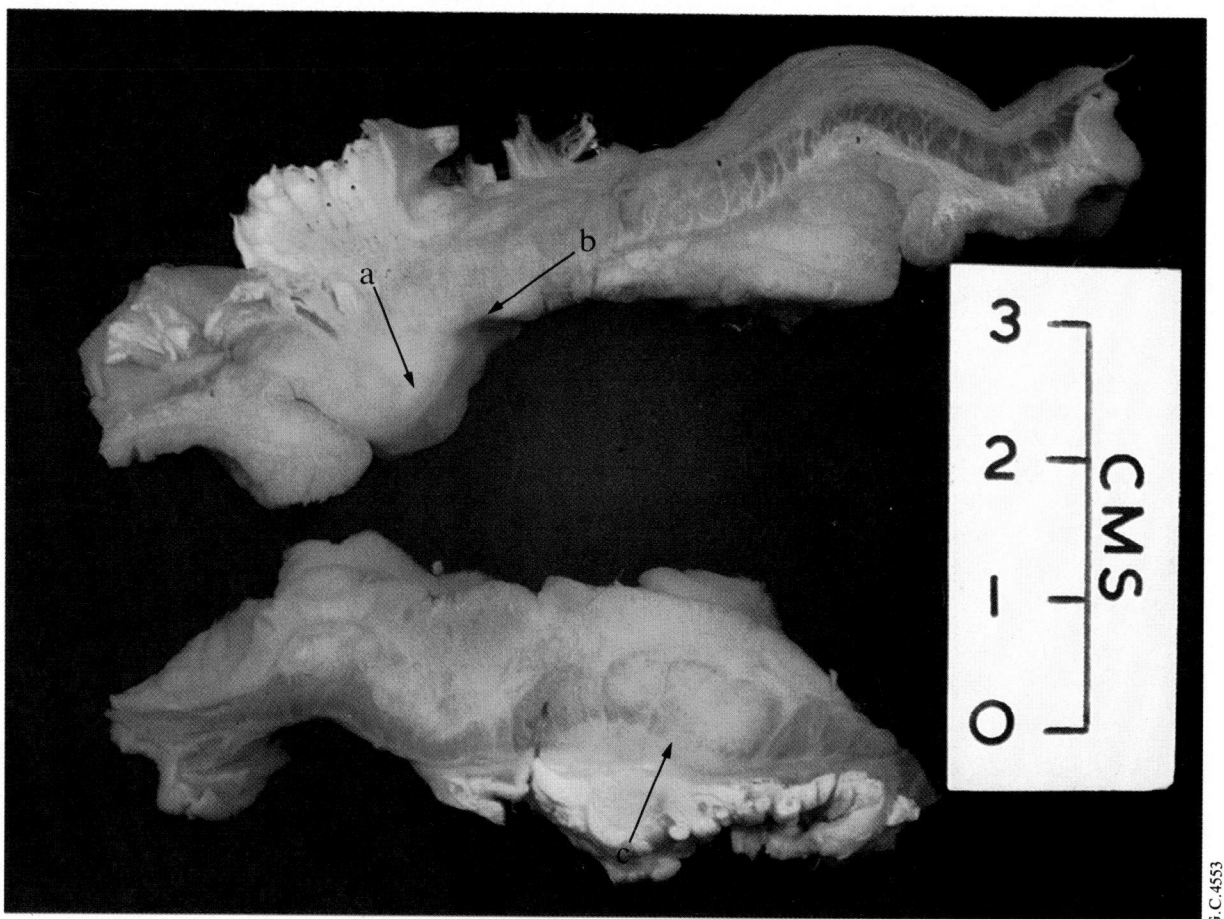

(c) Commencing malignant penetration of the great omentum at the greater curvature.

21

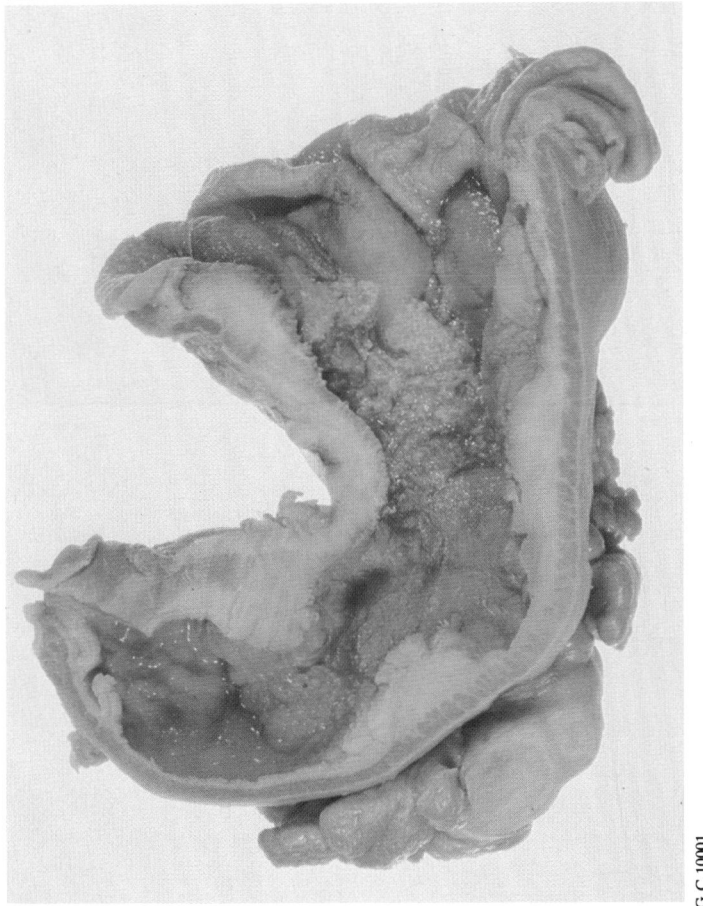

G.C.10001

21 An extensive ulcerating carcinoma of the antrum and body of the stomach involving both the greater and lesser curvatures. The special features to note in this specimen are the indurated and nodular character of the ulcer surface and the extensive invasion along the lesser curvature with destruction of the muscle coat. Along the greater curvature the tumour lies mostly in the submucosa and the muscle layer although penetrated is retained throughout its length. The gastro-colic omentum is the site of invasion, the tumour being present as a large nodule probably in a lymph node.

22

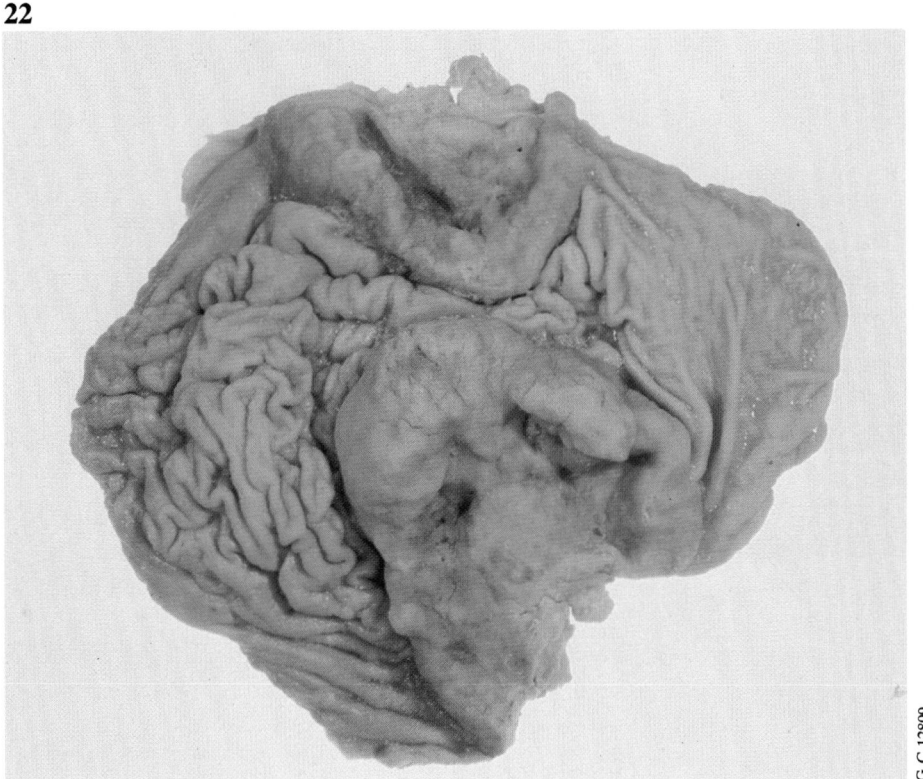

G.C.12809

22 From a male aged 63 years. Six month history of dyspepsia and increasing ill health. The specimen obtained at operation shows a large ulcerating carcinoma with projecting and everted edges situated on the lesser curvature and almost encircling the viscus. The base of the ulcer shows sloughing.

On sectioning the specimen there is evident destruction of the muscular coat by infiltration of malignant disease. In the more normal part, the rugae are prominent and the mucosa shows no signs of atrophy.

Histologically the tumour is a very cellular active glandular carcinoma with evident destruction and infiltration of the muscularis.

Form II (polypoid)

23   The characteristic feature is the great and rapid proliferation of the cancer cells internal to the muscle layer forming a soft projecting mass into the lumen of the viscus. The base of the tumour may be wide, in which case there is a protruding mass, or the base may be comparatively narrow in which case there is a pedunculated type of tumour. Spread beyond the submucosa is slow and extension to the peritoneal surface and lymph nodes relatively late.

(a) Mass protruding into the lumen of the stomach.

(b) Ulcerating surface.

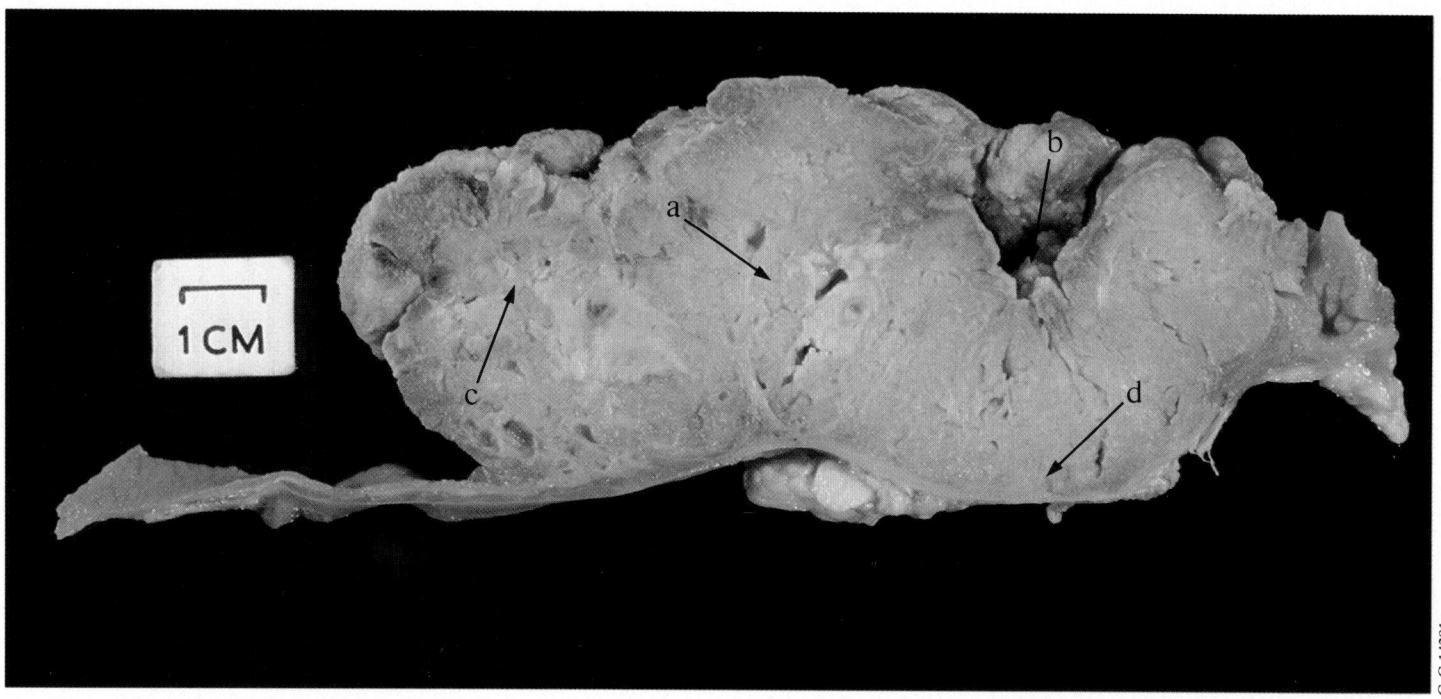

(c) Overhanging margin of protruding mass giving a pedunculated appearance in this area.

(d) Gross invasion of gastric wall.

24

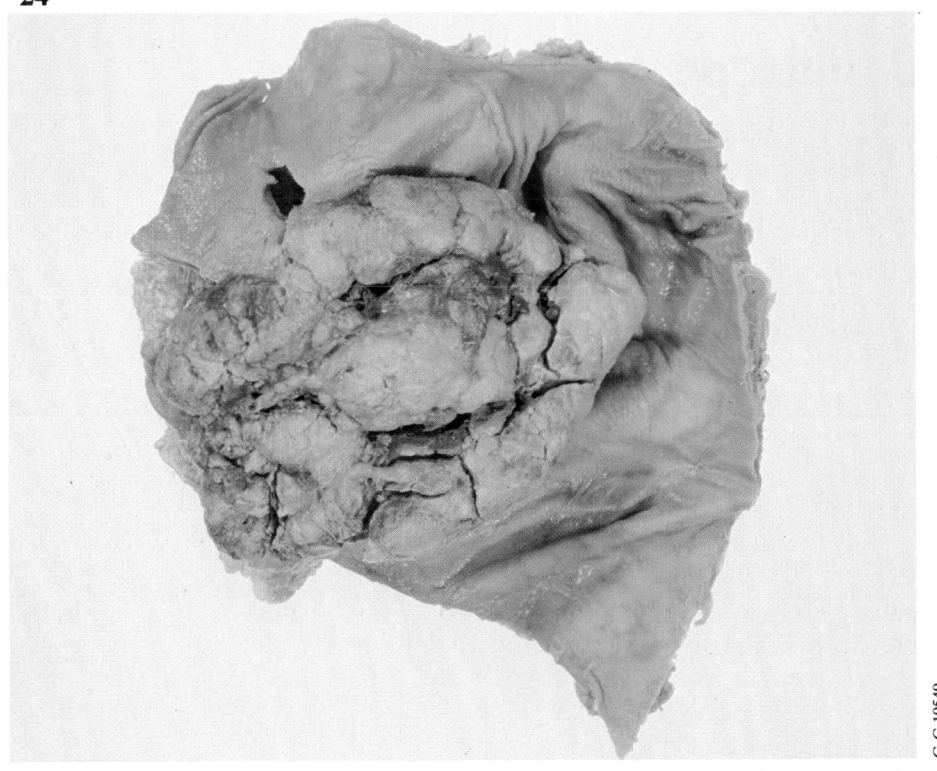

G.C. 10549

24 From a male aged 50 years, a diabetic with associated hypochromic anaemia. At operation there was no evidence of spread through the wall of the stomach and no metastases were found.

This specimen illustrates a tumour projecting into the lumen of the viscus. Surface ulceration has occurred and become extensive. It has penetrated deeply. The mass has become an ulcerated elevated plateau. Haemorrhage is a common feature.

Histological examination showed a papillary carcinoma with well differentiated glandular structure. The tumour did not spread beyond the submucosa.

25

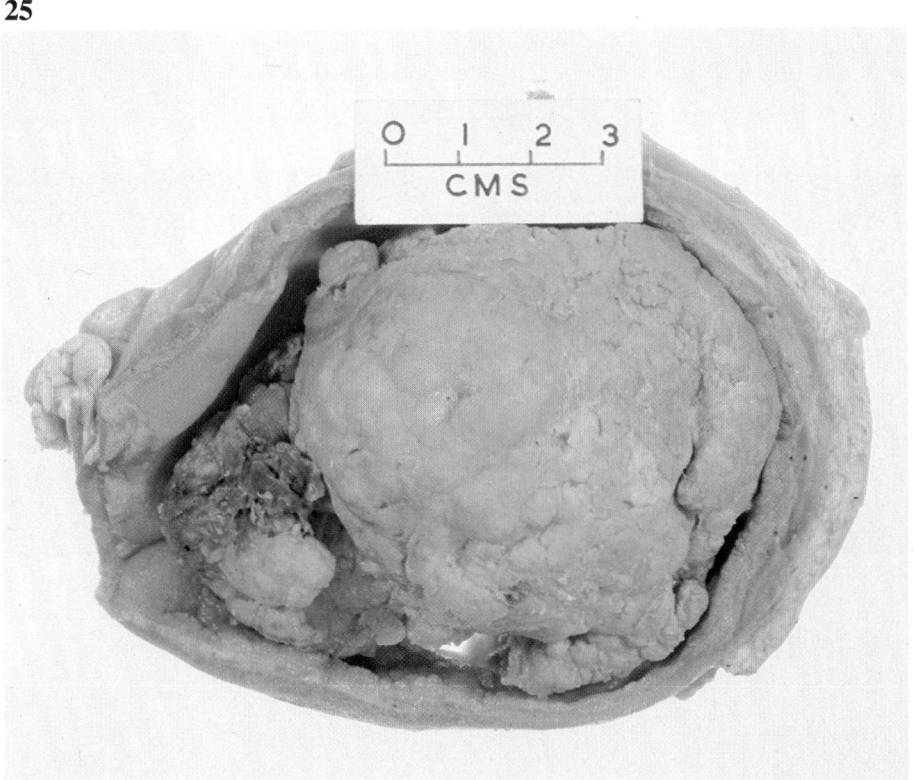

G.C. 14285

25 From a male aged 71 years. Six month history of anorexia and loss of weight. In spite of its size the tumour removal was comparatively readily accomplished and it was noted that there was no evidence of tumour spread. Many bulky tumours of the stomach are found to be readily amenable to surgical treatment and the prognosis is often remarkably good.

This specimen demonstrates a large polypoid tumour projecting into the body. The neck of the tumour is hidden in the picture but formed an attachment to the wall of the stomach narrower than the diameter of the projecting mass.

The surface is relatively smooth and shows no gross ulceration.

Form III (obstructing)

26 This form is characterised by a tumour which is infiltrating and associated with proliferation of stromal type elements. It encircles the wall including the muscularis causing occlusion, partial or complete, of the lumen. This form is typically seen involving the pyloric canal. Occasionally saddle-type carcinoma of the lesser curvature may cause a mid-gastric deformity due to stromal proliferation. Radiologically this deformity is described as an 'hour-glass' stomach and is comparable to mid-stomach constriction associated with simple chronic ulceration.

Note the narrow tubular appearance of the lumen of the pyloric canal. Extension of the disease in the wall of the antrum.

26

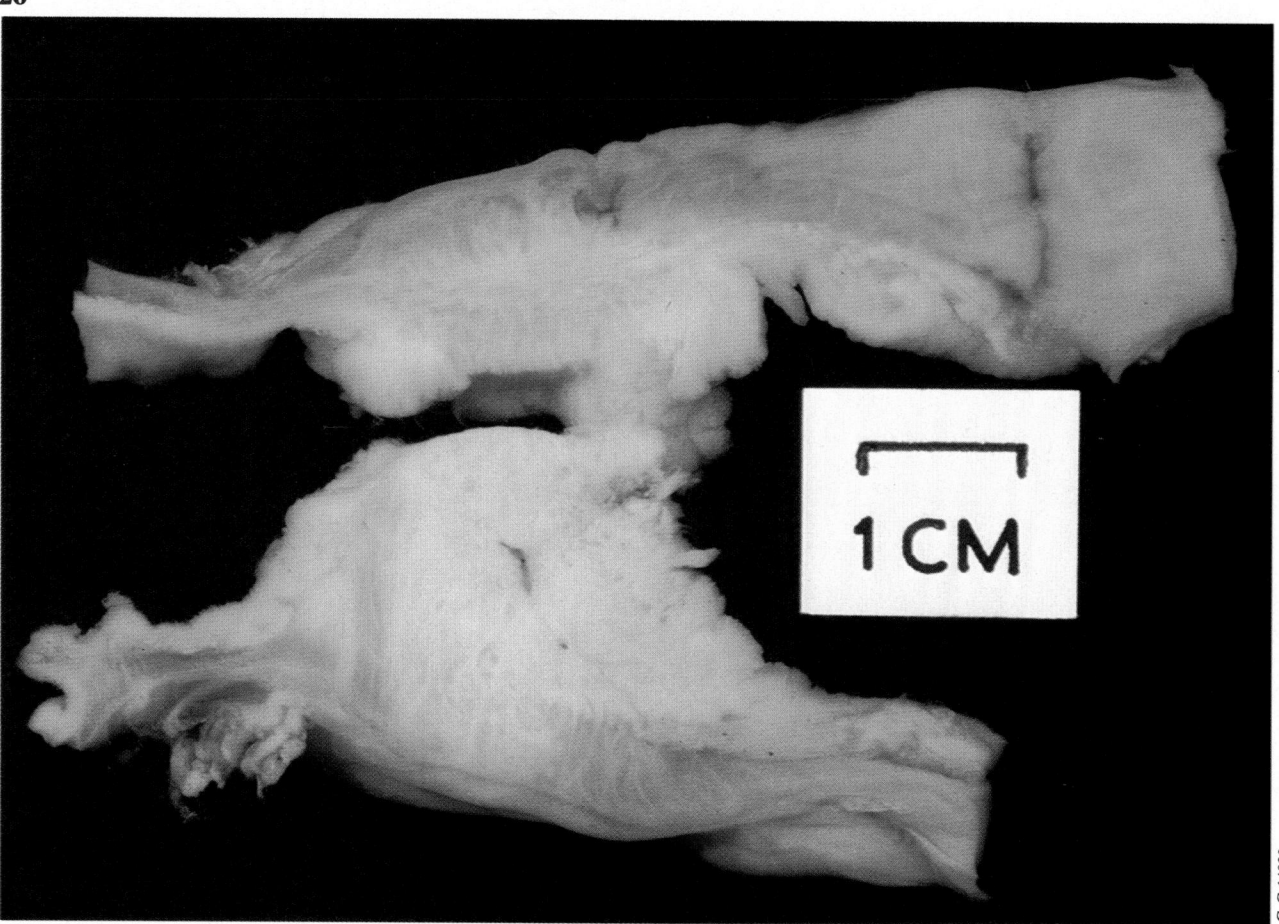

The tumour grows inwards towards the lumen but also shows considerable infiltration of the muscle.

27

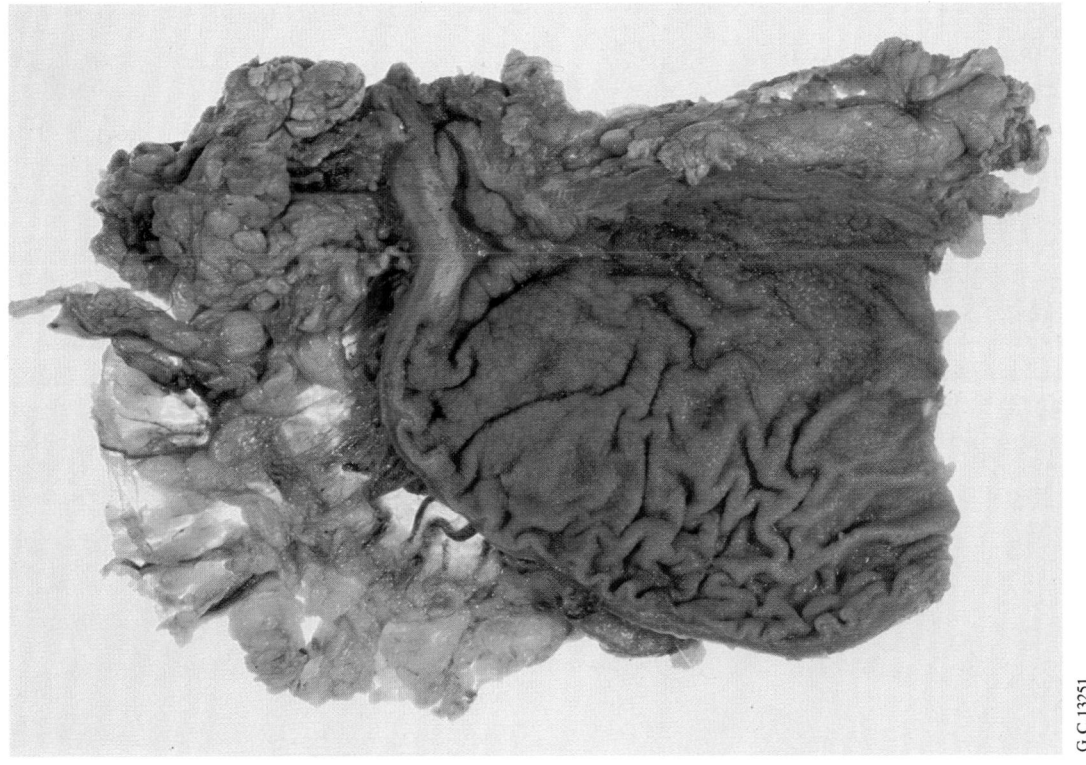

G.C.13251

27 From a male aged 66 years. Perforated duodenal ulcer 4 years previously. The specimen illustrates an ulcerating carcinoma of the pylorus with obstruction. The cut surface shows the carcinomatous involvement of the mucosa and submucosa but the muscularis is not deeply invaded. The tumour has spread proximally in the sub-mucosa and the antrum but has not extended distally into the duodenum.

Histologically the tumour is a glandular carcinoma with marked dedifferentiation in some areas and occasional evident areas with mucin formation. Evident lymph node involvement

28

G.C.6863

28 Male aged 83 years. Marked vomiting and haematemesis.

On the posterior wall of the pyloric antrum is a circular ulcer about 6mm in diameter, with smooth regular edges and a floor devoid of mucous membrane. The submucosa and muscular coats of the pylorus and its antrum are infiltrated and thick. At the junction of the antrum with the body of the stomach is a raised nodule which on section shows a grey homogeneous infiltration.

Histologically, the tumour is an infiltrating carcinoma.

This is a specimen of a carcinoma which at the time of operation could not be differentiated from a chronic ulcer from the exterior.

Form IV (diffuse)

29 This form is characterised by the extensive involvement of the wall of the stomach both longitudinally and circumferentially converting the organ into a rigid tube, the 'leather-bottle' stomach or 'linitis plastica'. Ulceration may be minimal and occurs at several separate areas. Spread through the muscular coat is diffuse. The disease usually occurs in patients of an earlier age group.

It was traditionally held that carcinoma of the stomach does not spread into the duodenum. Histological studies show the spread into the duodenum is lymphatic in character and the duodenal mucosa is not involved. In linitis plastica, however, involvement of the duodenum is found in 50% of cases.

29

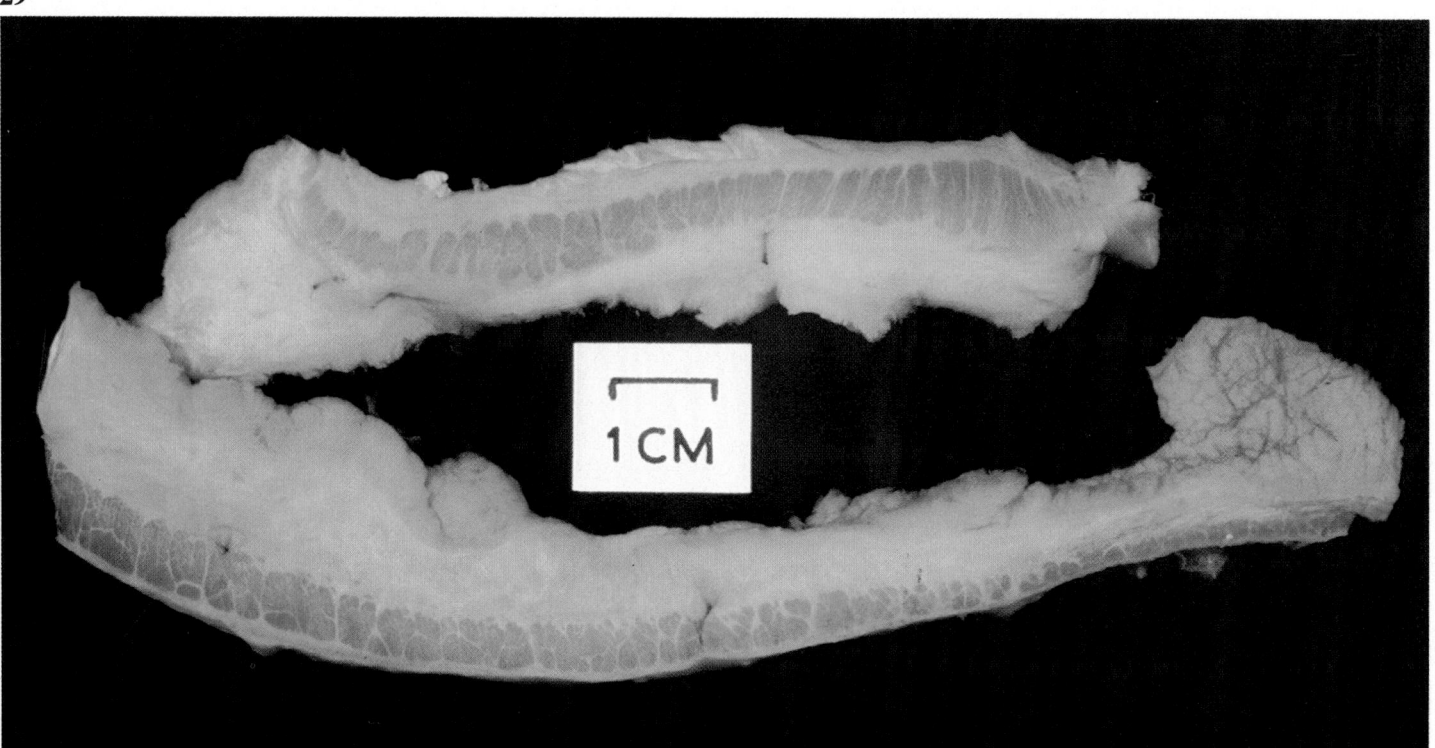

G.C.6867

The main bulk of the tumour is in the pyloric antrum, both on the greater and lesser curvatures. There is a uniform infiltration of carcinoma extending along the whole length of the specimen. This lies in the submucosa. The muscularis remains visible but shows, especially on the greater curvature, strands of infiltration. The stomach wall is thickened throughout.

30

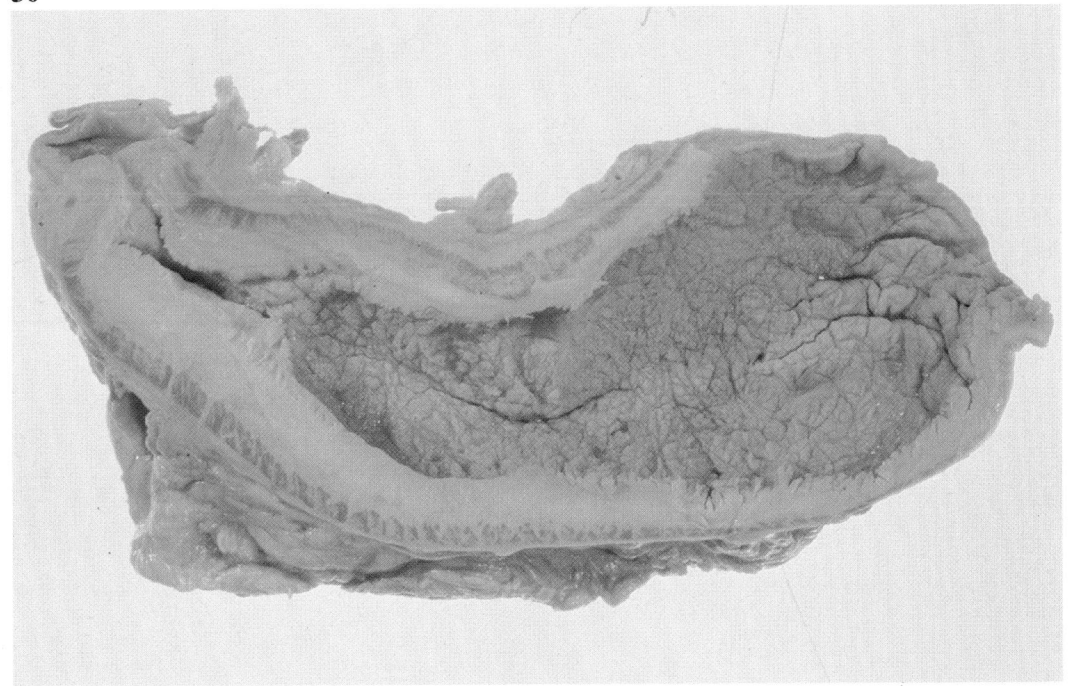

G.C.10027

30 From a male aged 66 years who 10 years previously had been operated on for gastric ulcer. Long history of dyspepsia and on examination complete achlorhydria was disclosed. The main tumour appears to have arisen in the pyloric canal and the tumour has spread extensively from there in the submucosa. This is clearly seen along both the greater and lesser curvatures. The whole stomach is converted into a rigid tube.

Microscopically a poorly differentiated carcinoma with only occasional acinar formation.

31

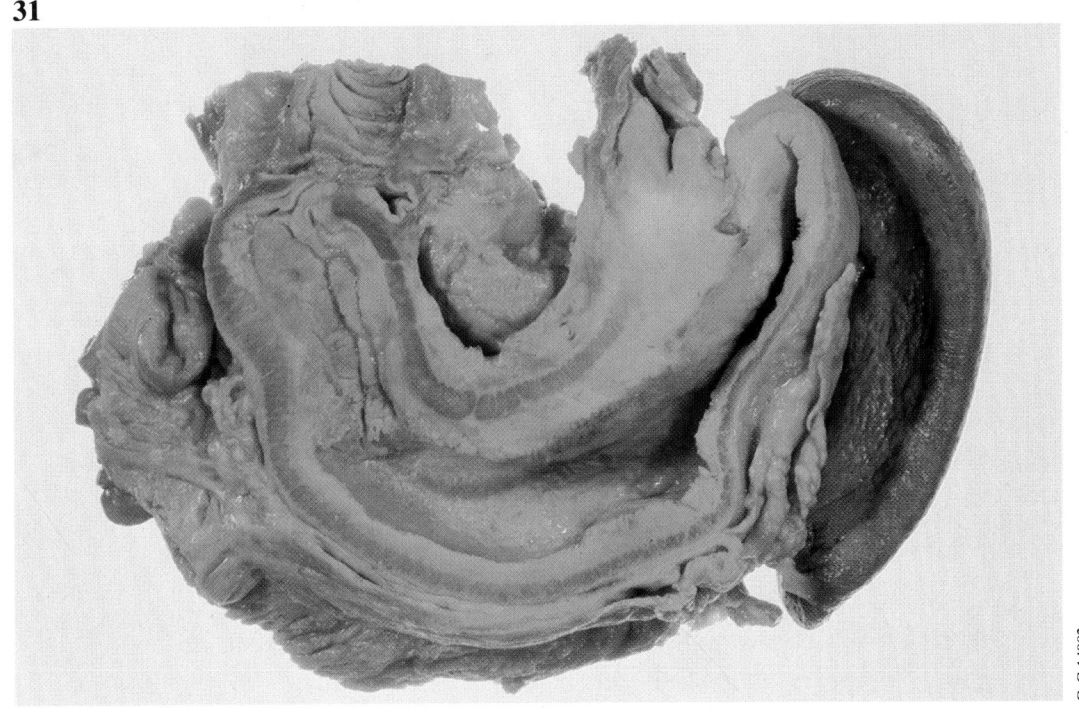

G.C.14902

31 From a male aged 40 years with an 8 month history of vomiting, pain and loss of weight. At laparotomy diffuse carcinoma of the stomach with involvement of adjacent organs and with metastases in the pelvis. The whole stomach wall is invaded by a carcinoma chiefly located in the submucosa but involving to an appreciable extent the muscularis especially at the cardio-oesophageal end of the stomach.

Microscopically a poorly differentiated carcinoma with marked fibrous reaction.

Form V (mucoid)

32   The distinct feature of these tumours is the gelatinous appearance. They may be bulky or diffuse with a rapid infiltration of all coats. Early involvement of the serosa is associated with widespread trans-coelomic metastases.

32

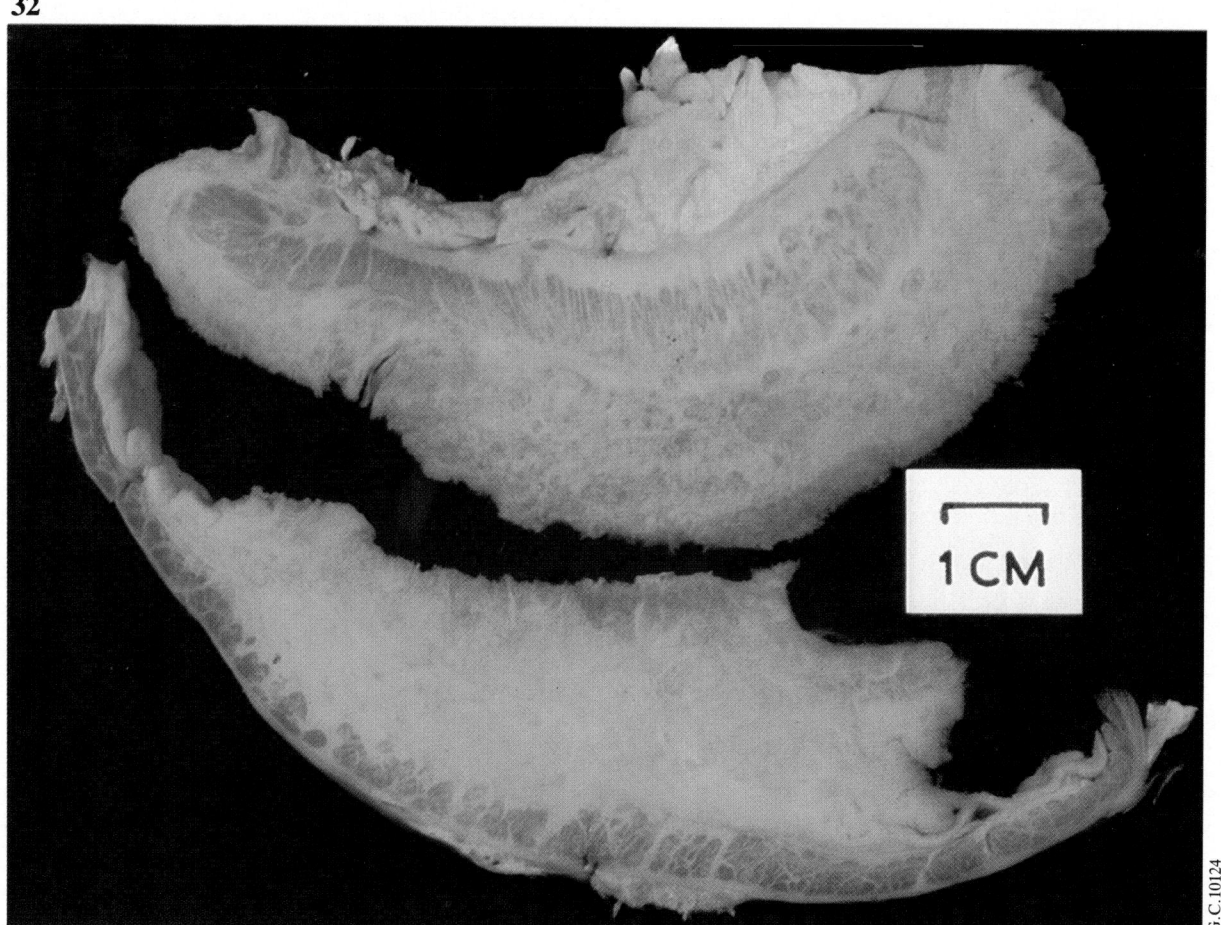

Note especially the ingrowth of tumour which causes narrowing of the pyloric canal leading to obstruction; gelatinous appearance of cut surface of the specimen and muscular infiltration by tumour.

33

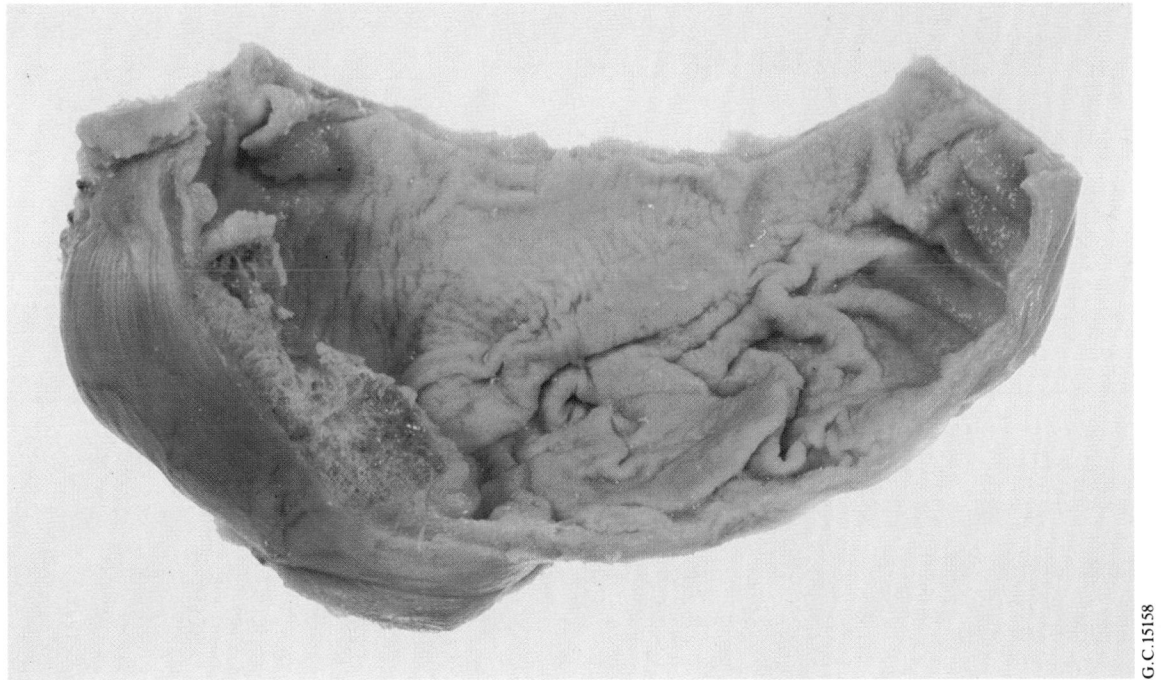

G.C.15158

33 From a female aged 53 years. A tumour in the pyloric antrum. The tumour protruded into the stomach and formed a mass 5.5cm in diameter. On the cut surface the tumour is gelatinous in texture and there is considerable micro cyst formation.

34 Above, the tumour forms large glandular spaces filled by mucin. Below, extracellular mucin containing only small groups of tumour cells separate strands of muscularis. *(H&E ×150)*

34

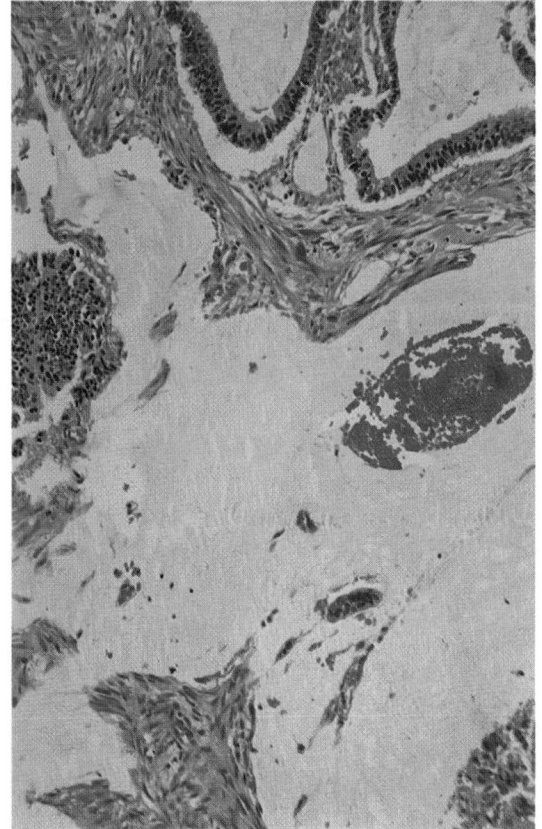

141

Form VI (atypical)

Papilliferous carcinoma

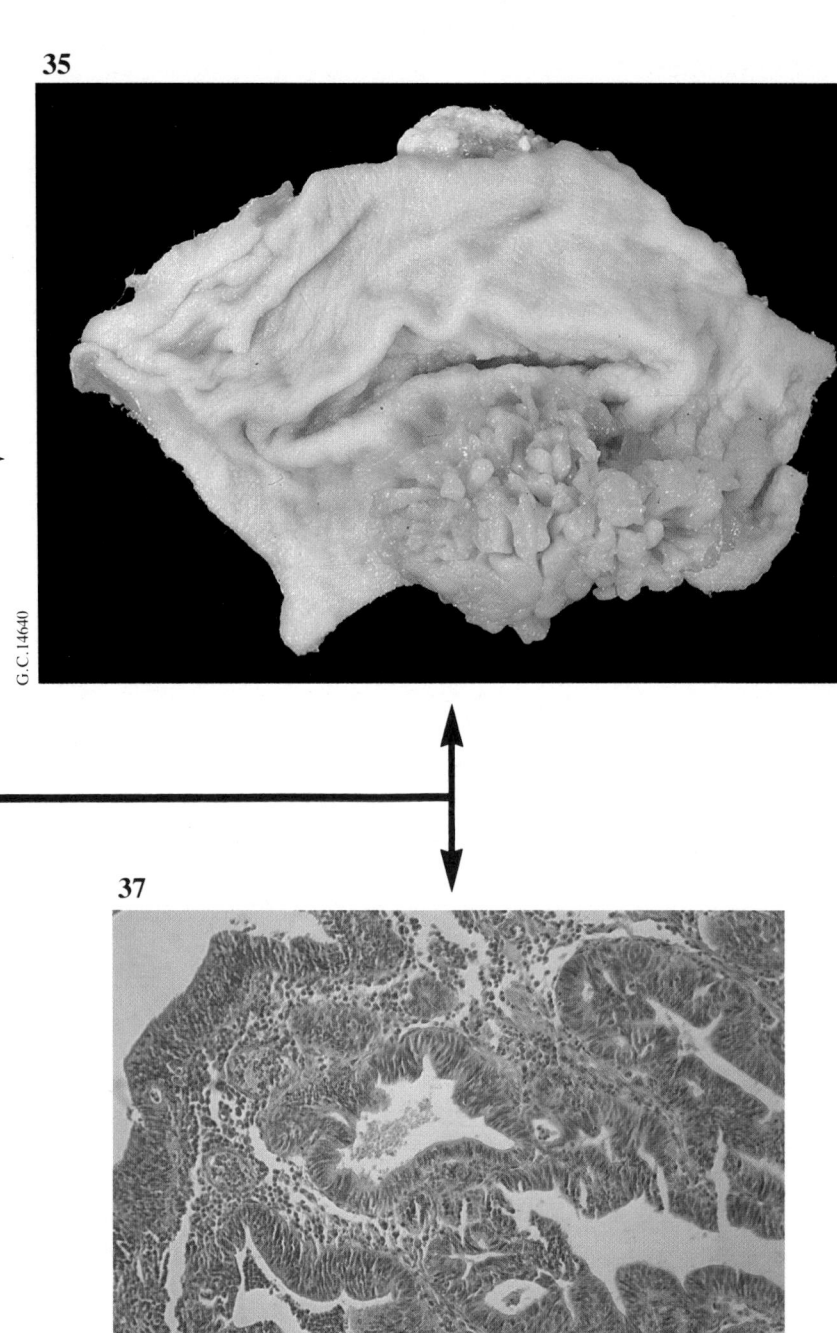

35 This is a rare type of carcinoma which has a multiple polypoid papillary formation.

Note how the tumour projects into the lumen of the viscus, has a pedunculated character and how on the surface of the main mass there is a multiplicity of small pedunculated outgrowths. The precise classification of this tumour is equivocal. It could result from a malignant change in a pre-existing adenomatous formation or it could be regarded as a multiple adenomatous type of carcinoma.

36 A section of an upper part of the above tumour showing the well differentiated papillary pattern. *(H&E ×40)*

37 A deeper portion of the same tumour. The infiltrating carcinoma now has a tubular or glandular pattern with stumpy papillary ingrowths. *(H&E ×125)*

Complications

Perforation

Frank perforation of carcinoma is rare. Occasionally, following perforation, localised abscess formation occurs.

38a **38b**

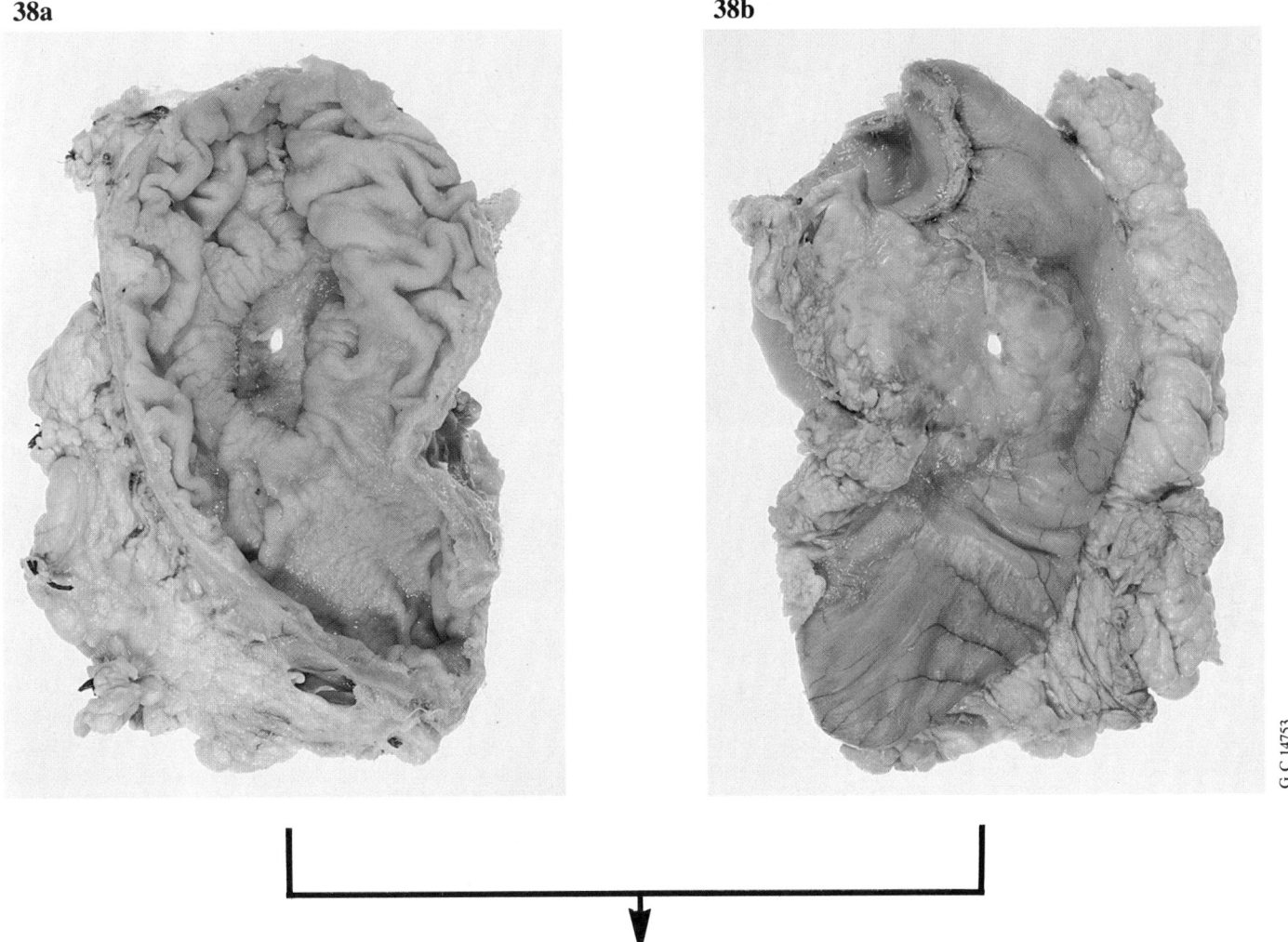

38a and **38b**   From a male aged 61 years who was admitted to hospital as a 'perforation'. An emergency gastrectomy was performed. There was a frank perforation in the anterior wall of the pyloric antrum which was the site of an evident carcinoma. The specimen demonstrates a penetrating carcinoma in the pyloric antrum of the stomach. The edges are inverted rather than rolled and there is a large central perforation. The remainder of the mucosa appears normal.

Histologically the tumour is a poorly differentiated, rapidly growing, adenocarcinoma with many mitoses. The antral mucosa shows some intestinal metaplasia. The fundic mucosa is thick and demonstrates numerous oxyntic and peptic cells. There was no involvement of the gastric lymph nodes.

Perforation appears to have resulted from the combination of a rapidly growing tumour associated with continued acid and pepsin production.

Cardio-oesophageal carcinoma

Carcinoma of the stomach at the cardiac orifice presents features closely similar to those of tumours at the lower end of the oesophagus. True carcinoma of the stomach will be an adenocarcinoma and frequently is a large bulky lesion.

39

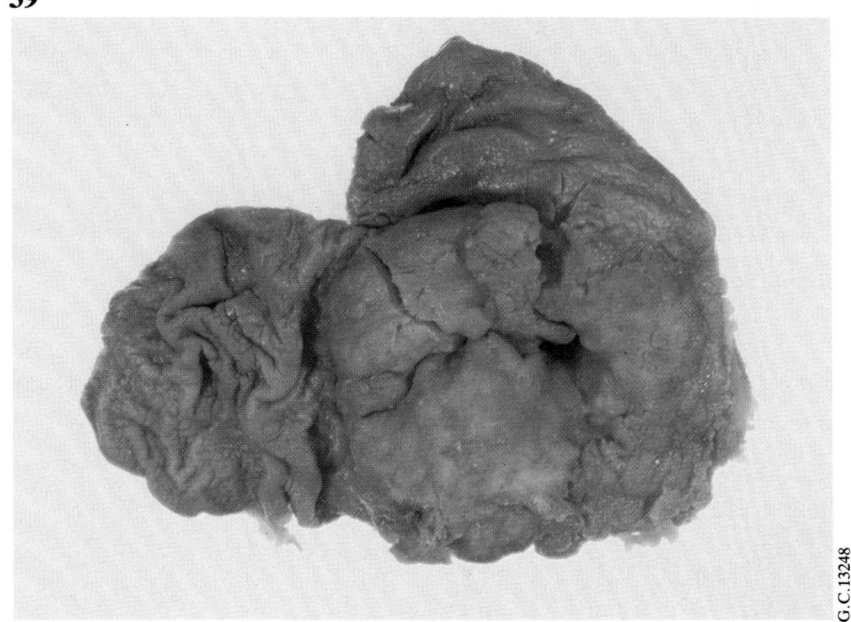

G.C.13248

39 From a male aged 50 years. Indefinite digestive symptoms for 5 years. Repeated examinations the last of which radiologically revealed evidence of a carcinoma at the oesophago-gastric junction. Resection performed.

The specimen has been opened by cutting from the oesophageal opening along the greater curvature of the stomach. A large ulcerating polypoidal carcinoma encircles the oesophago-gastric orifice and extends distally along the gastric wall, especially anteriorly. Microscopically the tumour is a rapidly growing anaplastic carcinoma of a colloidal type. There is deep infiltration. Some acinar formation is present and there is marked pleomorphism. Numerous cells of the signet-ring variety are present.

1 Carcinoma at the cardiac end of the stomach may spread proximally into the lower end of the oesophagus and thereby simulate closely a primary carcinoma of the oesophagus. The distinction, however, is made histologically. Carcinoma of the stomach is an adenocarcinoma but carcinoma of the oesophagus is an epidermoid carcinoma.
2 Following reflux oesophagitis squamous epithelium at the lower end of the oesophagus may be replaced by an upward extension of a gastric type of mucosa. Alternatively a congenital islet of gastric mucosa may be present in the lower oesophagus. In both instances a primary adenocarcinoma of the lower end of the oesophagus may develop.
3 In hiatus hernia part of the cardia together with the cardio-oesophageal orifice is displaced upwards. If a carcinoma develops in this segment of the stomach it simulates clinically and radiologically a carcinoma of the oesophagus (see Section 13 U 2).

Carcinoma subsequent to previous simple gastric operation

Following operative treatment of duodenal or gastric ulcer which involves gastroenterostomy either alone or with partial resection of the stomach it is now recognised that there is a subsequent increase in the incidence of gastric carcinoma. This incidence is variously reported as 3 to 6 times greater than that in the normal stomach. A suggested explanation is that reflux of bile and pancreatic and intestinal juices induces a chronic gastritis and metaplasia which is prone to undergo carcinomatous change. The interval between the time of operation and the development of carcinoma is frequently very long even up to 50 years.

Stomal carcinoma

The carcinoma arises in the gastric mucosa at the margin of the anastomosis and typically is an adenocarcinoma. The adjacent mucosa may show evidence of atrophic gastritis. The disease may extend largely into the gastric wall and may involve the adjacent colon leading to gastrojejunocolic fistula.

40

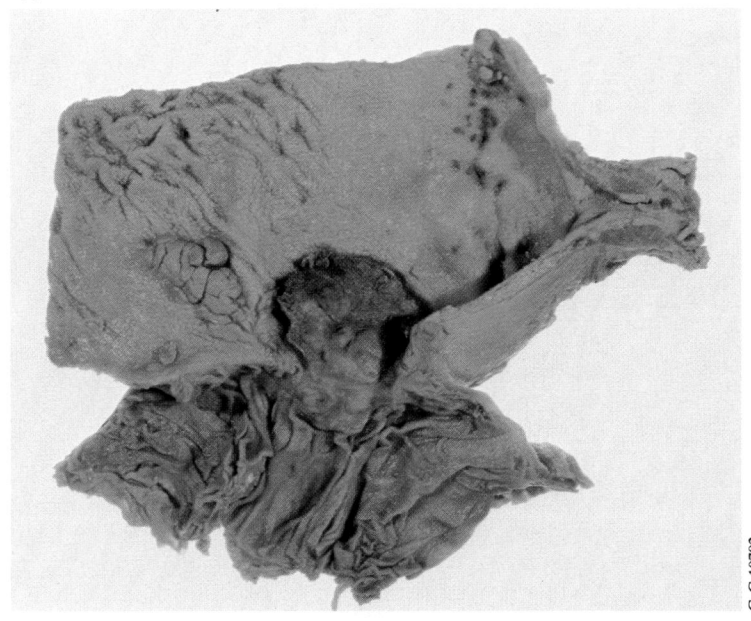

G.C.10702

40 From a male aged 72 years. Gastrojejunostomy performed for a simple gastric ulcer 35 years previously. The specimen shows the anterior wall of the distal portion of the stomach, the pylorus and the loop of jejunum to which the stomach had been anastomosed. Polyps are present and there is a raised almost circular tumour 4cm in diameter with typical elevated and everted margins situated at the stoma. The major portion of this tumour lies in the wall of the stomach but it has extended distally into the wall of the jejunum. The tumour has extended into the wall of the stomach which shows elevation with flattening of the rugae. Histologically the tumour is an adenocarcinoma. (*Vide infra.*)

Note that primary carcinoma of the stomach along the greater curvature is rare when there has been no previous operation yet it is in this area that the stomal carcinoma develops.

Gastric carcinoma associated with gastrojejunostomy

In some patients on whom a gastrojejunostomy or partial gastrectomy was carried out for a simple ulcer and in whom no evidence of malignant disease was found, a carcinoma subsequently develops in the stomach wall at some distance from the stoma. This is not therefore a true stomal carcinoma. The interval between the first operation and the subsequent development of carcinoma is often prolonged. It is held that only if the period between the operation and the onset of carcinoma is less than 5 years can it be assumed that tumour was present at the time of operation. This type of lesion is included in the statistics dealing with the incidence of carcinoma following simple operation and apparently shows a higher occurrence rate than that of neoplasms in the normal stomach.

41

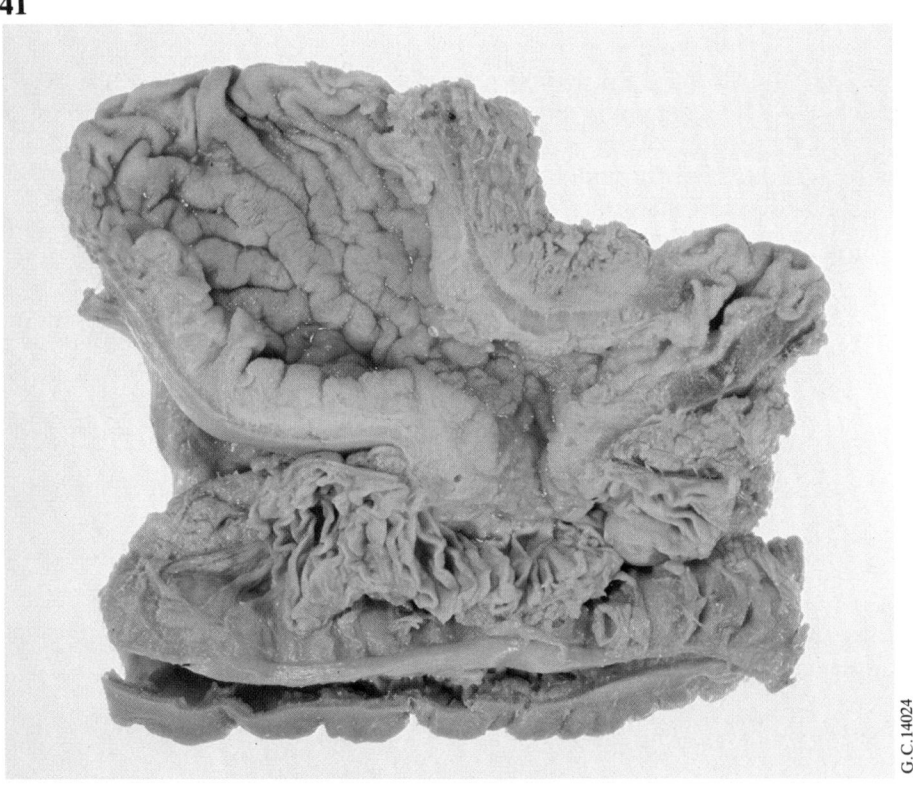

G.C.14024

41 From a male aged 59 years. 40 years previously a gastrojejunostomy had been performed. Following operation had intermittent dyspepsia. Re-examination disclosed the presence of a neoplasm. The specimen shows the anterior wall of the stomach and the pylorus is therefore on the right side of the illustration. The tumour is of the ulcerative type with gross involvement of the submucosa and much infiltration of the muscularis. It appears to have arisen in the pyloric antrum which is extensively involved. The carcinoma extends proximally along the lesser curvature for some 6 cm from the pylorus and on the greater curvature for approximately 10 cm from the pylorus and involves the margins of the stoma.

Gastric carcinoma subsequent to partial gastrectomy

Following partial gastrectomy a carcinoma may develop at the line of anastomosis or in the fundus of the stomach and not overtly associated with the anastomosis. This latter type is illustrated.

42

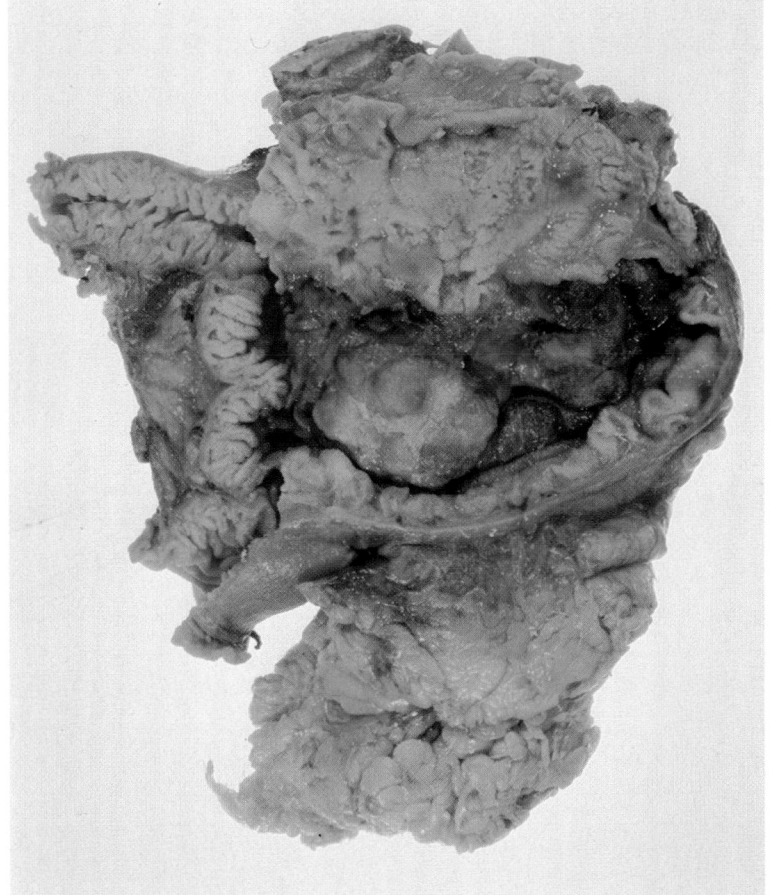

G.C.13667

42   From a male aged 44 years. At the age of 23 years the patient was admitted with a severe haematemesis and a partial gastrectomy (Polya) was performed. Twenty years later the patient developed weakness and loss of weight associated with dyspepsia.

Radiological examination disclosed a carcinoma of the gastric remnant.

The specimen shows the cardiac half of the stomach and the anastomosed loop of jejunum. There is a large polypoid carcinoma with a central ulceration occupying the whole of the upper half of the stomach. The tumour extends down to and has begun to encroach upon the stomal wall but clearly is a gastric neoplasm which is expanding beyond the line of anastomosis. Lymph nodes were palpable both at the cardia and in the mesentery of the jejunum. These were hard and appear to be involved by carcinoma – a feature confirmed histologically.

At the operation of partial gastrectomy the distal half of the stomach and lesser curvature are removed. It might be assumed therefore that since the most common site of carcinoma in the stomach (73%) has been excised the risk of the patient subsequently developing carcinoma of the stomach would be materially reduced. In fact, the incidence of carcinoma is not reduced, which indicates that there has been a true increase in the incidence of tumours in the fundic segment of the stomach.

Histology of gastric cancer

Virtually all carcinomas of the stomach are adenocarcinomas. Their microscopic appearances vary between one tumour and another and often between different parts of the same tumour. The histology of gastric carcinomas is modified according to:

    1   Degree of differentiation
    2   Amount of mucin secretion
    3   Extent of fibrosis
    4   Degree of invasion

Combinations of these variants produce an infinite variety of histological patterns, and only a number of the more characteristic forms are illustrated.

A number of gastric carcinomas secrete intestinal-type mucin and some authorities distinguish between tumours of gastric mucosal type (diffuse) and those showing intestinal affinities (intestinal type).

Well differentiated tumours commonly have a glandular pattern. Less often they are frankly papillary or show an admixture of the two patterns.

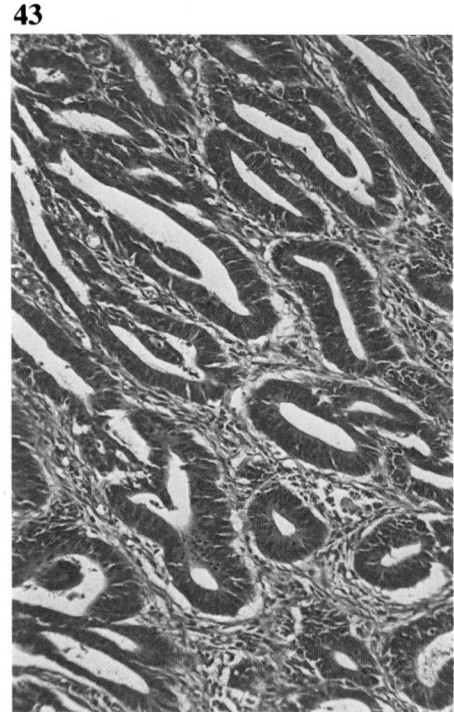

43 Well differentiated gastric carcinoma with a resemblance to colonic carcinoma. *(H&E ×125)*

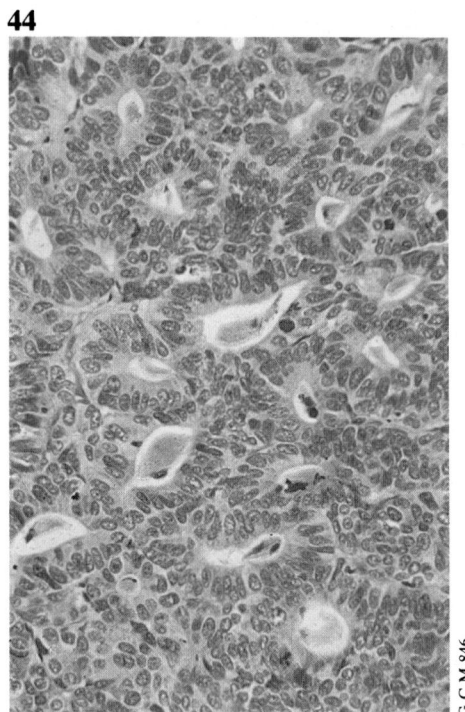

44 Differentiated gastric carcinoma with a glandular pattern becoming solid in some places. *(H&E ×250)*

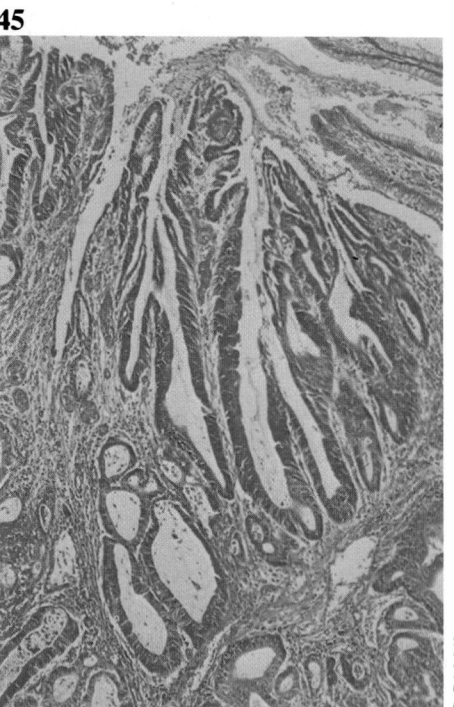

45 Adenopapillary gastric carcinoma. Note the change from papillary to glandular pattern as the tumour infiltrates. *(H&E ×62.5)*

46

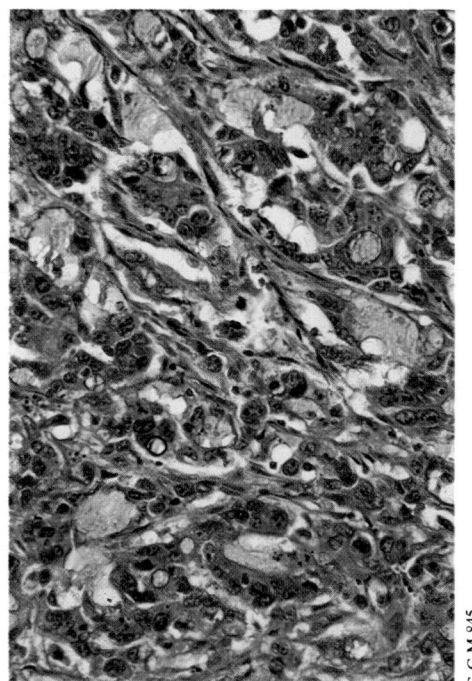

46 Gastric carcinoma. Tumour with poorly formed glandular pattern, secreting intestinal-type mucin. *(Alcian green, phloxin, tartrazine ×250)*

47

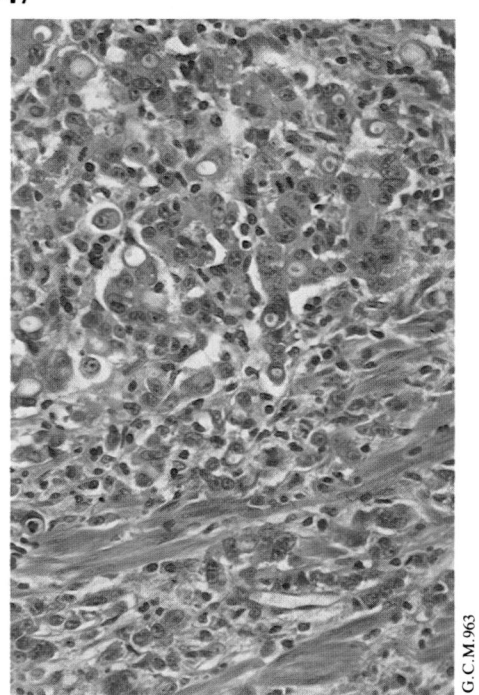

47 Gastric carcinoma. Poorly differentiated. High mitotic activity. *(H&E ×312.5)*

48

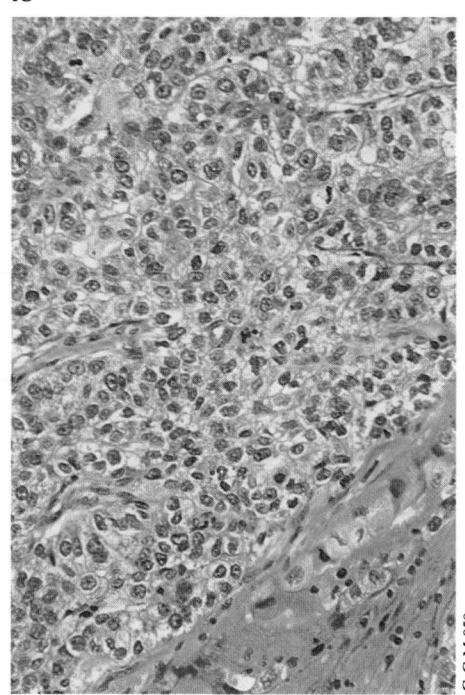

48 Gastric carcinoma. Diffuse type invading muscularis. *(H&E ×250)*

49

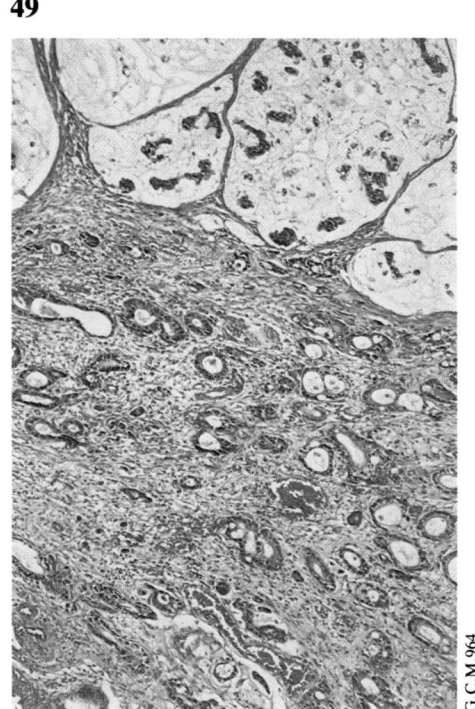

49 Gastric carcinoma. The upper part of the tumour shows marked mucoid change, small groups of tumour cells lying in large pools of mucin. *(H&E ×62.5)*

50

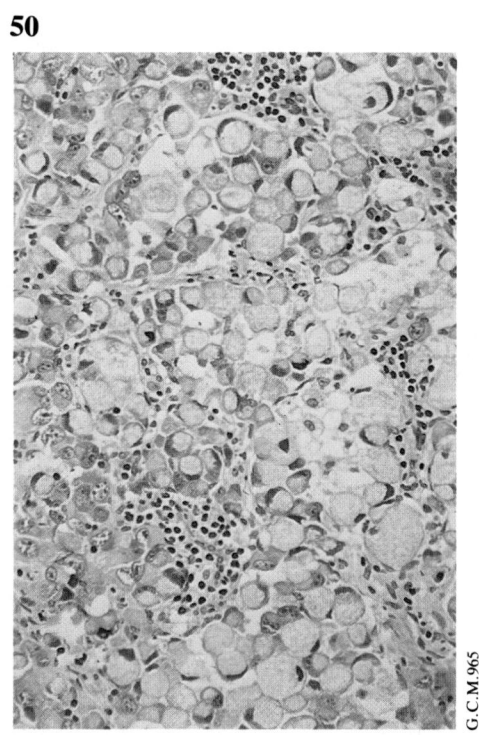

50 Gastric carcinoma. Closely packed tumour cells are distended by intra-cytoplasmic mucin (signet ring cells). *(H&E ×250)*

51

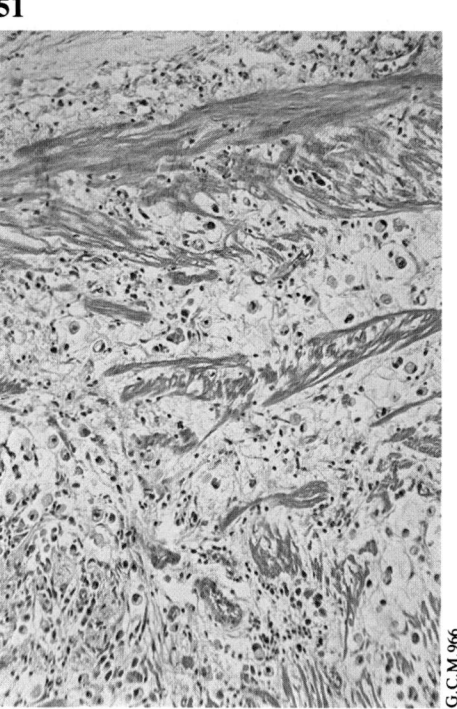

51 Gastric carcinoma. Strands of muscle in outer muscularis are separated by mucoid tumour. *(H&E ×125)*

Histology *(Continued)*

52

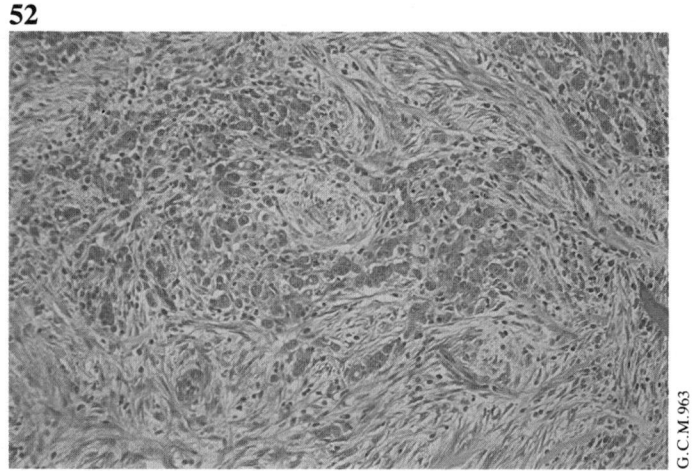

G.C.M.963

52 Scirrhous carcinoma. A poorly differentiated gastric carcinoma with marked fibrosis. *(H&E ×125)*

53

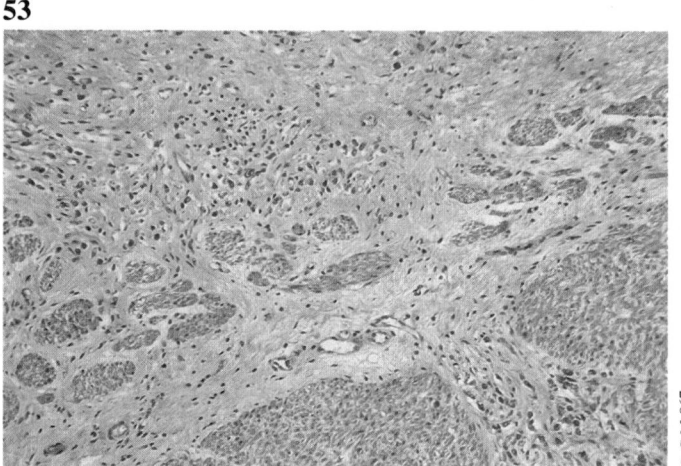

G.C.M.967

53 Linitis plastica. Gastric carcinoma. Inconspicuous, darkly-staining tumour cells lie in the abundant fibrous tissue lying between muscle bands. *(Alcian green, phloxin, tartrazine ×125)*

54

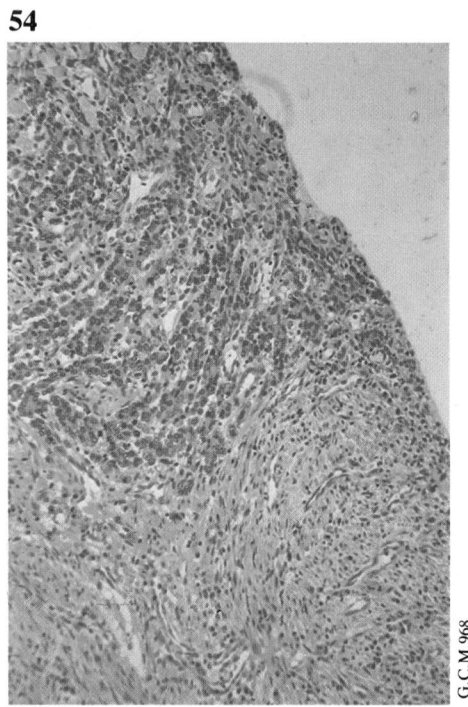

G.C.M.968

54 Gastric ulcer cancer. Poorly differentiated carcinoma infiltrates the margin of a chronic gastric ulcer. *(H&E ×125)*

55

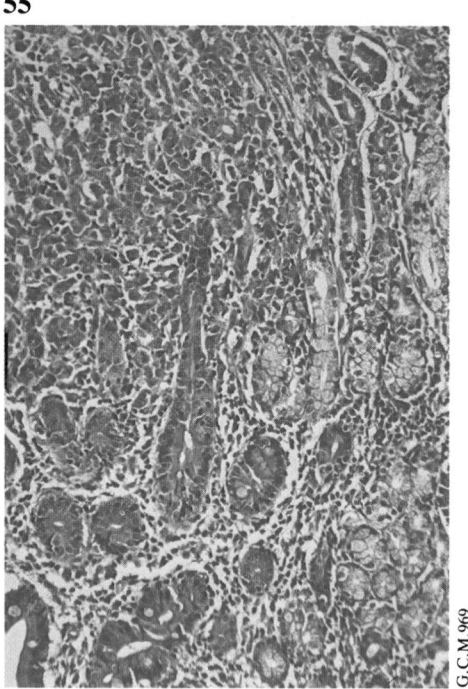

G.C.M.969

55 Carcinoma at gastroenterostomy stoma. In the upper part of the illustration, poorly differentiated carcinoma cells infiltrate the stoma. Intestinal glands lie to the left and gastric glands to the right. *(P.A.S. ×150)*

Early gastric cancer

Endoscopy in recent years has led to the diagnosis of gastric carcinoma before deep invasion has occurred.

Surface carcinoma – partial gastrectomy specimen

56

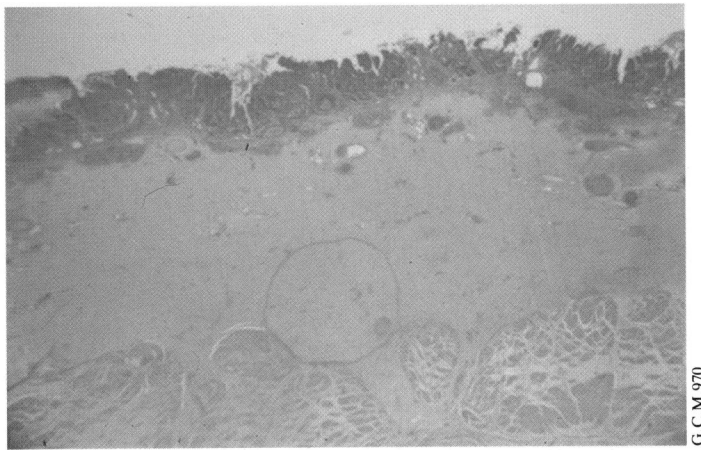

57

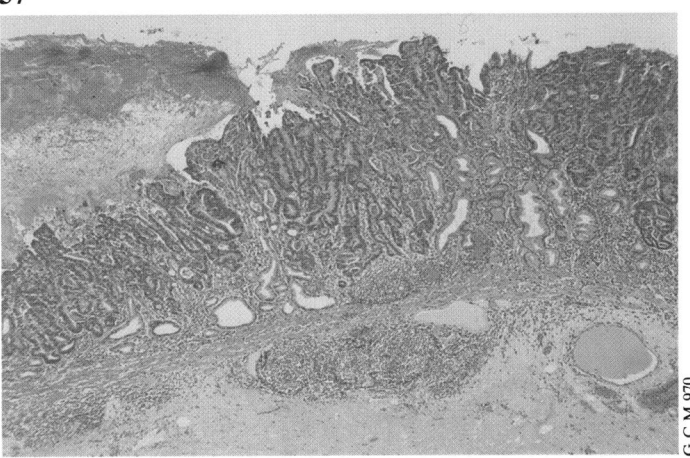

56 A portion of gastric wall including mucosa, submucosa and inner muscularis. The mucosa shows extensive carcinomatous infiltration but there is no invasion of the thickened submucosa. *(H&E ×10)*

57 A higher power view of the left-hand end of the previous illustration. There is early ulceration of the surface carcinoma, but no invasion beyond muscularis mucosae. *(H&E ×40)*

Surface carcinoma – endoscopy specimen

58

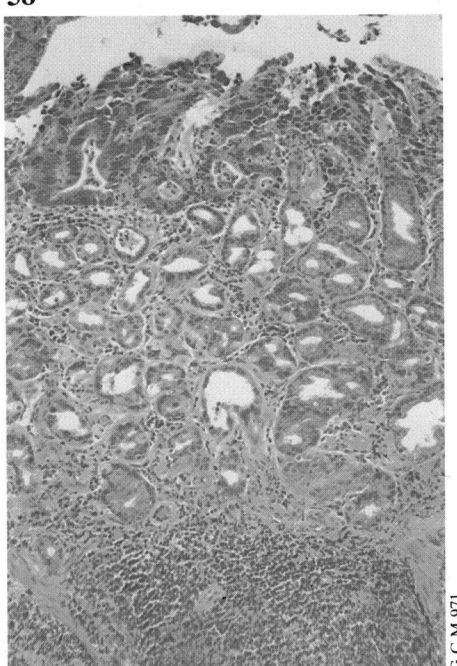

59

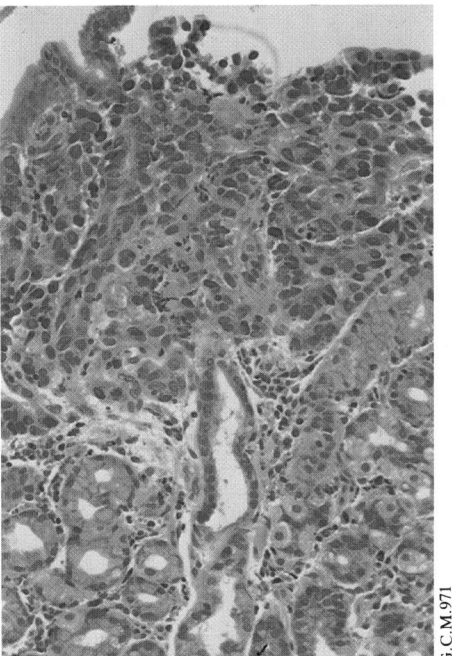

58 The tumour is confined to the upper layers of the mucosa. *(H&E ×125)*

59 Same case. Different field. The surface tumour contrasts with deeper gastric glands containing parietal and chief cells. *(H&E ×250)*

Local spread

Submucous spread is a common feature around the tumour and may extend for a considerable distance. The overlying mucosa is stretched and elevated. Rugose formation is lost and the mucosa often presents with a roughened tongue-like surface but without frank ulceration.

Direct invasion of the muscle is common and frequently early. The overlying peritoneum then becomes involved. In some specimens it is noteworthy that submucosal spread may be extensive while the muscular invasion remains minimal.

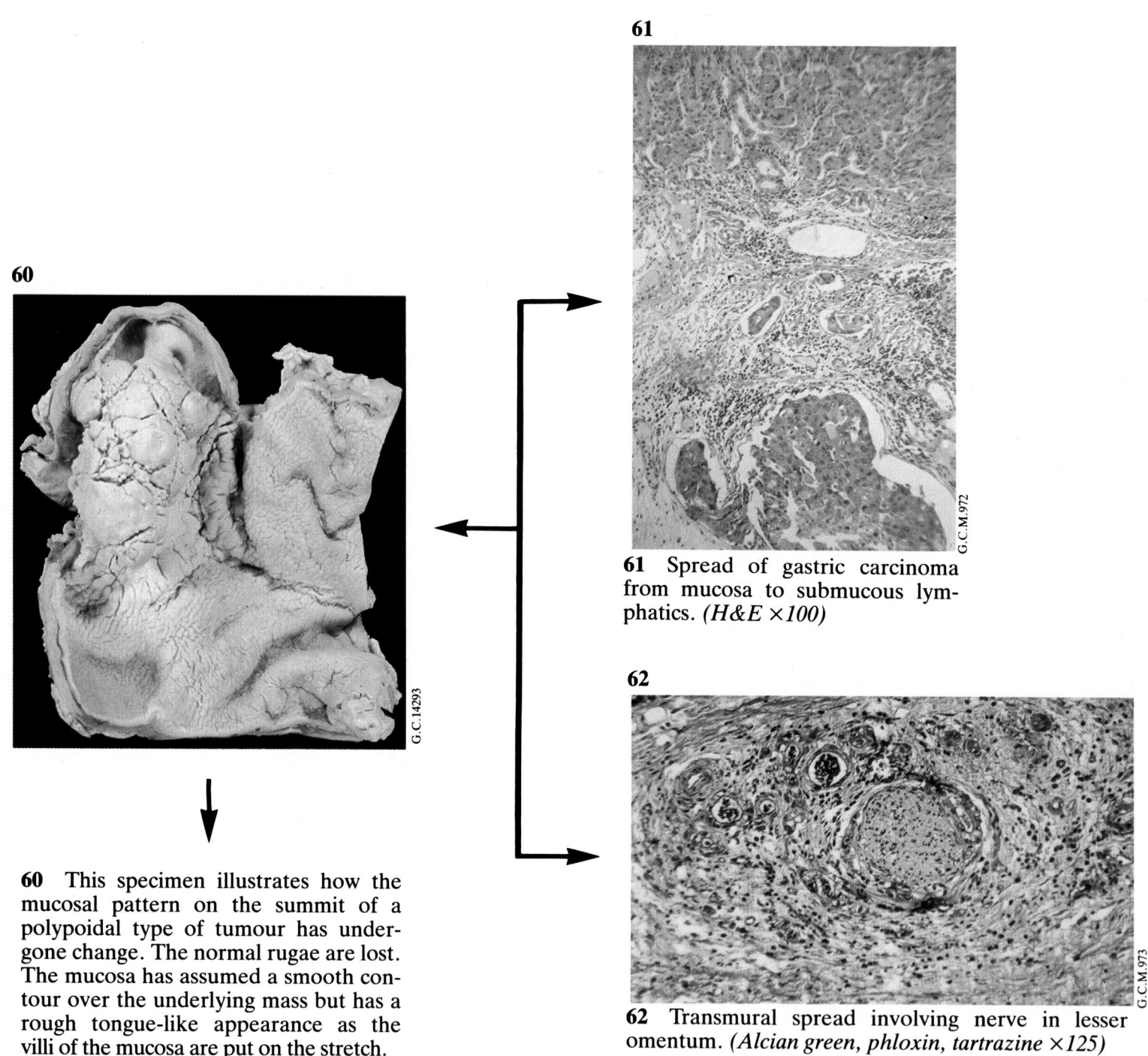

61 Spread of gastric carcinoma from mucosa to submucous lymphatics. *(H&E ×100)*

60 This specimen illustrates how the mucosal pattern on the summit of a polypoidal type of tumour has undergone change. The normal rugae are lost. The mucosa has assumed a smooth contour over the underlying mass but has a rough tongue-like appearance as the villi of the mucosa are put on the stretch.

62 Transmural spread involving nerve in lesser omentum. *(Alcian green, phloxin, tartrazine ×125)*

The affected peritoneum becomes adherent to adjacent viscera notably the transverse colon, pancreas, omentum, liver and spleen in that order of frequency and later malignant invasion occurs. Where the transverse colon has been invaded a gastro-colic fistula may follow.

Distant and late involvement of the intestine may occur with the formation of strictures – sometimes multiple and occasionally of some length. Tumours arising in the cardia commonly extend upwards into the lower oesophagus. A feature of gastric carcinoma located in the pyloric region is the apparent rarity of distal spread beyond the pylorus with duodenal involvement (Rokitansky, 1861). More recent work has demonstrated that limited spread does occur and may be shown by histological studies even where naked-eye appearances are apparently normal. Generally only the first 2 cm beyond the pylorus are involved.

Duodenal involvement appears to follow lymphatic spread in a retrograde manner from the subpyloric lymph nodes.

Lymphatic spread

There is a diffuse rich network of lymphatics in the submucosa. Early involvement of this plexus is common. It is difficult to differentiate between direct local spread and submucous lymphatic spread.

63

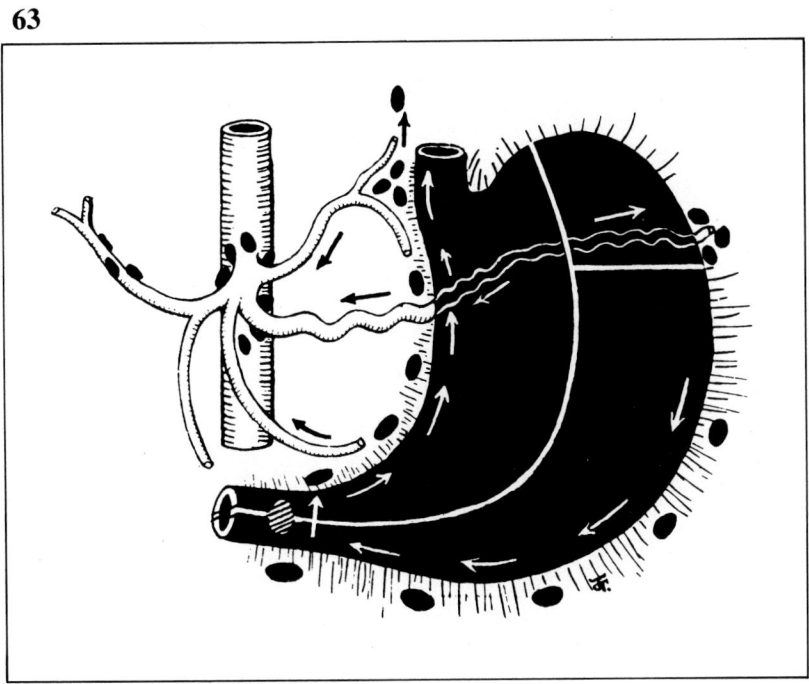

Overt lymphatic spread

63 Overt lymphatic spread is found in 70% of surgical resections. Lymphatics pass from the stomach wall to the lymphatic chains along the greater and lesser curvatures and the three fields of drainage are illustrated here. Eventually the lymphatics drain into the lymph nodes located about the coeliac axis from which further extensive spread occurs, notably to the porta hepatis and through the posterior mediastinum. The classical picture of this is the involvement of the supra-clavicular (Virchow) lymph node.

Haematogenous spread

Haematogenous spread initially to the liver is common. Later more widespread dissemination of the carcinoma, especially to the lungs, occurs.

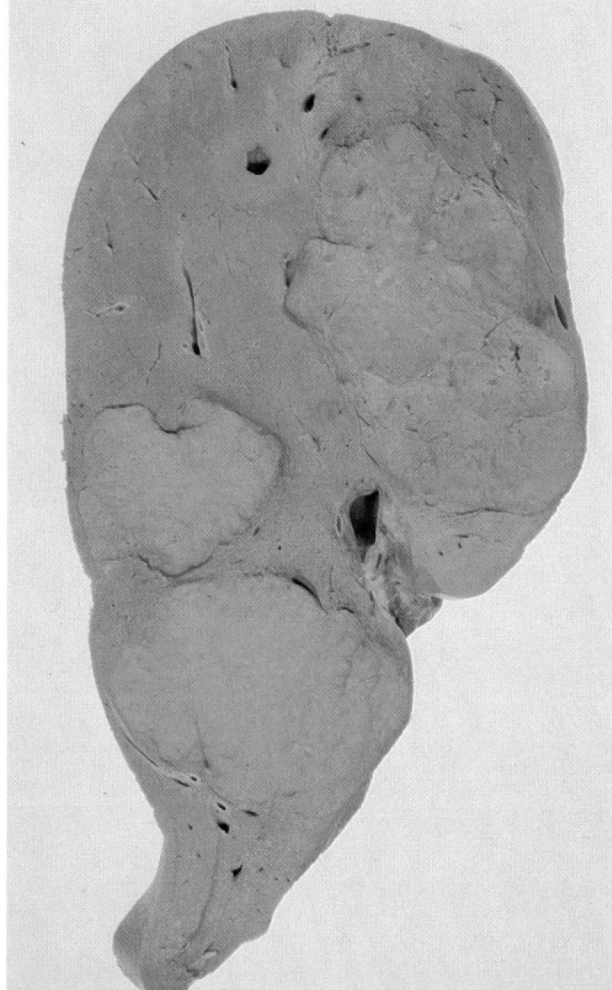

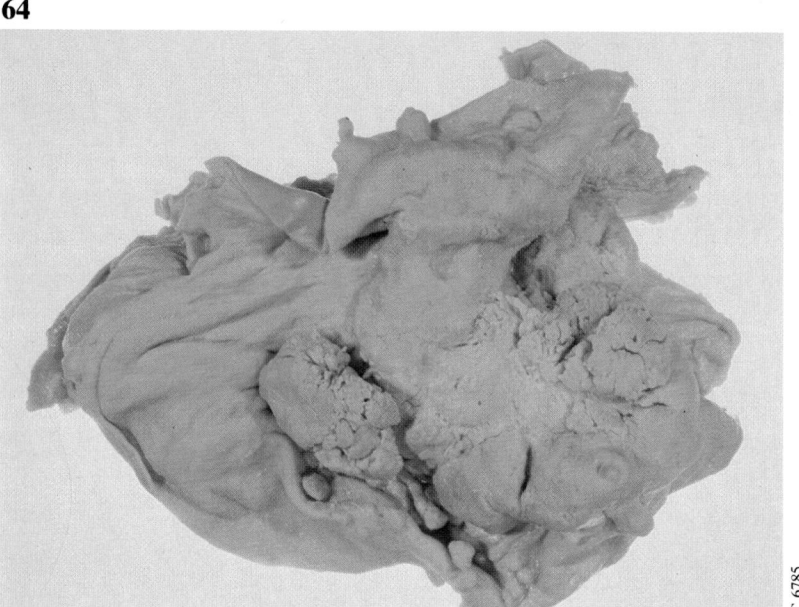

64 From a male aged 43 years. At post mortem examination the primary tumour of the stomach was identified and metastases were present in the liver and pancreas.

The specimen illustrates a large ulcerated carcinoma with typical raised edges involving the cardia of the stomach.

65 The liver has been sectioned and several large deposits of carcinoma are present. Note how these have projected on the surface giving a typical bossing appearance. The tumour was an adenocarcinoma.

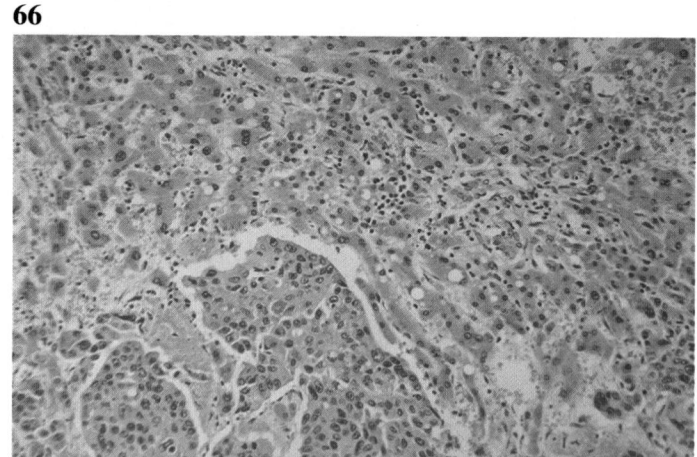

66 The liver parenchyma is invaded by poorly differentiated carcinoma (bottom left). *(H&E ×125)*

Implantation metastases

Implantation metastases in the abdominal wall are an occasional sequel to operation for gastric carcinoma.

67a

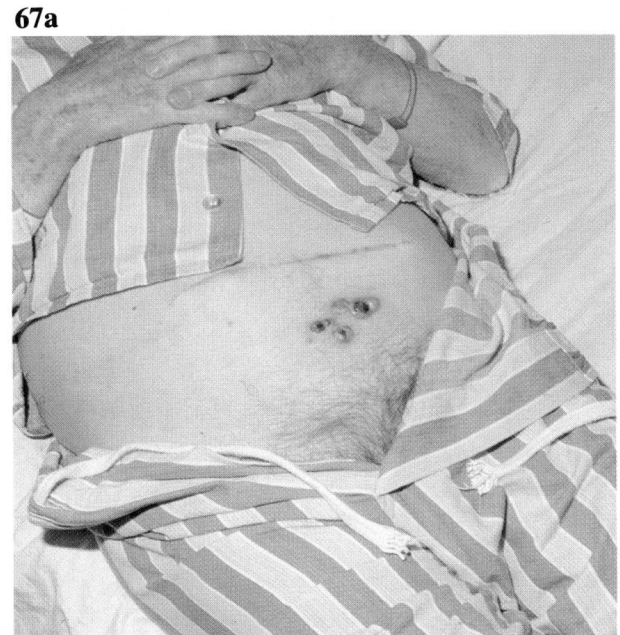

67b

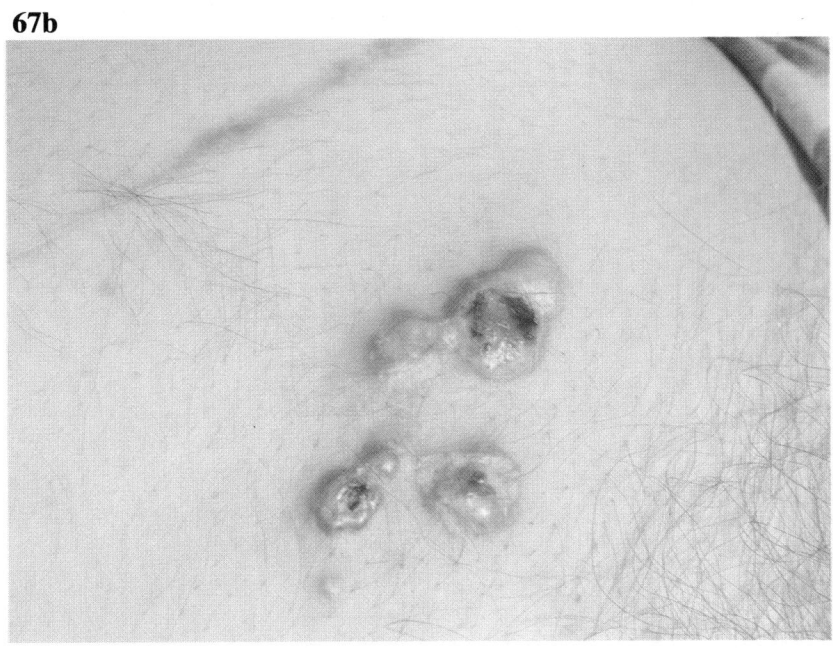

67a and **67b**   Male aged 81 years. This patient had had a palliative gastrectomy performed for carcinoma involving the pyloric antrum. The illustrations show metastases in the abdominal wall 6 months after the initial operation.

Peritoneal metastases

When the peritoneal surface overlying a malignant tumour of the stomach has become invaded individual cells may become detached and spread through the peritoneal cavity. Malignant peritoneal deposits develop and are associated with ascites.

68

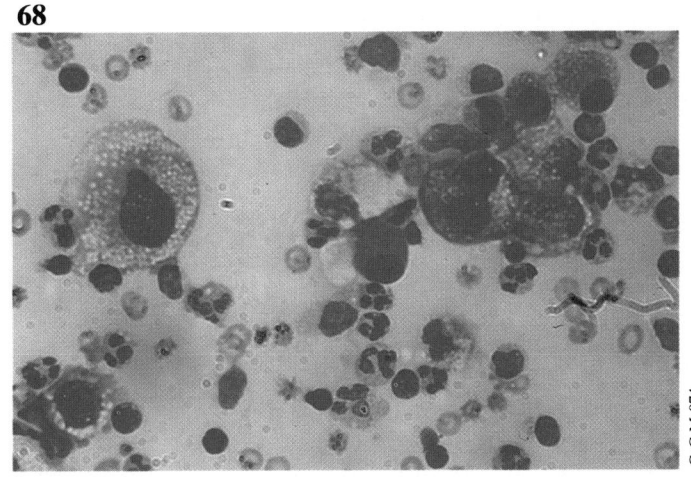

68   Ascitic fluid. Mucoid tumour cells from gastric carcinoma. *(Leishman ×500)*

Transcoelomic spread

Implantation metastatic growths of the ovary have long been recognised and may give rise to symptoms before the primary lesion is diagnosed. These tumours are most frequently seen in association with mucoid carcinoma of the stomach and the deposits are multiple and bulky, both ovaries being affected (Krükenberg tumours).

Krükenberg tumour

69

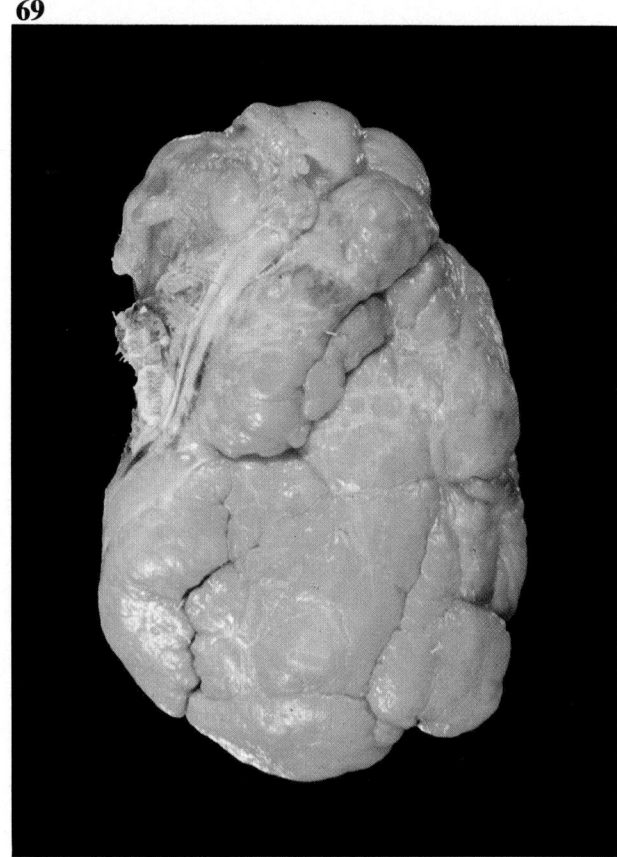

G.C.15102

69 From a female aged 56 years. Gastrectomy was performed two years previously for carcinoma of the stomach. Returned to hospital on account of lower abdominal pain. A palpable, mobile, firm mass was evident in the lower abdomen. At laparotomy bilateral ovarian neoplasms of similar character were found. The illustration is of the outer surface of one of these tumours and demonstrates the smooth but lobulated surface. The cut surface showed areas mainly of compact, homogeneous tissue with intervening areas where mucoid tissue was present.

70

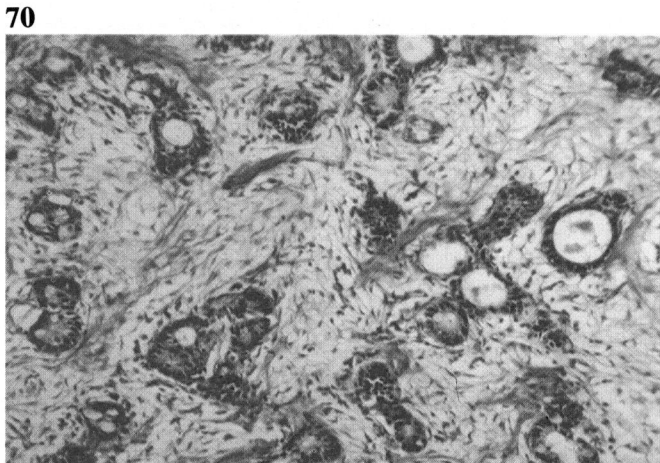

70 Microscopic examination showed a well differentiated adenocarcinoma set in loose mucinoid stroma. *(H&E ×125)*

71

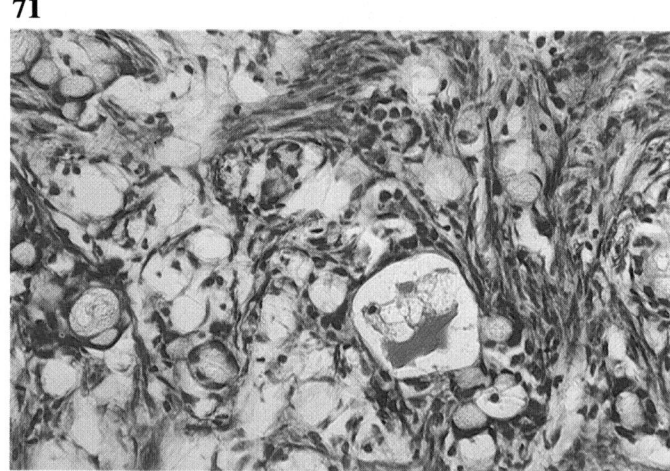

71 Same case. Numerous tumour cells distended by mucin are present in the ovarian stroma. *(H&E ×250)*

Radiology

The outline and motility of the oesophagus, stomach and duodenum can be best studied by a <u>barium meal.</u> The examination is carried out with the patient standing or supine. With the head tipped downwards it is possible to demonstrate the fundus and cardia and the competence of the oesophago-gastric junction. The movements of the stomach can be examined by direct fluoroscopic screening or indirectly using image intensification. Representative areas of abnormality are recorded on film.

72

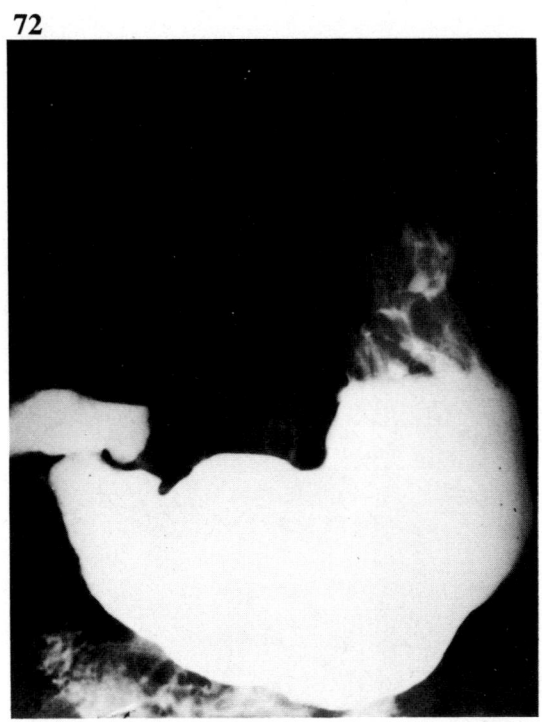

72 A filling defect of the fundus of the stomach which is not occasioning oesophageal obstruction. Note the character of the shadow proximal to the main mass of barium in the stomach showing the irregular surface of the tumour.

73

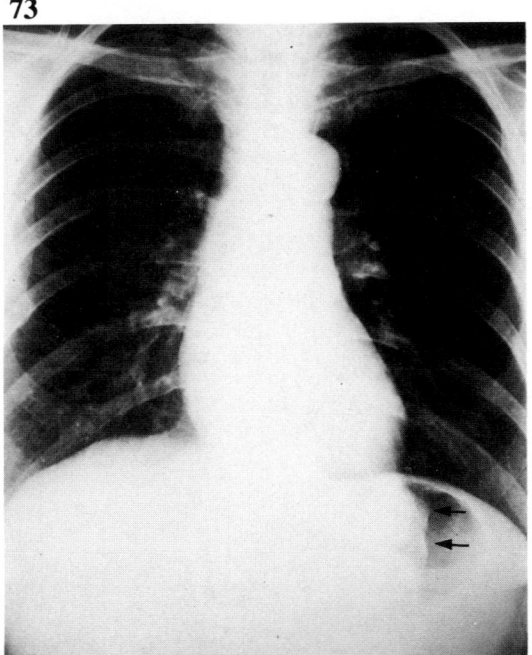

73 A rare picture from a straight X-ray demonstrating a filling defect of the air bubble in the fundus of the stomach. The tumour obviously arises in the vicinity of the cardio-oesophageal orifice and its irregular outline is clearly demonstrated. The picture is that of a carcinoma.

Radiology *(Continued)*

74

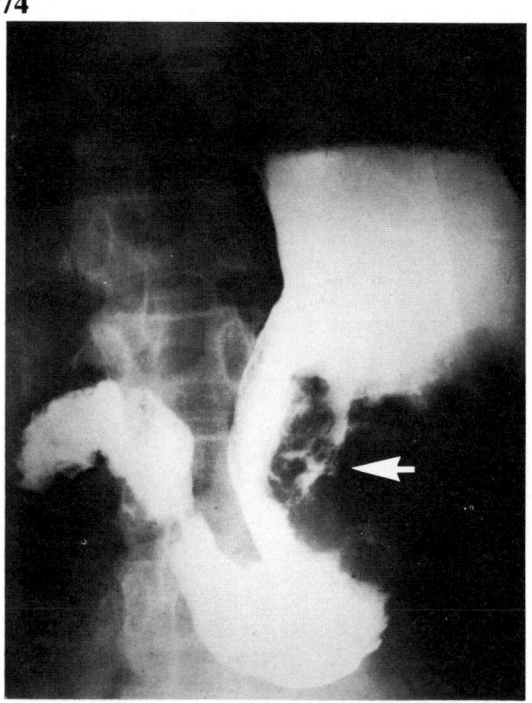

74 A large proliferating carcinoma of the body of the stomach. The filling defect extends from the greater curvature towards the lesser curvature, which is distorted.

75

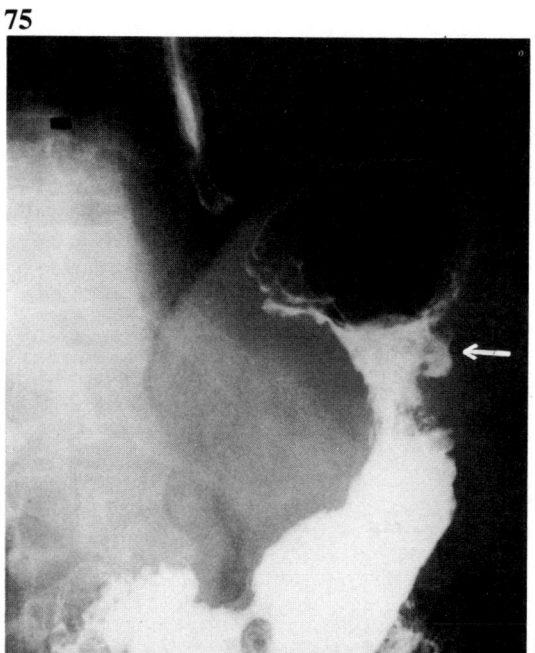

75 A large gastric ulcer is present on the greater curvature with associated irregularity and deformity of the stomach. The appearances are highly suggestive of malignancy. The remainder of the stomach and duodenum is normal. This is the type of case in which radiology is not conclusive and biopsy should be undertaken.

76

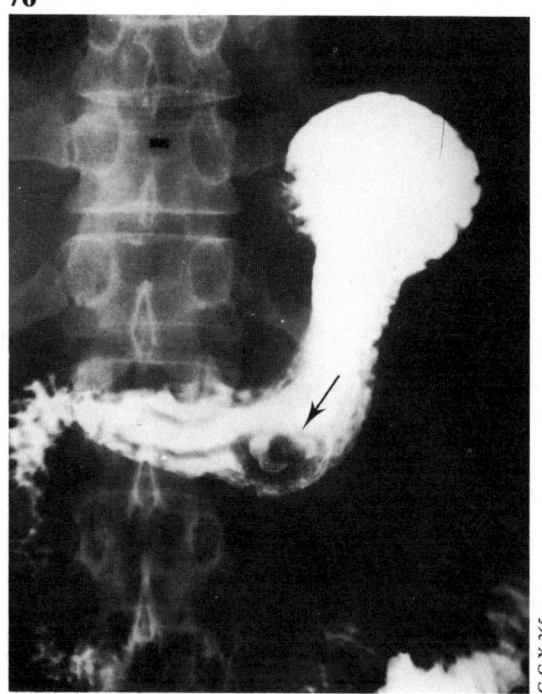

76 The picture is that of an ulcer *en face* at the mid point of the body of the stomach. The stomach has contracted and shows considerable irregularity. The picture is that of an extensive ulcerating tumour.

77

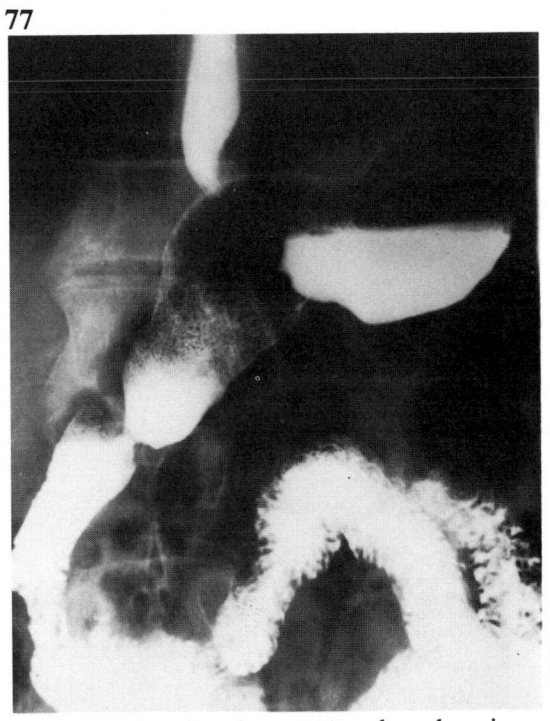

G.C.X.374

77 Leather-bottle stomach showing distortion, the absence of rugae and the impression of smoothness and rigidity in the gastric wall.

78

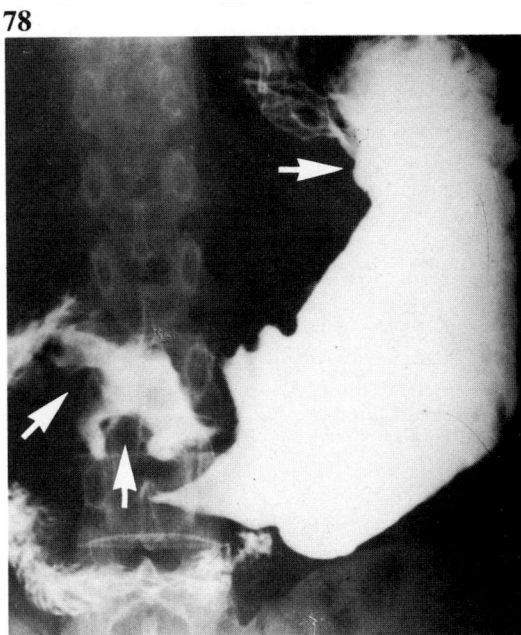

G.C.10598

78 The X-ray shows an ulcer crater high up on the lesser curvature and a filling defect in the pyloric antrum indicating the presence of a bulky, fungating type of tumour which is causing obstruction to the outflow of gastric content.

79

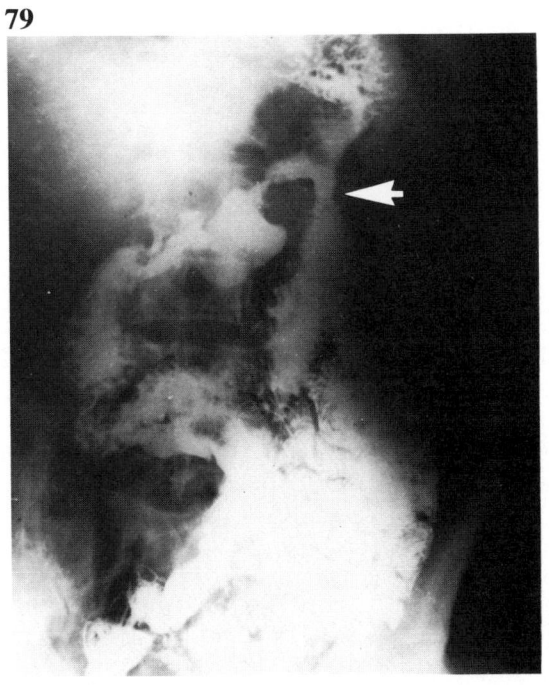

G.C.10217

79 Stomal carcinoma.

The X-ray shows a rigid deformity of the body of the stomach with escape of barium through the gastroenterostomy and also through the pylorus.

The operative specimen shows a carcinoma arising at the stoma.

Gastroscopy

With the introduction of fibreoptic instruments it is now easy and safe to inspect the lining of the stomach, obtain biopsy material to establish the diagnosis and secure photographs for permanent record.

Illustrative cases

Benign lesion

80

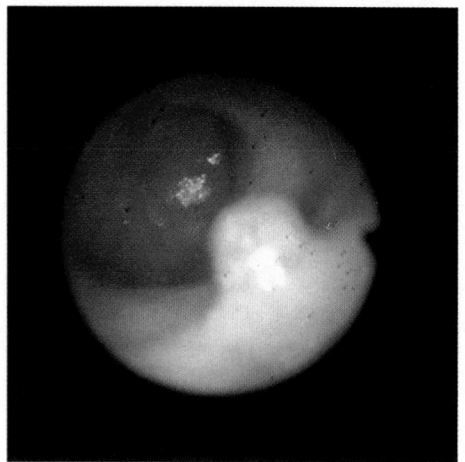

G.C.P.220

80 A benign gastric polyp is visualised. In the far distance the pyloric antrum is observed and the entrance into the duodenum.

81

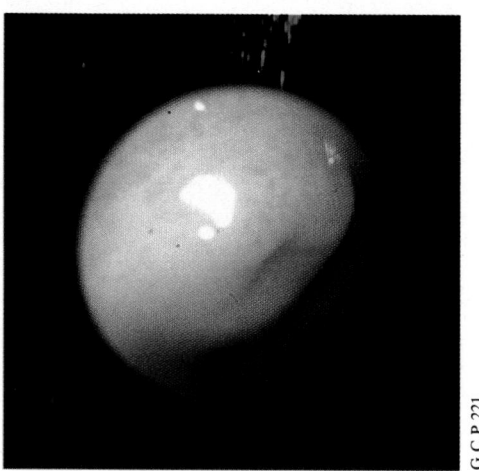

G.C.P.221

81 An ulcerating, smooth lesion is seen which is a central ulcer crater in a leiomyoma.

82

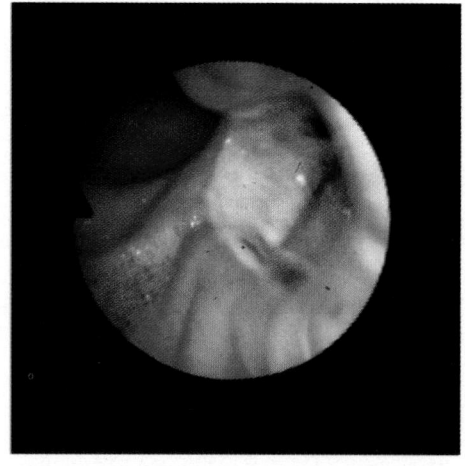

G.C.P.222

82 The appearance is that of a very chronic lesser curve gastric ulcer in the region of the incisura.

Carcinoma

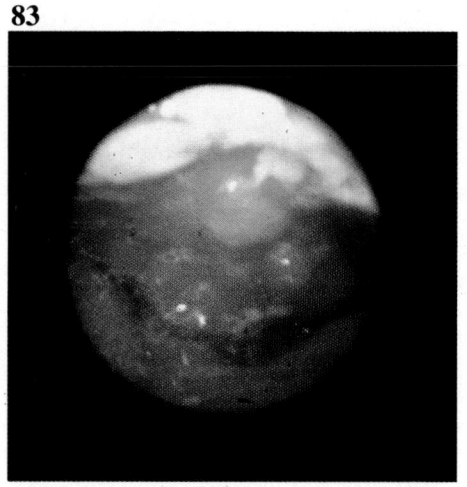

G.C.P.223

83 An ulcerating lesion with proliferative rolled edges is visualised. The appearance is that of a carcinoma.

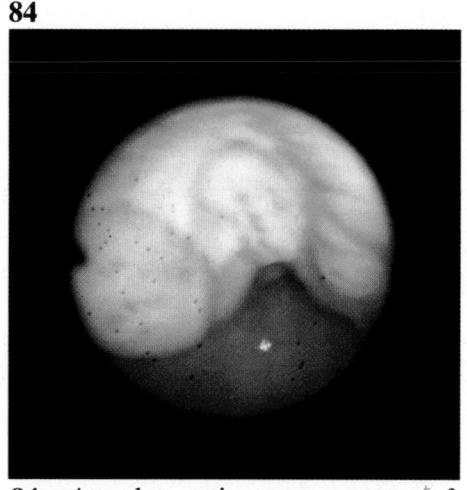

G.C.P.224

84 An alternative appearance of a carcinoma characterised by proliferative mass associated with infiltration into the submucosal region.

Endoscopic biopsy

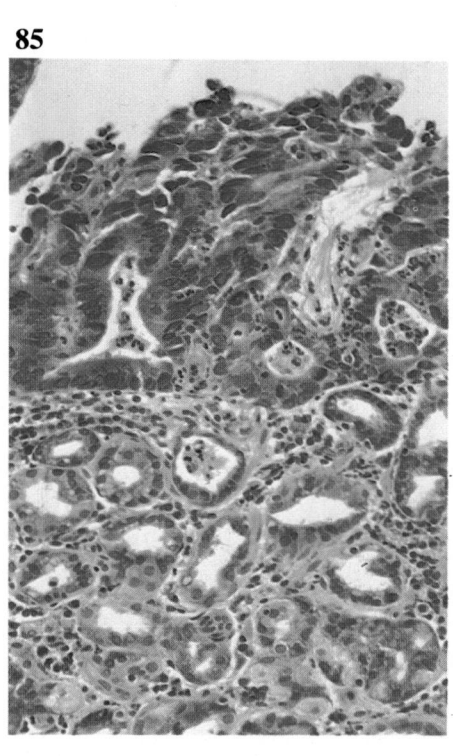

G.C.M.971

Where a proliferative lesion is observed biopsy specimens are secured from the evident margins of the lesions.

85 From a case in which early carcinoma was suspected.

Carcinomatous change has occurred in the upper portion of the mucosa. The large hyperchromatic cells which form the tumour are clearly distinguishable from those of the more normal glands below.

This may be defined as a surface carcinoma. *(H&E ×250)*

Diagnostic cytology and biopsy

Cytology

Cytology is now widely employed in the diagnosis of suspicious gastric lesions. Specimens are obtained either from centrifuged deposits of gastric lavage or from brushings made at fibreoptic examination. The cell morphology will have undergone change as the result of the action of gastric acid and pepsin and in consequence recognition of malignant cells may be difficult. A high degree of accuracy is obtained in the most experienced centres. Brush biopsies should however be complemented by biopsy.

86

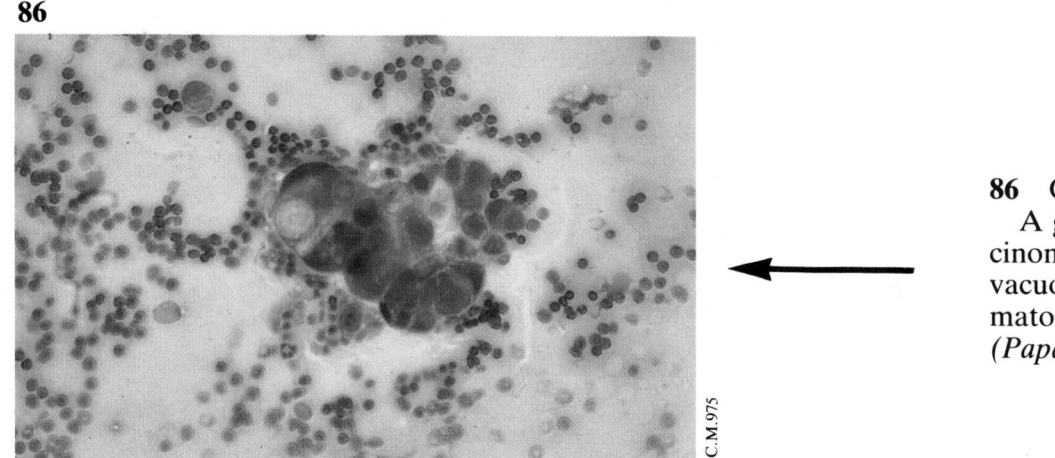

G.C.M.975

86 Gastric washing.
  A group of large hyperchromatic carcinoma cells, some with mucoid vacuoles, with surrounding inflammatory cells and erythrocytes.
(Papanicolaou ×312.5)

Biopsy

Where an ulcer is present and the differentiation by simple endoscopy between carcinoma and simple chronic ulcer is equivocal multiple specimens for histological purposes are taken. The samples selected should include any suspicious areas showing mucosal hyperplasia. In general tissue should be taken from at least the four quadrants of the ulcer, and when possible from the floor of the ulcer.

Illustrative case

From a female aged 81 years with a short history of loss of appetite, vague indigestion and epigastric tenderness. A barium meal demonstrated a large ulcer high on the lesser curvature. The appearances were not diagnostic of either a simple or malignant ulcer. Gastroscopy revealed an ulcer which appeared to be benign. Biopsy specimens from the margin of the ulcer and brushings from the floor of the ulcer were taken. The brushings from the floor of the ulcer revealed malignancy. The ulcer was excised and the patient made a satisfactory recovery.

The case illustrates an example of the value of the cytological examination. This was an elderly patient in whom, had the diagnosis of simple ulcer been assumed, treatment by drugs would have been undertaken in view of her age and condition.

87

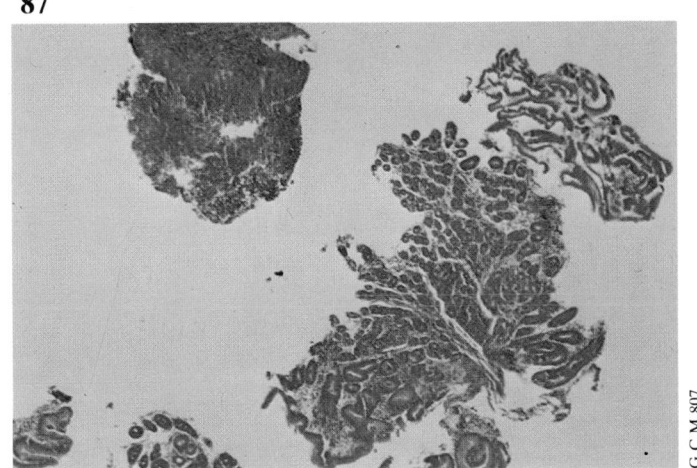

87 Biopsy from margin of ulcer showing only normal gastric mucosa. No evidence of malignancy. *(H&E ×37.5)*

88

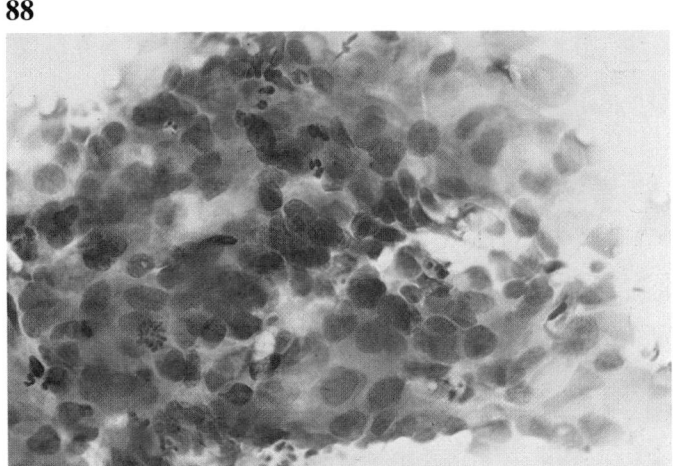

89

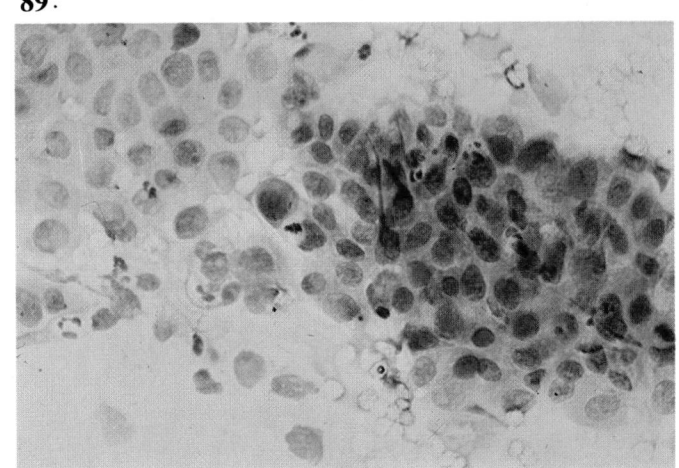

88 and **89** Brushings from floor of ulcer showing poorly differentiated tumour cells. *(Papanicolaou ×375)*

Histological studies from operative specimen

90

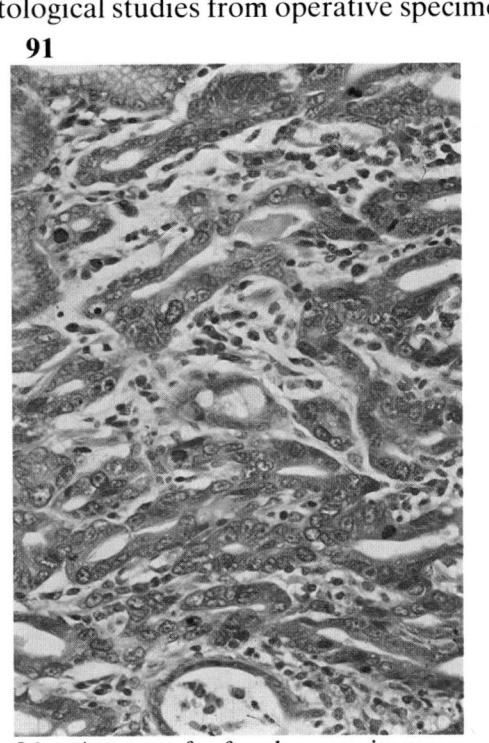

90 Margin of carcinomatous lesion both normal and neoplastic elements present. *(H&E ×100)*

91

91 Area of frank carcinoma. *(H&E ×250)*

92

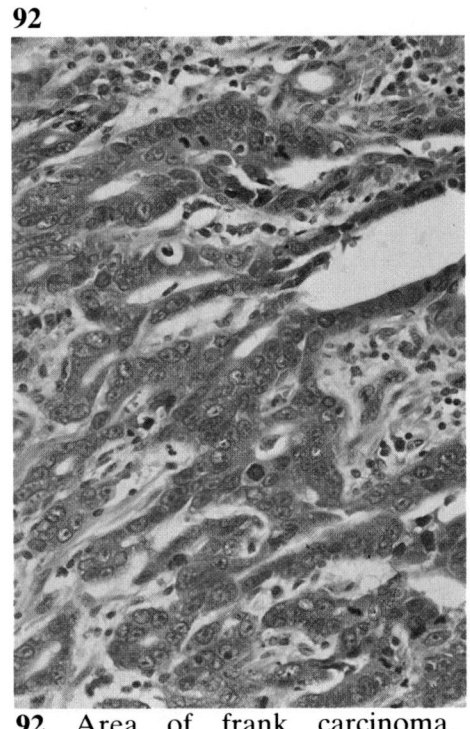

92 Area of frank carcinoma. *(H&E ×250)*

J.W.W. Thomson

Carcinomas of the duodenum are generally considered as intestinal neoplasms rather than related to gastric carcinoma. They are very rare and only short series of cases have been reported. These tumours are most usually found in patients in the 6th decade and there is a male preponderance.

———

These tumours are described as occurring in three sites:
1 Carcinoma of the 1st part of the duodenum is rare and early writers related the carcinoma in some instances to preceding duodenal ulcer but proof of duodenal ulcer directly leading to malignant change is lacking.
2 Carcinoma of the 2nd part of the duodenum is generally found in relation to the ampulla of Vater and is the most common site of malignancy. It is difficult to differentiate between tumours arising in the duodenal mucosa and those which arise from the biliary duct mucosa. It is held that those of duodenal origin tend to be circumferential ulcerative lesions with evident spread in the wall of the intestine (see Section 16 UE).
3 Tumours of the 3rd part of the duodenum are excessively rare.

Duodenal carcinoma represents 4% of all intestinal tumours and in a series reported of 40 cases, the site distribution was 1st part – 8, 2nd part – 24 and 3rd part – 3.

Haemorrhage is a recognised complication and where the tumour is located at the ampulla, biliary obstruction with jaundice occurs.

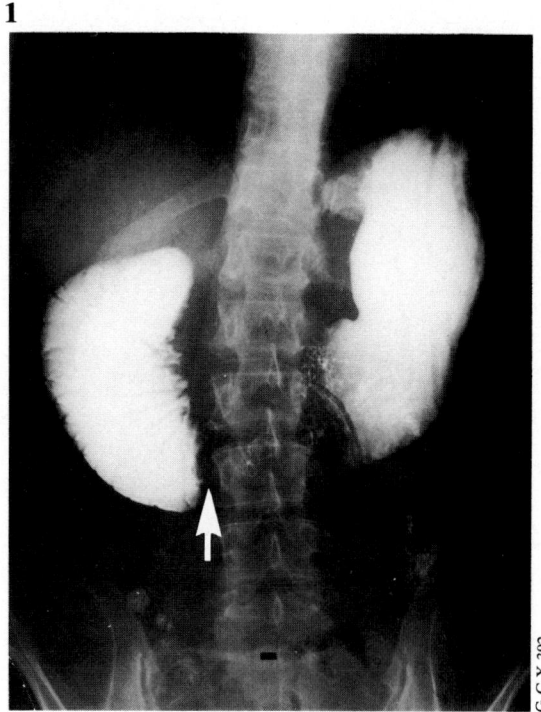

1

1 From a female aged 54 years. Three month history of nausea and flatulence – not related to meals.

The barium follow through shows an incomplete obstruction in the third part of the duodenum with gross proximal dilatation. The picture is that of a stenosing lesion and most probably a carcinoma.

———

Lymphatic spread is usually evident by the time of diagnosis.

G.C.X.392

2

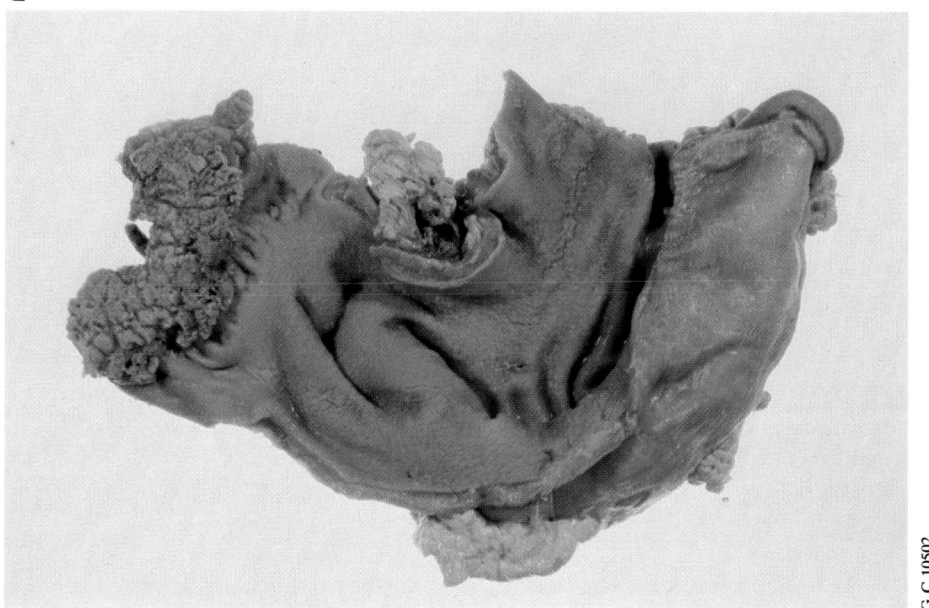

G.C.10502

2 From a female aged 59 years. Two year history of vomiting which became progressively more frequent and finally daily. Palpable tumour right hypochondrium. Achlorhydria present. Radiology – obstructing lesion first part duodenum. Treated by partial gastro-duodenectomy.

The specimen has been opened anteriorly and demonstrates a papillary tumour of the first part of the duodenum. It extends from a point 2 cm distal to the pylorus and in its long axis measures 3 cm. Histologically the tumour is a papillary adenocarcinoma with much mucus secretion. There is invasion of all coats of the duodenal wall. There was no evidence of lymphatic spread.

3

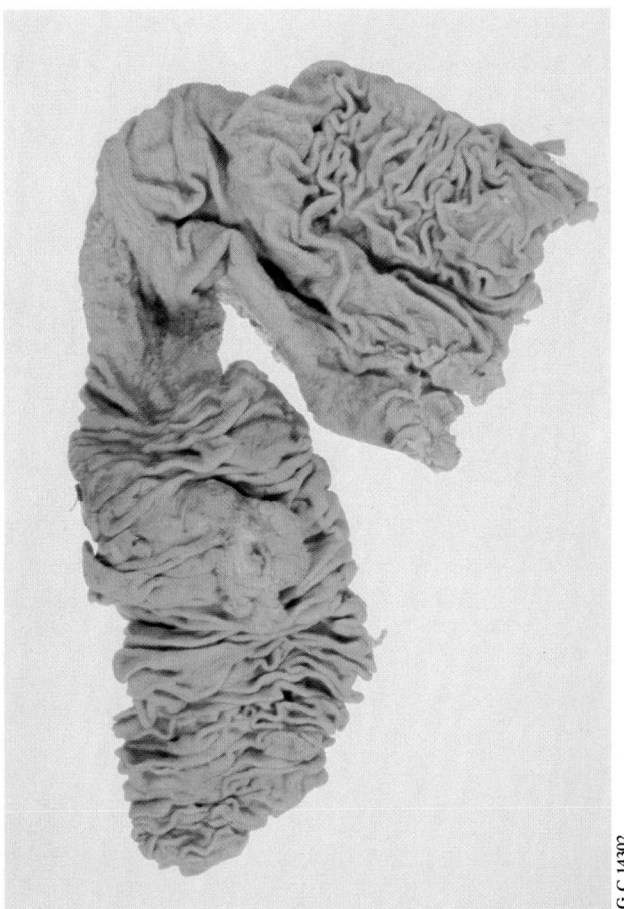

G.C.14302

3 From a male aged 67 years. History of painless and increasing jaundice for over 4 weeks. Radiographs demonstrated an indentation in the second part of the duodenum on the medial side. A duodenectomy and partial pancreatectomy (Whipple) was performed. At the ampulla of Vater a small ulcerating and projecting tumour is present. The aperture of the biliary duct is seen lying in the centre of the mass.

Histologically the tumour is a typical papillary carcinoma with rather long fronds and the cells show a uniformity of type. There is no evidence of any pleomorphism nor are mitotic figures a common feature – the evidence is of low malignancy.

Trichobezoar

The ingestion of hair is usually seen in young girls who have formed a habit of nibbling the ends of their pigtails. The hair is retained in the stomach and ultimately forms a matted mass. After a time it may form a complete cast of the stomach. It is largely symptomless but may impair the appetite and ultimately forms a palpable mass in the upper abdomen. When removed the bezoar is a slimy, malodorous firm mass from which on pressure, mucus extrudes.

Two complications occur:
1 Ulceration on the lesser curvature of the stomach which is associated with haematemesis but rarely with perforation.
2 Detached fragments of the hair ball pass down the intestine and may lead to obstruction either of the duodenum or terminal ileum.

1

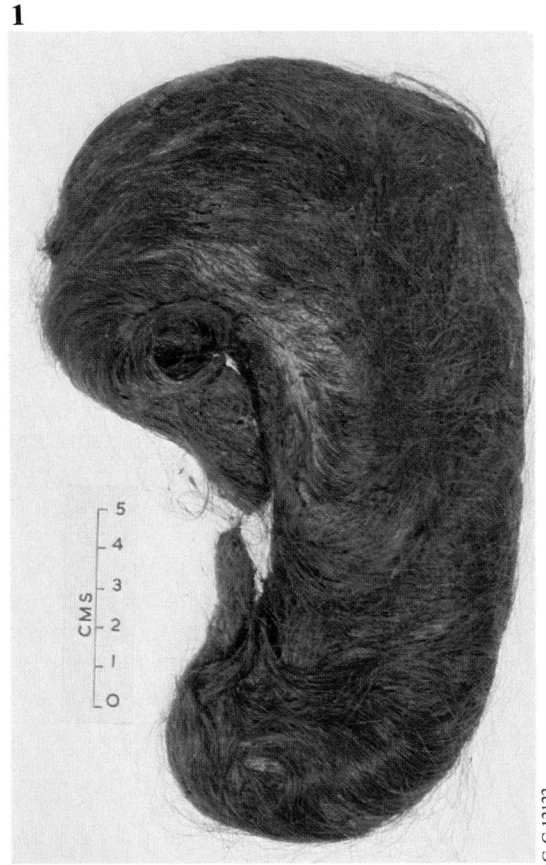

1 From a female aged 15 years who was admitted to hospital for severe upper abdominal pain and vomiting. On examination there was evidence of marked abdominal rigidity and loss of liver dullness.

At operation a small anterior gastric perforation was found. Further examination showed the whole of the stomach to be filled with a hard mass. A large trichobezoar was removed and the ulcer excised.

2

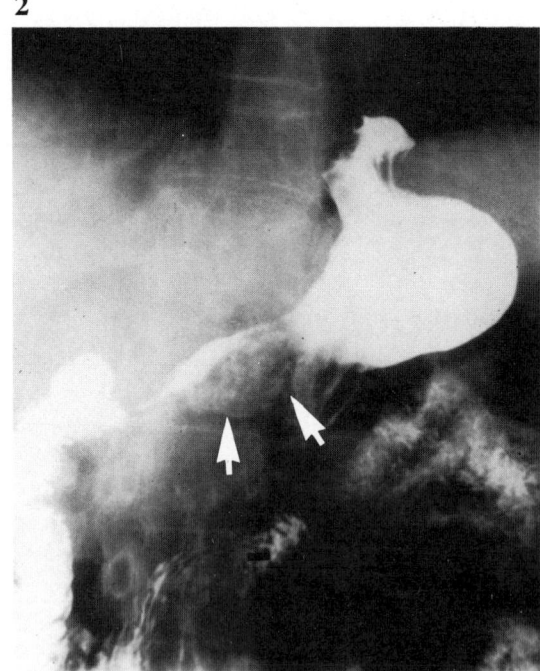

2 These lesions may be diagnosed radiologically, the bezoar causing a filling defect in the stomach.

3

3 Hair balls are occasionally found in animals. This example is from an aged donkey which was found to have several similar rounded masses in its stomach.

G.C.4415

Phytobezoar

The ingested material in this condition is vegetable fibres. As in the previous type a mass develops which constitutes a cast of the gastric lumen. The colour of the mass varies depending on the vegetable material which has been ingested. Occasionally bezoars pass into or are formed in the intestine.

4

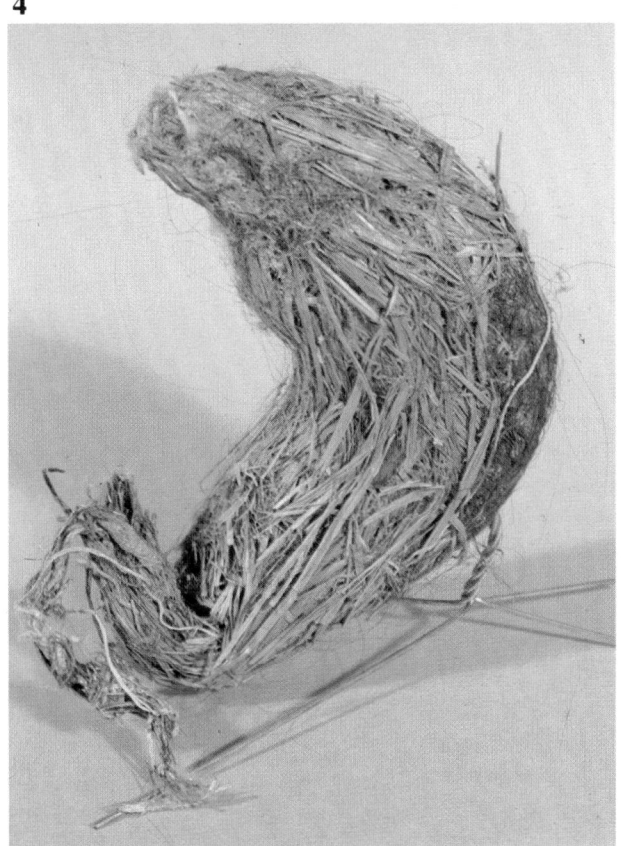

G.C.6307

4 Phytobezoar from a female aged 10 years.

This child was admitted for acute umbilical abdominal pain of unknown origin but not associated with abdominal rigidity or tenderness.

The mass was present in the upper abdomen and at operation this proved to be a phytobezoar. In this case it appears to be composed mostly of straw, with pieces of string and thread and some coarse hair or bristles.

Obstruction to the forward flow of intestinal contents is a common and often fatal complication of many lesions of the gut. It occurs in a variety of forms depending on the degree and level of the obstruction, the character of the bowel content and the pathology of the causal lesion.

Causal lesions

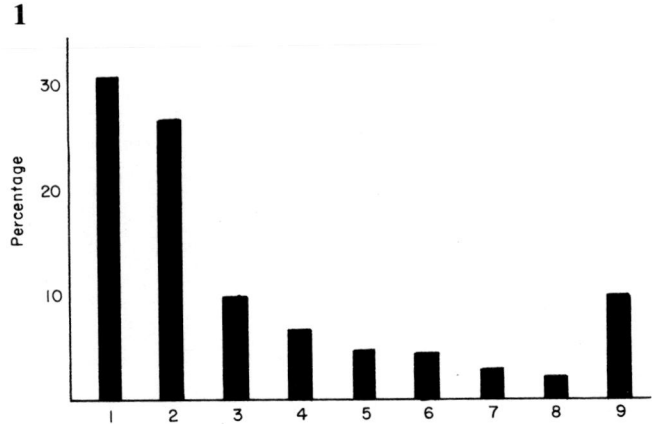

1	Adhesions	31%
2	Neoplasms	27%
3	External hernia	10%
4	Operative complication	7%
5	Congenital lesions	5%
6	Inflammatory strictures	4%
7	Volvulus	3%
8	Intussusception	2%
9	Miscellaneous	11%

Mortality

The mortality associated with intestinal obstruction at the beginning of this century was exceedingly high (50%).

This stimulated much intensive research resulting in an improved knowledge of the pathology, an understanding of the part played by bacteria and an appreciation of the biochemical changes which ensued from obstruction.

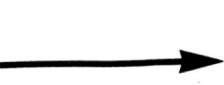

These advances led to improved techniques of management – introduction of gastro-intestinal decompression, correction of electrolyte imbalance, development of surgical techniques and the introduction of antibiotics.

These innovations resulted in a progressive improvement of the prognosis to the present mortality rate of 10%.

Classification

Four forms of intestinal obstruction are described depending upon the nature of the obstruction, the presence of vascular impairment and the dynamic activity of the musculature. Within each group systemic disturbances may arise as the result of biochemical change or bacterial activity, resulting in a difference in the lethal factor arising in these cases. An understanding of these factors depends upon experimental work and is the basis of management.

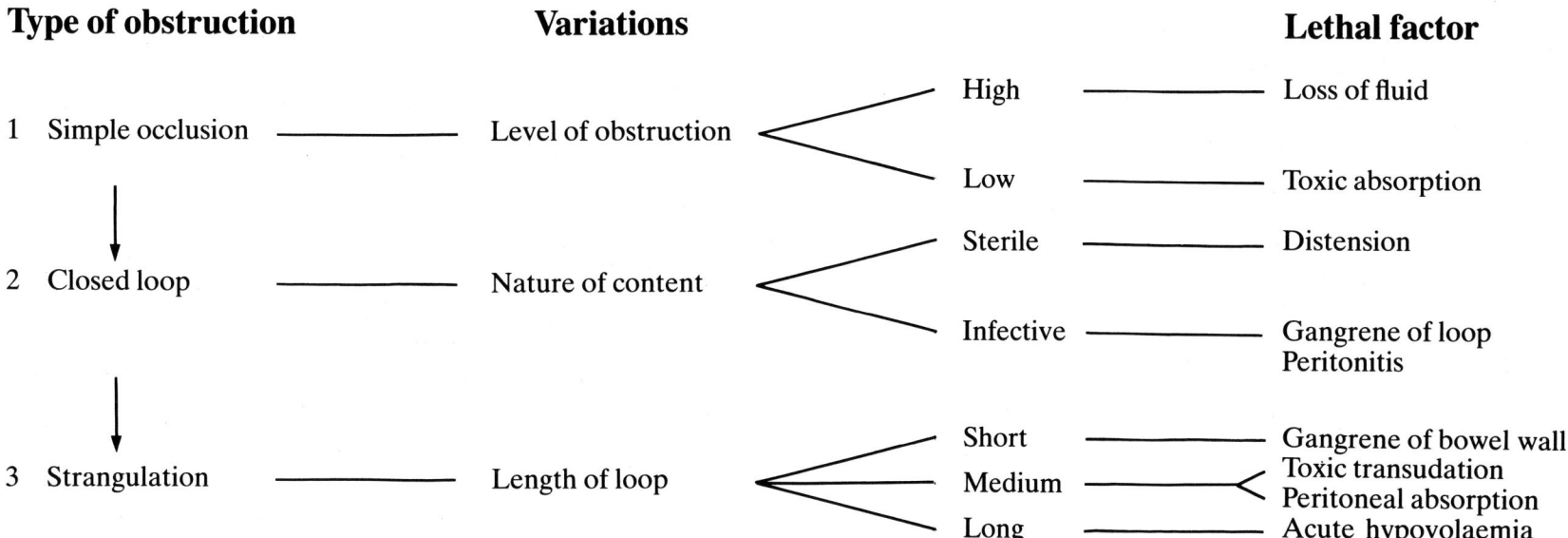

Type of obstruction	Variations		Lethal factor
1 Simple occlusion	Level of obstruction	High	Loss of fluid
		Low	Toxic absorption
2 Closed loop	Nature of content	Sterile	Distension
		Infective	Gangrene of loop Peritonitis
3 Strangulation	Length of loop	Short	Gangrene of bowel wall
		Medium	Toxic transudation Peritoneal absorption
		Long	Acute hypovolaemia

4 Functional obstruction

Simple occlusion

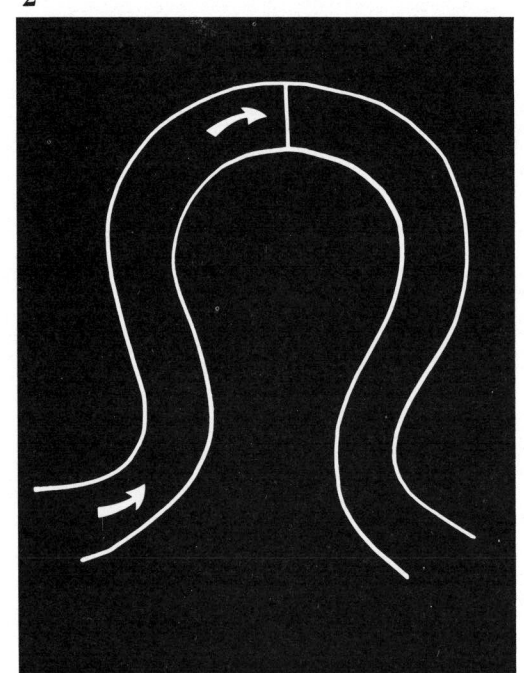

2 Simple occlusion occurs where the lumen of the gut is narrowed at one point and there is cessation of forward movement of the intestinal content. This may be partial or complete.

Mechanical effects

(a) Proximal

Periodic bursts of exaggerated peristalsis proximal to the obstruction are the cause of early colic and quiescent intervals vary depending on the level of the obstruction: 3 to 5 minutes in high obstruction and 10 to 15 minutes in lower ileal obstruction.

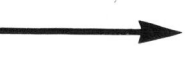

The occurrence and severity of vomiting also depends on the site of the obstruction. When the obstruction is high (jejunum/duodenum) vomiting is early, frequent and copious. When the obstruction is low (ileum) the onset of vomiting is delayed and it is commonly malodorous and faeculent.

(b) Distal

The bowel distal to the obstruction empties by evacuation and absorption. Thereafter it lies collapsed.

(c) Distension

The bowel proximal to the obstruction progressively dilates, with accumulation of fluid and gas.

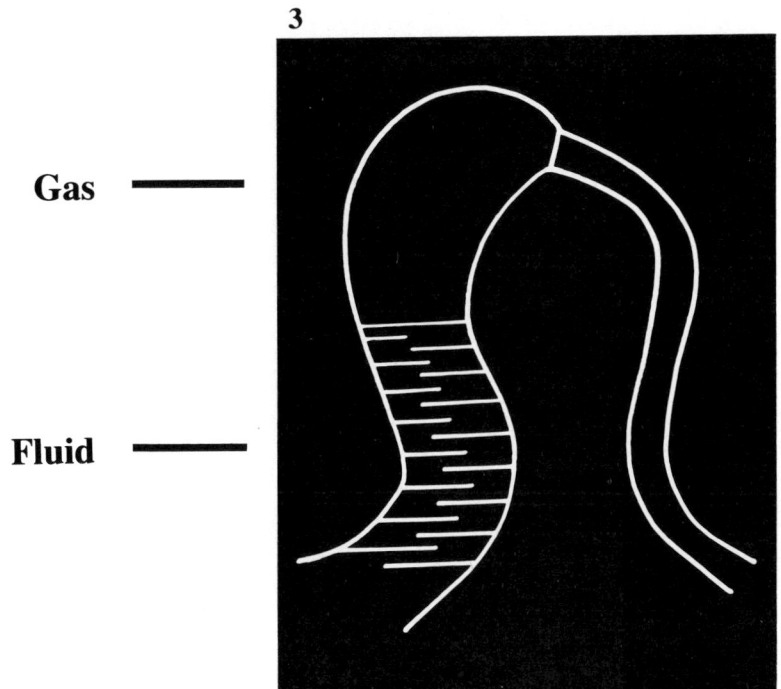

3

Gas ——————

Fluid ——————

Gas

The gas is derived from:

1   The digestion of food – formation of CO_2 from carbohydrates
    – putrefactive action of bacteria.

2   Interchange of gas from blood – occurs across the permeable bowel wall normally and maintains the O_2/CO_2, equilibrium. N is absorbed only slowly from the gut.

3   Swallowed air.

    In acute high obstruction:
    70% of the gas originates from swallowed air.
    20% from diffusion of blood gases (especially N).
    10% from digestive and bacterial fermentation. In colonic obstruction 20 to 25% of the gas is due to fermentation.

Effect on gut wall

Stretching of the muscle leads to paralysis of the gut wall.
   Distension of the gut alone can prove fatal as shown experimentally by balloon distension of isolated loops. Denervation of the loop prolongs survival.

Fluid

The fluid which accumulates consists of saliva, gastric, biliary and pancreatic secretions and succus entericus (8–10 l/day). In the presence of obstruction there is also secretion of fluid into the intestinal lumen. Decreased absorption in varying degrees depending on the level of the obstruction also results in an increased volume of intraluminal fluid but plays a less important role than increased secretion.

Simple occlusion *(Continued)*

Radiology

4 In the presence of obstruction radiological examination confirms the diagnosis and may indicate the level of the causal lesion. Gas and fluid may be limited to one segment of the intestine as in high obstruction but more frequently multiple fluid levels and gas-filled loops are present.

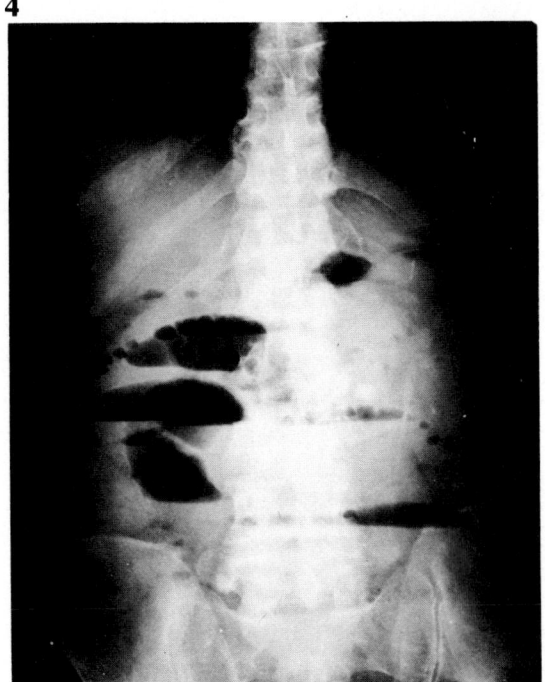

G.C.X.950

(d) Vascular change

There is no initial interference with the blood supply to the gut wall until the intraluminal pressures reach 30 mmHg. (Normal 2 to 4 mmHg.)

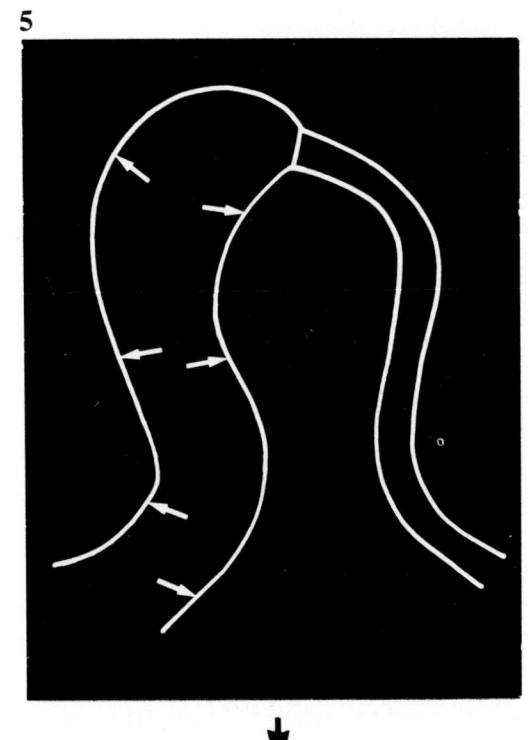

The tension within the lumen rises but is modified by the degree of dilatation. A much greater relative increase in pressure develops in the wall of the gut than in the lumen.

5 Tension within the lumen of the gut leads to:
1 Impairment of the mucosal capillary circulation (intraluminal pressures greater than 30 mmHg).
2 Submucous venous occlusion (intraluminal pressures greater than 50 mmHg).
3 Eventual arterial occlusion (pressures greater than 90 mmHg).

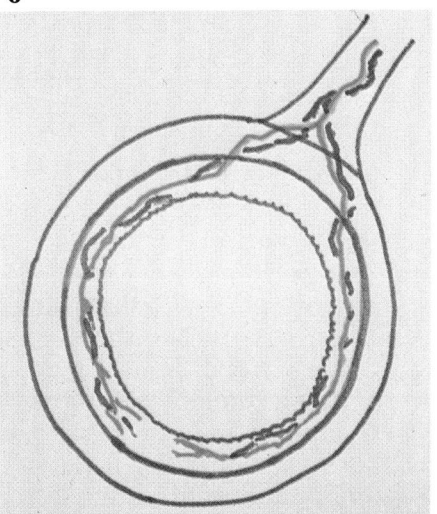

6 Jejunum.

Vessels supplying the bowel wall on leaving the mesentery run for a variable distance in the subserosa before penetrating the muscle coat, after which they run in the submucosa.

The vulnerability of the vascular supply is dependent upon the anatomical course of the vessels in different segments of the intestine. The longer the submucous course of the vessels, the earlier and greater are the effects of intraluminal tension.

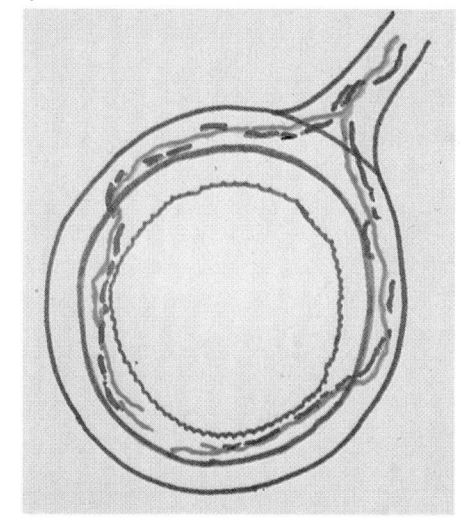

7 Ileum.

In consequence the intestinal mucosa shows progressive changes:
1   Oedema
2   Congestion
3   Devitalisation
There is abnormal permeability of the bowel wall and perforation may occur.

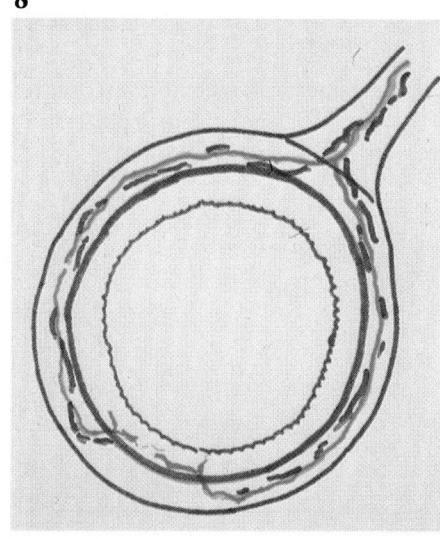

8 Colon.

Simple occlusion *(Continued)*

Level of obstruction

The effects of obstruction vary according to the level of the causal lesion. It has been established by experimental work that the most lethal forms of obstruction are those occurring at a point immediately below the ampulla of Vater (Draper Maury line). In consequence the secretions of stomach, pancreas and liver are ejected by vomiting and there is no reabsorption of these fluids below this point. In clinical practice it is recognised that lesions of the upper small intestine (jejunum) result in early systemic disturbance (hypovolaemia with peripheral circulatory failure) chiefly attributable to fluid loss. To these the term 'high obstruction' is given.

Where the obstruction is in the lower small intestine or colon the toxic effects resulting from fermentation and bacterial growth predominate. The systemic effect is slower in onset and associated with greater distension. Vomiting is less. To this form of obstruction the term 'low' is given.

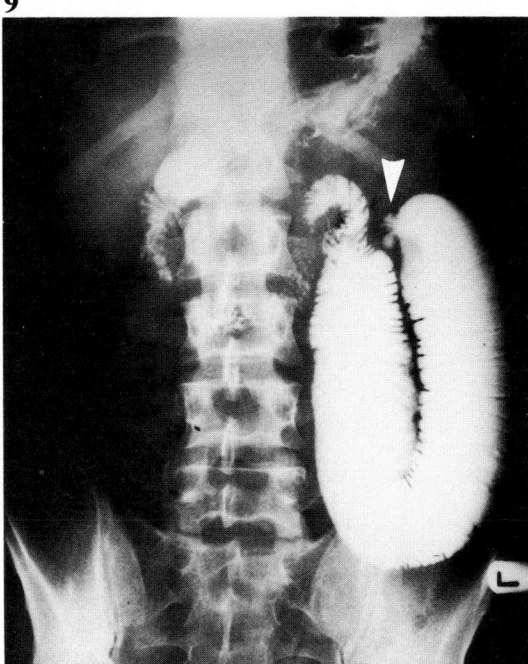

9 From a male aged 43 years. Admitted to hospital for upper abdominal pain and vomiting. A barium follow-through disclosed a high obstruction in an upper loop of the jejunum and demonstrated that this was due to an adenocarcinoma. Ordinarily a barium follow-through is only carried out in a non-acute (chronic) obstruction.

Post-operative shock

An operative hazard of serious significance is the sudden onset of shock and toxaemia following the operative relief of the obstruction. This is held to be due to the rapid absorption of toxins from the bowel lumen as the mucosa becomes congested following the relief of the intraluminal pressure. This risk is lessened by pre-operative aspiration and antibiotics.

Systemic effects

From early in the 19th century it was recognised that intestinal obstruction was associated not only with mechanical occlusion of the gut but that there was also systemic disturbance which indeed was the eventual cause of death. The cause of death in intestinal obstruction was variously ascribed to 'shock' or 'toxaemia'. It was not until the earlier decades of this century that some understanding of the true nature of the problem was evolved.

The three factors which have been identified all play a part in patients with intestinal obstruction and occur in varying degree synchronously. For purposes of analysing the subject it is desirable to study each factor separately.

Fluid loss

The earliest observers recognised that fluid loss, which they chiefly attributed to vomiting, was a prime factor.

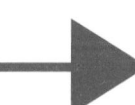

Electrolyte loss

Further observation indicated that loss of sodium chloride (salt) was of particular significance. Depletion of potassium also played a part although this was of less and later significance.

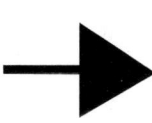

Toxic absorption

It was recognised that there was an additional (toxic) factor although the origin of the toxin and its route of absorption into the blood stream were at first obscure and subject to much investigation.

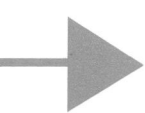

Simple occlusion *(Continued)*

Fluid loss

Loss of fluid occurs through sequestration into the bowel lumen, oedema of the bowel wall, and by vomiting or therapeutic gastrointestinal suction. This leads to a reduction in the volume of the extracellular fluid, with particular emphasis on the plasma volume. A compensatory movement of extracellular fluid into the intravascular compartment then occurs.

Electrolyte loss

Electrolyte composition of gastric, biliary, pancreatic, jejunal and ileal secretions:

	Na^+	K^+	Cl^-	HCO_3^-
	mmol/l			
Stomach	60-90	10	90–130	–
Bile	145	5	100	35
Pancreas	140	5	75	115
Jejunum	105	5	100	–
Ileum	115	5	105	30

Secretion of fluid into the bowel causes increased loss of potassium, which is 3 to 6 times the normal. This acute loss is not reflected in the level of serum potassium.

Toxic absorption

The content of the normal intestine is toxic but not usually absorbed. Bowel contents, when stagnant in a distended loop, show an increase in the number of bacteria as compared with normal bowel. This remains harmless so long as the mucosa and peritoneum of the intestine are intact and viable.

Hypovolaemia leads to peripheral circulatory failure, renal insufficiency and death, unless treatment is initiated urgently. Only in the late stages is there transfer of intracellular fluid to the interstitial spaces.

Clinical assessment of fluid loss (depending on site of obstruction):
(a) signs of obstruction but without vomiting: 1 to 3 litres.
(b) persistent vomiting with evidence of dehydration: 3 to 4 litres.
(c) persistent vomiting with hypotension: 4 to 6 litres.

Metabolic alkalosis

Metabolic alkalosis will result from the loss of H^+ from the stomach (e.g. pyloric stenosis). Following surgery increased output of adrenocortical hormones will cause further loss of potassium in urine.

Metabolic acidosis

Metabolic acidosis occurs with loss of small bowel fluid containing both biliary and pancreatic secretions.

Increased intraluminal pressure may produce patchy areas of necrosis sufficient to permit the escape of putrid intestinal contents into the peritoneal cavity. It has been shown that the venous and lymphatic systems draining a loop of obstructed bowel are not the routes whereby the lethal contents gain access to the circulation. Absorption of this fluid from the general peritoneal cavity is more important.

It is still uncertain exactly which bacterial product causes the fatal outcome but endotoxin is important. Experimentally, germ-free animals survive obstruction longer than conventional animals and the lethal effect of intraperitoneal infections of strangulation fluid can be reduced by similar injections of antibiotics. In the clinical situation antibiotics reduce the mortality.

Simple occlusion *(Continued)*

Chronic obstruction

The bowel proximal to the obstruction shows dilatation and compensatory muscular hypertrophy. If there is stasis of content, fermentation and bacterial overgrowth occur. The mucosa is inflamed with outpouring of secretion and may even ulcerate. Faulty absorption may become evident leading to a malabsorption syndrome with steatorrhoea.

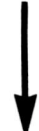

10 The gut lumen is narrowed but not completely occluded. The effect of the narrowing will depend on the nature of the gut content. If fluid, the obstruction will be incomplete and systemic effects are therefore less. Acute obstruction may supervene.

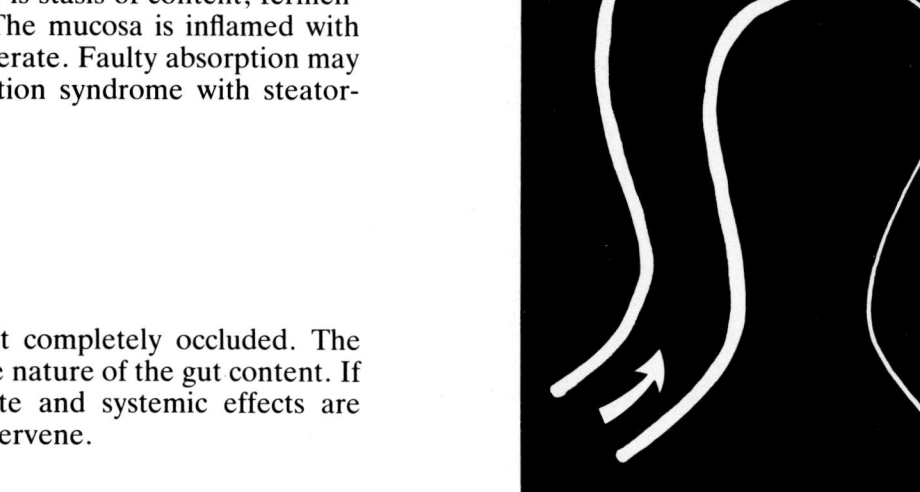

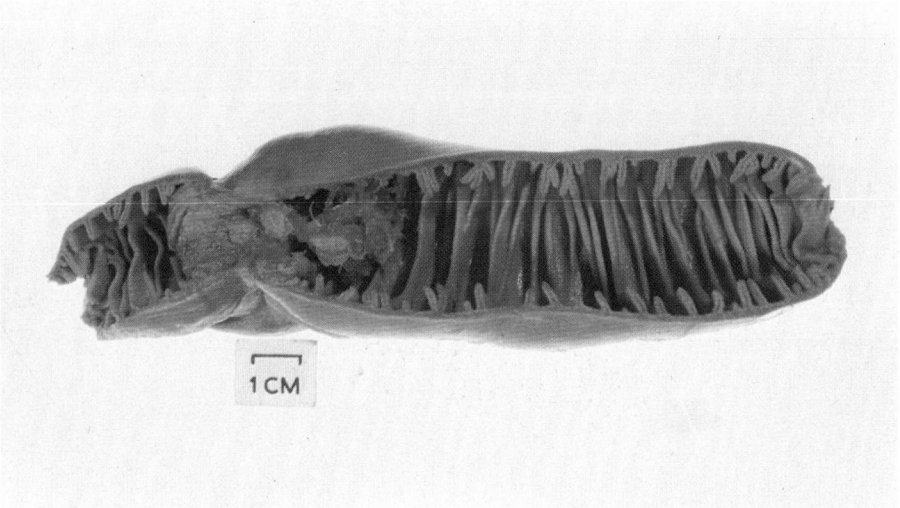

11 This specimen, from a female aged 71 years, illustrates the presence of a carcinoma of the intestine which has caused a partial chronic obstruction. Subsequently the lumen has become acutely blocked by a plug of vegetable debris leading to total occlusion of the lumen – acute obstruction.

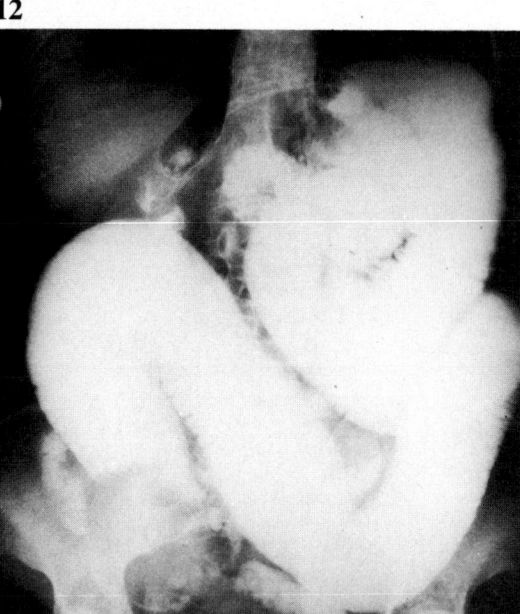

12 From a patient suffering from an obstructing lesion at the ileocaecal junction.

The radiograph illustrates the resulting gross dilatation of the lower ileum.

Causal lesions

Lesions causing simple obstruction fall into three groups:
1 Intraluminal
2 Mural
3 Extramural

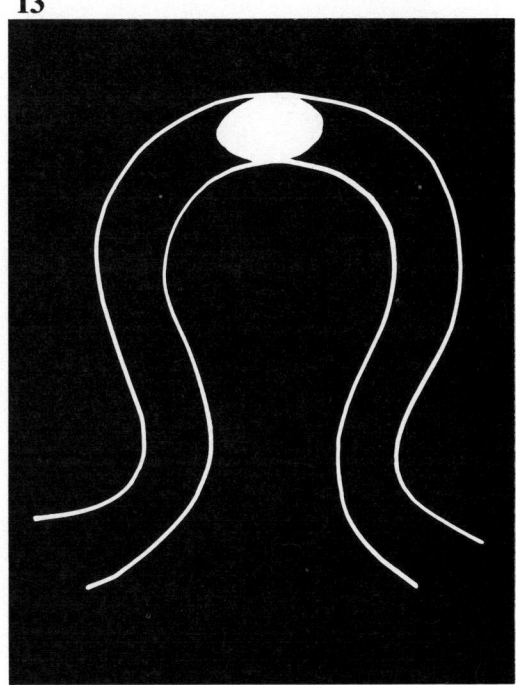

13 Intraluminal e.g. gallstone or enterolith.

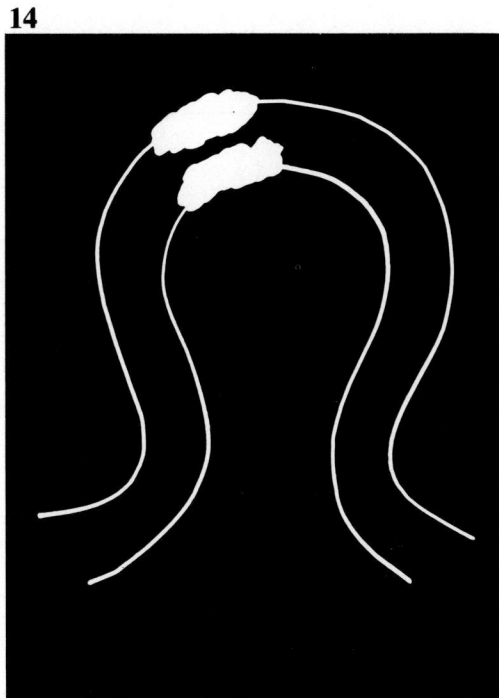

14 Mural e.g. stricture, carcinoma.

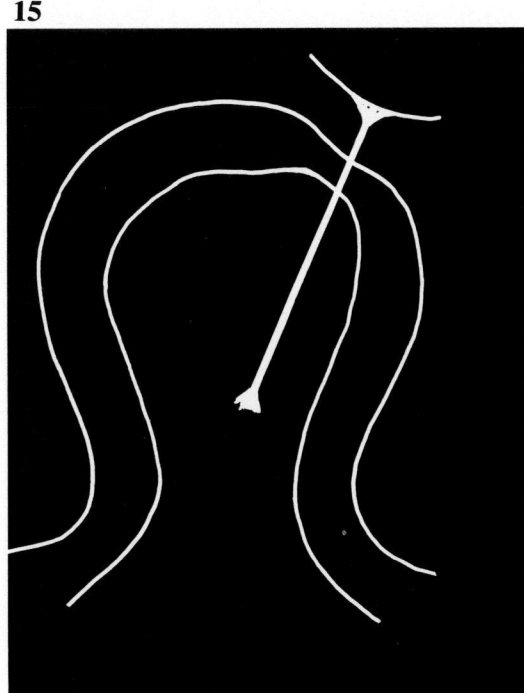

15 Extramural e.g. peritoneal band constricting underlying loop.

Closed loop

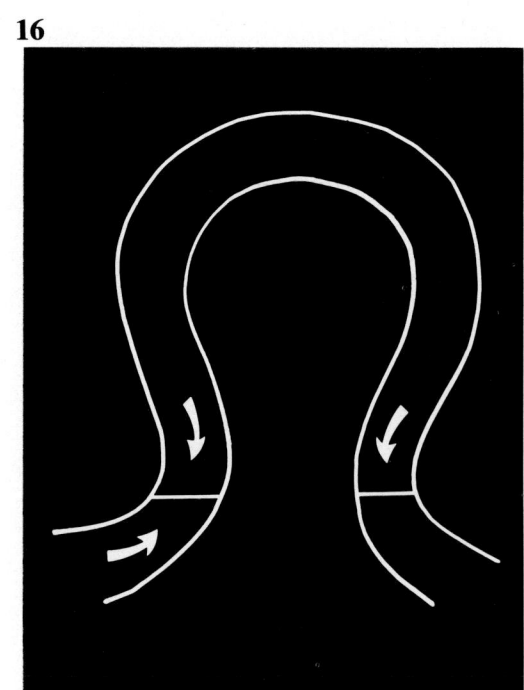

16 The term 'closed loop' obstruction signifies that there is a double occlusion of the lumen between which the bowel contents cannot pass proximally or distally.

The changes within a 'closed loop' depend upon the nature of the content of that loop, the nature of the bacterial flora and the degree of tension which develops within the loop.

In clinical practice a simple obstruction exists above the proximal occlusion and the picture is therefore a complex one except in the appendix or in a diverticulum of the intestine.

Experimental studies

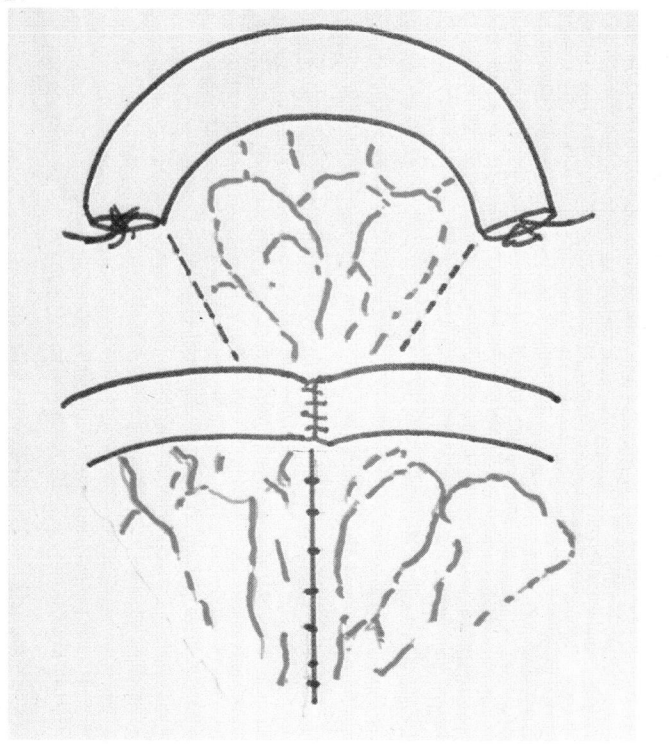

17 In order to study the complex features of a closed loop obstruction of the intestine it is necessary to differentiate between the combined effects of the pathological process above the proximal point of occlusion – a simple obstruction as already described – together with the features of the pathological changes within the closed loop, and the effects of the latter situation on its own. This has been achieved experimentally by studies of an isolated closed loop. A segment of intestine is isolated, both ends being occluded, with no interference to its blood supply. The continuity of the intestine is then restored. It is thus possible to study the changes which occur in the isolated loop.

Bacterial content

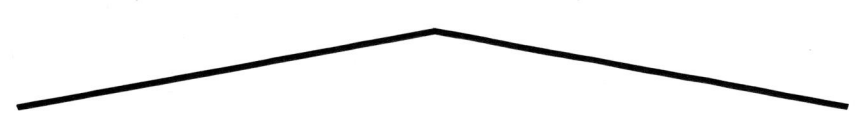

If sterile, mucus accumulates and there is a limited rise in the intraluminal pressure with distension – mucocoele. Occasionally this may rupture leading to myxoma peritonei.

If infected, an acute inflammation develops. There is marked proliferation of organisms especially anaerobes. Thrombosis of the mural blood supply leading to gangrene rapidly supervenes. Rupture then occurs. This is a rapidly fatal condition.

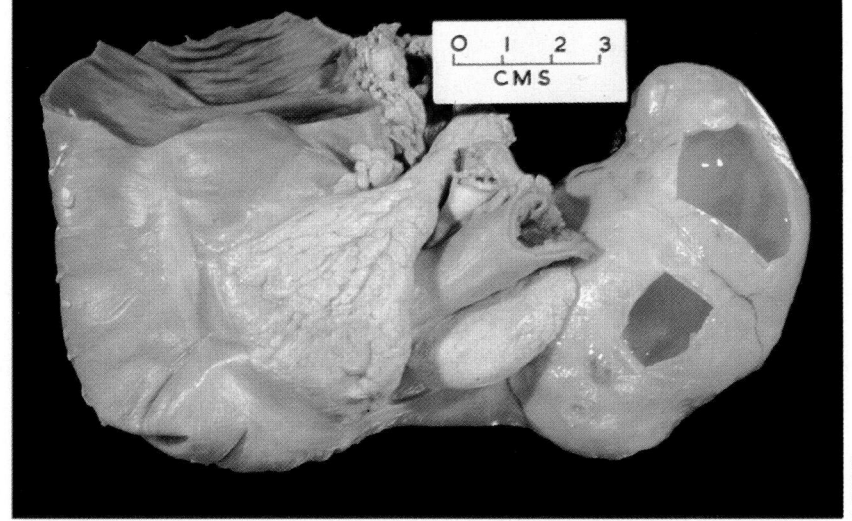

18 Female aged 55 years. The appendix was grossly distended and the appendicular wall shows absence of epithelial elements. The content is entirely mucin.

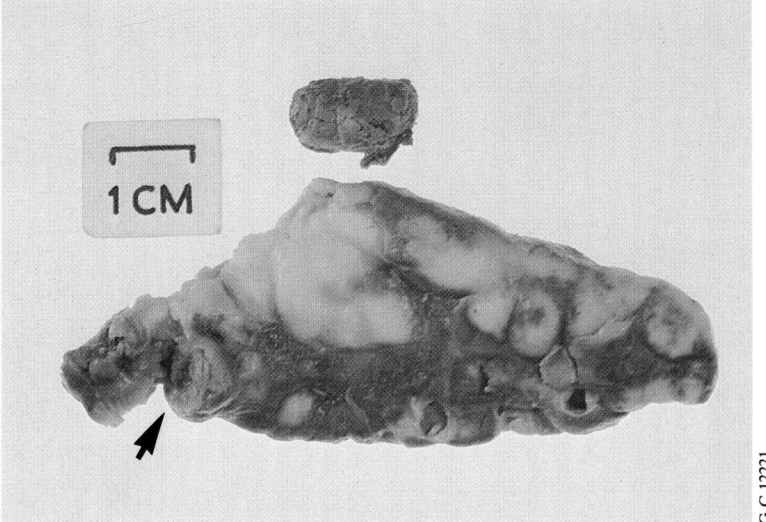

19 Female aged 47 years. Onset of acute lower abdominal pain which later became generalised. At operation diffuse purulent peritonitis. The appendix was gangrenous and had perforated close to the base and a faecolith was lying free in the peritoneal cavity. The site of perforation was the point at which the faecolith had pressed on the wall.

Length of loop

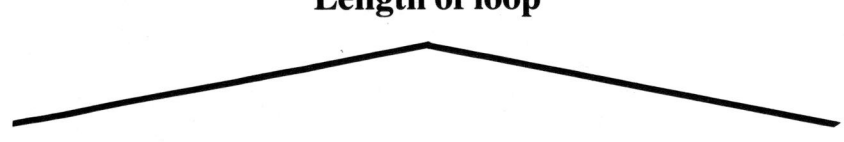

Short – distension causes a rapid rise in intraluminal and mural pressure with early necrosis.

Long – the rise in tension is slower and the onset of necrosis delayed.

Closed loop *(Continued)*

The bowel lumen may be occluded at two or more points by adhesions or by inflammatory or neoplastic strictures or in non-acute hernias.

In colonic obstruction competency of the ileo-caecal valve leads to the formation of a 'closed loop'. In gross distension of the caecum (usually greater than 12 cm in diameter) the anterior wall of the gut may become ischaemic leading to tension gangrene and perforation.

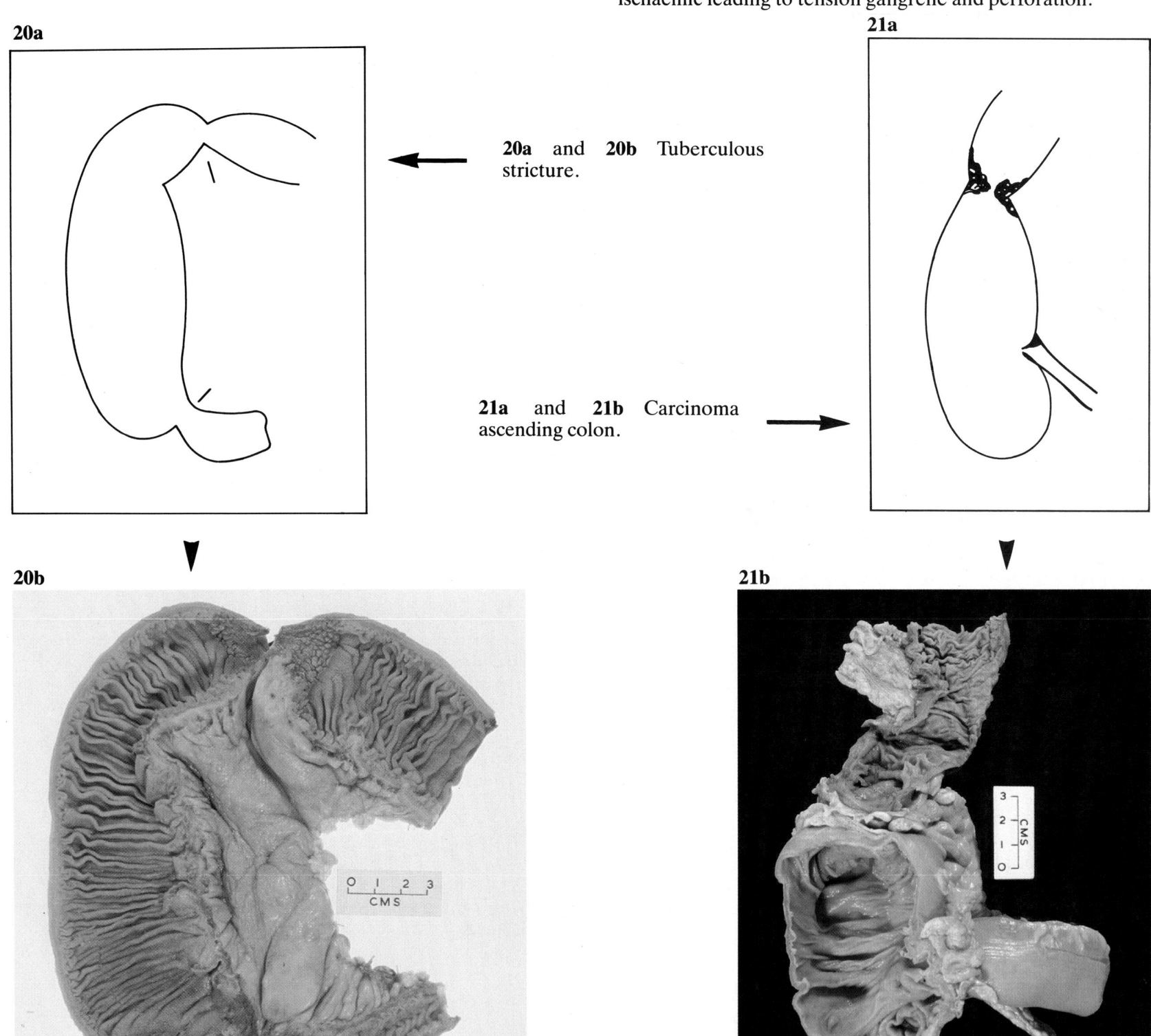

20a and **20b** Tuberculous stricture.

21a and **21b** Carcinoma ascending colon.

Obstructive appendicitis

22a

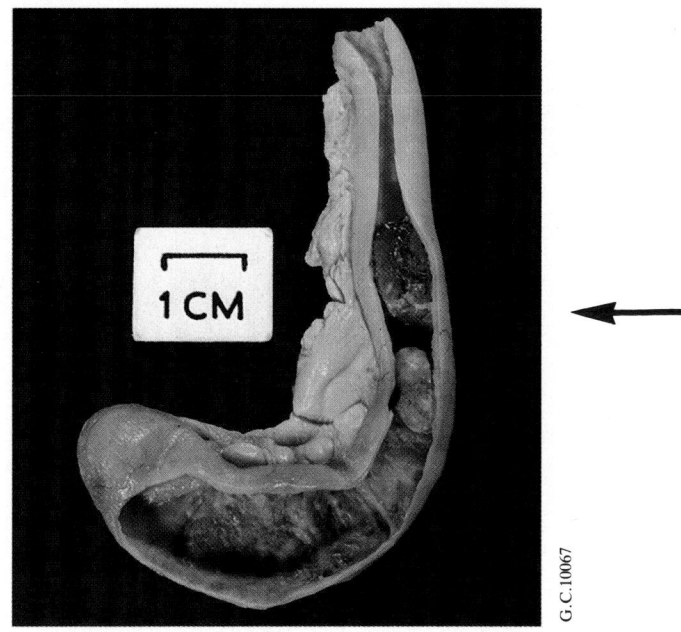

G.C.10067

22a and **22b** In acute obstructive appendicitis a concretion which has formed within the lumen of the appendix becomes impacted close to its base. Thereafter when the contents are infective an acute inflammatory process results leading to devitalisation of the appendix wall. At the point where the calculus is impacted there is additional pressure exercised on the wall and at this point rupture occurs early leading to peritonitis.

22b

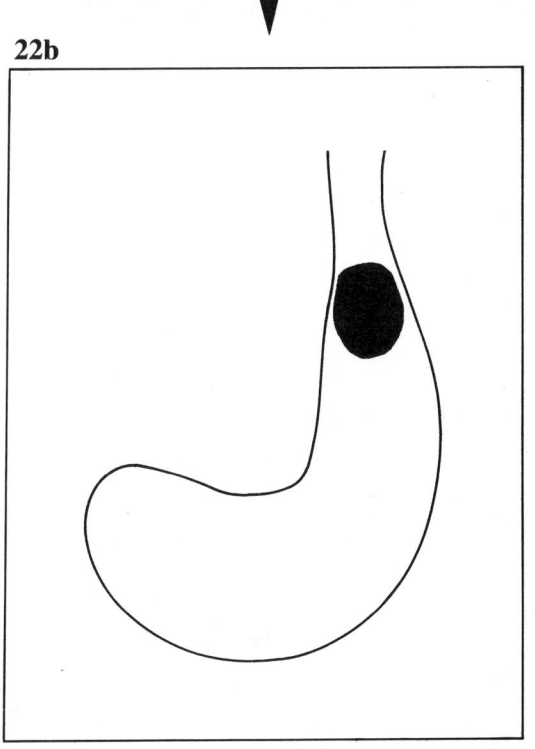

In 1914 D.P.D. Wilkie demonstrated that appendicitis occurred in two forms – the simple catarrhal variety which might result from a surface mucosal inflammation or a haematogenous infection settling in submucous lymphoid tissue. The lumen remained patent. The second form was an acute inflammation consequent upon the blockage of the lumen of the appendix by a concretion (constituting a closed loop intestinal obstruction). This form was rapidly and frequently fatal due to the development of gangrene of the wall of the appendix and rupture at the point where additional pressure was exercised by the concretion. In his experimental work, to simulate the conditions in the appendix, Wilkie used the technique of an isolated closed loop of small intestine. While his primary interest was in appendicular disease he was demonstrating fundamental changes in one form of intestinal obstruction.

Reference

WILKIE, D.P.D. (1914) *British Medical Journal* **2**, 959.

Strangulation

23

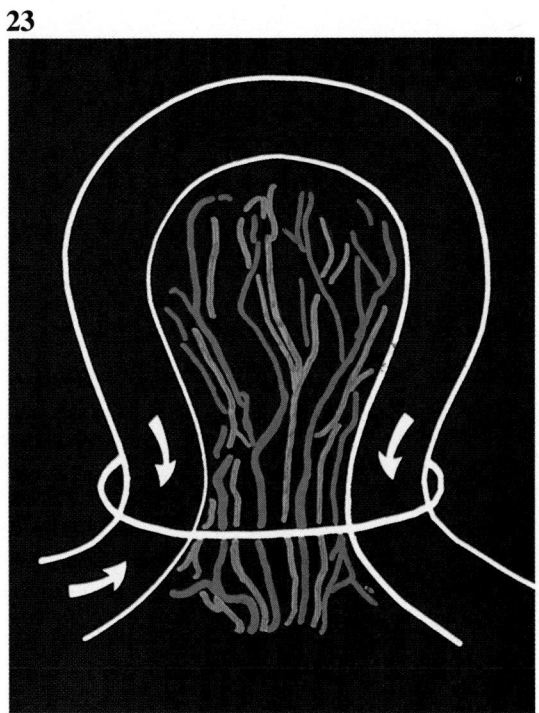

Strangulation is the most serious and lethal form of intestinal obstruction, carrying with it a mortality of 35%. The essential feature is interference with the blood supply in combination with simple obstruction and the formation of a closed loop.

The obstructing agents may be:
    Adhesions (60%)
    External herniae (26%)
    Volvulus (12%)
(The vascular changes resulting from mesenteric embolus or thrombosis produce a condition in many ways comparable to strangulation.)

Radiology

24a

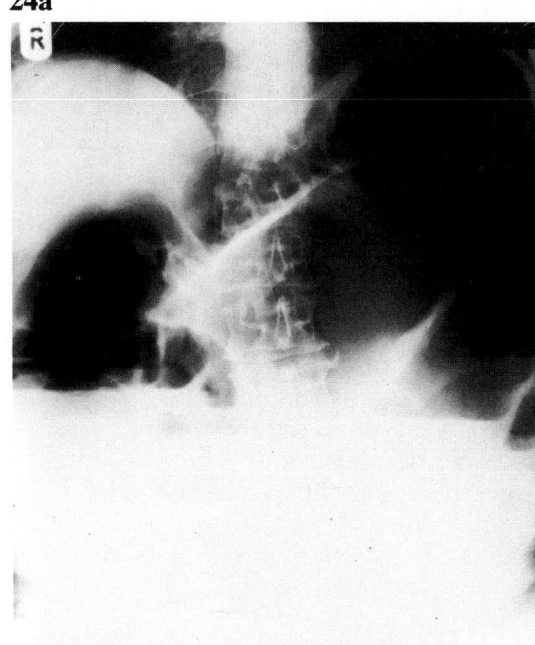

24a and **24b** Male aged 54 years. Acute volvulus of the sigmoid colon.

24b

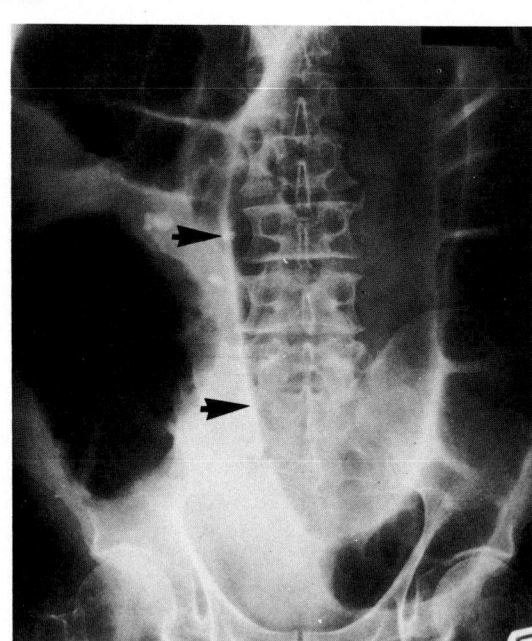

24a Radiograph (erect) showing gross gaseous distension of intestine and numerous fluid levels.

24b Radiograph (supine). The pelvic colon is seen as a large ovoid swelling filled with gas and clearly demarcated.

Length of loop

The cause of the high mortality has been the subject of much experimental research using isolated strangulated loops and by specific techniques studying outflow from these loops which would escape into the peritoneal cavity. It has been discovered that the cause of death varies according to the length of loop involved. The distinction is drawn between short, medium and long loops.

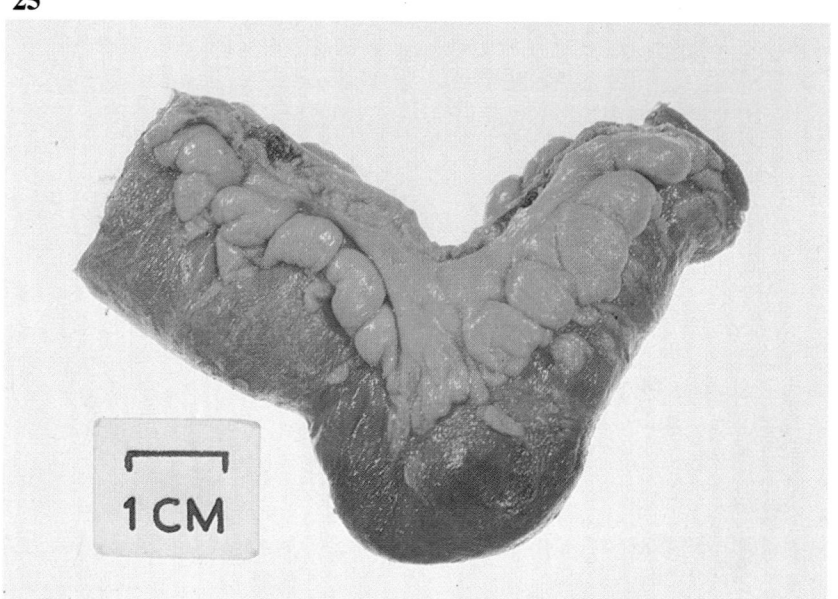

Short loop

25 The strangulation involves a very short segment of the intestine or it may involve only part of the circumference of the bowel as seen in a Richter's hernia. Gangrene of the wall occurs rapidly with perforation leading to a peritonitis. The cause of death is therefore perforation with peritonitis.

Medium loop

26 In a strangulated hernia a toxic transudate collects within the hernial sac from which there is little absorption. If at operation this fluid escapes into the general peritoneal cavity there is rapid absorption often with a fatal outcome.

Following operation there may be direct absorption from the bowel wall following restoration of the circulation of the gut.

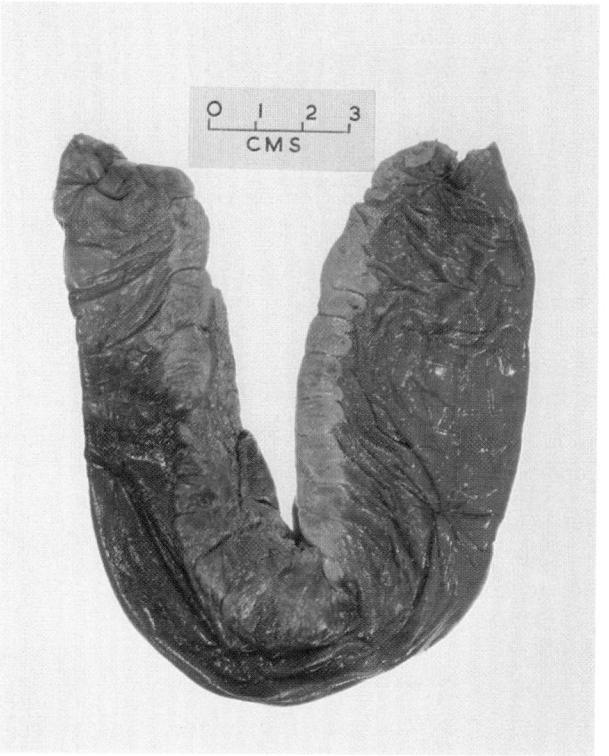

The cause of death is toxaemia, which produces acute circulatory failure and rapid death. Following strangulation the transudation of bacteria and toxins from the affected loop to the general peritoneal cavity increases progressively as the devitalisation of the mucosa and muscularis develops consequent upon ischaemia.

Strangulation *(Continued)*

Long loop

The cause of death is hypovolaemia due to sequestration of blood within the strangulated loop. This is a rapid and early phenomenon which has been shown experimentally to be of greater significance in early mortality than the toxaemia, but if this phase is effectively treated there remains the risk of a later fatal outcome from toxaemia.

27 Intussusception Occurring in childhood may present the features of long loop obstruction. The quantity of blood sequestrated in intussusception represents a relatively high proportion of the circulating blood volume of the child.

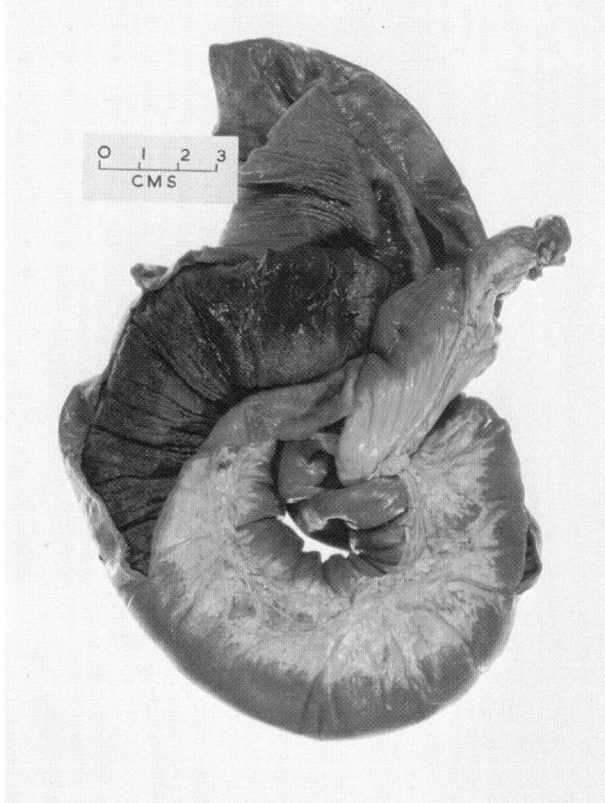

In major thrombosis of the mesenteric vessels a very large volume of blood is sequestrated and the effects are comparable to those of a long loop strangulation. The cause of death in these cases is acute hypovolaemia. If the patient survives this phase infarction of the intestine with escape of contents and peritonitis occurs.

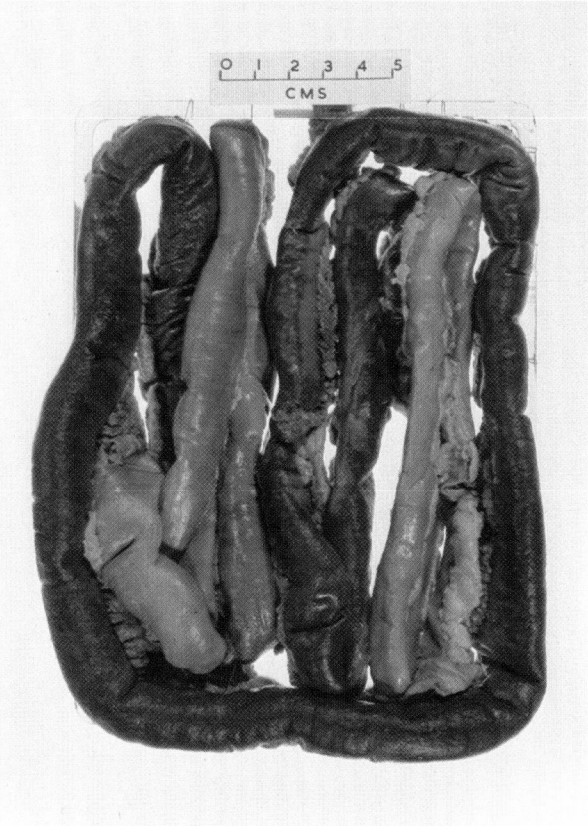

28 Mesenteric thrombosis From an elderly female admitted to hospital with the features of acute intestinal obstruction. At operation thrombosis of the mesenteric veins was found.

The affected segment of the small intestine was congested with subperitoneal haemorrhages. The bowel was not distended. The patient died 10 days after resection and at post mortem examination thrombosis of some terminal radicals of the portal vein within the liver was discovered.

Bowel viability

The differentiation between viable and non-viable bowel at laparotomy can be difficult. Even in the presence of obvious gangrene the line of demarcation between strangulated and viable intestine may be ill defined.

	Viable	Non-viable
Colour	Pink Red Purple	Purple Black Green
Mesenteric pulsation	Present	Absent
Visceral surface	Bright, glistening	Dull, lustreless
Peristalsis	Transmitted through damaged segment	Absent from damaged segment.

Reduction of intraluminal pressure by decompression will considerably reduce resistance to blood flow. Warm, moist packs concomitant with the inhalation of 100% oxygen will after a short time produce a bright pink colour to damaged but viable bowel.

Additional lesions

Hernia

Internal herniation especially of the small intestine occurs when a loop of intestine intrudes into a preformed pouch of the posterior parietal peritoneum. These pouches, which are congenital, most commonly are found to the left side of the 4th part of the duodenum. The protrusion lies beneath the inferior mesenteric vein and the left colic artery. Other posterior fossae are found behind the caecum and at the apex of the attachment of the pelvic mesocolon.

Intestinal strangulation may also result from the passage of a loop of intestine through the epiploic foramen. Foramina, possibly acquired, occasionally occur in the mesentery and through these also a loop of intestine may pass.

Other peritoneal abnormalities may arise as a result of a previous inflammation and the formation of adhesions by which a loop of intestine may be compressed or strangulated. The pathological sequelae of strangulation have already been noted.

Details of the congenital herniae will be found in text books of anatomy.

29

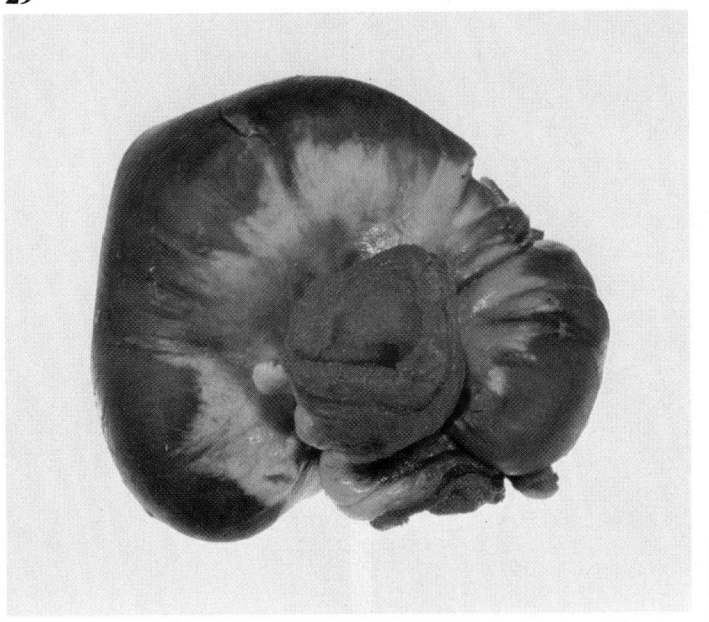

G.C.14341

29 From a female aged 32 years. The patient gave a 48 hour history of abdominal colic, vomiting and complete constipation. The abdomen was distended and radiologically multiple fluid levels were observed. It was found that a loop of terminal ileum had intruded itself through a gap in its own mesentery and thereafter undergone rotation with resulting strangulation.

J. Anderson

Additional lesions (*Continued*)

Volvulus

Volvulus is defined as the twisting or torsion of a loop of bowel around its related mesentery in such a way as to obstruct the lumina of both the proximal and distal limbs of the loop. Torsion of this nature can only occur where the intestine is normally mobile and attached by a long mesentery or where it is abnormally mobile and with an atypical mesenteric attachment. Volvulus neonatorum and essential features of strangulation of the gut have already been described (see Sections 15 and 15B). In this section attention is directed to those forms of volvulus which occur in the colon in later life.

In the large intestine the classical sites of volvulus are the sigmoid colon, the caecum and more rarely the transverse colon.

Sigmoid colon

There is wide variation in the incidence of volvulus throughout the world. In North America and Europe the incidence is relatively low. The lesion is much commoner in Africa, Asia, especially India, and in some parts of South America. It is believed that the explanation lies in the differing dietary habits. Where the incidence of volvulus is high the diet has a high carbohydrate content, a bulky residue and is customarily consumed in one large meal per day. Where the incidence is low the diet is highly refined with a low residue and a high protein content.

The length of the pelvic colon varies and may be increased by a persistent bulky content such as would be produced by a high residue diet or by inadequate bowel clearance.
It is believed that an abnormally long sigmoid loop is at increased risk of undergoing volvulus and there is some evidence to suggest that in certain African races the sigmoid loop is congenitally longer than in the Caucasian races.

In Europe and North America there is an increased incidence amongst inmates of psychiatric and geriatric hospitals. It is assumed that the difficulty of regulating bowel action in such patients leads to chronic faecal overloading of the sigmoid colon, and that this predisposes to volvulus.

Another factor of significance is the character of the root of the sigmoid mesentery. The attachment is described as 'V' shaped with the apex of the V pointing upwards and to the right. Rotation of the attached colon is facilitated when the two limbs of the V approximate closely. It may be that the limbs are unduly close congenitally or become approximated as the result of inflammation and fibrosis or adhesion formation – the omega (Ω) loop.

The final precipitating factor is probably some abnormal peristalsis which may be occasioned by a wide variety of causes.

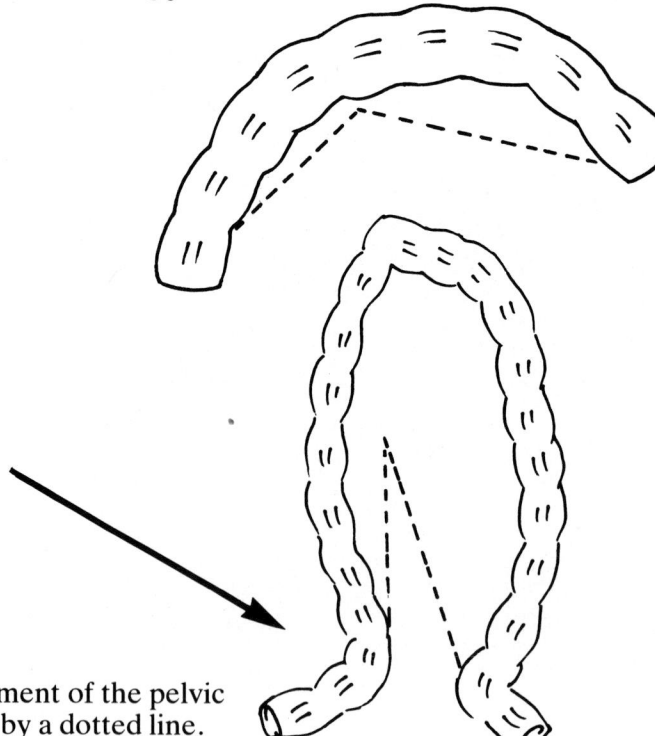

30

30 The line of attachment of the pelvic mesentery is indicated by a dotted line.

The affected loop most frequently shows a clockwise rotation of 180° but rarely exceeds 360°. In certain individuals the sigmoid loop may be permanently twisted through 180° and anything which causes distension of the colon will tend to straighten out the loop and in turn to increase and tighten the twist so that obstruction supervenes.

In addition, recurring minor episodes of volvulus may take place. This leads to a branching pattern of fibrosis in the mesentery which in turn may be the cause of a final complete volvulus.

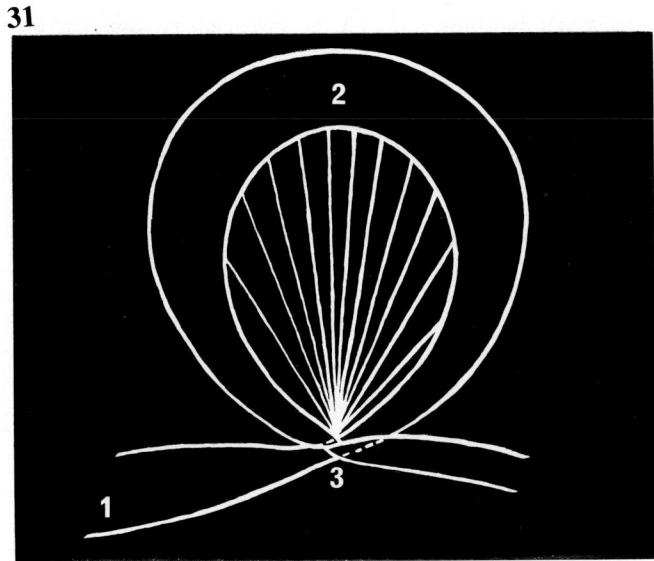

31 The three features of strangulation as already described now become apparent:
1 Simple occlusion proximal to the point of rotation
2 A closed loop obstruction
3 Strangulation of the blood supply to the loop

There is very gross gaseous distension of the closed loop due to a combination of swallowed air trapped within the volvulus and the gases produced by bacterial fermentation. As the torsion of the mesocolon tightens the sigmoid veins are partially occluded and the bowel wall becomes congested and oedematous. The accumulation of secretions increases intra-luminal tension and this in turn interferes with the blood flow through the small vessels of the bowel wall. Finally the sigmoid vessels become totally obstructed and strangulation ensues. The incidence of complete strangulation with gangrene of the twisted loop is 7 to 10% but it is believed that this occurs less readily in individuals who have a thicker and more vascular sigmoid colon.

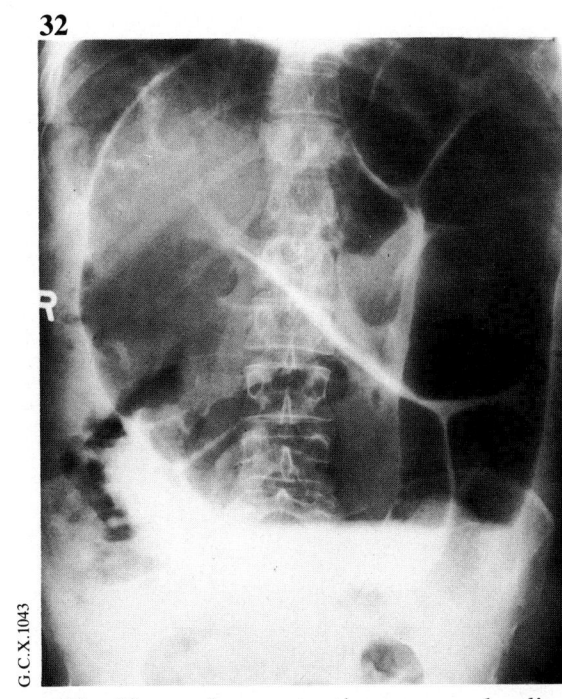

G.C.X.1043

32 X-ray demonstrating a grossly distended pelvic colon containing air projecting upwards on the left side of the abdomen. The fundus of the loop is pressing upwards under the diaphragm.

Additional lesions *(Continued)*

Sigmoid colon *(Continued)*

There is evidence from the clinical history that initially an intermittent partial rotation may take place and recur. Alternatively there may be some degree of obstruction from persistent partial rotation.

When complete strangulation occurs the diagnostic features are:

1 Short history and severe lower abdominal pain
2 Evidence of constitutional disturbance with tachycardia and possibly hypotension
3 Abdominal tenderness, guarding, and absent bowel sounds
4 Pneumoperitoneum on plain abdominal X-ray if perforation has occurred
5 Some blood stained fluid may be passed per rectum and there will be purple discoloration of the colonic mucosa at the highest level which can be reached by sigmoidoscopy

Radiology

The important radiological features are as follows:

1 Gross gaseous distension of sigmoid loop which extends upwards as far as the liver and may elevate the left dome of the diaphragm (**33**)
2 There are wide fluid levels in both limbs of the closed sigmoid loop (**33a**)
3 There are usually three dense curved lines on the supine films running downwards and converging upon the site of the torsion. The middle line is the most constant and the most prominent and is produced by the two walls of the loop lying pressed together

33
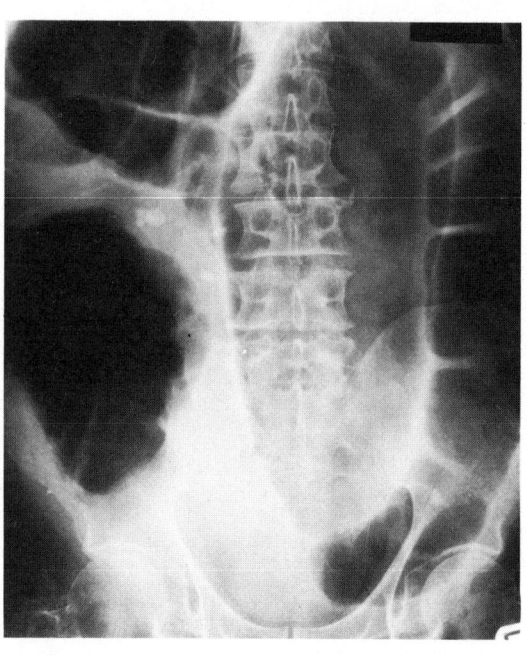
G.C.X.952

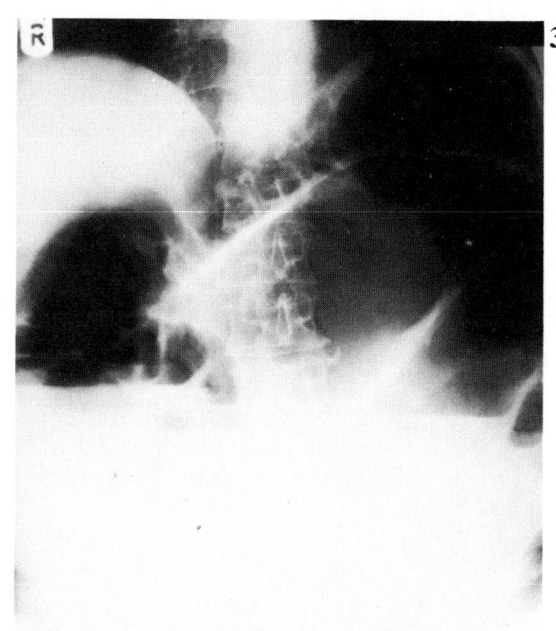
33a

33 and **33a** Male aged 54 years. Acute volvulus of the sigmoid colon

Ileo-sigmoid knotting

Cases sometimes occur in which there is a sigmoid volvulus around which a loop of ileum has become coiled and twisted. The sigmoid loop may carry with it a loop of ileum but it is more usual for an ileal loop to wrap itself around the narrow base of a long redundant loop of sigmoid colon. The condition carries a high mortality because of the early onset of strangulation.

Ileocaecal volvulus

As a result of incomplete fixation during the third stage of intestinal rotation (see Section 15B), the terminal ileum, caecum and ascending colon are unduly mobile. Volvulus of this part of the intestine can occur in later life. It is a relatively rare condition in all parts of the world and dietary factors play little part in its aetiology. In Western Europe and North America it constitutes less than 25% of all cases of volvulus and an even lower proportion in those countries where volvulus is a common condition.

Precipitating factors

Other factors which determine the incidence of right colon volvulus in persons who have the anatomical predisposition have been identified as follows:
1   Pregnancy and parturition
2   Congenital intra-abdominal bands and adhesions
3   Acquired adhesions following abdominal operations
4   Distension of the caecum due to an obstructing lesion of the left colon

Ileo-caecal volvulus is prone to early strangulation and gangrene.

Radiology

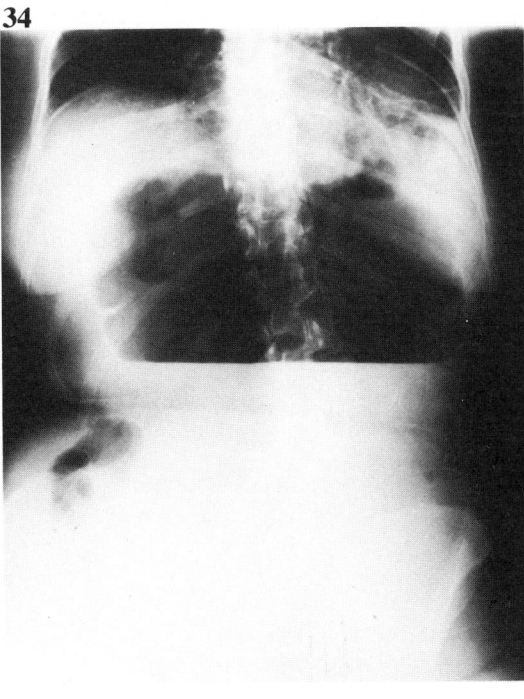

34

G.C.X.866

The radiographic appearances of right colon volvulus are as follows:
1   A large spherical, oval or kidney-shaped translucency lying towards the middle of the abdomen
2   The distended right colon loop differs from that of a sigmoid volvulus in that the two limbs do not rise out of the pelvis
3   A single very broad fluid level may be seen as distinct from the sigmoid volvulus which gives rise to two fluid levels.
4   Loops of distended small bowel lie to the right side of the grossly distended caecum and the distal colon will be empty

Transverse colon

This is the rarest form of volvulus. It may arise if adhesions develop between proximal and distal limbs of a long redundant loop of transverse colon or if there happens to be a congenital or acquired intra-peritoneal band around which the transverse colon becomes twisted.

I.F. MacLaren

Intussusception – additional notes

In infancy

Intussusception in infancy results from disordered peristalsis possibly due to viral infection as it is always associated with lymphoid hyperplasia of the Peyer's patches and mesenteric lymphadenitis. It is usually encountered between the ages of 6 months and 1 year.

Occasionally a Meckel's diverticulum may lead to intussusception in older children.

35

35   From a child.

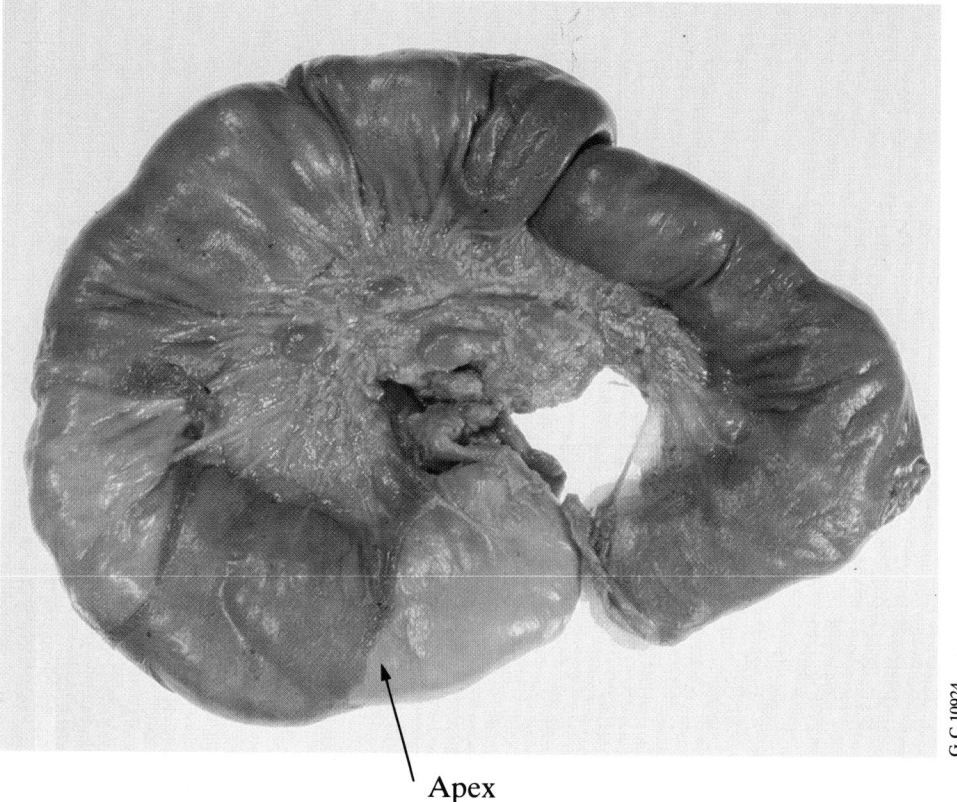

Apex

G.C.10924

This specimen illustrates well the distinctive anatomical parts of the lesion. The apex represents the first part of the intestine to undergo invagination and remains the leading point of the intussusceptum however much further invagination occurs. The intussusceptum grows at the expense of the sheath. Occasionally the apex of the intussusception may present through the anal canal and simulate a prolapse of the rectum.

The neck of the intussusception is the point of danger. It is here that the entering arteries and veins become compressed leading to necrosis of the bowel wall (intussusceptum). Eventually, infected material leaks back through the neck causing peritonitis.

Very rarely the intussusceptum becomes completely separated and may be passed per rectum. If sufficient adhesions have been formed at the neck before separation occurs spontaneous cure may result.

Functional obstruction

Adynamic ileus

This lesion is an obstruction due to failure of the propulsive contractions of the intestinal muscles and is caused by:

1 Peritonitis – bacterial or chemical
2 Retroperitoneal irritation – haemorrhage, ureteric stone
3 Drugs – tricyclic antidepressants, ganglion blocking agents
4 Postoperative ileus
5 Electrolyte imbalance – including uraemia
6 Miscellaneous – spinal cord injuries, blunt abdominal trauma

The pathogenesis of adynamic ileus has been the subject of much experimental study. There is no actual paralysis of the gut. The impaired motility is thought to be due to reflex inhibition mediated via sympathetic nerves. Section of the splanchnic nerves abolishes this inhibition. However, direct irritation of the bowel wall also results in inhibition of contraction and this is not abolished by splanchnic nerve section. Various workers have implicated the local neuromuscular apparatus in the gut wall but final conclusive evidence of this has not been achieved.

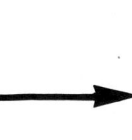

In the presence of impaired motility swallowed air will cause distension and there is intraluminal fluid accumulation with loss of electrolytes. Distension and electrolyte loss will further impair motility setting up a vicious spiral of events. The mainstay of treatment is overcoming the distension by nasogastric suction – this removes swallowed air and gastric secretions and allows removal of small intestinal gas and fluid by retrograde passage into the empty stomach.

Spastic ileus

This is a rare form of functional obstruction caused by severe spasm of the bowel wall. It may be initiated by irritating causes within the lumen e.g. worms, or by reflex causes via the coeliac plexus, following blunt abdominal trauma or via the central nervous system. In many cases there is no apparent mechanism.

The extent of the spasm varies from short ring-like bands of contraction to long segments, occasionally involving the whole colon. The constrictions are usually single and there is a sharp delineation with non-contracted bowel. The contracted segment is hard and pale but histologically is normal.

J. Anderson

The gastrointestinal tract is the gateway through which the foodstuffs, minerals, vitamins and water enter the body. Carbohydrates, fats and proteins are largely digested in the small intestine, and the products of digestion, the minerals, vitamins and water cross the intestinal mucosa and enter the blood or lymph. Substances are absorbed from the lumen of the gastrointestinal tract by diffusion, facilitated diffusion, solvent drag, active transport and endocytosis.

Infoldings of mucosal tissue (the valvulae conniventes) increase the surface area × 3.

Transport rate = area × flux. A large surface area makes for increased transport.

The intestinal surface is adapted for absorption by its anatomical and histological structure which greatly increases the apparent surface area.

The mucous membrane is covered by villi (20 to 40/mm^2 of mucosa), which are finger-like processes 0.5 to 1 mm long projecting from the mucosal tissue into the lumen. These villi increase the surface area a further 10 times. Each villus is covered by a single layer of columnar epithelium (enterocytes) and contains a network of capillaries and a lymphatic vessel (lacteal).

The apical surfaces of the enterocytes have numerous microvilli (brush border) which increase the surface area for absorption a further 20 times. The enterocytes are connected to each other by tight junctions. The brush border is rich in digestive enzymes such as disaccharidases and peptidases and is lined on its luminal side by an amorphous layer, the glycocalyx, consisting of sulphated weakly acidic mucopolysaccharides. The glycocalyx subserves a number of functions in that it is a protective mechanical barrier and filter against bacteria and foreign materials, and selectively binds substances to aid digestion and absorption. Outside the glycocalyx is an unstirred water layer 100 to 400 μm thick. Solutes must diffuse across this layer to reach the mucosal cells.

The mucosal cells are formed from mitotically active cells in the crypts of Lieberkühn and migrate up to the tips of the villi where they are shed. The average life of a mucosal cell is approximately 2 to 5 days.

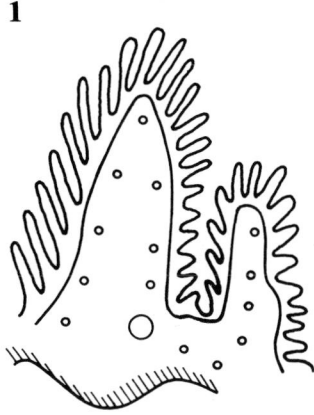

1 Low power section of small intestine showing two valvulae conniventes.

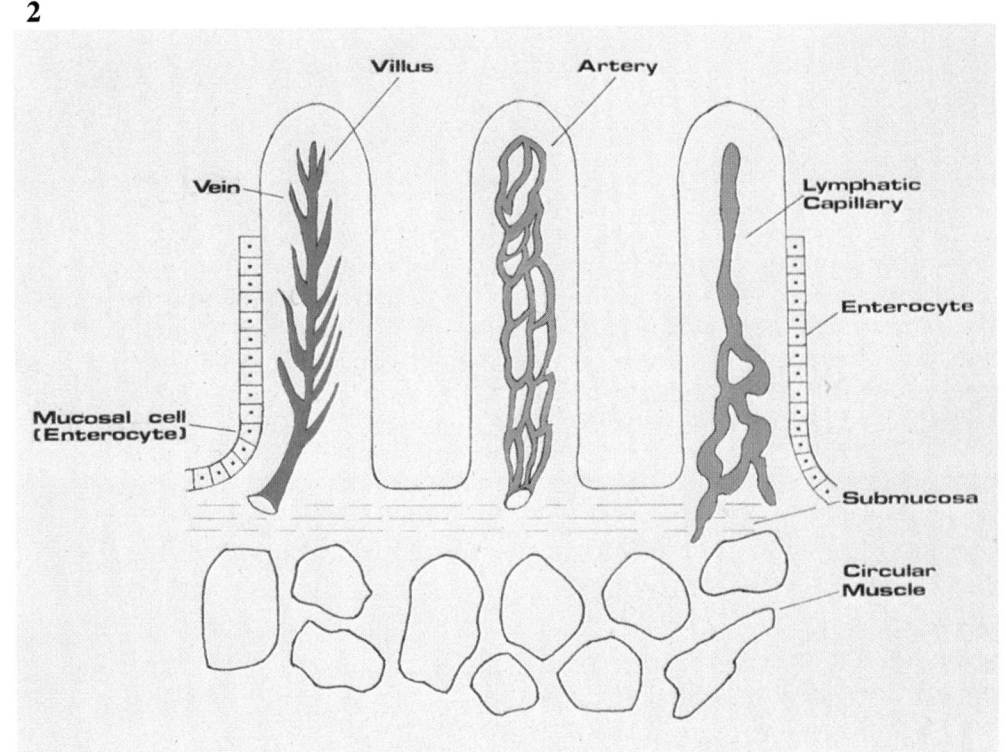

2 Three villi covered with mucosal epithelium (enterocytes).

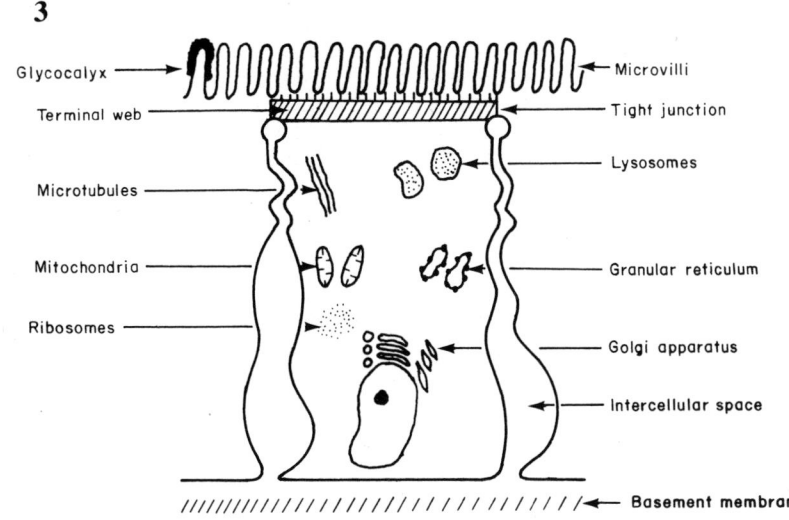

3 Mucosal cell showing microvilli.

The small intestine normally absorbs large amounts of digested foodstuffs, water, minerals and vitamins per day and has considerable functional reserve.

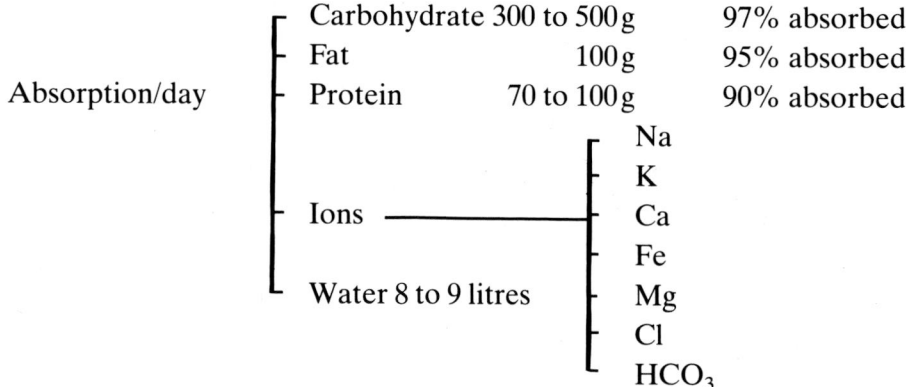

Absorption is not uniform throughout the small intestine. Ninety per cent of the absorption occurs in the first 120 cm of the small intestine where the contents are rich in digestive enzymes and the mucosa has a large surface area and active transport mechanisms for most of the digestive products. Substances absorbed by passive transport are absorbed where their intestinal concentration is highest, and their absorption is closely correlated with the rate of intestinal transit.

Substance	Site of absorption in small intestine		
	Upper	Mid	Lower
Monosaccharides	++	+++	++
(Monoglycerides, fatty acids)			
(Cholesterol, fat soluble vitamins)	+++	++	+
Amino acids	++	++	+
Bile salts	0	0	+++
Vitamin B_{12}*	0	0	+++
Water soluble vitamins	+++	++	0
Na^+	+++	++	+++
Cl^-	+++	++	+
Ca^{++}	+++	++	+
Fe^{++} (Absorbed in ferrous form)	+++	++	+

*Absorption requires presence of intrinsic factor produced by gastric parietal cells.

Carbohydrate digestion and absorption

The principal dietary carbohydrates, the enzymes required for their digestion and their digestion products are shown below:

Polysaccharides		Disaccharides and other breakdown products	Monosaccharides	
			Brush border oligosaccharidases	
Starch Glycogen	Salivary and Pancreatic Amylase	$\propto$ limit dextrins	$\propto$ limit dextrinase	
		Maltotriose Maltose Maltose	Maltase Maltase	Glucose Glucose
		Lactose	Lactase	Glucose Galactose
		Sucrose	Sucrase	Glucose Fructose

Salivary and pancreatic amylase initiate the digestion of starch and glycogen to produce a mixture of maltose, maltose triose and $\propto$ limit dextrins. Oligosaccharidases located on the brush border of the intestine complete the digestion.

The monosaccharides, glucose, fructose and galactose are absorbed from the intestinal lumen, glucose and galactose by active transport and fructose by facilitated diffusion. Cellulose cannot be broken down in the human small intestine, and this passes on to the colon where it is acted on by the colonic bacteria to produce gases and organic acids.

Carbohydrate digestion and absorption *(Continued)*

4 Glucose and Na$^+$ share the same carrier molecule. Intracellular sodium is low and Na$^+$ moves into the enterocyte along its concentration gradient. Glucose and Na$^+$ pass into the cell on the carrier and are released intracellularly. Na$^+$ ions are actively extruded into the lateral intercellular spaces and glucose diffuses into the interstitium and then to the capillaries. By pumping Na$^+$ out of the cell the intracellular (Na$^+$) is maintained at low levels so that more Na$^+$ and thus more glucose enters the cell. Glucose and galactose are transported by the same mechanism.

Fructose has a different carrier which does not require Na$^+$ for cotransport. Its uptake is by facilitated diffusion.

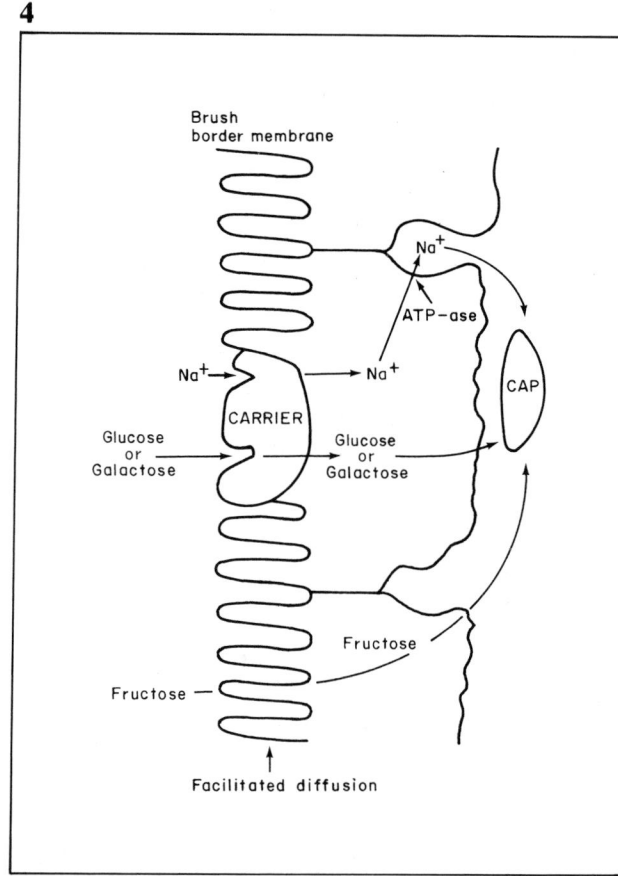

Protein digestion and absorption

The diet contains approximately 100g of protein to which are added digestive enzymes and shed mucosal cells. Proteins are hydrolysed by proteolytic enzymes present in the gastric, pancreatic and intestinal juices.

Source of secretion	Enzyme	Substrate
Stomach	Pepsins	Proteins and polypeptides
Pancreas	Trypsin	Proteins and polypeptides
Pancreas	Chymotrypsin	Proteins and polypeptides
Pancreas	Carboxypeptidase	Proteins and polypeptides
Pancreas	Elastase	Elastin and other proteins
Intestinal mucosa	Enterokinase	Trypsinogen $\rightarrow$ Trypsin
Intestinal mucosa	Aminopeptidase	Polypeptides
Intestinal mucosa	Dipeptidase	Dipeptides

Some free amino acids are produced within the gastrointestinal tract lumen but others are released at the brush border by amino peptidases and dipeptidases present in this area. The free amino acids in L form are actively transported out of the intestinal lumen into the enterocyte by at least four different transport mechanisms which are sodium dependent. The absorbed amino acids diffuse passively into the capillaries and thence to the portal blood. Some di- and tri-peptides are actively transported into the enterocyte and are digested to amino acids intracellularly, the amino acids then passing into the bloodstream.

Lipid digestion and absorption

Fat globules present in the chyme are finely emulsified in the intestine by the detergent action of the bile salts and phospholipids (lecithin).

Pancreatic lipase hydrolyses the 1 and 3 ester bands of the triglyceride yielding monoglycerides and free fatty acids. Dietary cholesterol (in the form of cholesterol esters) is hydrolysed by pancreatic esterase to free cholesterol.

When the concentration of bile salts in the intestine is high, lipids and bile salts form micelles which are particulate aggregates 3 to 10nm in diameter. Micelles contain Free Fatty Acids (FFA), monoglycerides, phospholipid and bile salt. Non-polar compounds such as cholesterol and the fat soluble vitamins dissolve in the lipid centres of these micelles. Micellar formation solubilises the lipids and gives a method for lipid transport to the mucosal cells. The micelles move down their concentration gradient through the barrier of the unstirred water layer to the brush border of the mucosal cells and pass into the space between the microvilli where they break up on reaching the mucosal cell surface. The monoglycerides, FFA and cholesterol then enter the cells by passive diffusion.

The fat soluble vitamins A, D, E and K are absorbed at the same time probably by specific transport mechanisms. The bile salts released are absorbed in the terminal ileum.

Within the enterocyte, FFA of less than 10 carbon atoms pass from the mucosa cells into the portal blood to the liver. Fatty acids of greater than 12 carbon atoms are re-esterified to triglycerides in the mucosal cells. The triglycerides are combined with cholesterol, cholesterol ester, phospholipid and protein to form an aggregate called a chylomicron which enters the lymphatics.

Water and electrolytes

Typical figures for water and sodium handled by the small intestine each day are shown below.

Source		Water (ml)	Sodium (mmol)
Diet	Beverages Water in solid food	2000	100
Salivary secretion		1500	50
Gastric secretion		2500	100
Pancreatic secretion		1500	150
Bile		500	200
Intestinal juice		1000	150
Total		9000	750
From ileum to colon		1500·	200

Of the 9 litres of fluid entering the small intestine, only 1½ litres pass through the ileocaecal valve, indicating an absorption of 7½ litres per day by the small intestine. The figures only indicate net absorption and do not take account of the rapid bidirectional movement of water and ions across the mucosa. Water is transported passively in a direction depending upon the osmotic gradient. As chyme entering the duodenum may be hypertonic with respect to blood, the initial direction of water movement will be blood to lumen, to render the chyme isosmotic. This isotonicity is maintained throughout the rest of the small intestine.

During passage of the chyme through the small intestine, the digested food particles and electrolytes are absorbed, creating an osmotic gradient between the enterocytes and the lumen of the gastrointestinal tract; water is thus absorbed into the enterocyte along the osmotic gradient produced. Sodium ions diffuse passively from the luminal chyme into the enterocytes along an electrochemical gradient, and are transported actively to the intercellular spaces. The osmotic pressure rises in these spaces, and water passes from the chyme into these spaces along the osmotic gradient.

Malabsorption

Because so many factors are involved in absorption, the causes of malabsorption are numerous.

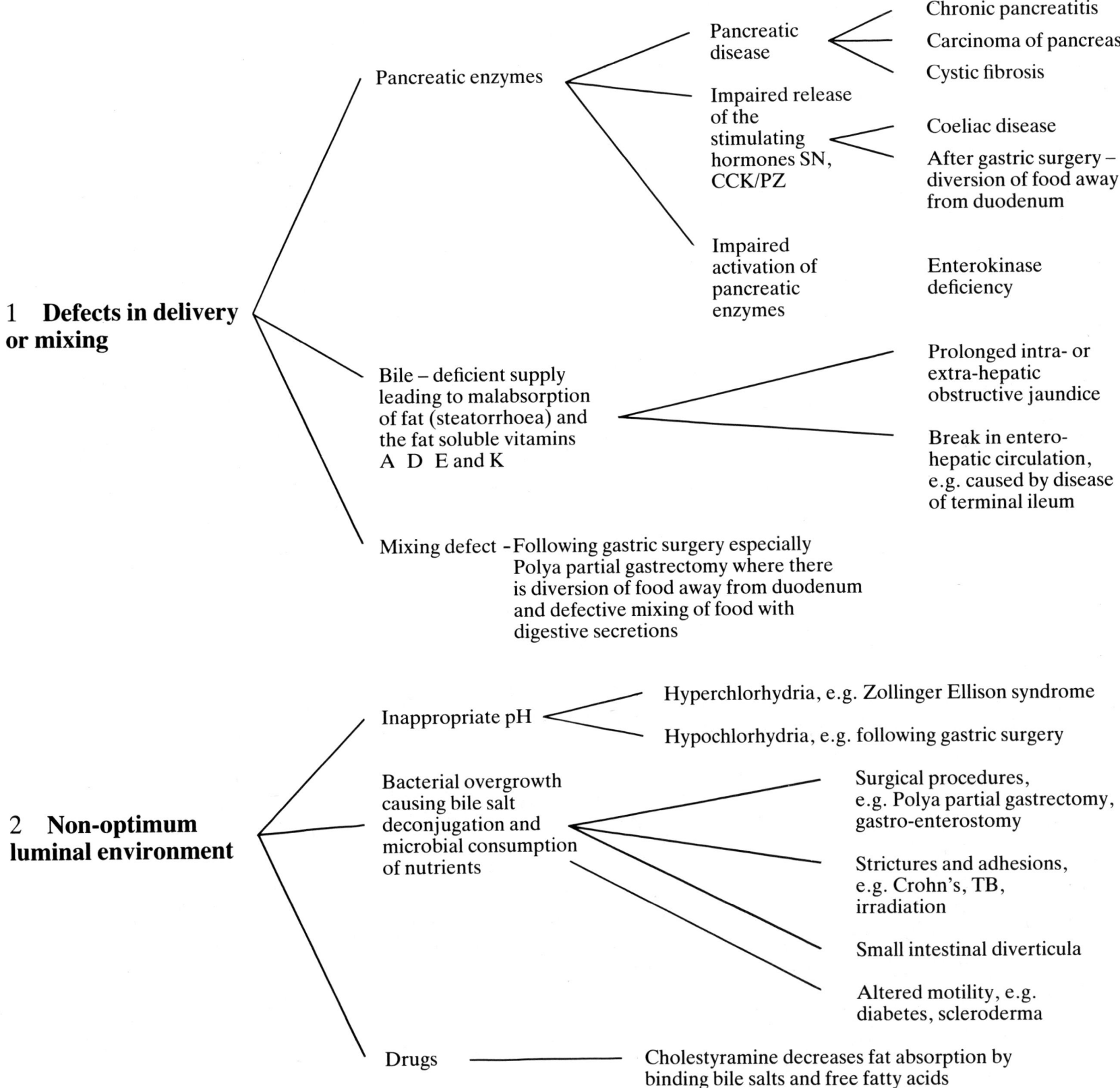

1 Defects in delivery or mixing

- Pancreatic enzymes
  - Pancreatic disease
    - Chronic pancreatitis
    - Carcinoma of pancreas
    - Cystic fibrosis
  - Impaired release of the stimulating hormones SN, CCK/PZ
    - Coeliac disease
    - After gastric surgery – diversion of food away from duodenum
  - Impaired activation of pancreatic enzymes
    - Enterokinase deficiency
- Bile – deficient supply leading to malabsorption of fat (steatorrhoea) and the fat soluble vitamins A D E and K
    - Prolonged intra- or extra-hepatic obstructive jaundice
    - Break in entero-hepatic circulation, e.g. caused by disease of terminal ileum
- Mixing defect – Following gastric surgery especially Polya partial gastrectomy where there is diversion of food away from duodenum and defective mixing of food with digestive secretions

2 Non-optimum luminal environment

- Inappropriate pH
    - Hyperchlorhydria, e.g. Zollinger Ellison syndrome
    - Hypochlorhydria, e.g. following gastric surgery
- Bacterial overgrowth causing bile salt deconjugation and microbial consumption of nutrients
    - Surgical procedures, e.g. Polya partial gastrectomy, gastro-enterostomy
    - Strictures and adhesions, e.g. Crohn's, TB, irradiation
    - Small intestinal diverticula
    - Altered motility, e.g. diabetes, scleroderma
- Drugs
    - Cholestyramine decreases fat absorption by binding bile salts and free fatty acids

Adapted from Sircus, W. and Smith, A.N. (1980)
Scientific Foundations of Gastoenterology

Malabsorption *(Continued)*

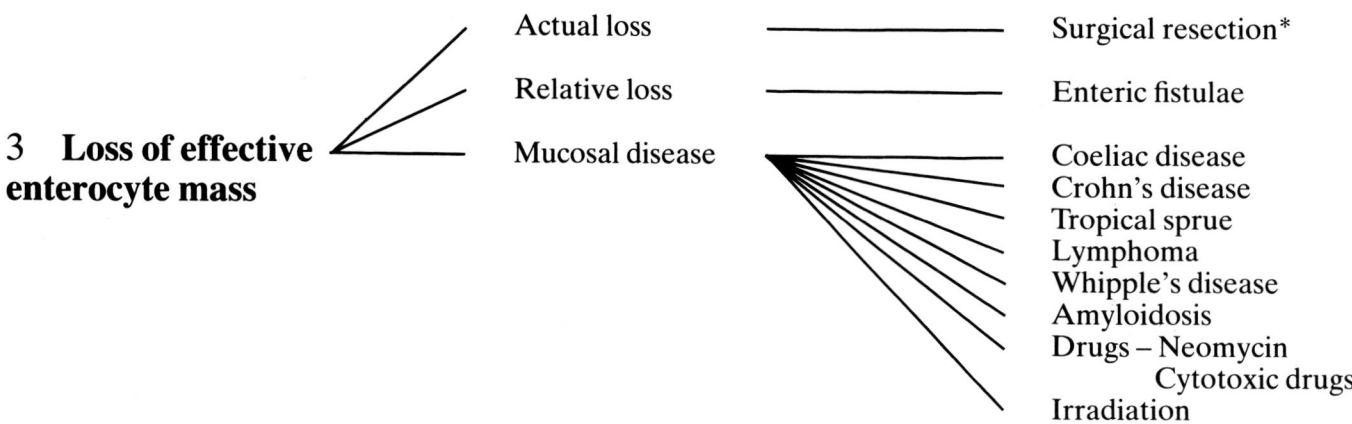

3   Loss of effective enterocyte mass

- Actual loss ——— Surgical resection*
- Relative loss ——— Enteric fistulae
- Mucosal disease
  - Coeliac disease
  - Crohn's disease
  - Tropical sprue
  - Lymphoma
  - Whipple's disease
  - Amyloidosis
  - Drugs – Neomycin
    - Cytotoxic drugs
  - Irradiation

*Note: The small intestine has considerable reserve capacity; half the total length can be resected without serious nutritional problems. Survival is possible with only 60 to 90 cm of small intestine.

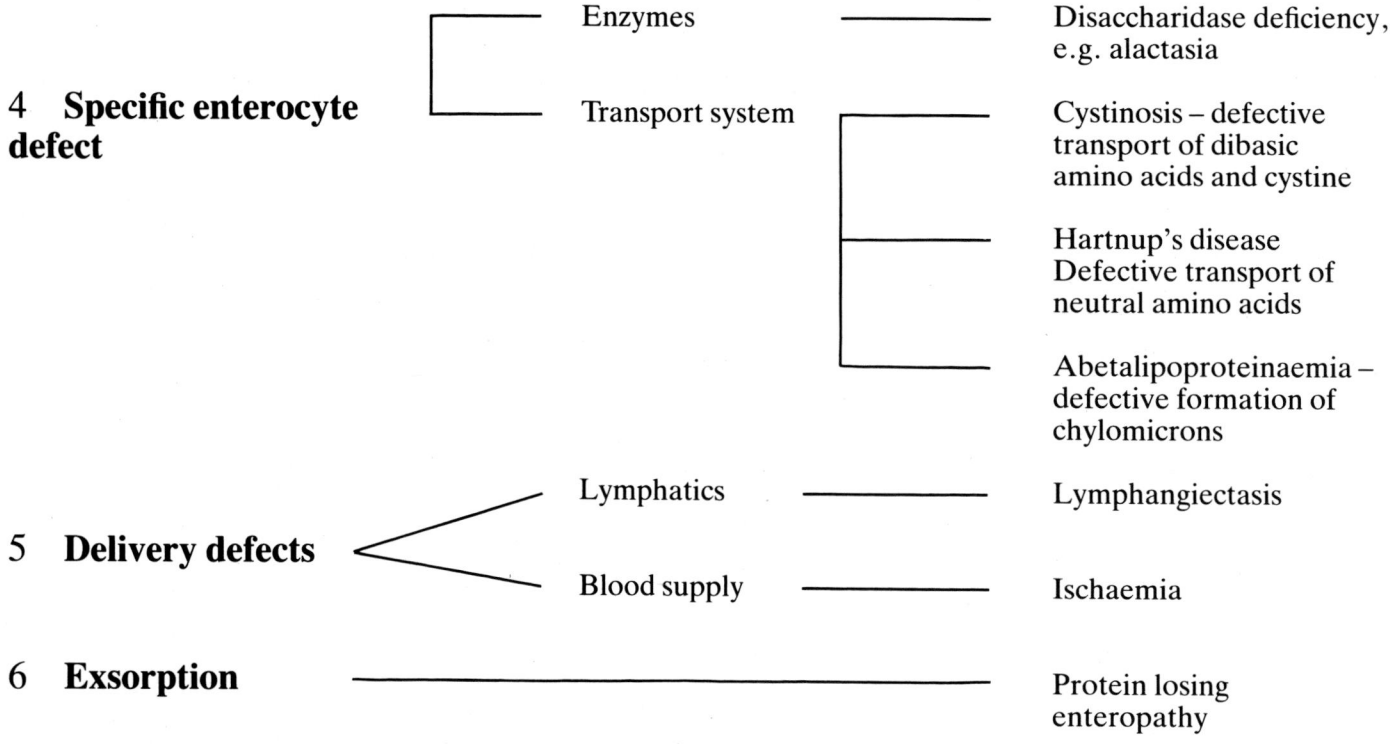

4   Specific enterocyte defect

- Enzymes ——— Disaccharidase deficiency, e.g. alactasia
- Transport system
  - Cystinosis – defective transport of dibasic amino acids and cystine
  - Hartnup's disease Defective transport of neutral amino acids
  - Abetalipoproteinaemia – defective formation of chylomicrons

5   Delivery defects

- Lymphatics ——— Lymphangiectasis
- Blood supply ——— Ischaemia

6   Exsorption ——— Protein losing enteropathy

Protein losing enteropathy

The serum proteins, albumin and globulin, are found in the gastro-intestinal tract secretions; 5 to 15% of the normal turnover of albumin and globulin is by enteric protein loss. In protein losing enteropathy, there is excessive loss of serum proteins into the gastrointestinal tract leading to hypoproteinaemia. It may be associated with malabsorption caused by the small intestinal abnormalities already mentioned. In addition it sometimes presents in its most severe forms in giant hypertrophic gastritis (see Section 14 S) and in ulcerative colitis (see Section 15E).

Post operative malabsorption

In many conditions the mechanisms of malabsorption are complex and several stages of the digestive absorptive process are abnormal. This may be illustrated by consideration of one of the commonest causes of malabsorption, viz. gastric surgery, especially following a Polya type operation.

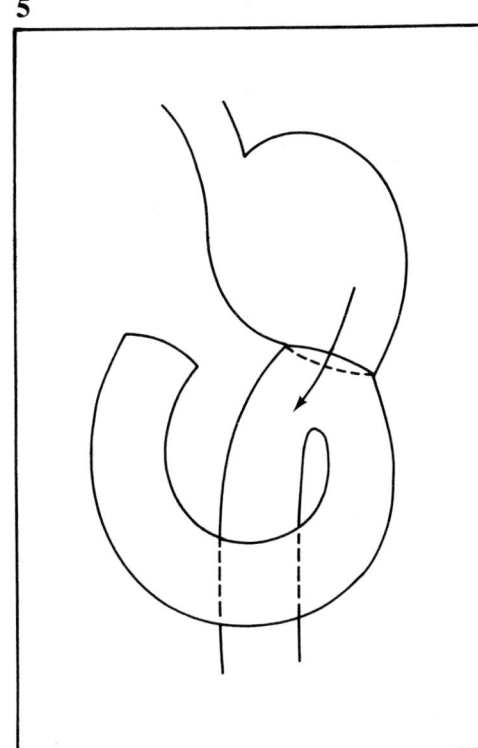

5 Partial gastrectomy (Polya)

1 There is reduced food intake, because the stomach is smaller. Food intake is reduced because of the fear of abdominal discomfort following meals.

2 By-passing the duodenum results in inadequate stimulation of secretion and CCK/PZ release with consequent reduction in pancreatic juice and bile within the intestine. Because of the modified anatomical arrangement there is poor mixing of food with the bile enzymes, and loss of absorptive area (**5**).

3 Hypochlorhydria leads to loss of optimum conditions for enzyme action; there may be impairment in the absorption of iron and of calcium. Iron deficiency leads to a hypochromic anaemia; calcium and protein deficiency to either osteomalacia or osteoporosis.

4 Hypochlorhydria and surgical alteration of intestinal continuity lead to stasis and alteration in the normal bacterial colonisation of the intestine (the blind or stagnant loop syndrome). The bacteria increase from normal 10^3/ml to $10^8 – 10^{11}$/ml of intestinal contents (*E. coli, Bacteroides fragilis, Cl. perfringans, Strep. faecalis*). Fat malabsorption results from deconjugation of bile salts to free bile acids which leads to deficient micelle formation. Dietary amino acids are converted by the bacteria to ammonia which is absorbed and converted to urea. Vitamin B_{12} malabsorption also occurs.

5 Removal of the pyloric sphincter leads to a more rapid entering of chyme into the small intestine. This chyme not having been properly mechanically mixed in the stomach, is not in a suitable form for digestion and absorption. The increased rate of entering of chyme into the intestine leads to a more rapid transport through the gastrointestinal tract and consequently less time for absorption.

6 Megaloblastic anaemia may occur due to mucosal atrophy of the gastric remnant with consequent loss of intrinsic factor.

M.O. Wright

During development the intestinal canal undergoes a series of changes of position, length and complex rotation. Anomalies of this process may lead to complications and are of surgical importance. The classical account of these changes was given by Norman M. Dott in 1924. The following description is largely drawn from this work and the diagrams are adapted from his original drawings.

Embryology

The alimentary canal arises from the entodermic vesicle which as the embryo enlarges becomes a tubular structure. The cephalic segment of the alimentary tract, as far caudally as the site of development of the pancreatic buds (later the ampulla of Vater), is derived from the foregut and from this segment the pharynx, oesophagus, stomach, the first, and a portion of the second part of the duodenum, arise. The caudal segment forms the hindgut and from this the distal part of the transverse colon, descending and sigmoid colon and rectum are derived. The intervening segment – the midgut – is initially a simple straight tube and from it arises the remainder of the duodenum, jejunum, ileum, caecum, ascending and proximal two-thirds of the transverse colon. The process of elongation, associated rotation and fixation are described as occurring in three stages.

First stage

Foregut

Asymetrical dilatation occurs – the primitive stomach and the gut assume an oblique position with deviation of the duodenal segment to the right.

The rudimentary pancreatic buds develop from the foregut in the area corresponding to the second part of the duodenum of later life. The dorsal of these buds grows into the mesentery leading to the fixation of the first and second parts of the primitive duodenum.

Hindgut

The proximal end of the hindgut becomes fixed in position to the posterior wall by a retention band close to the origin of the superior mesenteric artery – colic angle. This point of fixation remains constant throughout subsequent development. Initially the hindgut follows a vertical course downwards to the anorectal junction but progressively lengthens and becomes displaced towards the left.

Midgut

Rapid elongation of the midgut occurs forming a sagittal loop, the mesentery of which is traversed by the superior mesenteric artery (a). The proximal and distal ends of the loop are fixed points by reason of the fore and midgut attachments (b) to the posterior abdominal wall and corresponds to the second part duodenum and (left) or splenic colic angle. These points of fixation lie closely together and form the isthmus of the midgut.

As the liver develops the capacity of the embryonic abdominal cavity becomes inadequate and herniation of the midgut loop through the umbilical orifice occurs. Close to the apex in the post-arterial limb dilatation occurs representing a primitive caecum. This becomes the leading part of the protruding loop and is commonly regarded as the 'apex'.

Fourth week

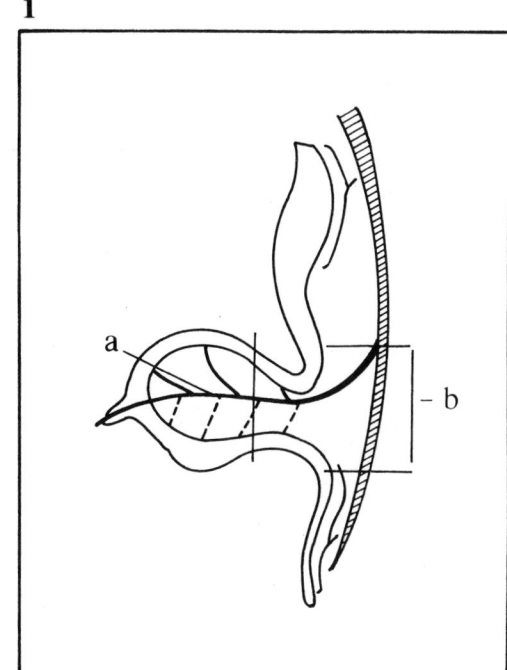

1 Formation of the midgut loop before rotation. Initial herniation through umbilical orifice (Indicated by a straight line crossing the loop).

Second stage

5th to 11th weeks

The second stage is characterised by rotation of the loop. Initially this is to accommodate the rapidly growing preaxial loop within the umbilical sac. The reduction of the herniated loop occurs during the 9th to 11th weeks.

Between the 5th and 10th weeks anti-clockwise rotation of the midgut loop occurs about its arterial axis within the umbilical cord and this rotation is continued during the reduction of the herniated loop between the 9th and 11th weeks.

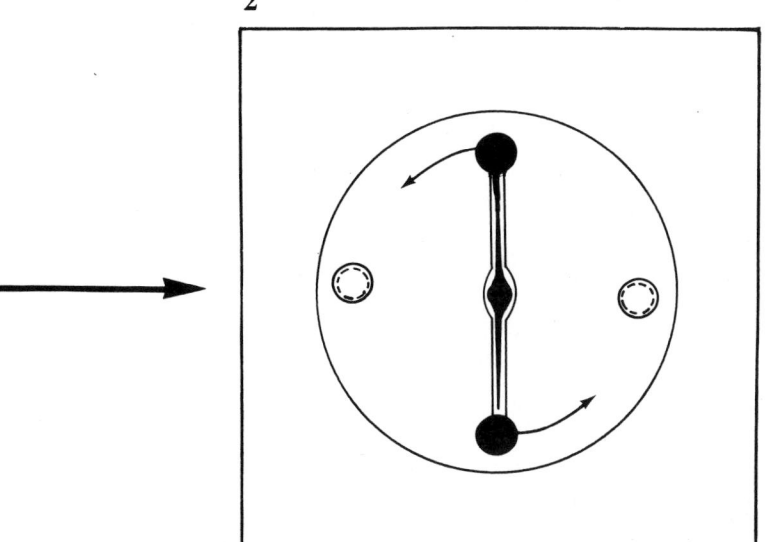

2 Initial rotation of the midgut at the umbilical orifice.

Second stage *(Continued)*

When rotation occurs the pre-axial limb, which includes the primitive caecum, moves downwards and to the right of the abdominal cavity of the embryo. The large intestine (post axial segment) moves upwards and to the left.

Eighth week

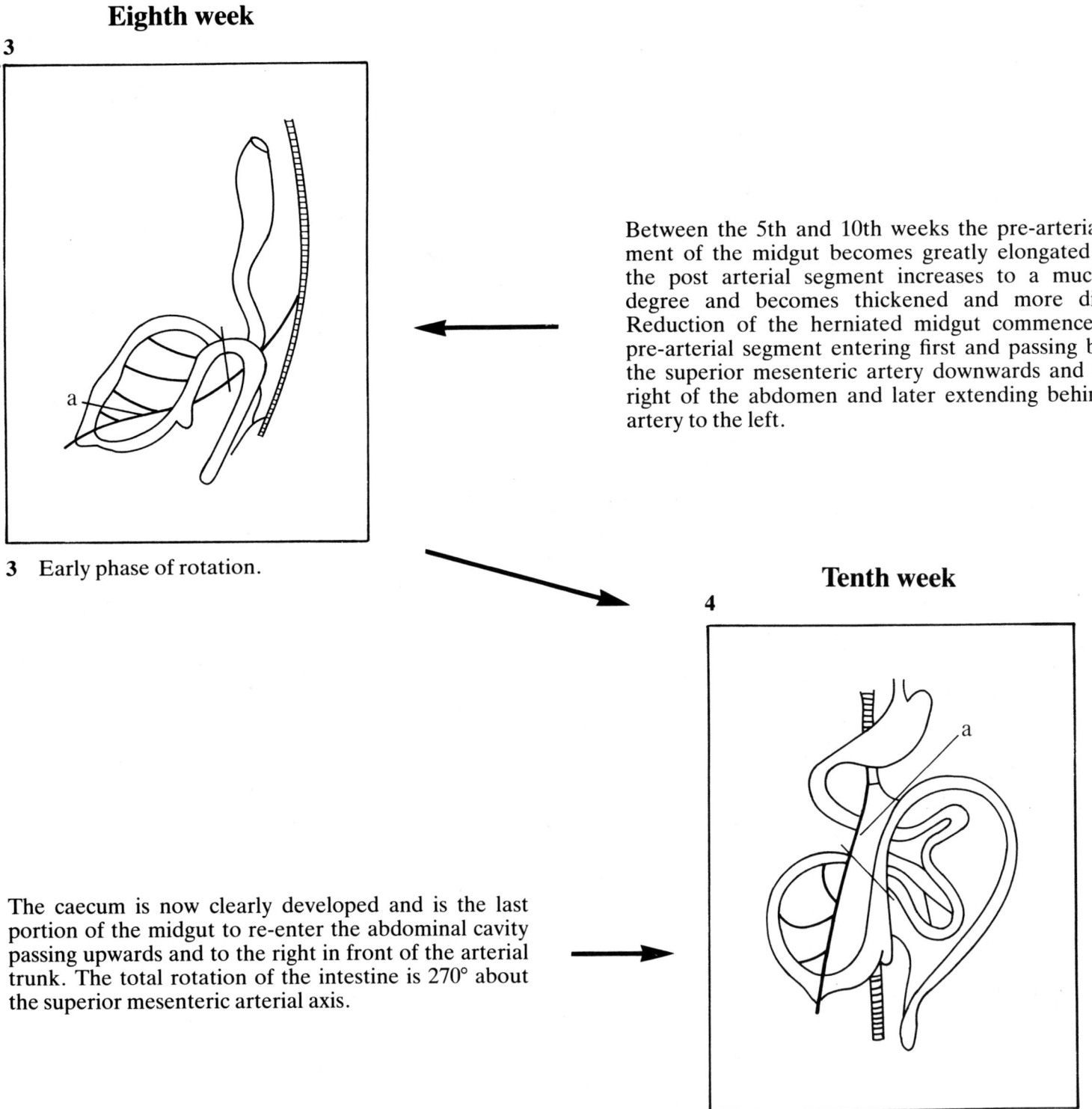

3

3   Early phase of rotation.

Between the 5th and 10th weeks the pre-arterial segment of the midgut becomes greatly elongated while the post arterial segment increases to a much less degree and becomes thickened and more dilated. Reduction of the herniated midgut commences, the pre-arterial segment entering first and passing behind the superior mesenteric artery downwards and to the right of the abdomen and later extending behind the artery to the left.

Tenth week

4

The caecum is now clearly developed and is the last portion of the midgut to re-enter the abdominal cavity passing upwards and to the right in front of the arterial trunk. The total rotation of the intestine is 270° about the superior mesenteric arterial axis.

4   Reduction of herniated midgut is nearly complete.

Third stage

The essential features of the third stage are:
1   Further migration of the caecum and colon into their final position
2   Fixation of gut to the posterior abdominal wall

The caecum moves first upwards and to the right (subhepatic) and then downwards into the right iliac fossa.

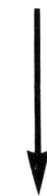

The mesentery of the midgut becomes fused along the line of the artery to the posterior abdominal wall running obliquely downwards and to the right. The caecum and ascending colon lose their mesentery and become attached to the posterior abdominal wall.

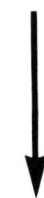

The descending and sigmoid colon are pressed to the left flank by the re-entering and enlarging midgut. The cephalic end of this segment is fixed at the colic angle.

5

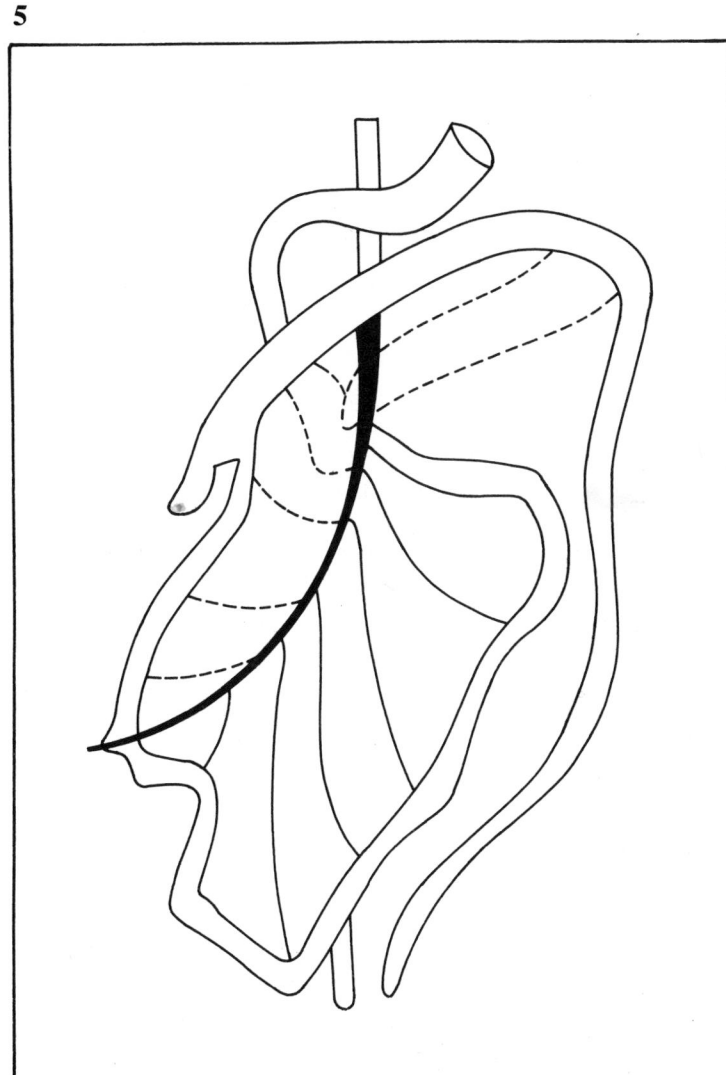

5   Eleventh week. Rotation is now complete except for the elongation of the right colon and the further descent of the caecum from the right subhepatic to the right iliac position. The hindgut (descending and sigmoid colon) has been pushed to the left by the expanding mass of small intestine.

Anomalies of rotation

First stage

Derangements of the first stage of rotation of the midgut are very rare, occurring only in the presence of extroversion of the cloaca.

There is failure of the gut distal to the vitello-intestinal duct to develop and rotation does not occur.

Second stage

Derangements of the second stage are well recognised but relatively uncommon. Norman M. Dott collected a series of 48 cases from the literature in 1924 showing a male preponderance of 3 to 1. An unduly large umbilical orifice appears to favour malrotation. The condition may be symptomless and un-recognised. It is found most frequently at operation for some lesion such as appendicitis but the symptoms in such event will have been anomalous, e.g. site of tenderness.

Reversed rotation

6

6 In this anomaly, during reduction of the herniated loop, the caecum and large intestine re-enter the abdomen first and are followed by the small intestine. The rotation of the gut is clockwise through 90°. The transverse colon lies behind the mesenteric artery. The duodenum crosses anterior to the artery.

The small intestine and its mesentery remain largely unattached to the posterior abdominal wall except by a narrow pedicle. The point of attachment corresponds to the isthmus noted during development between the fixed duodenum and the colic angle. The post-arterial segment is not attached to the posterior abdominal wall but the degree of mobility varies.

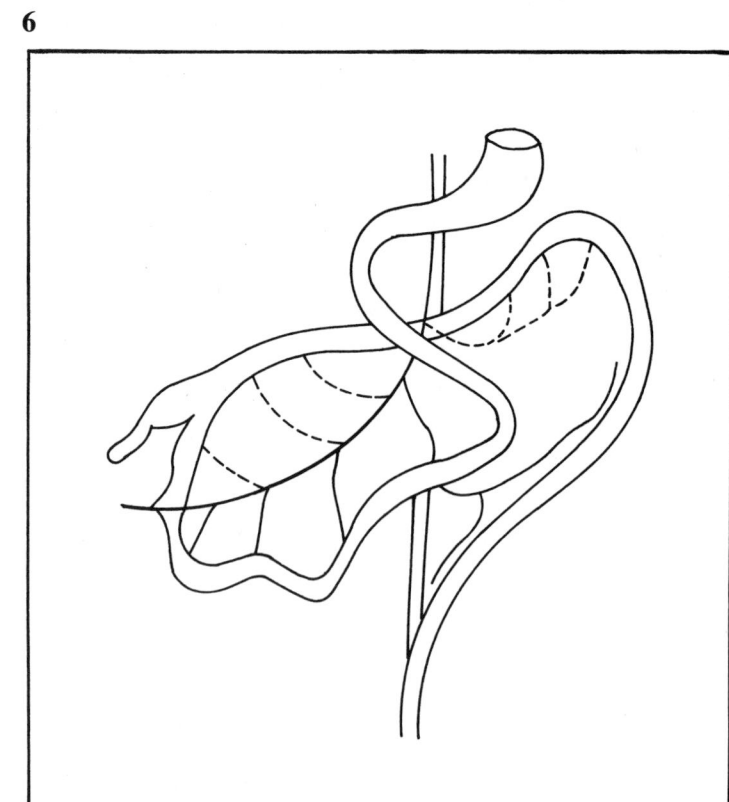

Non-rotation

7 The returning small intestine occupies the whole of the right side of the abdomen, the terminal ileum crossing the midline to enter the caecum from the right.

The caecum, which may lie in the left iliac fossa or in the pelvis, together with the whole of the large intestine lies on the left side. The ileocaecal valve lies on the medial (right) side of the caecum.

In the later (*vide* 3rd) stages when mesenteric fixation should occur, in this form of malrotation, the process may be wholly absent. A variety of anomalous types of fixation may also result.

7

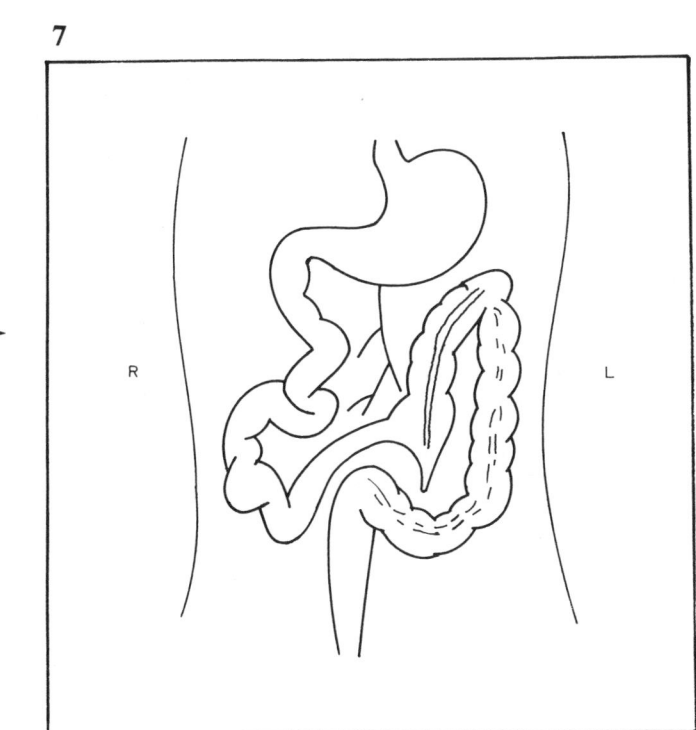

8

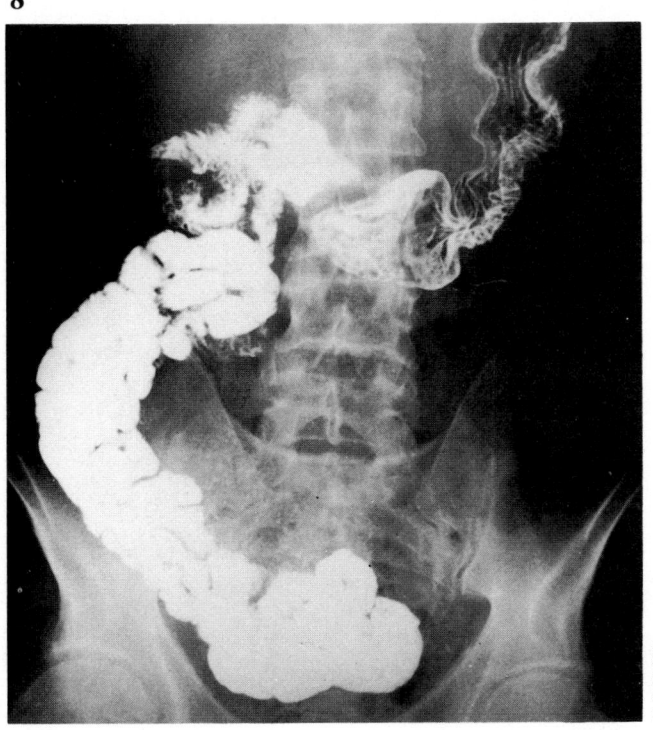

G.C.X.389

8 From an adult male. Symptomless. The duodenum and the jejunum lie to the right of the midline. The ileum is in the pelvis. The caecum and colon (gas filled) lie in the left half of the abdomen.

Volvulus

9

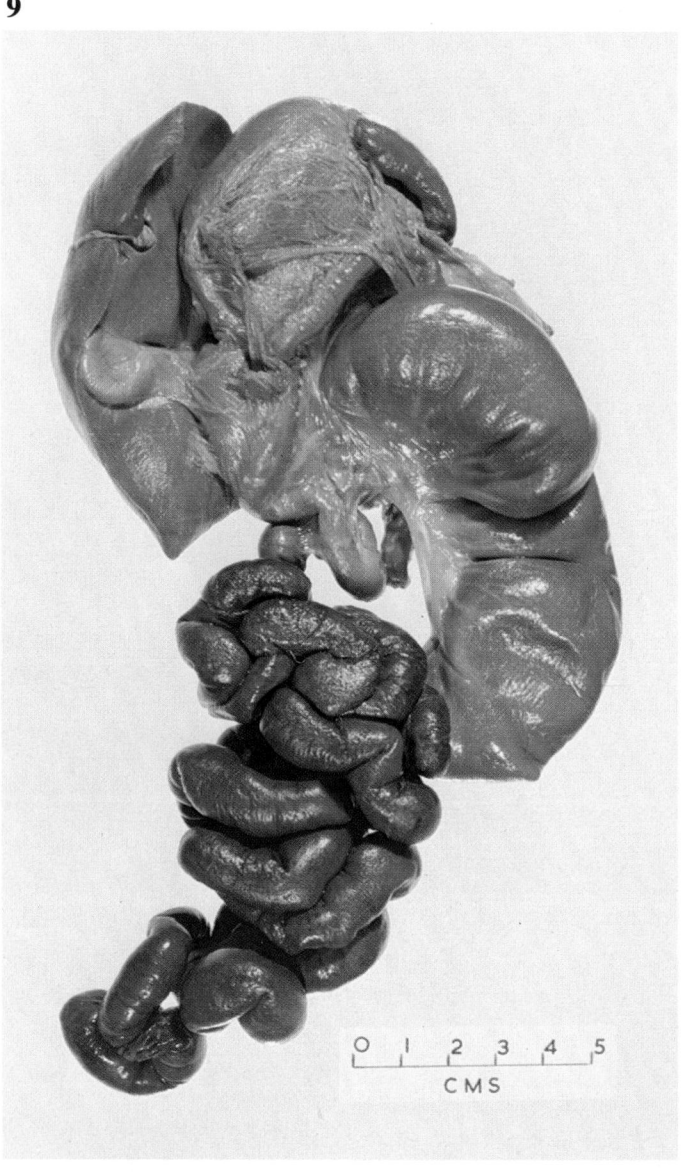

G.C.9509

9 Volvulus Neonatorum. From a neonate – 6 days persistent vomiting.

In the newborn the precipitating factor is the increase of peristalsis following first feeding. The strangulated loop includes the small and large intestine and carries a very high mortality. In Dott's series of 13 cases of malrotation, torsion occurred in 11.

10 When there is a mobile loop of midgut with a narrow pedicle as the result of malrotation, torsion is liable to occur. The risk is enhanced when the remnant of the vitello-intestinal duct remains attached to the anterior abdominal wall.

10

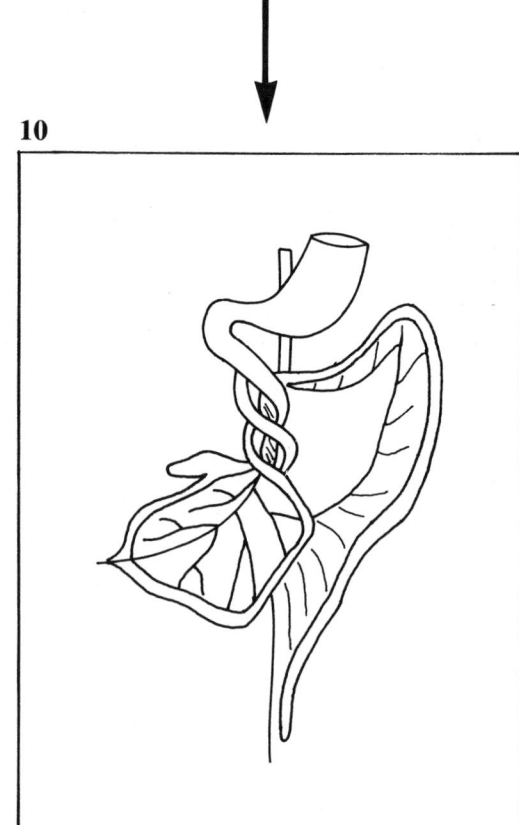

In the adult

When torsion occurs in later life, usually the caecum and terminal ileum are alone involved.

Other forms of malrotation

In addition to the two main types of malrotation already described other irregularities of rotation and fixation can occur. These follow when the caecum and large intestine re-enter the abdomen first and are followed by the small intestine as in reversed rotation but the pre-arterial segment only partially crosses to the left in front of the artery. The caecum remains in the subpyloric region. The resulting irregularity in rotation and fixation increases the risk of intestinal obstruction and volvulus.

Third stage

Derangements of the third stage are relatively common and characterised by abnormality of the intestinal attachment to the posterior abdominal wall and the formation of abnormal bands.

Faulty fixation or failure of fixation of the terminal ileum, caecum and ascending colon occurs due to either failure of elongation or excessive elongation of the colon.

Pressure on the intestine by abnormal bands or kinking of the intestine may cause intermittent or acute obstruction.

11

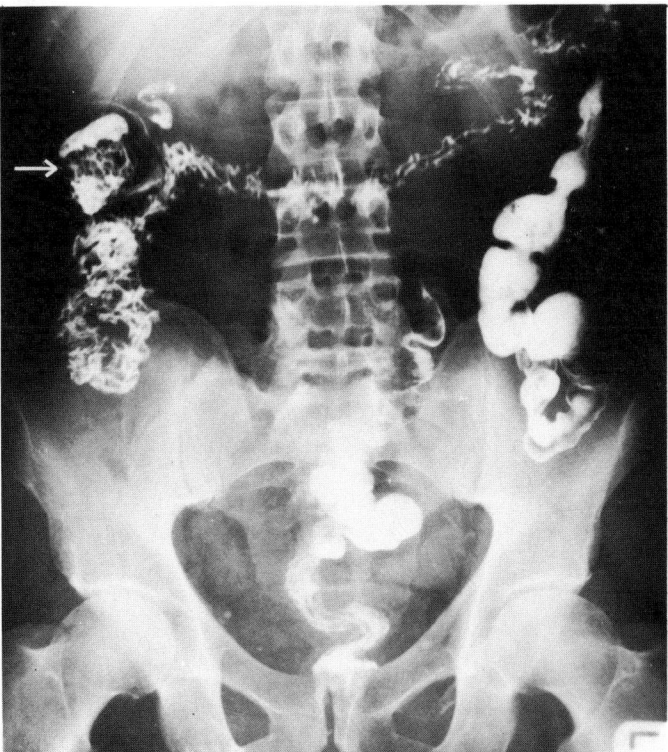

G.C.X.424

11   Caecum in the undescended position. From an adult.

Reference

DOTT, N.M. (1924) *British Journal of Surgery* XI 251.

I. S. Kirkland

This is the most common congenital anomaly of the alimentary tract and cause of intestinal obstruction in the newborn. In 33% of these infants other congenital anomalies are present. If untreated death ensues due to vomiting, dehydration or rupture 4 to 10 days after birth according to the level of obstruction.

Theories of causation

1 Between the 5th and 10th week of foetal life there is a proliferation of the intestinal epithelium which wholly occludes the previously existing lumen of the primitive gut. Thereafter, vacuoles appear in the cells. These coalesce and ultimately restore the continuity of the gut lumen by the 12th week
2 The condition is a true failure of development of the intestine occurring between the 6th and 12th week
3 There has been a localised interference with the blood supply to the intestine

In contradistinction to atresia of the intestine, oesophageal and anorectal atresias are certainly primary mal-developments.

12

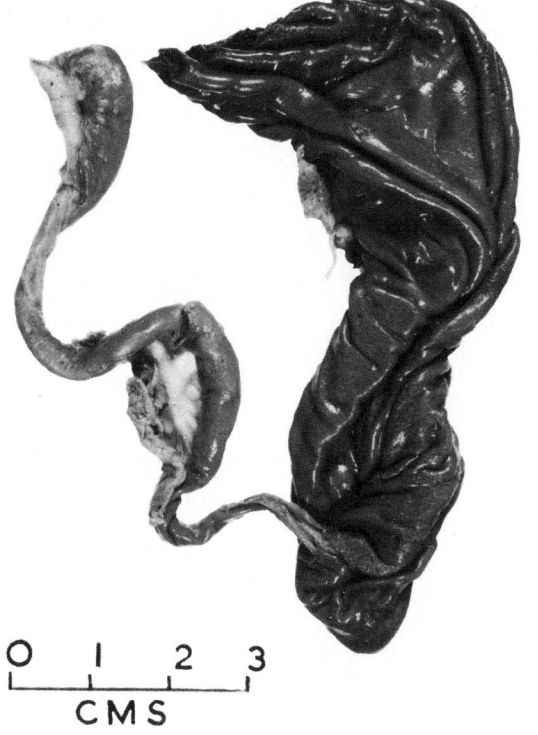

O 1 2 3
CMS

G.C.10122

12 From a full term male. There was severe vomiting and death occurred 84 hours after birth.

Post mortem specimen shows atresia of the mid ileum. The proximal intestine is distended and the distal ileum is small in calibre.

13 The malformation is of varying degree:

(**a**) The atresia is complete and there is occlusion of the lumen. The proximal segment ends as a distended blind sac connected by a cord to the distal segment which is minute in calibre

(**b**) Similar to the previous type but without a connecting cord and with a discontinuity of the mesentery

(**c**) Where the maldevelopment is of less degree resulting in only partial occlusion of the lumen, the condition is known as congenital stenosis

(**d**) The defect may be limited to the presence of a mucosal diaphragm which may be complete or more frequently has a central aperture.

The lesion may affect a solitary segment or may be multiple.

13

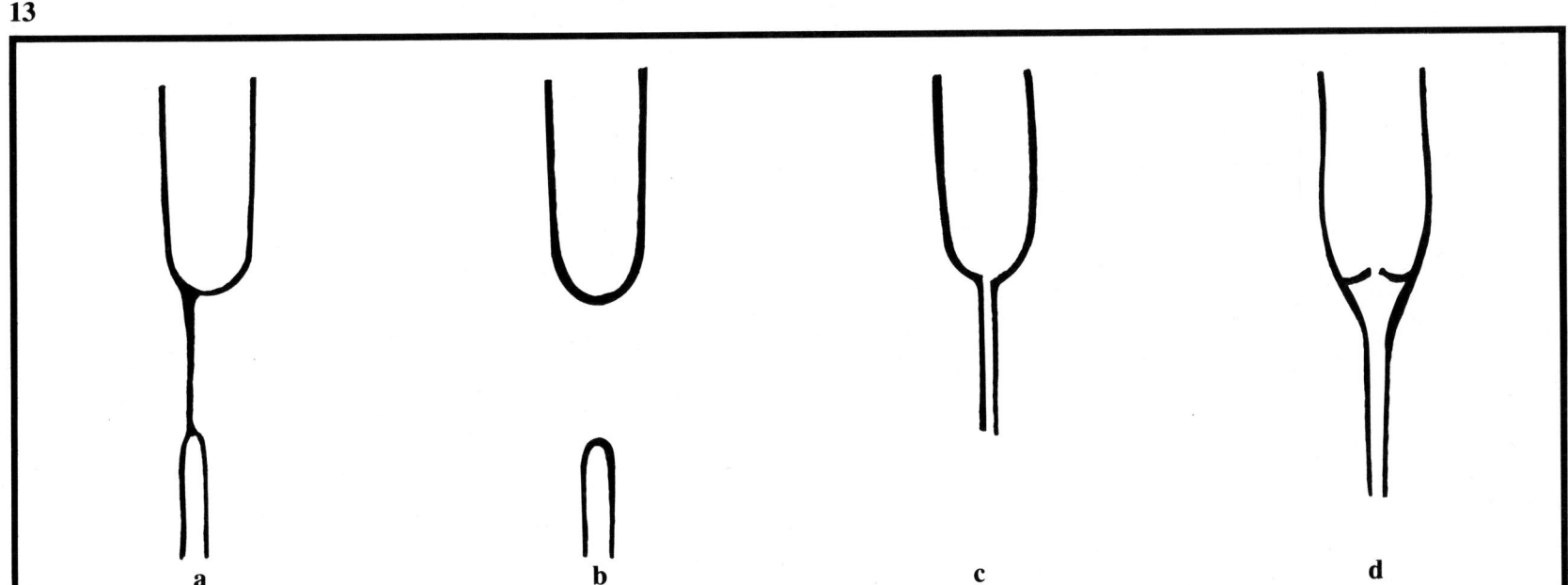

The proximal loop is distended. The wall shows hypertrophy of the musculature but due to the distension may appear to be thin. Ischaemia leading to rupture may occur. The distal segment is always minute but of normal structure and possesses a lumen.

In multiple lesions the picture presents as a succession of distinct swellings between the most proximal and most distal segments. The distal distended segment contains only mucus and a few desquamated cells.

———

Meconium consists of the secretions of the intestine, pancreas and bile with detached cells of the intestine. It also contains swallowed amniotic fluid and desquamated cutaneous cells from the skin of the foetus (vernix caseosa). The absence of cornified cells in the bowel content passed per rectum by the infant is evidence of intestinal atresia – Farber's Test.

The aetiology of the condition is unknown:
1   The error has been held to arise during the period of epithelial proliferation and revacuolation of the mucosal lining of the intestine (5 to 10 weeks)
2   It has alternatively been stated that pouching of the mucosa through the muscularis can be observed in the period of early development. If sequestration of such pouches occurs this could explain duplication or cyst formation

———————

This congenital anomaly may be present as:
1   A localised cyst or
2   A long tubular structure lying in relation to a segment of gut
Any portion of the alimentary tract from the base of the tongue to the anal canal may be affected, but most frequently the error is located in the ileum.

Whether cyst-like or tubular in character the anomalous structure is intimately attached to the normal canal and shares with it a common muscular coat. Because of this, separation of the two elements is rarely possible.

The mucosal lining of the duplicated segment is comparable to that normally found in the affected segment of gut. The occurrence of small islets of 'gastric mucosa' is associated with the risk of the development of 'peptic ulceration' (See also Meckel's diverticulum).

Where there is no communication with the alimentary canal the content is clear mucoid fluid which sometimes is under tension and may cause destruction of the lining membrane. Haemorrhage may occur into the sequestrated segment or, by causing congestion of the mucosa of the normal channel, lead to overt haemorrhage.

The duplicate loop frequently communicates with the main lumen at one or both ends and the contents will therefore be those of the alimentary canal. There may be retention with consequent complications including obstruction, anaemia and blind loop syndrome.

Cyst formation

14

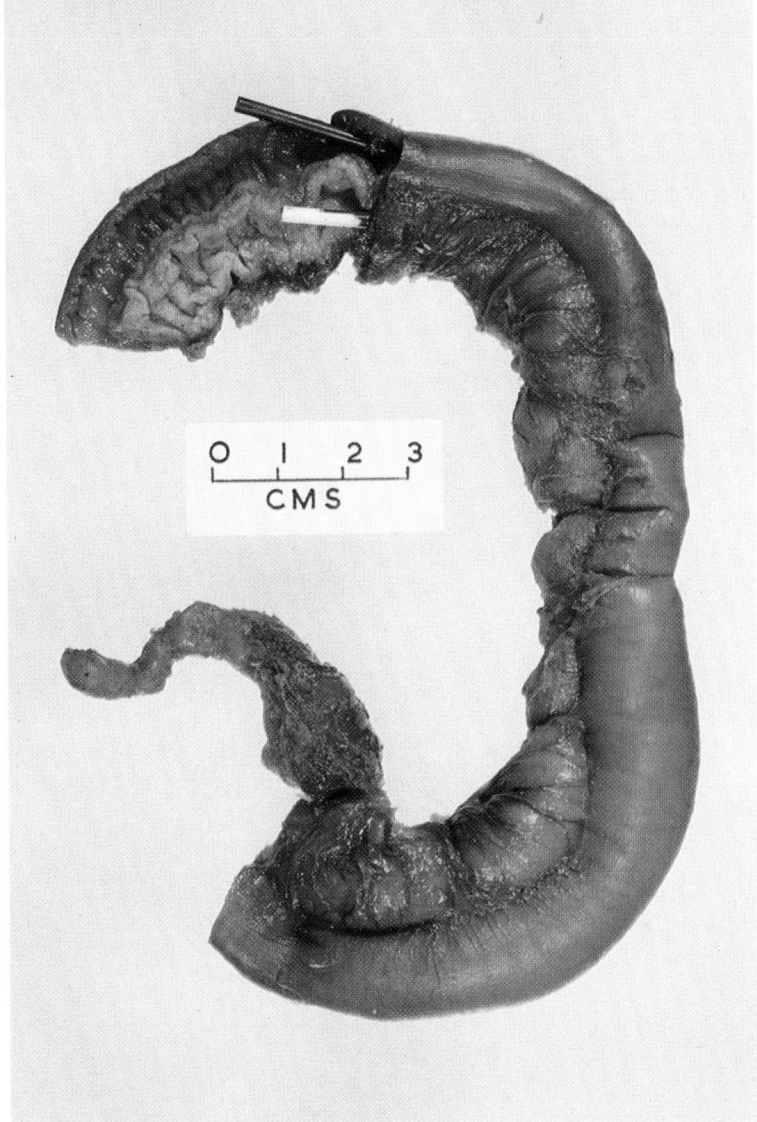

G.C.10603

Tubular formation

15

G.C.11907

14 From an infant aged 5 weeks. There was immediate postnatal vomiting but this subsided. Five weeks later vomiting returned after feeds and there was evidence of intestinal obstruction. An exploratory laparotomy revealed a volvulus of the lower segment of the small intestine. In the mesentery of the volvulus an enterogenous cyst was present.

This is a typical duplication of gut in which no communication exists between the cyst and the lumen of the gut. Note the absence of any inflammatory change in the mucosa of the cyst.

15 From a male child aged 8 weeks. At operation a loop of ileum with a narrow tubular duplication was removed. It communicates at its proximal end with the main lumen and, as is characteristic, lies on the mesenteric border of the gut. Glass rods have been inserted into the lumen of each portion at the proximal end.

Enterogenous cyst

Certain cysts found in the mesentery or lying in relation to the intestine, which are lined with mucosa of gastrointestinal type, are believed to be alternative forms of the same developmental anomaly.

In longstanding lesions such as are found in adults the mucosa within the cyst may have degenerated completely and the cyst appear only to have a fibrous wall. These features are seen in the specimen shown.

16

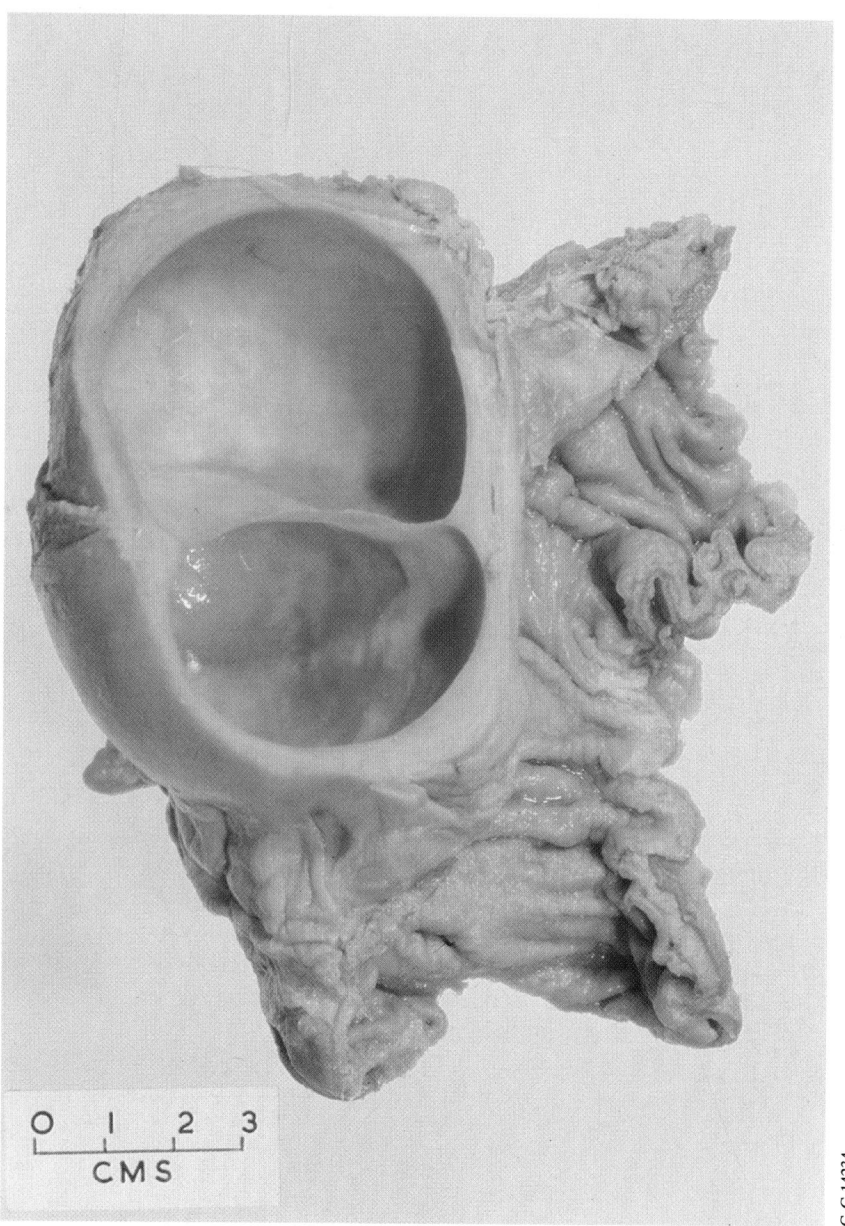

16 From a female aged 56 years in whom a palpable swelling was present in the right hypochondrium and extended into the iliac fossa.

The ascending colon shows no abnormality of its mucosal lining or other pathological change. Attached to this segment of gut is a bilocular cystic swelling the wall of which is some 2 to 5 mm thick and the external surface is smooth and the outline is ovoid on opening. Where it is attached to the wall of the intestine, the wall of the cyst and the wall of the gut appear to form an integrated tissue without any line of cleavage. The cyst measures 9 cm in its long axis.

The cyst, on histological examination, was found to have a fibrous wall without a mucosal lining. The epithelial lining has degenerated probably as the result of distension within the cyst. There is no communication with the gut. This appears to be an end result of a duplication of the ascending colon.

G.C.14234

Twinning

Complete duplication with the formation of two totally separate canals each with an independent blood supply most commonly affects the colon, rectum and anus but may involve the small intestine. This anomaly may be associated with duplication of other viscera – uterus, bladder, vagina, urethra and with gross spinal anomalies. Clearly this anomaly results from an entirely different mechanism from that resulting in the localised duplication already demonstrated. It is evidence of twinning.

17

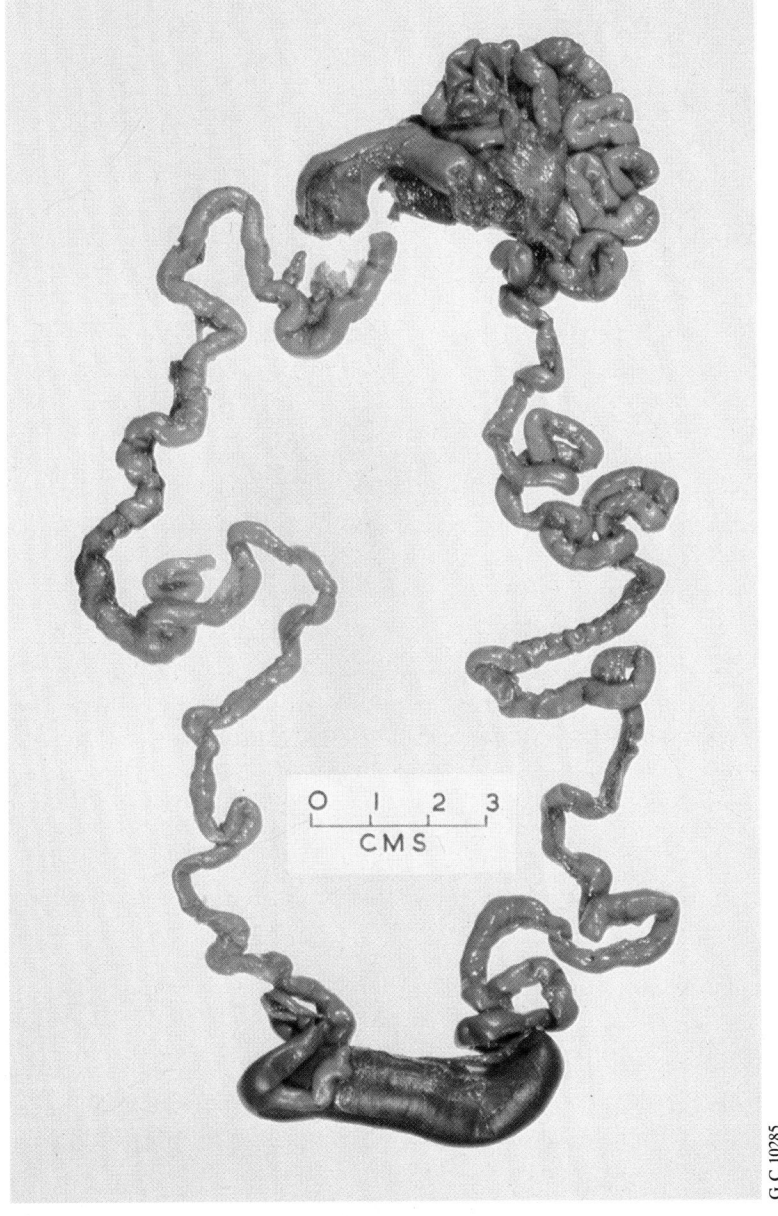

G.C.10285

For such gross malformation a disturbance in a very early stage of development must be postulated (Willis).

In certain limited duplications of the alimentary tract, e.g. oesophagus and in the lower gut, there is a linked anomaly of the notochord. This results in vertebral abnormalities including duplication.

17 From a diencephalic monster.

Reference

WILLIS, R.A. (1958) *The Borderland of Embryology and Pathology*. London, Butterworth.

I.S. Kirkland

Defects of closure

The vitello-intestinal duct is the communication between the yolk sac and the alimentary tract extending from the apex of the midgut loop. The duct normally becomes occluded during the 7th week of foetal life and the connection between the gut and umbilicus disappears. Failure of closure of the duct in whole or part results in a series of developmental anomalies including Meckel's diverticulum illustrated overleaf.

1

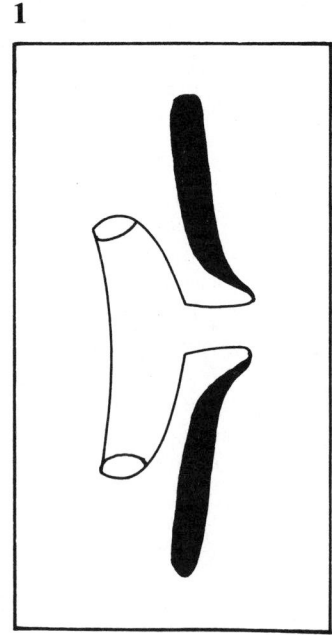

2

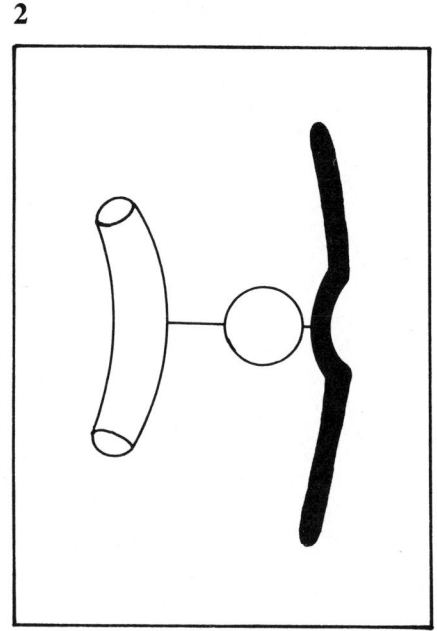

1 The duct remains patent as a fistula from which there is a discharge of meconium.

2 A segment of the tract becomes isolated and persists but retains an attachment both to the umbilicus and to the ileum. The cyst may undergo strangulation.

3

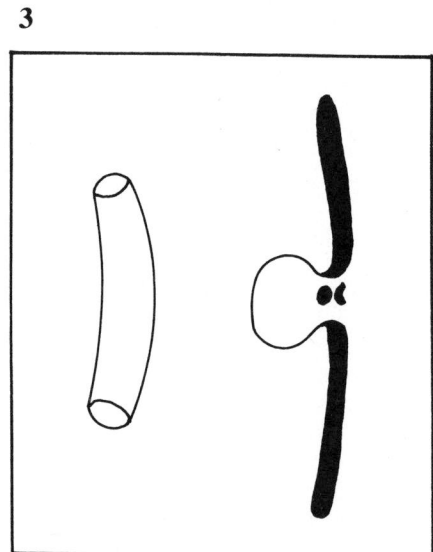

4

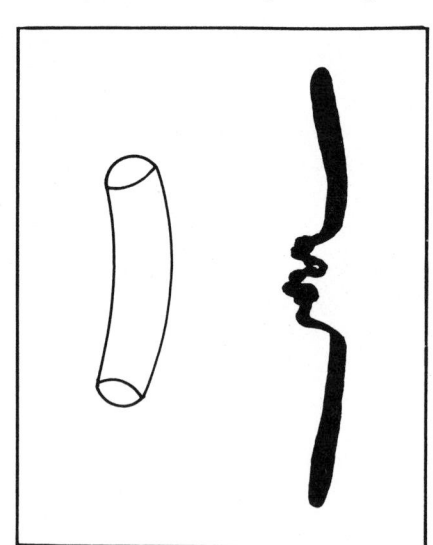

3 The distal portion of the duct may persist and form a sinus with a persistent mucus discharge. Alternatively a subumbilical cyst has ruptured and a fistulous channel is formed.

4 A small patch of residual mucosa may persist at the umbilicus and have the appearance of a granuloma or an aggregation of small mucous polyps.

Cyst formation

Persistence of peripheral portions of the duct is commonly associated with delayed separation of the umbilical cord.

5

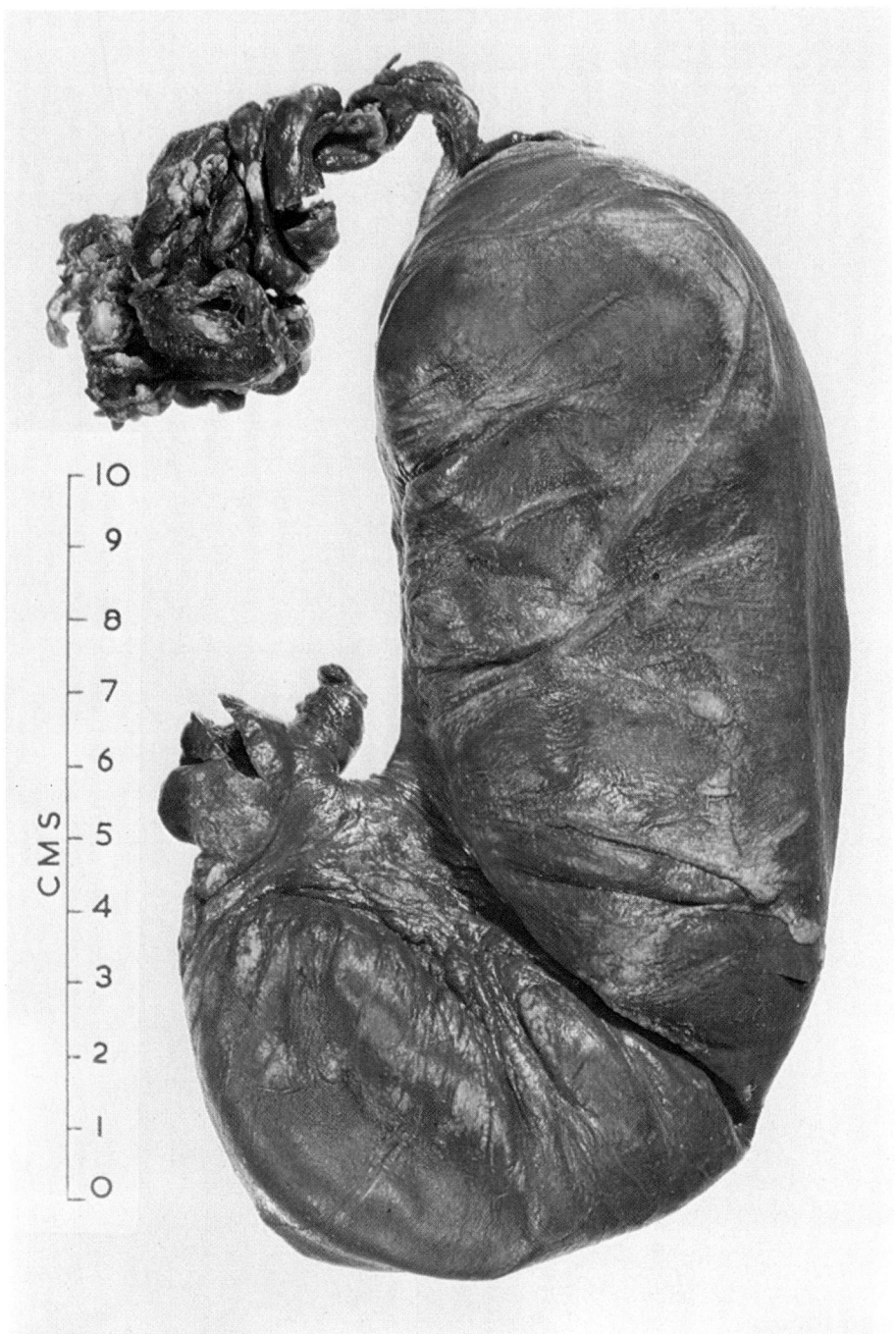

5 Male aged 10 years. Five day history of abdominal pain, distension and vomiting. At operation blood-stained fluid was found in the peritoneum. The cyst was found to be attached to the distal ileum and had undergone torsion. There was no communication with the gut and the cyst was successfully removed.

The presence of a persistent vitello-intestinal tract may lead to torsion of the intestine (volvulus), or cause strangulation of a loop of intestine.

Meckel's diverticulum

6

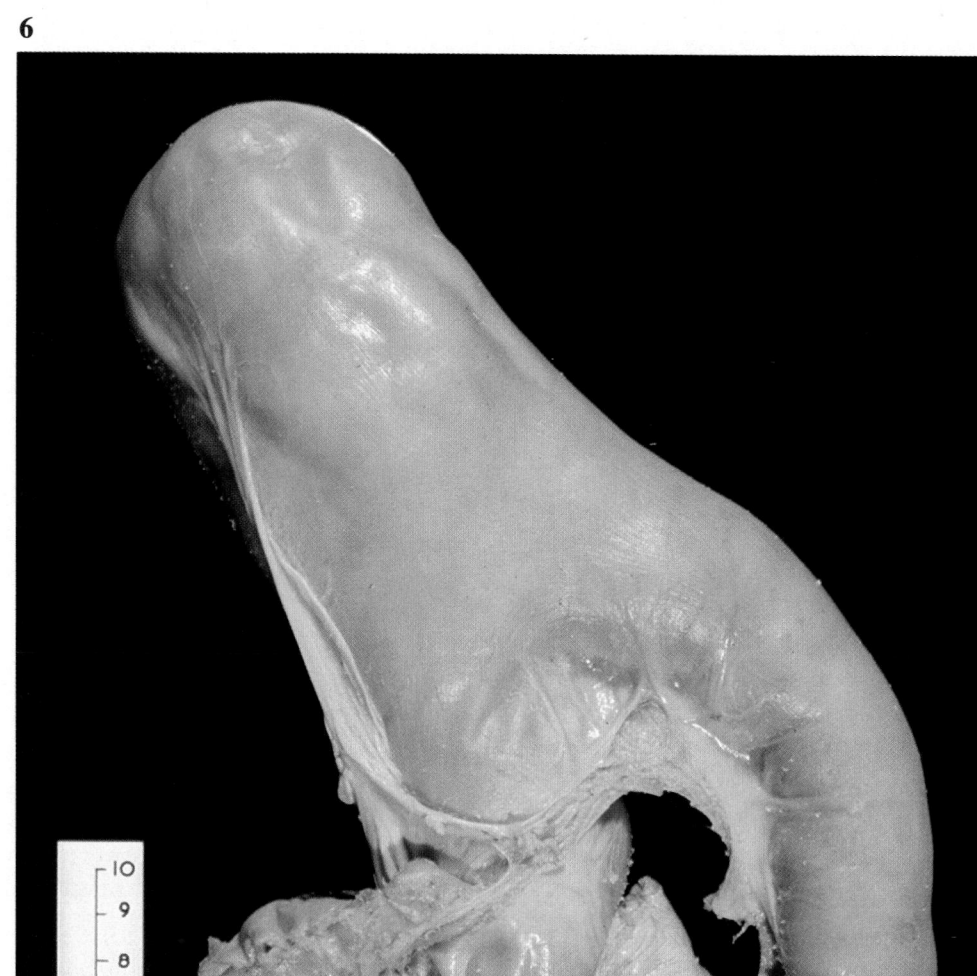

G.C.13230

6   From an adult male. This specimen was obtained at autopsy from a patient who had had a lobectomy for long-standing tuberculosis. His general condition was poor. At no time were there any clinical features suggestive of an abdominal lesion. The Meckel's diverticulum is 5cm in diameter, 10cm long, and possesses a rudimentary mesentery. Note the enormous size of the stoma.

The description of this diverticulum was made by Meckel in 1809 but it had been recorded by John Hunter in 1763.

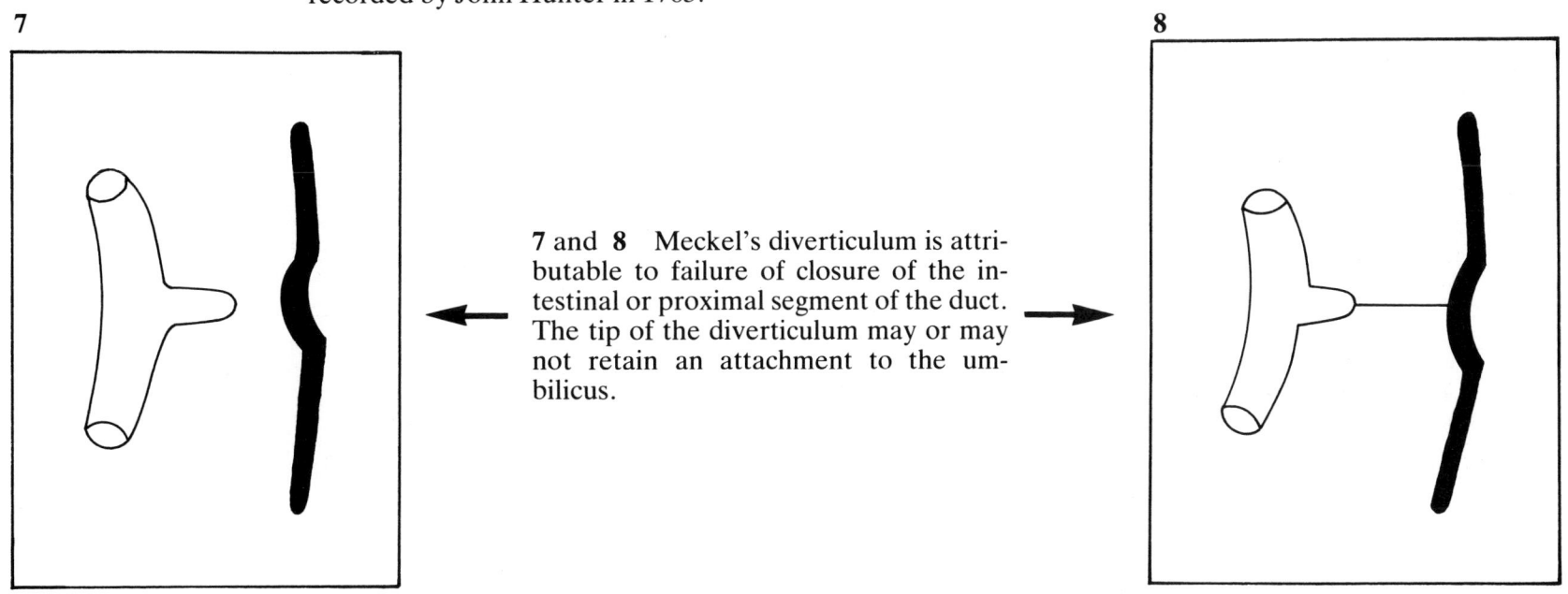

7 and **8**   Meckel's diverticulum is attributable to failure of closure of the intestinal or proximal segment of the duct. The tip of the diverticulum may or may not retain an attachment to the umbilicus.

This diverticulum is found on the antimesenteric border of the lower ileum – in the adult approximately 75 cm proximal to the ileocaecal junction. The diverticulum varies in size from a small pouch to a giant 'cystic' swelling. The stoma of the diverticulum is usually wide so that contents pass in and out freely. It possesses the same structure as the normal ileum.

Torsion

Rarely the apical adhesion to the umbilicus predisposes the diverticulum to torsion.

9   From an adult. (Clinical notes are not available.) The Meckel's diverticulum had retained its attachment to the anterior abdominal wall and undergone torsion and strangulation.

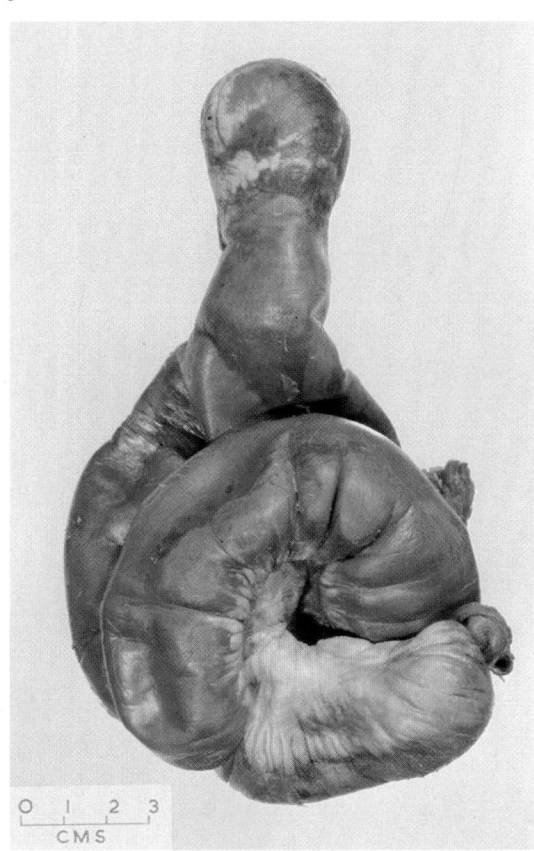

221

Meckel's diverticulum *(Continued)*

Inflammation

The Meckel's diverticulum may be the site of inflammation and become adherent either to adjacent loops or to the mesentery. The inflammation may be acute and proceed to abscess formation or peritonitis. This is comparable to and often misdiagnosed as appendicitis.

10

10   Male aged 43 years. History of 3 days acute abdominal pain mimicking appendicitis. The Meckel's diverticulum is adherent to the under surface of the mesentery of the ileum. The apex of the diverticulum is inflamed and an abscess has formed. Arrow marks the site of biopsy.

Obstruction

11

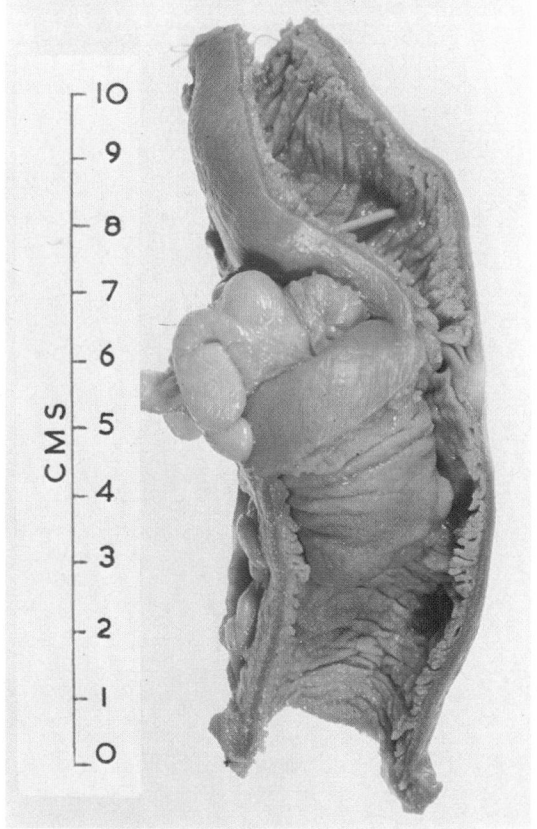

When a Meckel's diverticulum is present either by reason of its primary attachment to the umbilicus or consequent upon secondary peritoneal adhesions from a localised inflammation, obstruction of adjacent loops of intestine by compression or kinking can occur. Obstruction may also arise as the result of an intussusception commencing in a Meckel's diverticulum.

11   Female aged 52 years. History of 1 year occasional abdominal pain and vomiting. Loss of weight. Achlorhydria. At operation only an intussusception commencing in a Meckel's diverticulum was found. Examination of the specimen shows an invagination of the diverticulum. There is hypertrophy of the gut proximal to the lesion thus indicating a chronic or recurrent partial obstruction. The actual cause of the intussusception was a small leiomyoma at the neck of the Meckel's diverticulum (not visible in the specimen).

Peptic ulceration

Islets of heterotopic gastric mucosa may be present in a Meckel's diverticulum – their secretions can cause peptic ulceration in the mucosa of the diverticulum or adjacent ileum (see Section 14 EA). Less frequently nodules of pancreatic tissue may be found in the wall.

Illustrative case

A female aged 42 years complained of pain in the right lower abdomen. At laparotomy a Meckel's diverticulum was found and was resected. Part of it was inflamed and covered by congested fibrotic peritoneum. Most of the 3 cm long diverticulum was lined by normal ileal mucosa, but there was an additional inflamed locule which also showed gastric mucosa and pancreatic tissue. In the locule acid peptic secretions had caused inflammation and ulceration of the adjoining ileal mucosa, whilst part of the pancreas was acutely inflamed and necrotic.

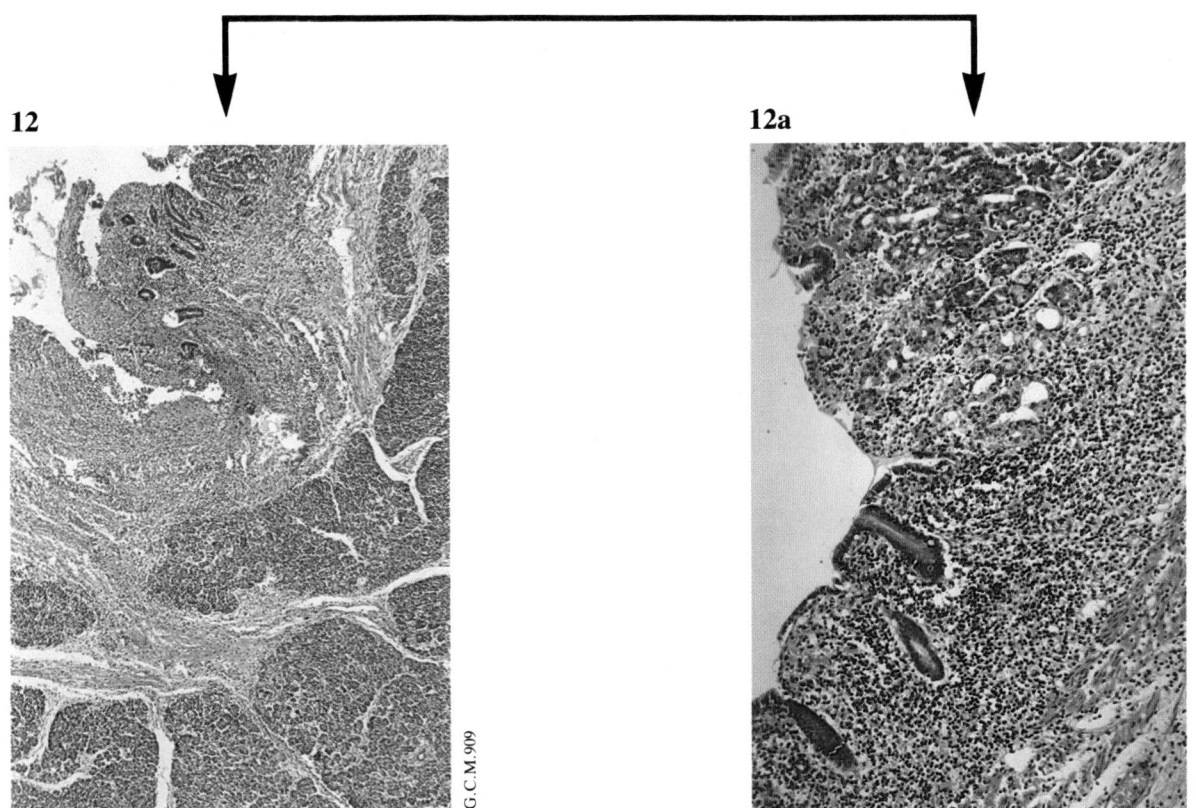

12 In this diverticulum both pancreatic tissue and gastric mucosa were present. The illustration shows peptic ulceration in a portion of the ileal - type mucosa overlying pancreatic tissue. *(H&E ×40)*

12a Junction of inflamed gastric and ileal-type mucosa. The secretions of the gastric mucosa have inflamed the intestinal mucosa and caused total villous atrophy. *(H&E ×100)*

Complications in Meckel's diverticulum are principally seen in childhood although the specimens illustrated have been obtained mostly from adult patients.

I.S. Kirkland

Congenital anomalies of the rectum, anus and bladder are amongst the most serious and grave malformations. They may lead to acute obstruction in the neonate. They present problems of greatest technical difficulty to the surgeon and all too often the end result is impaired function and incontinence associated with life long social embarrassment.

Congenital malformations are variously estimated to occur once in every 5000 to 10000 births and show a slight male preponderance. It is important that each newborn child should be examined with care so that the lesion is recognised immediately.

These anomalies may either be diagnosed or suspected antenatally from the 16th to the 20th weeks by:
1 The presence of hydramnios.
2 Ultrasonic screening.
3 Maternal serum or amniotic fluid levels of alpha foetoprotein.

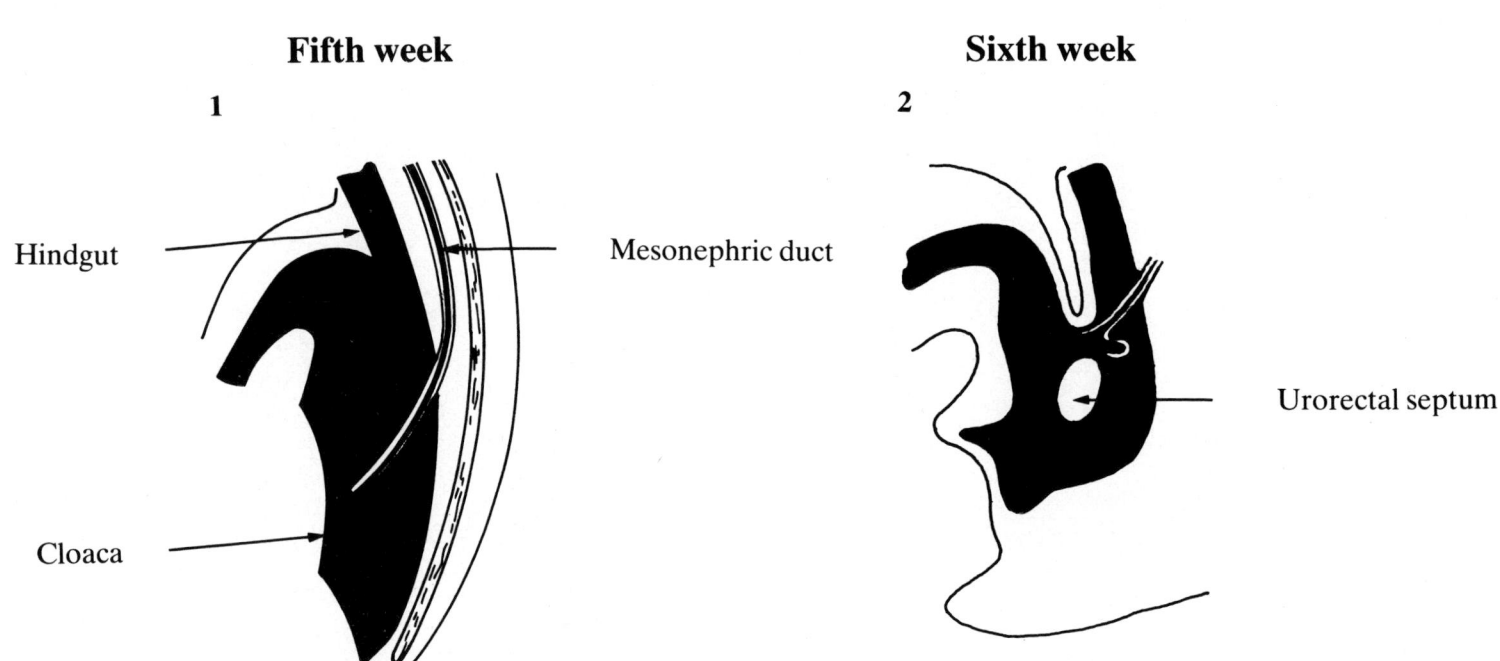

Fifth week

1

Hindgut

Cloaca

Mesonephric duct

Sixth week

2

Urorectal septum

1 By the end of the 5th week a cloaca is present. There is a wide communication between the cloaca and the hindgut. The mesonephric (Wolffian) ducts open into the cloaca. There is no external communication between the cloaca and the exterior.

2 During the 6th week there is commencing separation of the hindgut and the primitive bladder by the formation of the urorectal (cloacal) septum. The ureteric buds are now present at the caudal end of the mesonephric ducts.

Cloacal division

The embryological changes leading to the development of the rectum, anus, bladder and urethra are complex, occurring chiefly between the 5th and 9ths weeks of foetal life. Initially the primitive urogenital tract and the hindgut communicate with a common cavity – the cloaca. The separation of the parts and the development of the individual structures – rectum, anus, bladder and urethra – occur synchronously.

Developmental anomalies are numerous and arise consequent upon either failure of development, persistence of foetal connection or abnormal growth during the 5th to 9th weeks of foetal life. For clarity of presentation the subject matter is set out in sections. It must be appreciated that this division is artificial and that combinations of anomalies occur.

Ninth week

Seventh week

4

3

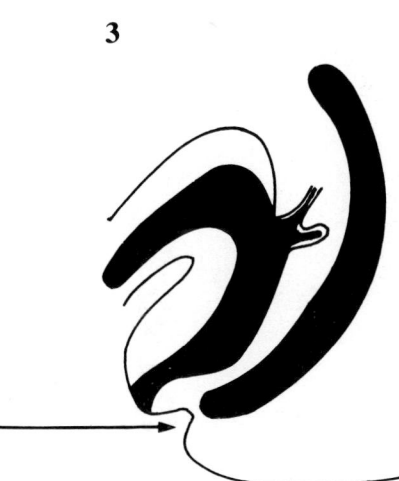

Proctodeum

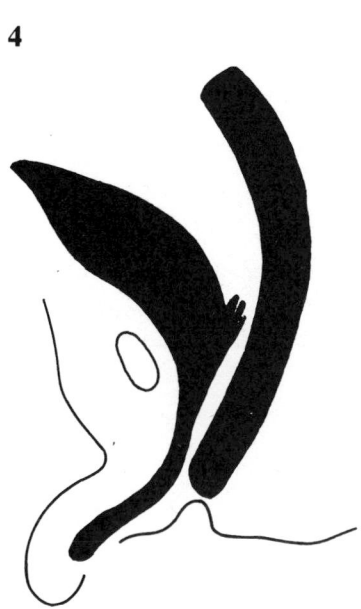

3 By the 7th week the hindgut has become separated from the urogenital sinus which also at this time establishes a communication with the surface (urethra).

4 By the 9th week the hindgut has established a junction with the proctodeum. A definite bladder has now been formed. The allantois has largely disappeared and the proximal urethra has developed.

225

Hindgut

Rectum

5

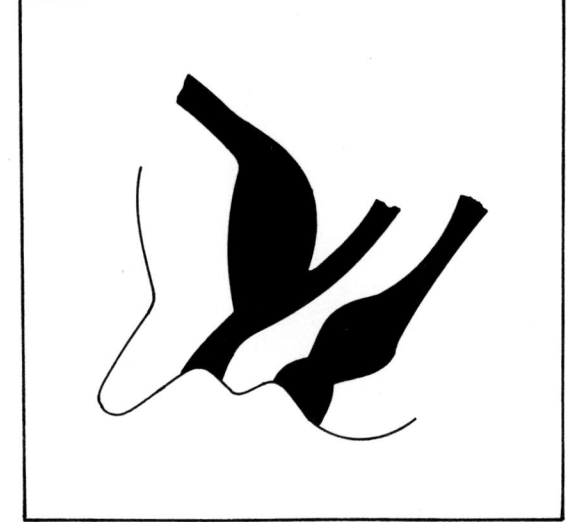

The terminal part of the hindgut is relatively dilated and between the 4th and 6th week communicates freely with the cloaca but separation is completed by the 7th week.

5 In the 7-week embryo the hindgut will be seen to extend caudally as the rectal tube. This prolongation shows two areas of spindle-shaped enlargement the first of which later develops into the rectal ampulla while the lower swelling corresponds to the upper part of the anal canal and lower rectum.

Proctodeum

6 During the 5th and 6th weeks development of the lower anterior abdominal wall occurs and the cloacal membrane passes caudally and dorsally to form the primitive perineum.

6 Point of future division

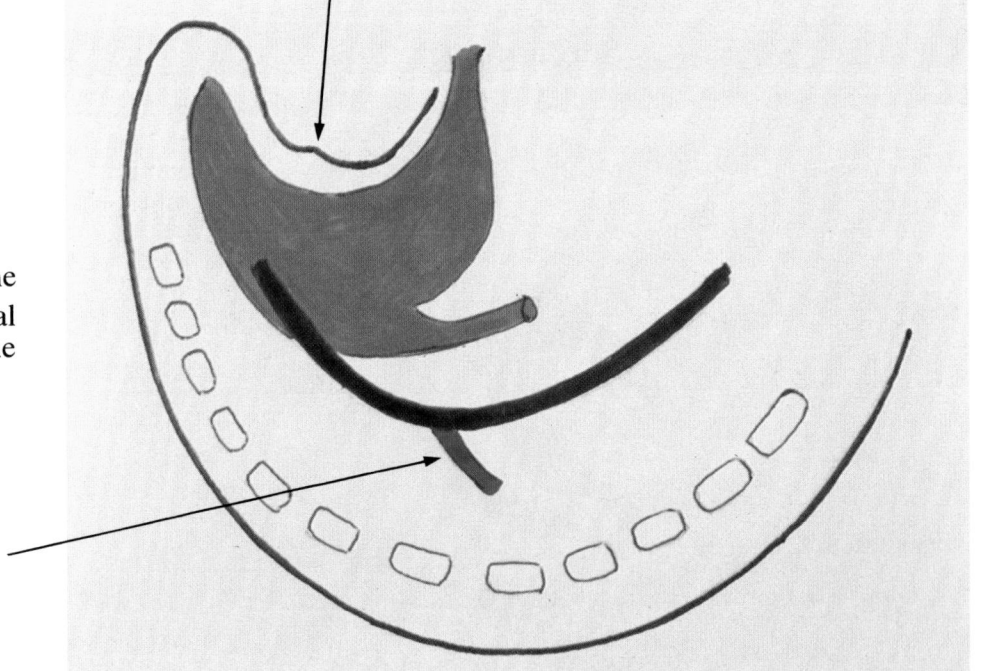

Ureter

By the 7th week the primitive perineum is divided into two parts (**6**). That portion lying anterior to the line of separation of the urogenital sinus and the rectum is concerned with the formation of the urethra. The area lying posteriorly is the site of development of the proctodeum. During the 8th week a localised area shows epithelial proliferation indicated on the surface as the anal dimple. Here this extends deeply and comes in contact with and then establishes communication with the hindgut during the 9th week of foetal life thus forming the anal canal.

Imperforate anus

Imperforate anus (ano-rectal atresia) occurs in a variety of forms depending on the precise nature of the developmental anomalies and the level of the obstruction. Ladd and Gross (1934) introduced a classification of these anomalies and described the four major varieties.

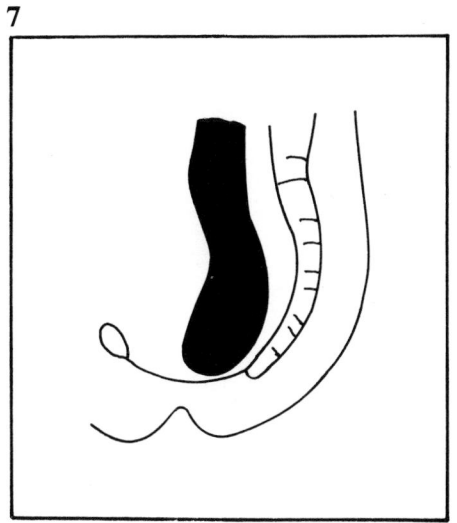

7 The hindgut may fail to descend ending blindly in the hollow of the sacrum above the level of the levator ani muscles. There is a mass of tissue between the blind end of the gut and the anal dimple.

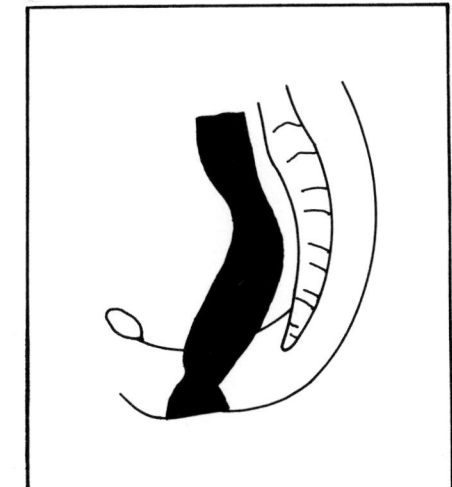

8 The rectal tube may fail to develop or show narrowing.

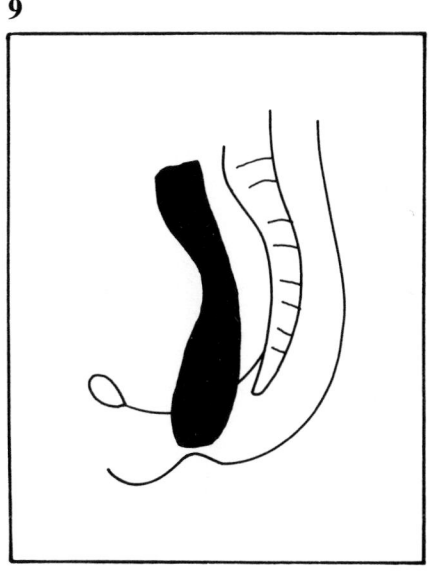

9 The proctodeum may fail to develop adequately or, if formed, fail to communicate with the rectum. In some instances a communication is established but is narrow.

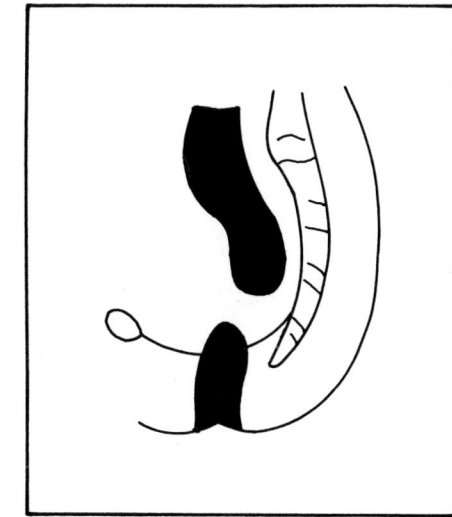

10 High rectal atresia with normal anal canal and lower rectum.

The concurrence of imperforate anus and fistula formation is found in over 50% of cases.
(45% male, 64% female – Ladd and Gross).
These cases show variations both of the degree of failure of development of the gut and the type of fistula present.

Fistula formation

6th and 7th weeks

11

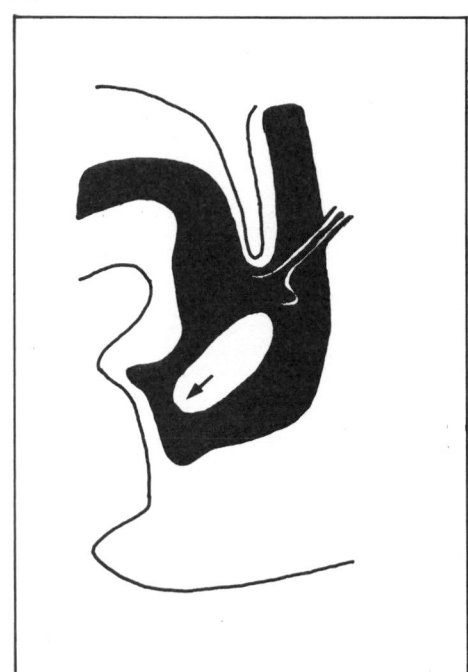

The cloaca is the cavity originally common to both the urogenital and alimentary tracts. During the 5th to 7th weeks separation of the primitive bladder and gut occurs. On the lateral walls of the cloaca ridges develop during the 5th week. These are joined above, at the point corresponding to the junction of the urogenital sinus and the intestine, by a transverse saddle-type ridge. By the approximation of these ridges a septum is formed closing the communication between the urogenital sinus and the rectum from above downwards. This is known as the urorectal or cloacal septum. A small residual communication, commonly termed the 'cloacal duct', may persist for a short further period. The process of closure is completed by the 7th week. Failure of closure of this duct is the explanation of congenital fistulae.

Residual duct

12

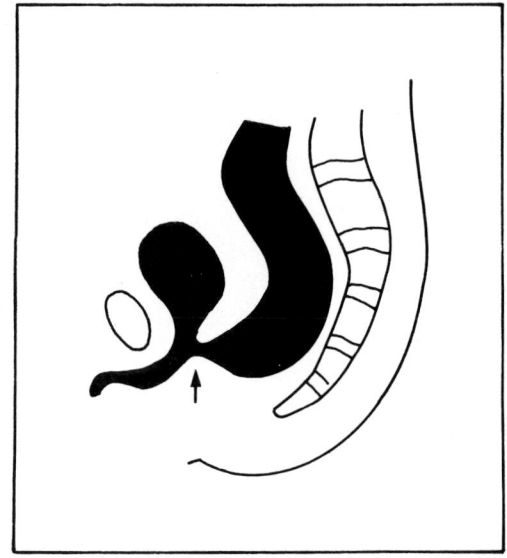

11   Caudal end of urorectal septum.

12   Cloacal duct.

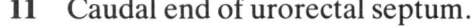

The fistulae may be between:

13

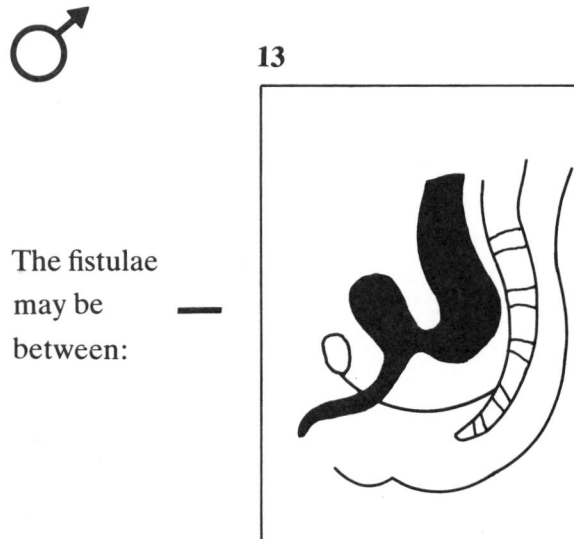

13   Rectum and bladder.

14

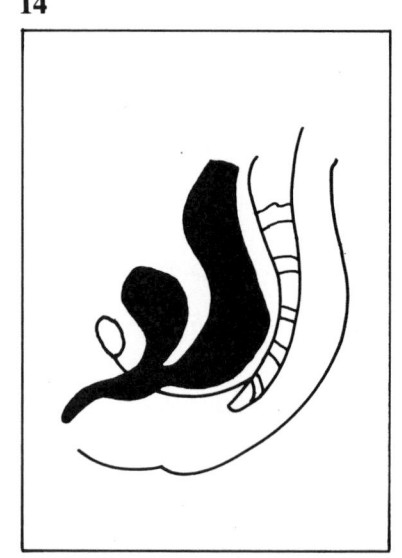

14   Rectum and prostatic urethra (most frequently encountered variety).

15

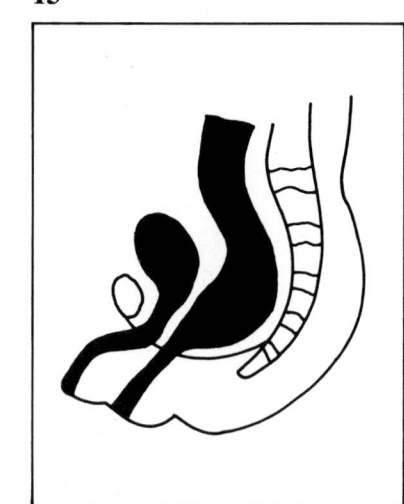

15   Rectum and perineum.

Fistulae of the bladder and urethra are commonly called high fistulae and lie above the plane of the levator ani muscles. Perineal fistulae (low) may open close to the anal orifice or, more frequently, lie adjacent to the scrotal–perineal angle.

In surgical practice the anomalies are classified according to whether the bowel ends above or below the level of the levator ani muscles – high and low. Anomalies ending above the levator ani require to be treated by a major combined technique (Abdomino-perineal). Those ending below the level of the levator ani may be corrected by a perineal operation. The external sphincter is always present and develops with the proctodeum.

16

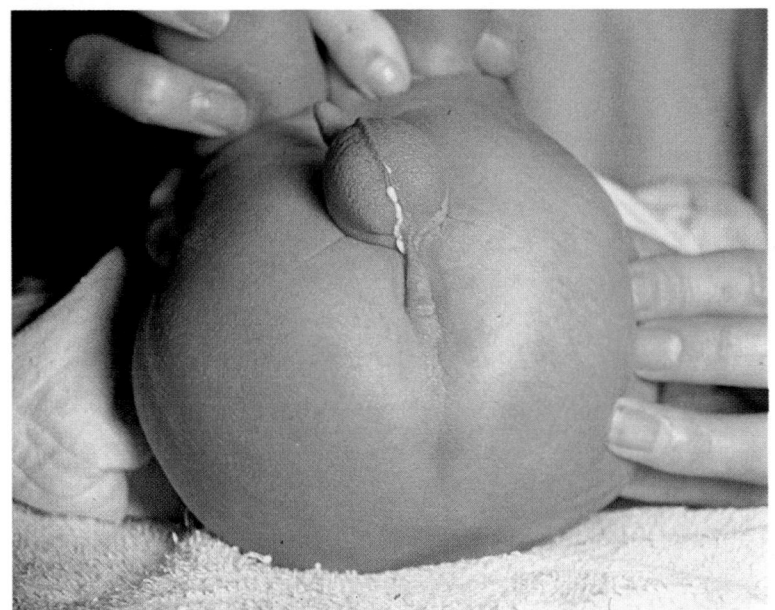

16 High anorectal atresia with a potential scrotal fistula.

17

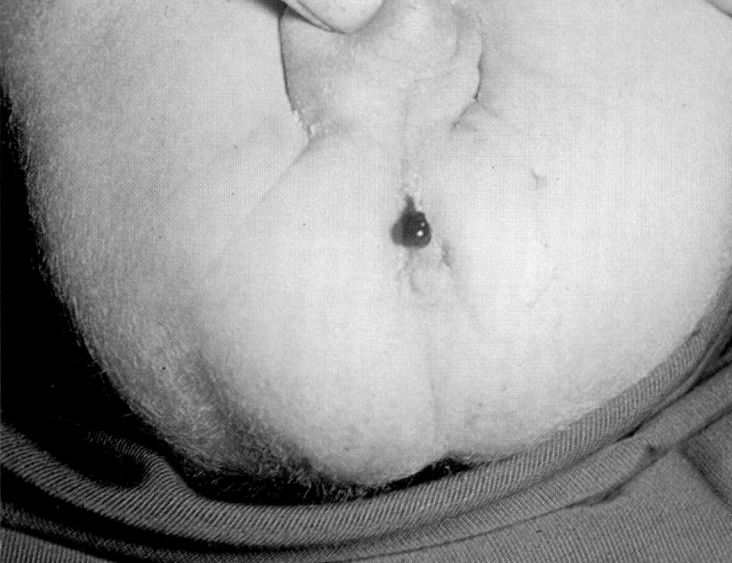

17 Low anorectal atresia with a perineal fistula.

Fistula formation *(Continued)*

♀ # Development and derivatives of the paramesonephric (Müllerian) duct

The paramesonephric (Müllerian) ducts first appear during the 6th week of foetal life and are derived from the coelomic mesothelium. The paramesonephric ducts are initially solid strands of cells lying adjacent to the mesonephric (Wolffian) ducts. They become attached to the urogenital sinus in the 8th week. The solid strands of paramesonephric tissue become canalised from above downwards (from the 8th week). The cephalic portions of the paramesonephric ducts give rise to the Fallopian tubes. Caudally the paramesonephric ducts are fused and by further development at this site the primitive uterus and vagina are derived and are interposed between the primitive bladder and rectum. The remnants of the mesonephric ducts may be seen in the broad ligaments and wall of uterus.

18

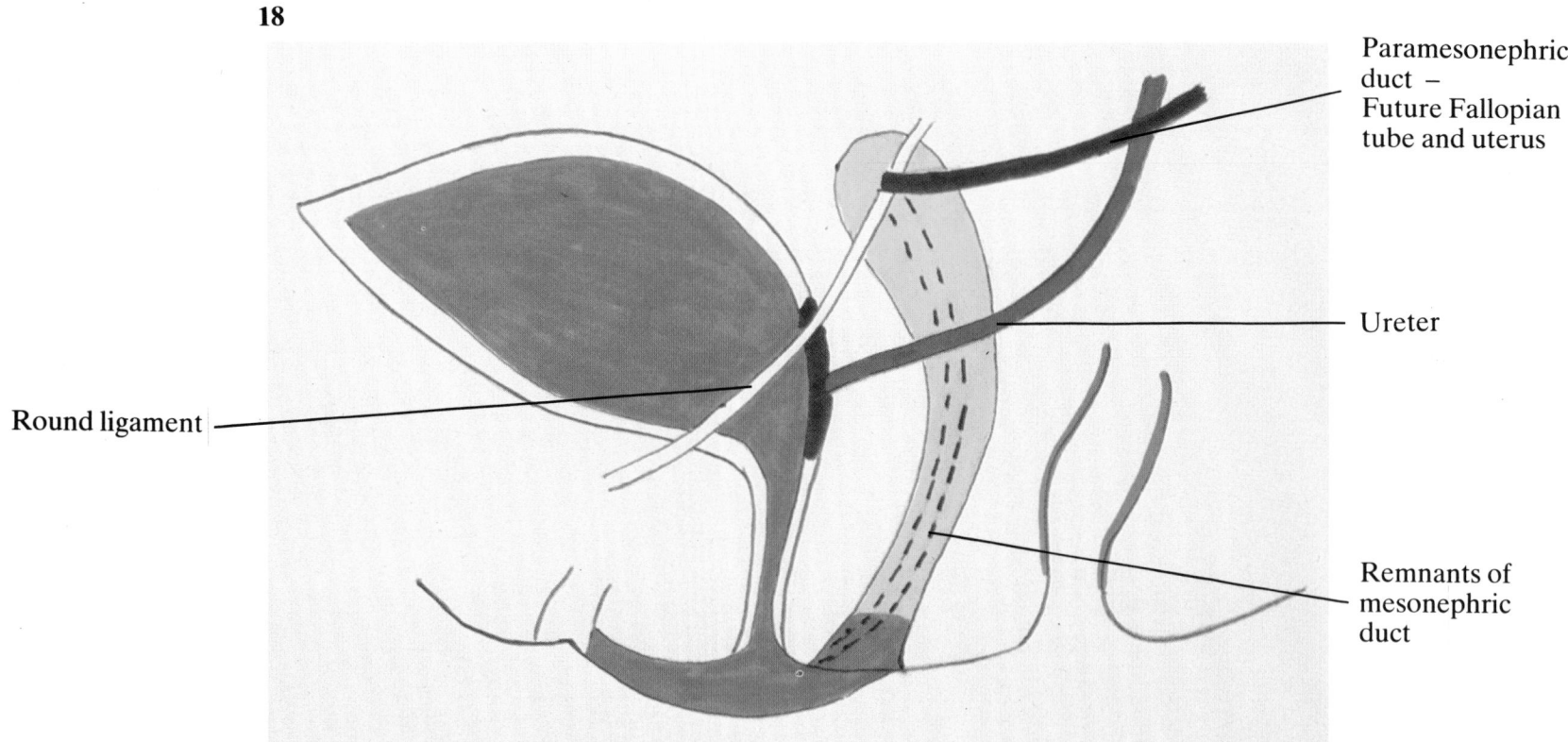

Paramesonephric duct – Future Fallopian tube and uterus

Ureter

Round ligament

Remnants of mesonephric duct

19

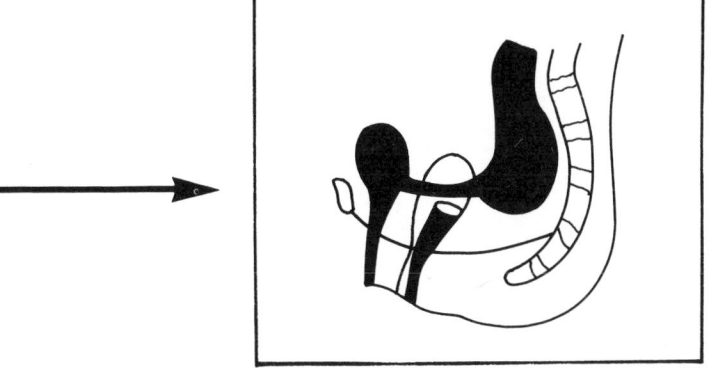

19 Since in the female the uterus and vagina are interposed between the rectum (posteriorly) and the bladder and urethra (anteriorly), rectovesical fistulae are rare, and only occur in the presence of a bifid uterus and vagina.

20

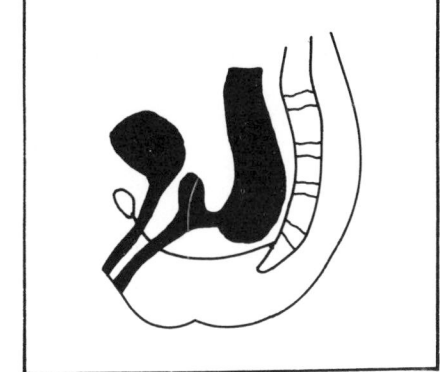

20 The more frequent lesion is the presence of a fistula between the rectum and vagina. The fistula may be high opening into the fornix.

Perineal fistulae rarely occur in the female.

21

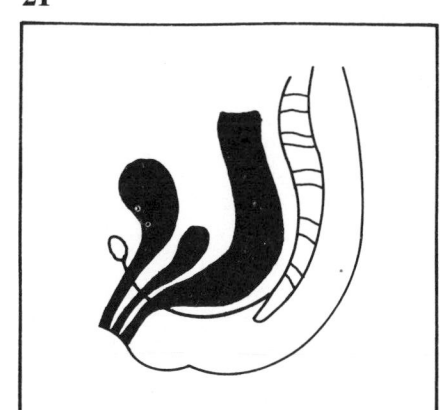

21 The fistula is more often at a lower level in the vestibule.

Rectovestibular fistula

22

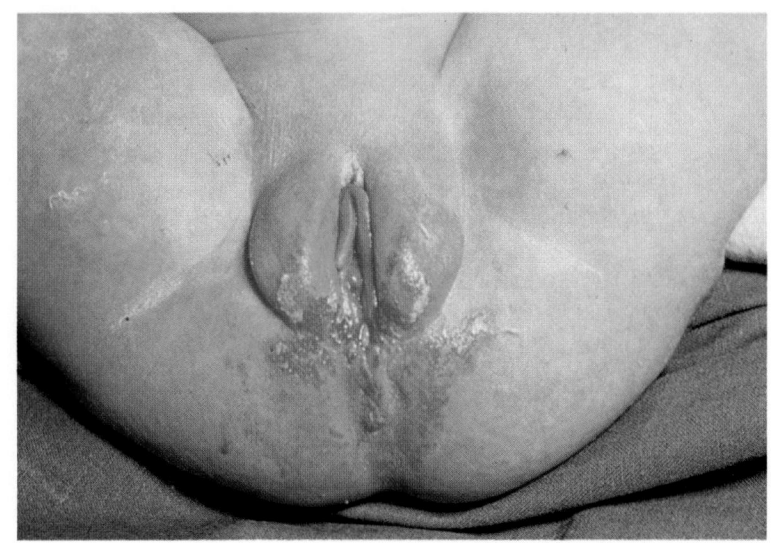

G.C.P.216

Associated lesions

Anomalies of the rectum and anus are frequently associated with congenital abnormalities in other systems (30%).

– Of the urogenital tract

23 In 20% of cases the anomaly of the rectum and anus is associated with an abnormality of the genito-urinary tract such as ectopia vesicae. These are discussed in congenital anomalies of the renal tract.

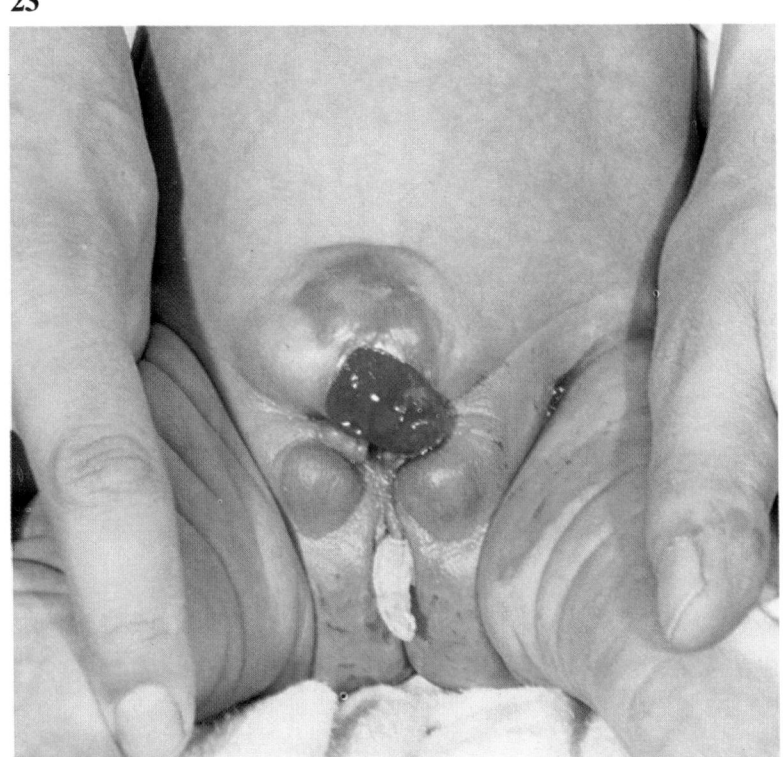

– Of the sacrum

24 An associated anomaly with hindgut maldevelopment is absence of part or all of the sacrum.

25 Where the sacrum is defective the levator ani muscle also is imperfect.

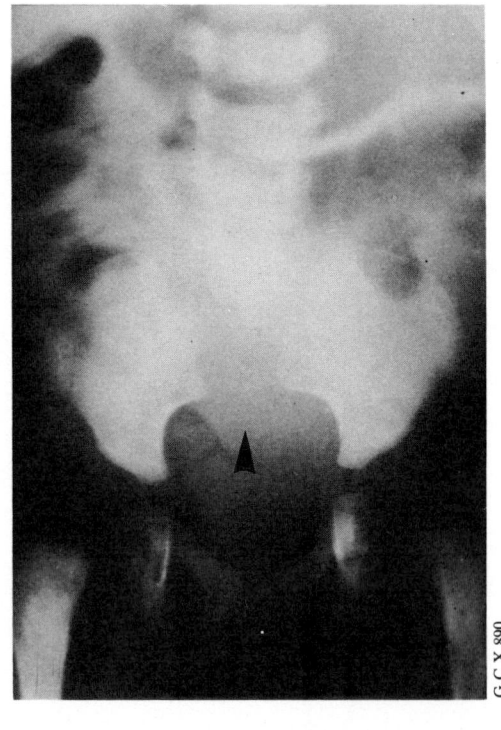

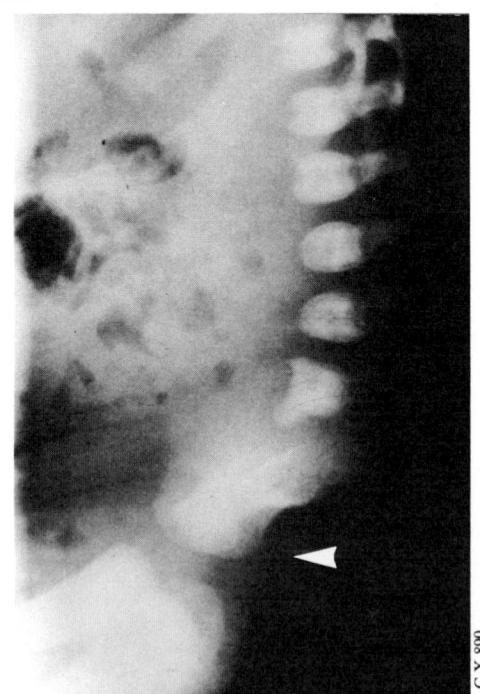

Classification

In 1970 a classification was introduced for international use by Santulli *et al.* (see below). This enabled variants and anomalies to be identified but the broad original classification of Ladd and Gross remains valid.

Male	Female
High (supralevator)	
(1) Anorectal agenesis	(1) Same
(a) Without fistula	(a) Without fistula
(b) With fistula	(b) With fistula
(i) Rectourethral	(i) Rectovaginal-high
(ii) Rectovesical	(ii) Rectocloacal
	(iii) Rectovesical
(2) Rectal atresia, miscellaneous Imperforate anal membrane Cloacal Exstrophy Others	(2) Same

Male	Female
Low (translevator)	
(1) At normal anal site	(1) Same
(a) Anal stenosis	(a) Same
(b) Covered anus-complete	(b) Same
(2) At perineal site	(2) Same
(a) Anocutaneous fistula (covered anus-incomplete)	(a) Same
(b) Anterior perineal anus	(b) Same
	(3) At vulvar site
	(a) Anovulvar fistula
	(b) Anovestibular fistula
	(c) Vestibular anus

References

LADD, W.E. and GROSS, R.E. (1934) Congenital malformations of anus and rectum. *American Journal of Surgery* **23,** 167.

SANTULLI, T.V., KIESEWETTER, W.B. and BILL, A.H. JR (1970) Anorectal anomalies: a suggested international classification. *Journal of Pediatric Surgery* **5,** 281.

Ian S. Kirkland

A diverticulum is an outward pouching of the wall of a hollow viscus. Diverticula occur throughout the alimentary tract and may be congenital or acquired.

Congenital ('true') diverticula

1 Congenital ('true') diverticula are outpouchings (extrusions) of the whole bowel wall, including all muscle coats. Their precise embryological origin is subject to speculation but is believed to occur during the early stages of development. They are allied to enterogenous cysts and duplications.

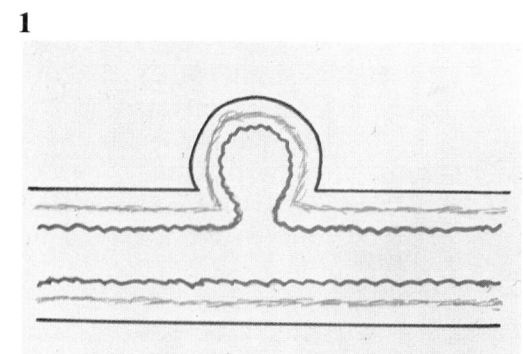

Acquired ('false' or pulsion) diverticula

2 In acquired ('false' or pulsion) diverticula the mucous membrane herniates through the circular muscle coat at a point of weakness, e.g. where a blood vessel passes through the muscle coat. The protrusion results from a raised intraluminal pressure. These diverticula are characterised usually by the absence of muscle elements but they may be covered by longitudinal muscle.

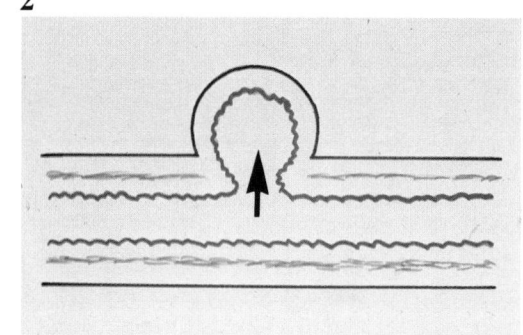

Acquired (traction) diverticula

3 Acquired traction diverticula are rare diverticula, the wall of the bowel having become attached by adhesions to an adjacent, usually inflammatory, lesion. Contraction of the adhesions produces the outward pouching. The wall of these diverticula contains all elements of the bowel wall.

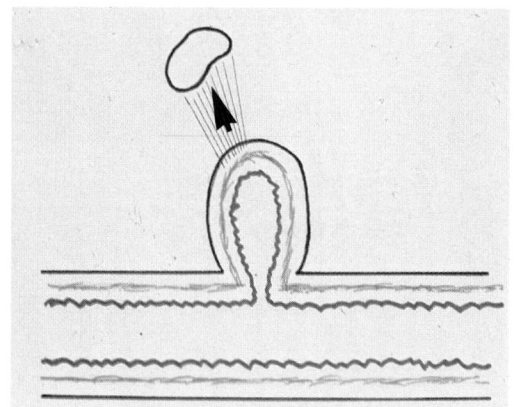

Many diverticula remain asymptomatic and are discovered incidentally either by radiology or at post mortem. Diverticula become clinically significant as a result of infection or mechanical complications. Diverticula may be associated with malabsorption syndromes, intussusception and simple obstruction, perforation or haemorrhage. Retention of contents, more common in colonic diverticula, is associated with infection leading to abscess formation, fistulae and stricture formation. The development of carcinoma within a diverticulum is recognised.

Pharynx

Pharyngeal diverticula or pouches were first recognised and described in 1767 and feature in William Hunter's Collection. A very typical case was illustrated by Sir Charles Bell in his Surgical Observations in 1816. This specimen is in the College Museum and the illustration is of the original engraving.

4

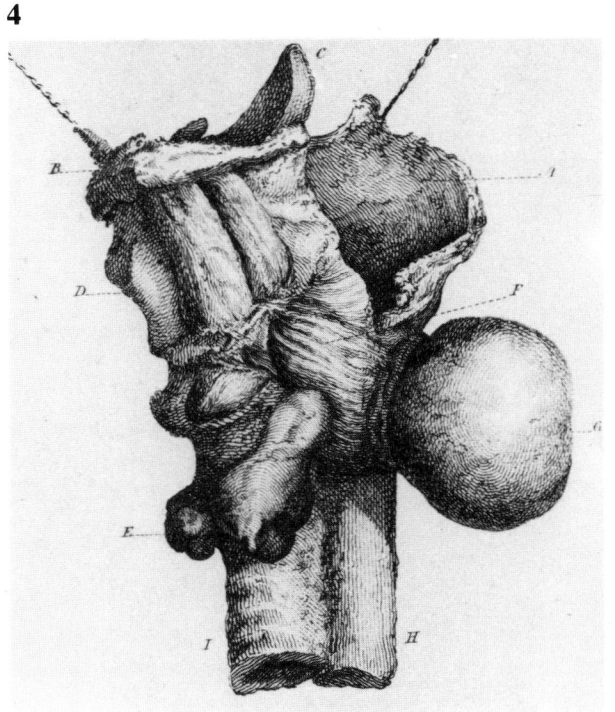

G.C. 10845

4 From an adult male who complained of dysphagia for one year and was treated by the passage of oesophageal bougies.

This lesion is characteristically seen in elderly males.

Pathology

An acquired diverticulum due to herniation of the mucosa through a weak area – the dehiscence of Killian – in the mid line of the posterior pharyngeal wall between the oblique and circular fibres of the crico-pharyngeus muscle (the lowest part of the inferior constrictor muscle). The sac wall consists of mucosa, a few attenuated muscle fibres and a zone of connective tissue.

Failure of normal coordinated relaxation of the crico-pharyngeus prevents the entry of swallowed food into the oesophagus. Consequent upon the build up of pressure the mucosa bulges posteriorly at the weak area of the pharyngeal wall. The cause of the incoordination is not known.

Pharynx *(Continued)*

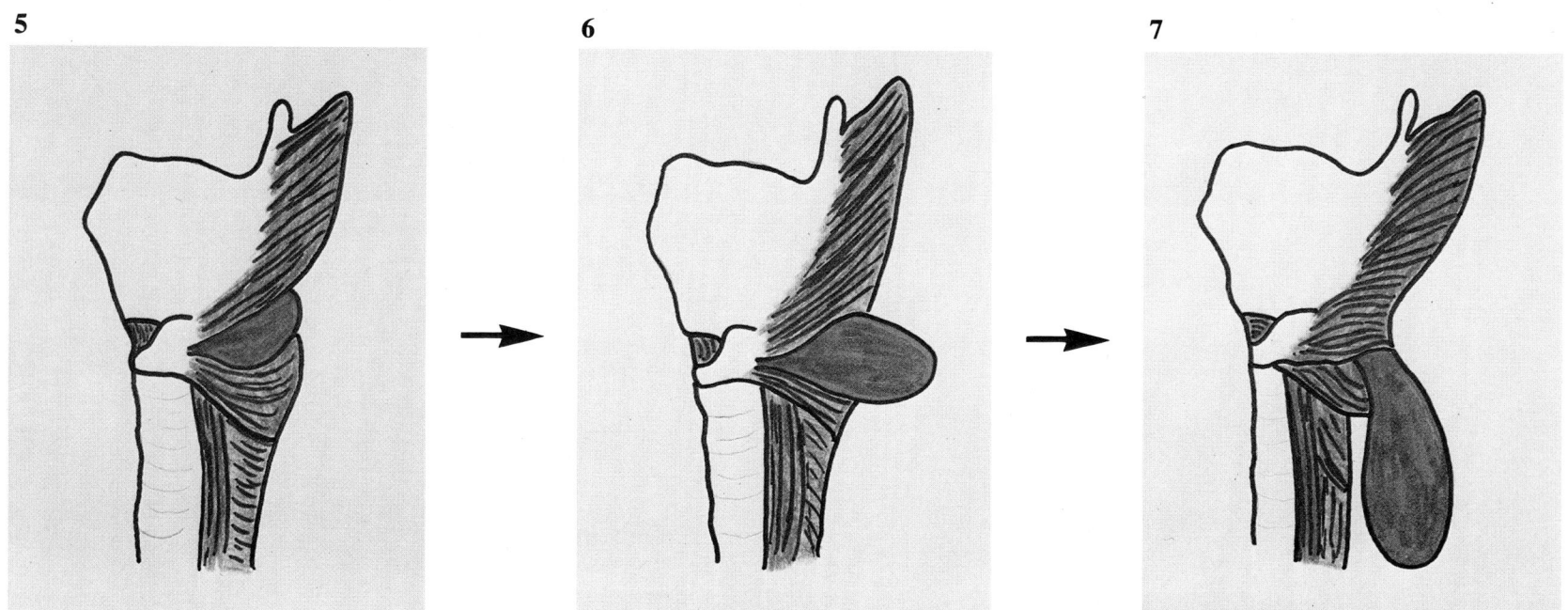

5, 6 and **7** The diverticulum is distended by retained food and gradually enlarges, passing downwards behind the oesophagus and then deviating usually to the left.

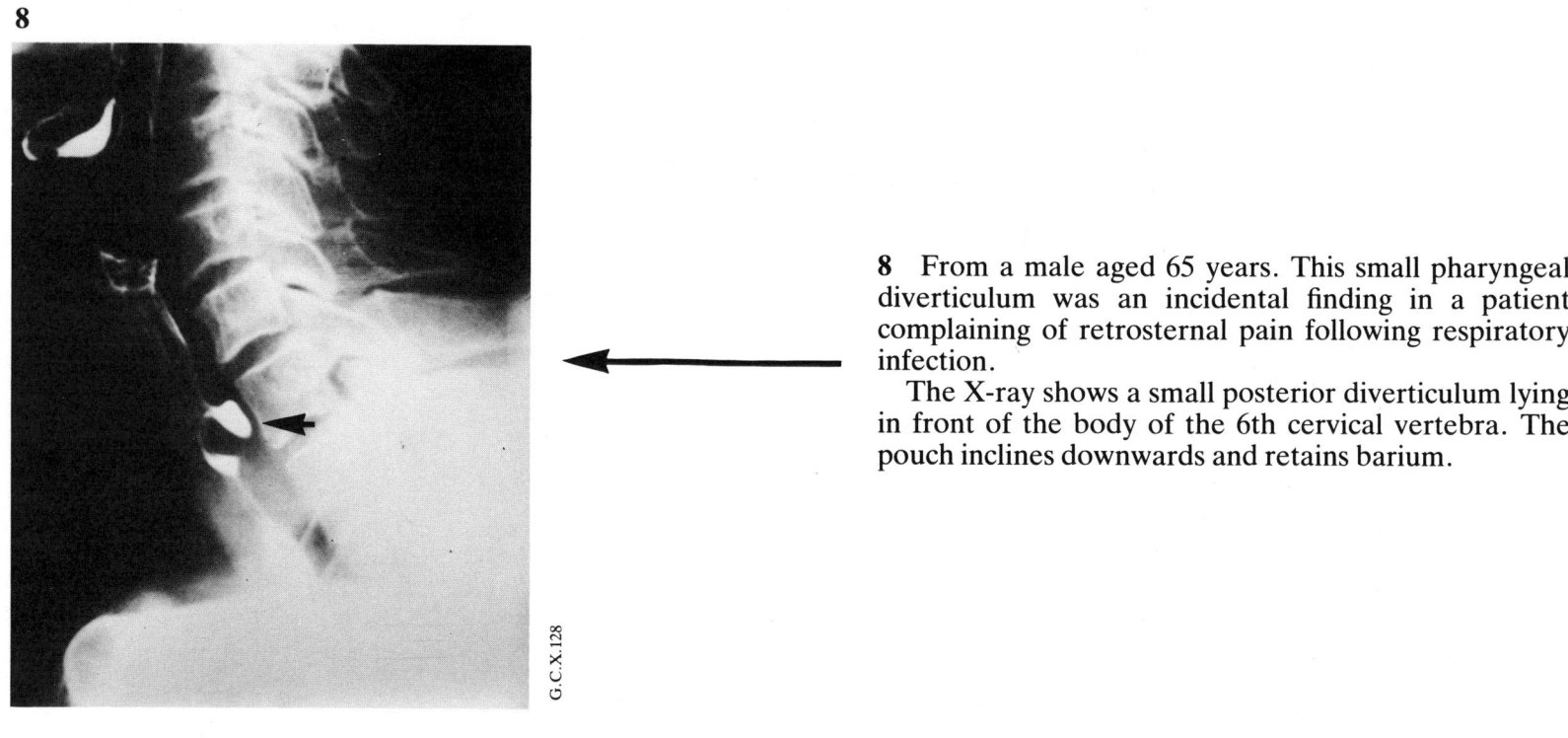

8 From a male aged 65 years. This small pharyngeal diverticulum was an incidental finding in a patient complaining of retrosternal pain following respiratory infection.

The X-ray shows a small posterior diverticulum lying in front of the body of the 6th cervical vertebra. The pouch inclines downwards and retains barium.

The oesophageal canal is distorted so that the mouth of the diverticulum comes to lie more directly in the line of the pharynx, whilst the opening of the oesophagus lies anteriorly and above. As the result of the distortion together with the incoordinated muscle action, food passes into the diverticulum (often referred to as a pharyngeal pouch) rather than the oesophagus. Dysphagia of a severe and persisting nature occurs and is the most serious aspect of the disease.

9

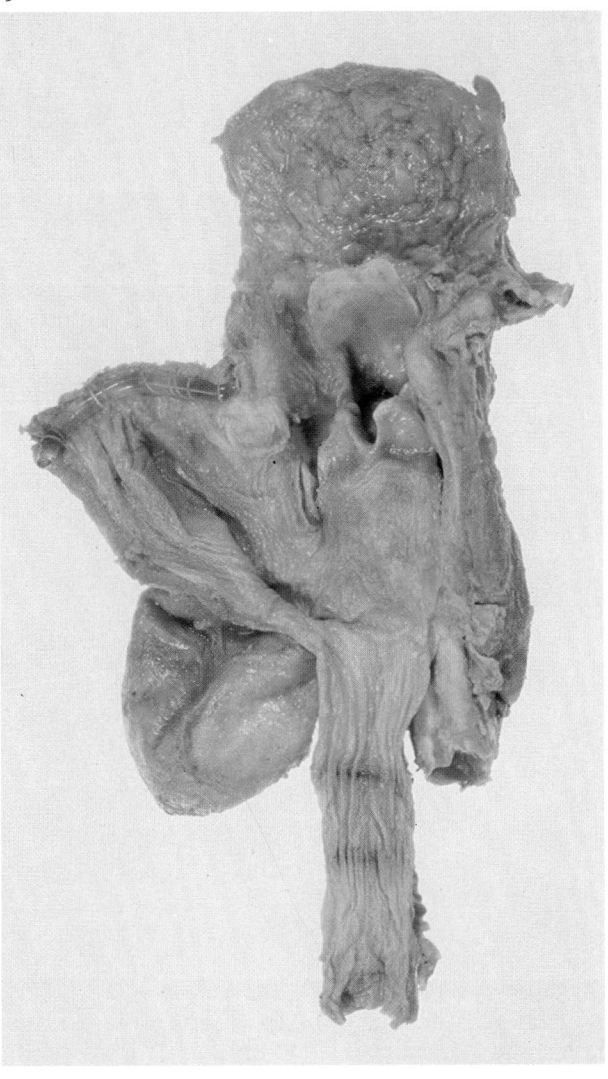

G.C.10942

10

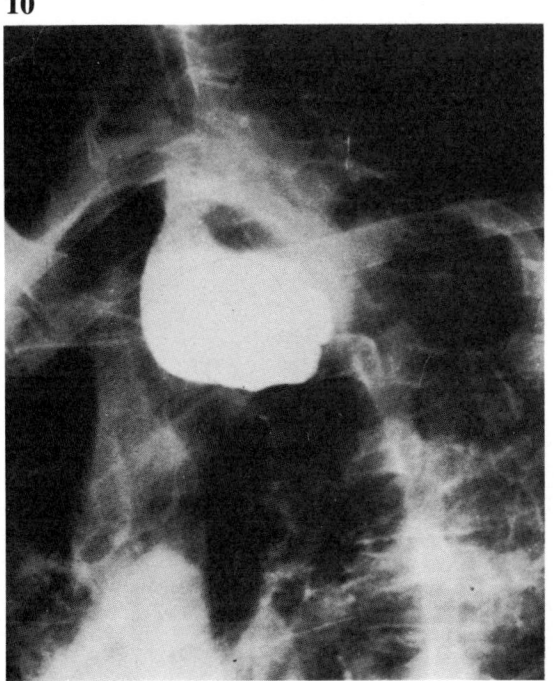

G.C.10946

9 Specimen of a pharyngeal diverticulum which has been opened along the right postero-lateral margin of the oesophagus. The posterior and left lateral walls of the oesophagus together with the diverticulum have been rotated to the left. The inferior aspect of the neck of the pouch lies above the cricoid segment (cricopharyngeus muscle).

10 From a male aged 65 years. Radiological examination of the oesophagus shows a large pharyngeal pouch arising in the usual situation. The base extends downwards to the level of the fourth thoracic vertebra.

Complications

Inflammation of the wall of the pouch results from putrefaction of retained contents. If of sufficient severity, perforation of the wall of the pouch leading to mediastinitis occurs. Respiratory infection – aspiration pneumonia – follows regurgitation of contents, especially during sleep. Carcinoma may develop in the pouch. Perforation during oesophagoscopy has been reported.

I.S.R. Sinclair

Oesophagus

Congenital

The origin of small congenital diverticula has been noted previously (see Section 13 B).

Acquired

Pulsion diverticula

11 Pulsion diverticula may arise in relation to dysfunction of peristalsis.

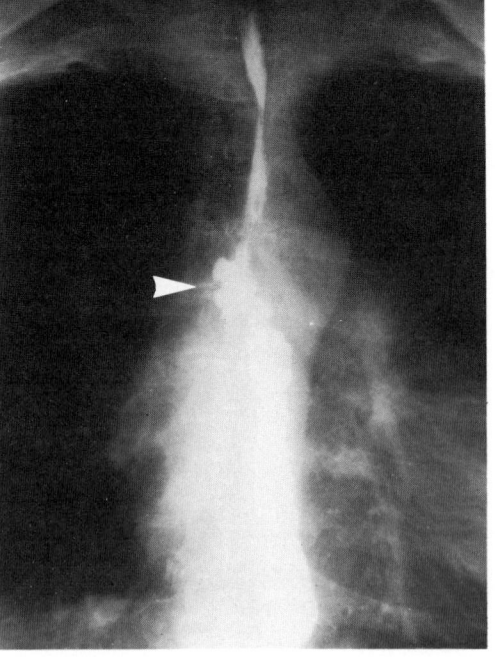

12 Pulsion or congenital diverticula occur rarely at the lower end of the oesophagus (epiphrenic) immediately above the diaphragm. Congenital diverticula may derive their blood supply from an aberrant branch of the aorta arising below the diaphragm.

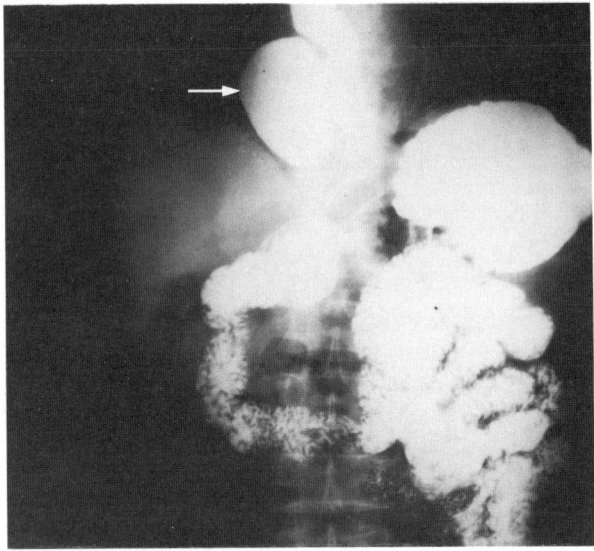

Traction diverticula

13 Traction diverticula occur in the middle third of the oesophagus, in the vicinity of the peribronchial and mediastinal lymph nodes which are often subject to inflammatory disease (e.g. tuberculosis). These diverticula are usually funnel shaped with the wide end at the normal lumen.

Occasionally, congenital diverticula result from faulty separation from the bronchus. There may be an associated bronchial fistula. Pulsion diverticula may occur with motility disorders of the oesophagus.

Stomach

A very rare condition. Usually a solitary diverticulum arises close to the cardio-oesophageal orifice on the posterior aspect of the stomach near the lesser curve. It occurs at a point of relative weakness between the diverging oblique muscle fibres where vessels penetrate the muscle coat. It is congenital in origin and has been described in the foetus. It may be associated with a hiatus hernia.

Very rarely a congenital diverticulum in the prepyloric region has been reported. Traction diverticula have been reported. Pseudodiverticula may be associated with peptic ulceration consequent upon scarring.

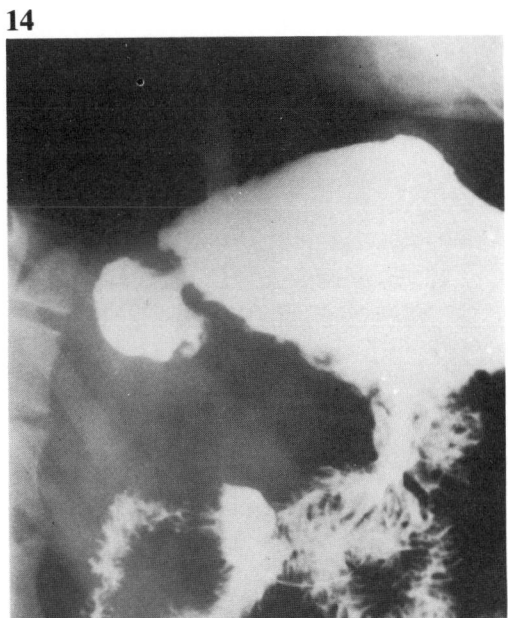

14 From a male aged 27 years.

Duodenum

Duodenal diverticula are pulsion and only occur with any frequency on the concave border of the second part of the duodenum, immediately adjacent to the ampulla of Vater. They are usually large (2 to 4 cm in diameter) and have a wide mouth which is, however, of smaller diameter than the sac. Many are symptomless but potential complications are numerous and include (a) enterolith formation, (b) infection with perforation or peridiverticulitis, (c) haemorrhage, (d) pressure effects occluding either pancreatic or common bile duct leading to pancreatitis or obstructive jaundice.

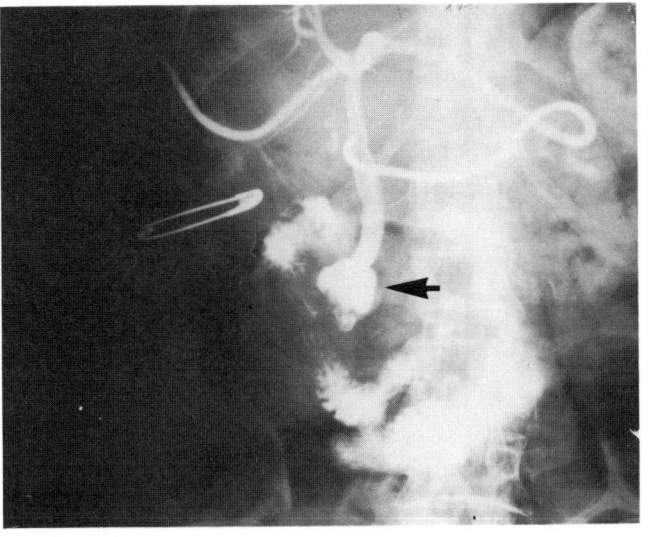

15 From a male aged 58 years.

16 From an adult female. Cholecystectomy and duct drainage. Post operative T-tube cholangiography.

Small intestine

These diverticula are acquired and are more frequent in the jejunum than ileum. They may be single or multiple and are usually asymptomatic. There is a preponderance of males. They lie along the mesenteric border of the bowel, in relation to the arterial branches.

Bacterial overgrowth within the diverticula may lead to malabsorption and disturbances of vitamin B_{12} metabolism (see Section 15A). Further complications include enterolith formation, perforation or haemorrhage and intestinal obstruction.

17 From a male aged 50 years who gave a history of dyspepsia over a considerable period. Radiological examination by barium meal revealed no abnormality but at an exploratory laparotomy multiple diverticula of a segment of jejunum were discovered and the segment resected. The patient made a complete recovery. The specimen consists of about 1 metre of jejunum. Along the mesenteric border are fourteen diverticula, ranging in size from 1.5 to 4 cm in diameter. The diverticula have extended into the adjacent mesentery and present on both surfaces.

17

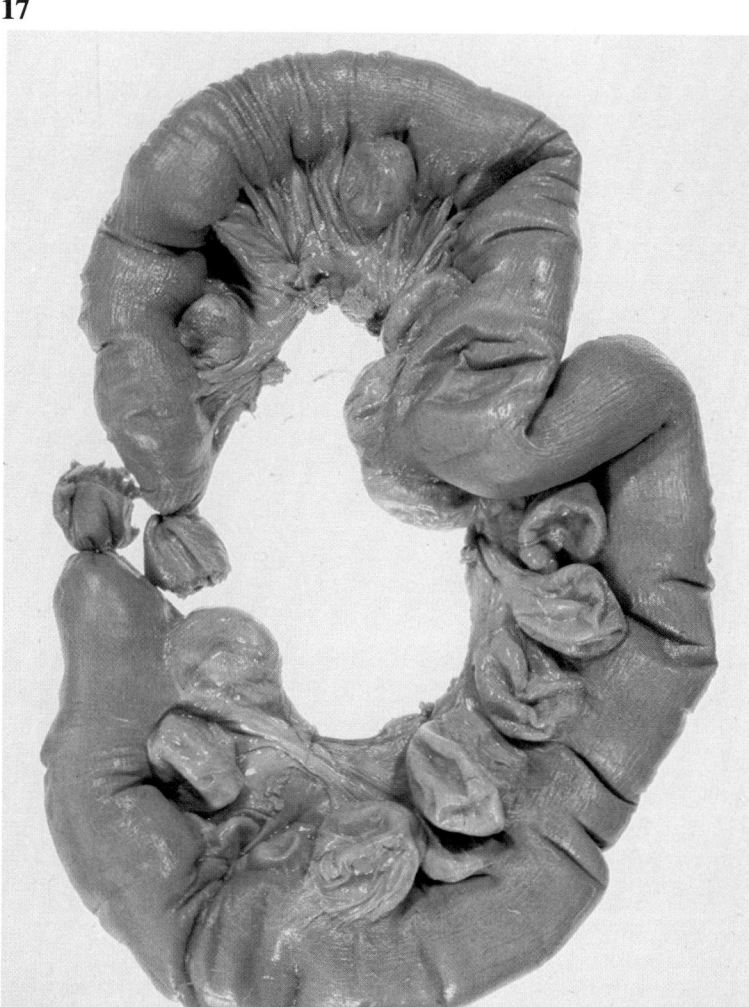

G.C.10194

18

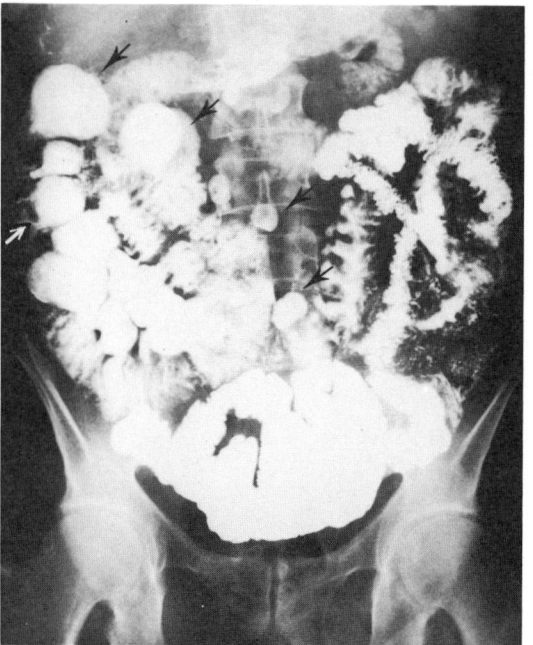

G.C.X.402

18 From an adult male. Prolonged history of loose stools and indigestion. The small intestinal pattern is abnormal and reflects enteropathy due to malabsorption of Vitamin B_{12}. The diverticula represent multiple small blind loops and this condition is one cause of the blind loop syndrome. Bacteria in the stagnant diverticula absorb Vitamin B_{12} at the expense of the host.

Meckel's diverticulum is fully described with other congenital anomalies. See Section 15 B.

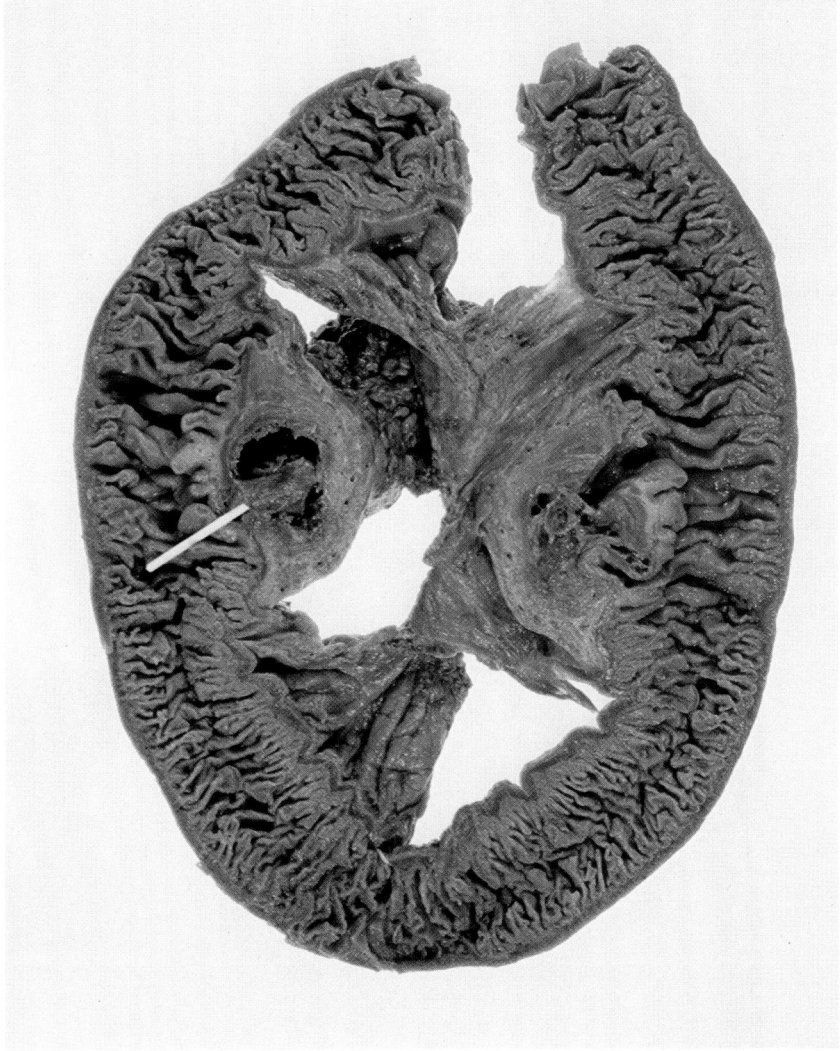

G.C. 10457

19 From a male aged 35 years. There was a 5 day history of abdominal discomfort followed by an acute exacerbation of the symptoms with elevation of pulse rate and temperature. The abdomen became rigid.

Exploratory laparotomy revealed general peritonitis with an oedematous purulent exudate. A loop of jejunum was swollen and congested and on its mesenteric border there was an inflammatory mass, to one surface of which was attached omentum and on the other a small perforation discharging pus. Approximately 50cm of jejunum with adjacent mesentery was resected and the remaining ends of jejunum were anastomosed. Recovery was smooth. The operative specimen has been sectioned in the mesenteric plane. On the cut surface (as illustrated) an abscess is seen in the mesentery adjacent to the bowel. The cavity, which was filled with pus, is about 2cm in diameter and is surrounded by a wall of inflammatory tissue about 1cm thick. A diverticulum, the apex of which has perforated, leads to the centre of the abscess. The white rod indicates the opening of the diverticulum. Another diverticulum 3cm distal, is seen protruding from the mesenteric border of the jejunum. The bowel is markedly congested and oedematous and likewise the mesentery.

On the outer surface (not illustrated) the bowel wall is swollen and congested. The peritoneal coat is acutely inflamed and is partly covered with a layer of coagulated purulent exudate. A hemispherical swelling about 5 cm in diameter extends from the bowel into the mesentery. On one surface of this mass there is a small sinus and to the other surface there is attached a portion of omentum.

Caecum/right colon

Usually solitary or few in number, diverticula of the right colon are rare. They are thought to be congenital in origin. Found most commonly on the posterior or anterolateral walls of the caecum. Acute inflammation of the diverticulum mimics appendicitis; chronic inflammation may simulate a carcinoma.

More recently diverticula of the right half of the colon have been increasingly recognised in Japan, the Philippines and Australia.

Appendix

Diverticulosis of the appendix is an occasional finding. It is of the secondary variety and is probably due to the occurrence of repeated episodes of elevated intraluminal tension whereby pouches of the mucosa pass through the muscularis and reach the subserosa. The condition is in all respects comparable with diverticulosis of the colon. Occasionally contents from the lumen of the gut will pass into these diverticula and a secondary inflammatory reaction may occur.

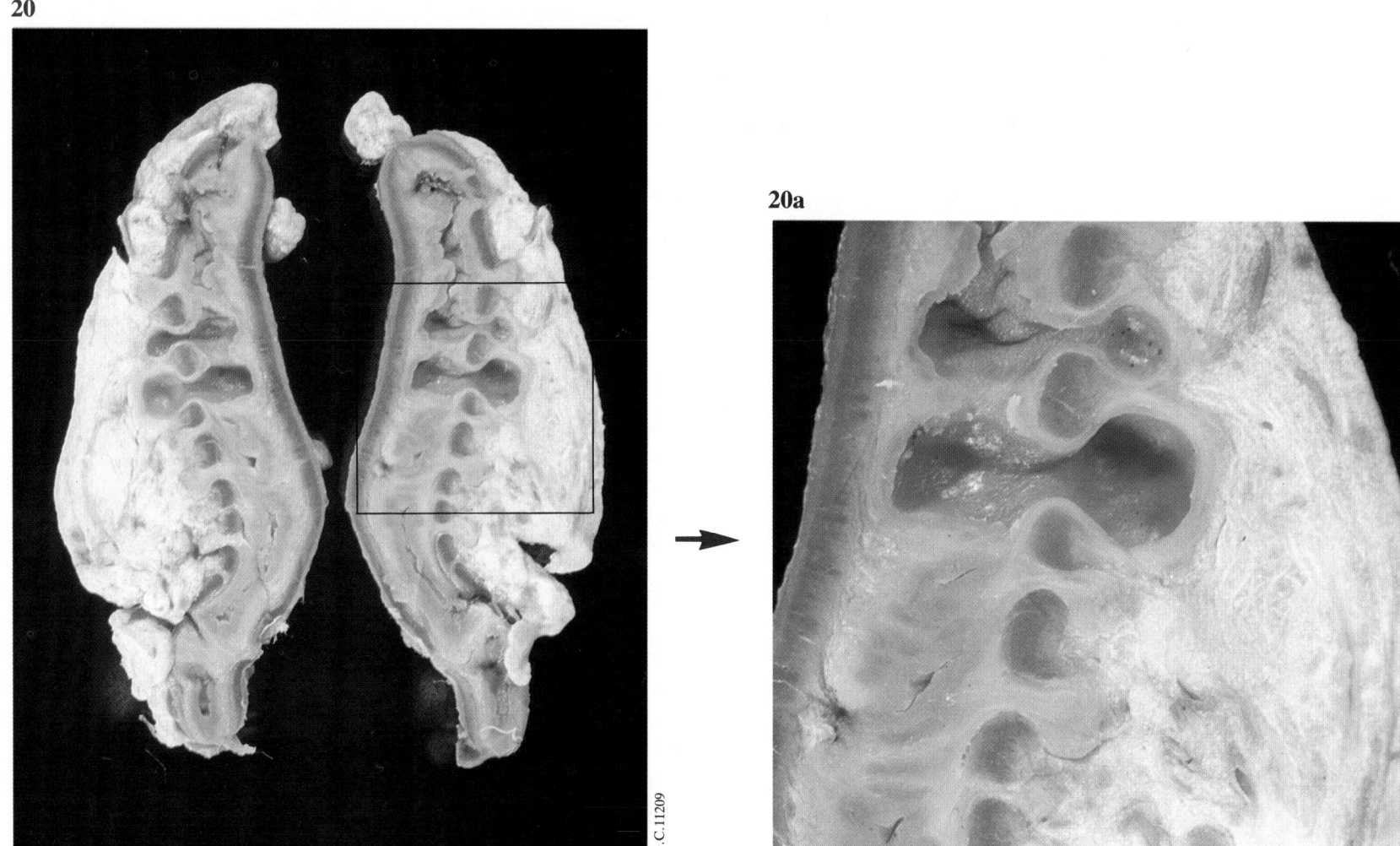

20

20a

G.C.11209

The patient was admitted to hospital as a case of typical appendicitis. At operation the appendix was seen to have a shaggy congested serosa. The mesentery was thickened. On section it is seen that there are numerous diverticula of the mucosa on the mesenteric border. These have transgressed the muscularis and in the subserosa have ballooned out forming cyst-like spaces but still communicating with the lumen of the appendix.

These illustrations deserve careful study because they demonstrate so clearly how the pulsion diverticula transgress the muscle layer and balloon in the subserosa at the attachment of the mesentery.

21

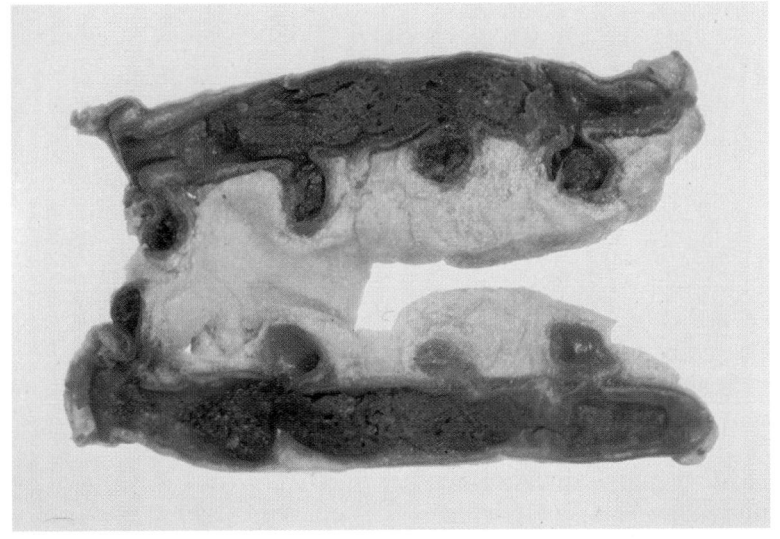

G.C.14016

21 Appendix – Diverticulosis. The illustration is of the appendix which has been sectioned to show the presence of four diverticula on the mesenteric margin of the viscus. The diverticula have passed through the muscularis and bulge into the mesentery. The diverticula are filled with faecal matter.

This specimen illustrates the manner in which diverticula become the receptacles of faecal matter. This is the source of inflammation and the condition is termed diverticulitis.

22

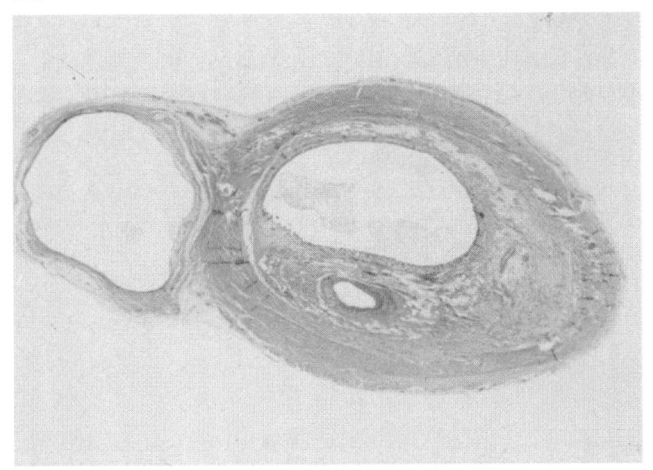

G.C.M.817

22 Appendix – Diverticulum. The diverticulum is thin-walled and its mucosa is atrophic. There is no evidence of inflammation. *(H&E ×5.25)*

23

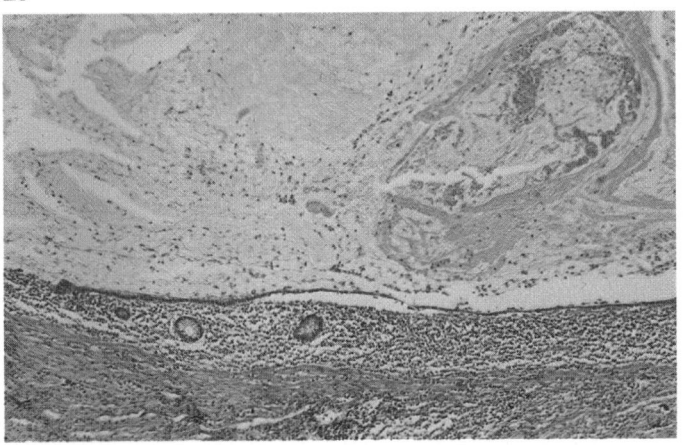

G.C.M.1001

23 Appendix – Diverticulum. The lumen is distended by mucin and the mucosa has undergone pressure atrophy. *(H&E ×62.5)*

Left colon

The muscular abnormality

Diverticula of the colon arise as part of an acquired disorder common in Western countries. It is rare in persons under 40 years of age but the incidence steadily increases with age. About one in three persons over 60 years has the condition.

It is now recognised that the process passes through three stages. The initial lesion (Stage I), is an abnormality of the musculature of the sigmoid colon associated with high intraluminal pressure.

This is followed by the development of pulsion diverticula (Stage II – Diverticulosis). These frequently become the site of inflammation (Stage III – Diverticulitis). When the disease was first recognised it was commonly confused with carcinoma. Clinically, while occasionally carcinoma and diverticulitis occur synchronously, it is not believed that diverticular disease is a precursor of carcinoma.

Stage I

It is recognised that diverticula of the left colon occur in those parts of the world in which the diet has a low roughage content. The incidence is low in those countries where the diet is bulky and has a large vegetable component.

The primary error appears to be in the muscle coat but the causation of this is unknown. It has been suggested that the apparent muscular hypertrophy is a response to excessive contraction to cope with the low residue mass in the colon – a form of work hypertrophy. Persistent contracture and a failure of the muscle to elongate has been recognised by radiological studies as the most characteristic feature.

Muscular spasm segments the colon into a series of almost isolated compartments within which the intraluminal pressure is greatly increased. The segmentation of the colon is often demonstrated best radiologically. There is evidence that muscular thickening or hypertrophy may be the initial stage of diverticular disease but later may return to more normal proportions. This view that the process of muscle thickening is reversible is disputed by some observers.

24

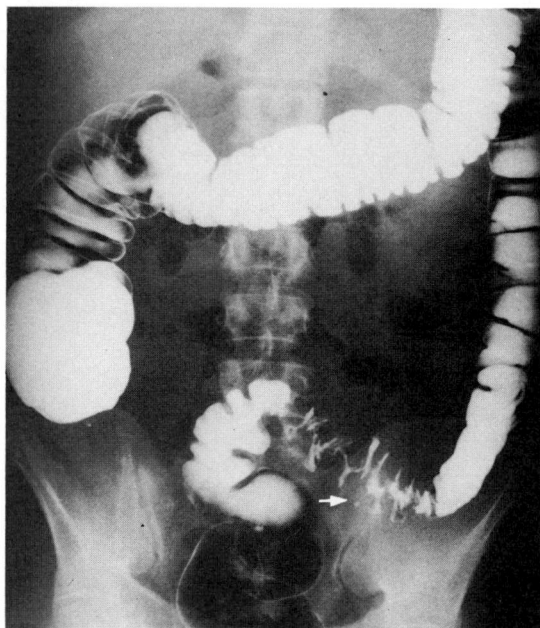

G.C.X.910

24 From an adult male who suffered from left-sided abdominal pain.

Barium enema shows marked circular muscle hypertrophy of the sigmoid colon with segmentation – the so-called 'saw tooth' sign. One small diverticulum has developed in the affected segment.

Muscle thickening is the most consistent feature of the disorder. The taeniae coli show thickening and in some cases become almost cartilaginous in consistency. Shortening of the colon occurs. The evidence of segmentation due to circular muscle spasm is less evident in other parts of the colon.

In some cases the lumen of the bowel is filled with redundant folds of mucous membrane. The lumen may become obstructed to a variable degree by these folds of mucosa. The excess of fat found around the sigmoid colon is probably due more to bunching of the pericolic and mesenteric tissues secondary to the bowel shortening than to a local response to chronic inflammation.

Histologically, the muscle shows thickening but no evidence of hyperplasia or hypertrophy of cells.

25

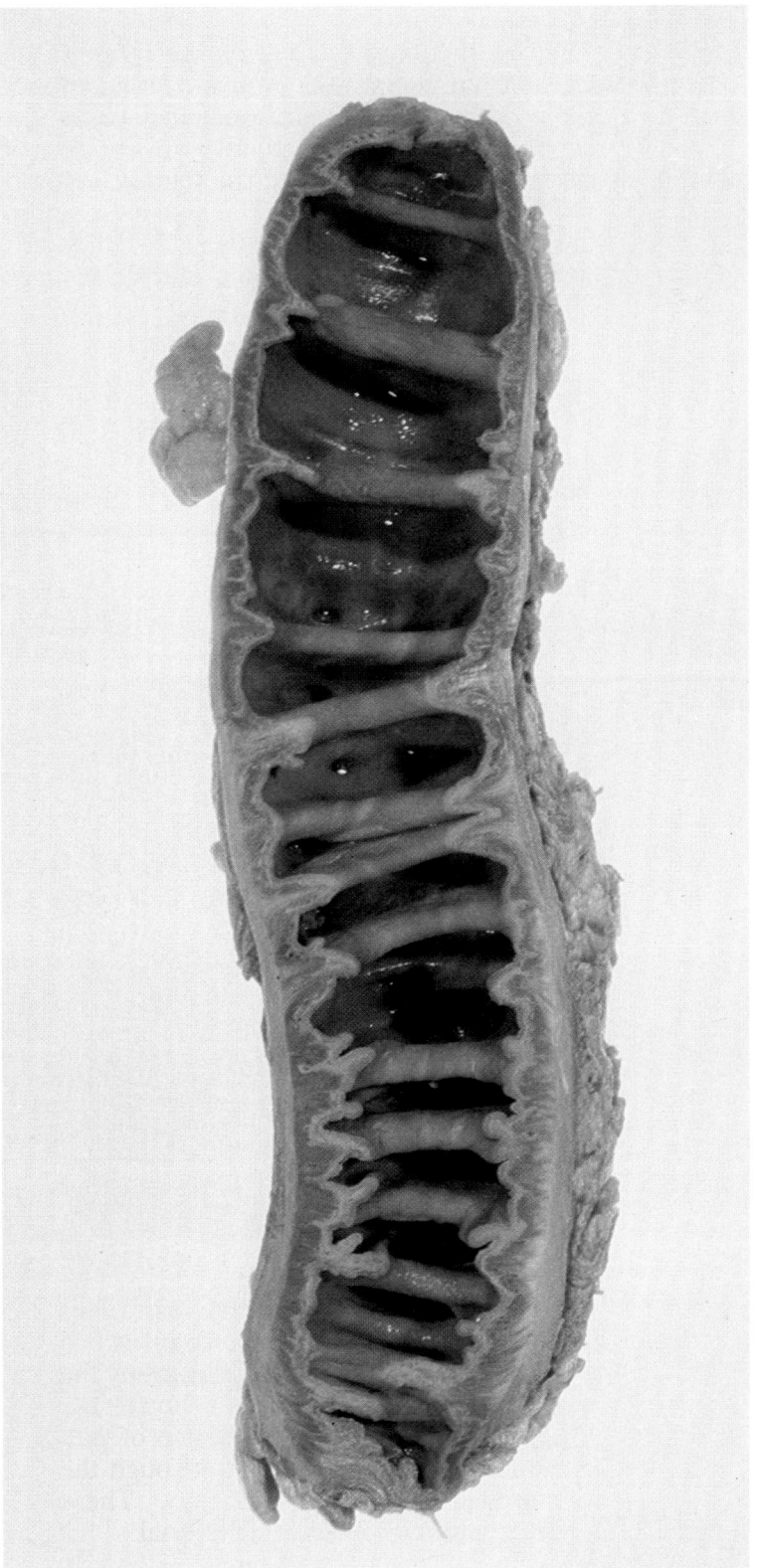

25 From a male aged 65 years. He gave a 5 year history of obstinate constipation and a five month history of left iliac fossa pain. The pelvic colon was resected. The patient made a good recovery.

The specimen shows the marked thickening of the muscle and the shortening of the colon which has resulted from spasm of the longitudinal muscles.

Note how the colon is segmented by mucosal folds resulting from the contraction of the circular fibres. The specimen has, however, passed into the next stage because small diverticula can be seen which have passed through the muscularis into the subserosa. This feature marks the development of the second stage – diverticulosis.

Diverticulosis

Stage II

The diverticula are of the typical pulsion type – a pouch of mucous membrane extending through the circular muscle into the pericolic fat and appendices epiploicae. The majority of diverticula pass through the bowel wall at points of weakness where the main blood vessels pass through the circular muscle coat to supply the mucosa. Usually two rows of diverticula are found between the taeniae. In the majority of cases diverticula are confined to the sigmoid colon but more proximal involvement may occur in addition. The rectum is never involved. The mucous membrane in the absence of complications is normal apart from an increase in the number and size of lymphoid follicles. The diverticula frequently contain faecal matter which may become inspissated. The diverticula may be demonstrated by endoscopy or radiographically.

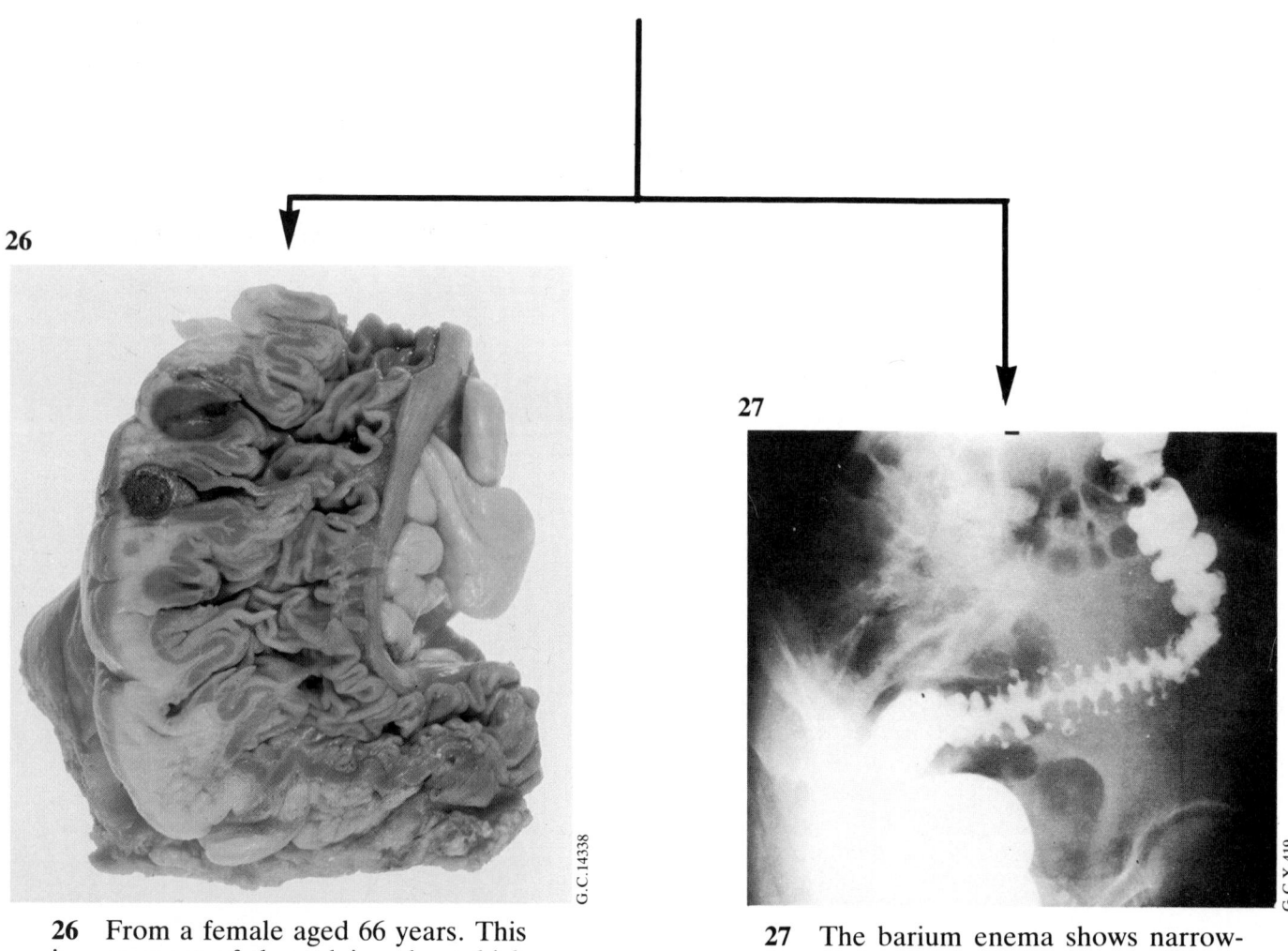

26 From a female aged 66 years. This is a segment of the pelvic colon which has been opened and demonstrates the characteristic features of shortening, segmentation and the presence of pulsion diverticula which pass through the muscularis to the subserosa. These diverticula contain faecal material.

27 The barium enema shows narrowing of the lower sigmoid colon due to marked hypertrophy of the circular muscle and muscularis mucosae with segmentation – the so-called 'saw tooth' appearance. There are also several small well developed diverticula. A relatively advanced but localised example.

Diverticulitis

Stage III

Diverticula become inflamed from abrasion of the mucosal lining of the diverticulum by the inspissated faecal matter that is not discharged through its neck. Commonly only one diverticulum is so affected and it is rare for more than 3 or 4 to be involved. The inflammatory process usually begins at the apex of the diverticulum and being extramural often involves only the pericolic fat. As a result of inflammation other abdominal organs may become adherent to the affected colon, e.g. small intestine or bladder. The inflammatory process may extend longitudinally immediately outside the bowel wall for some distance.

28

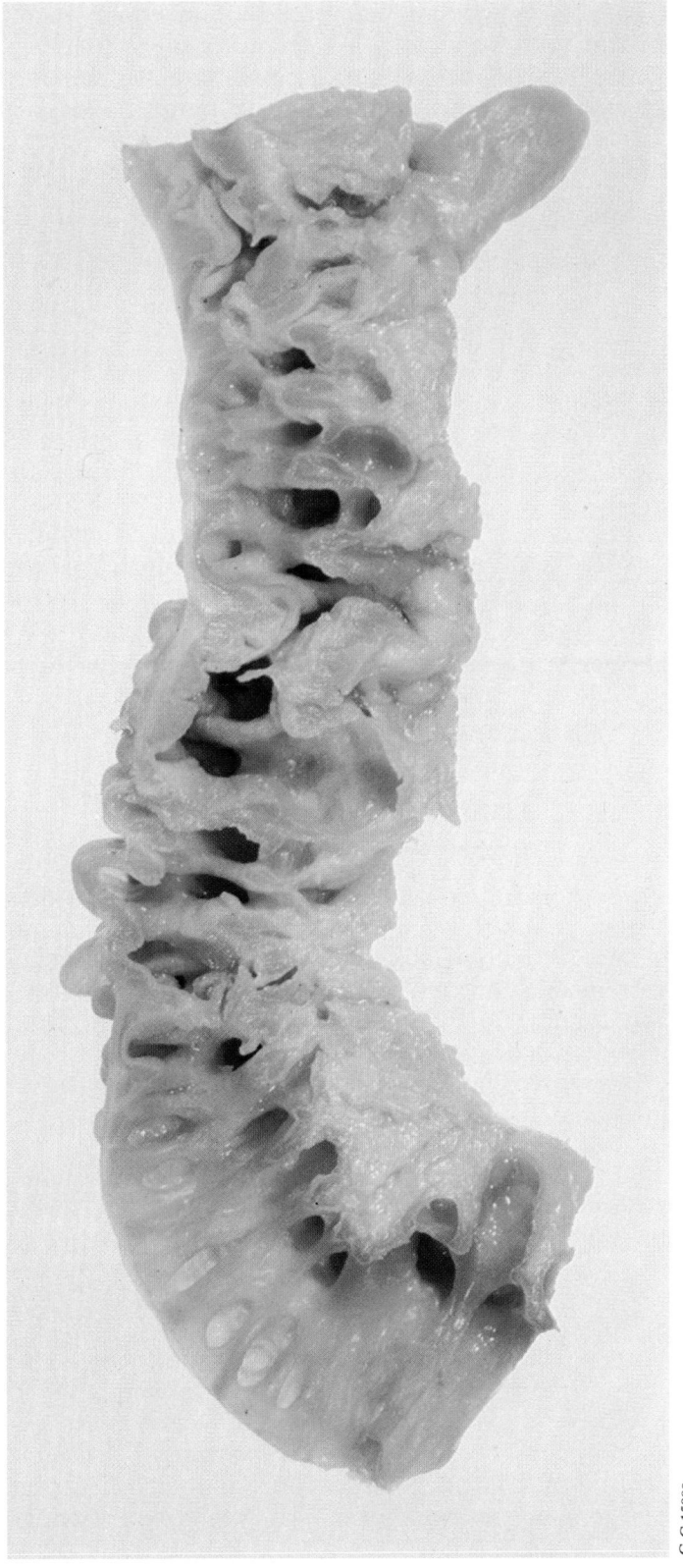

28 This specimen was obtained at post mortem examination from a woman aged 77 years who died from a subarachnoid haemorrhage.

Numerous thin-walled diverticula project between thickened muscle bands and these contained faecal masses which were removed during preparation of the specimen. At the mid point of the specimen is an area around a diverticulum which shows an inflammatory reaction with corresponding thickening of the bowel wall.

G.C.15009

Complications

Pericolic abscess

These abscesses are composed of pus and necrotic matter and often show a foreign body giant cell reaction. In most cases the abscesses are walled off by fibrous tissue and are chronic in nature. Dense adhesions between colon and bladder or small intestine are frequent.

29 From a female. The specimen is that of a 10cm length of sigmoid colon demonstrating a chronic abscess lying in its mesentery. This has arisen from infection of a diverticulum. The abscess cavity is surrounded by dense thickening of the colonic wall with fibrous tissue and with fibrosis in the fat of the pelvic mesocolon and peritoneal tissues.

29

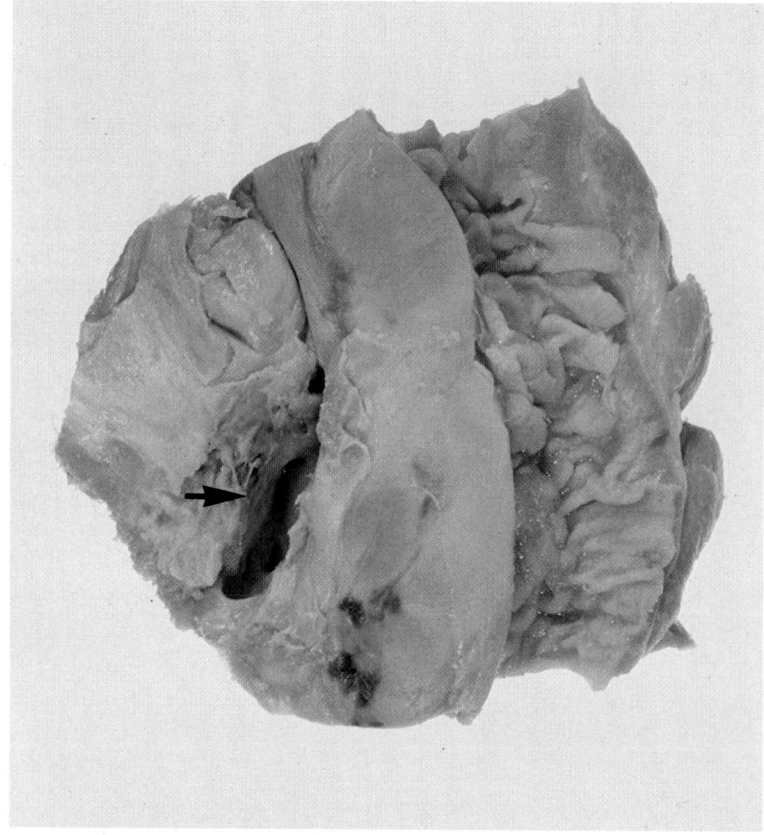

G.C.14900

Perforation with peritonitis

Frank perforation and communication between bowel lumen and the peritoneal cavity is uncommon; oedematous bowel wall seals off the diverticulum responsible or a well formed pericolic abscess supervenes. In these cases only seropurulent fluid is found at laparotomy.

Anaerobic gangrenous cellulitis of the colon wall and mesocolon is a serious complication.

Haemorrhage

Haemorrhage is generally slight or moderate. Severe haemorrhage with clinical shock is uncommon. The commonest source is an area of granulation tissue around the neck of a diverticulum. A prominent feature of diverticula of the right colon is haemorrhage and is an occurrence particularly common in South East Asia.

Fistula formation

This may result from the spontaneous rupture of an abscess into the bladder, vagina or small intestine or by direct rupture of one diverticulum into these organs (the so-called 'silent' form). Colo-cutaneous and colo-ureteric fistulae are usually seen following operation.

Intestinal obstruction

Obstruction may occur where the small intestine has become adherent to the affected segment of colon especially if there is a pericolic mass or abscess. The small intestine has become secondarily oedematous and kinked. Complete colon obstruction secondary to circumferential pericolic fibrosis is uncommon.

Diverticulum and carcinoma

Clinically, radiologically and even on exposure of the colon at operation it may be difficult to differentiate between diverticulitis and carcinoma of the colon. Both conditions are common in the pelvic colon and it is not infrequent to find coincidentally a carcinoma and diverticulitis. It is not, however, considered that diverticulitis is a precancerous lesion.

30

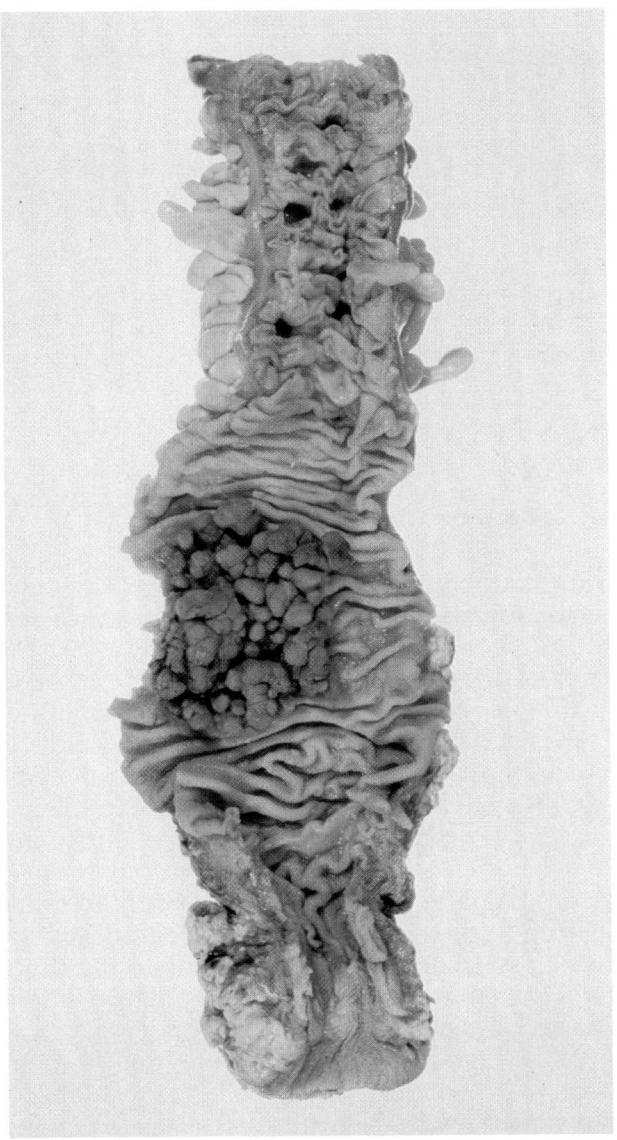

G.C.14679

31

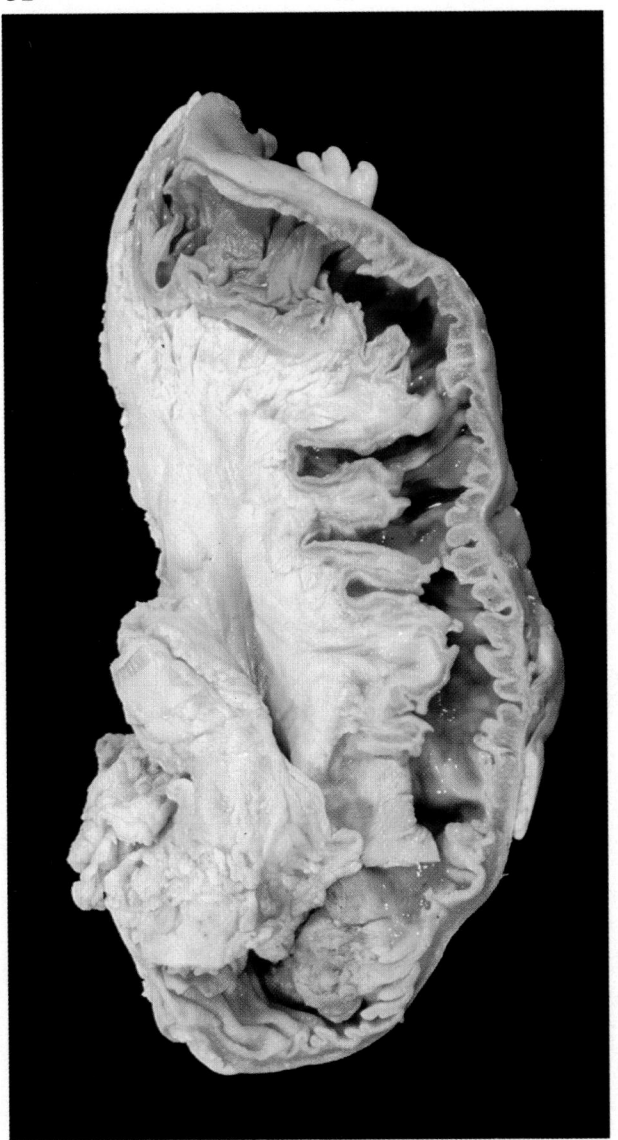

G.C.14337

30 From a female aged 34 years who had a 3 month history of rectal bleeding. Carcinoma of the ampulla of the rectum was observed and an abdomino–perineal resection carried out. The specimen shows clear evidence of two entirely separate lesions:

1 A polypoidal type of carcinoma in the rectum separated by a segment of normal rectal mucosa from
2 The pelvic colon showing diverticular disease associated with hypertrophy of the longitudinal muscle.

31 From a male aged 84 years. This specimen also shows the presence of advanced diverticular disease associated with carcinoma. In the upper part of the specimen are the clear manifestations of muscular thickening and deep segmentation and diverticula. At the lower part of the specimen is seen a carcinoma projecting into the lumen and causing partial intestinal obstruction.

Microscopically the tumour is an adenocarcinoma with infiltration of the muscle coats.

J. Anderson   A.N. Smith

Hirschsprung's disease is a functional obstruction of the bowel caused by congenital aganglionosis of the distal bowel. The condition is thought to result from a failure of neuroblasts from the cranio-cervical neural crest to migrate distally into the bowel.

Incidence

One in 5000 live births. No racial difference. Male to female ratio 4:1, but equal sex incidence in those cases where there is total aganglionosis. There is a familial incidence, which is commoner in total colonic aganglionosis.

1

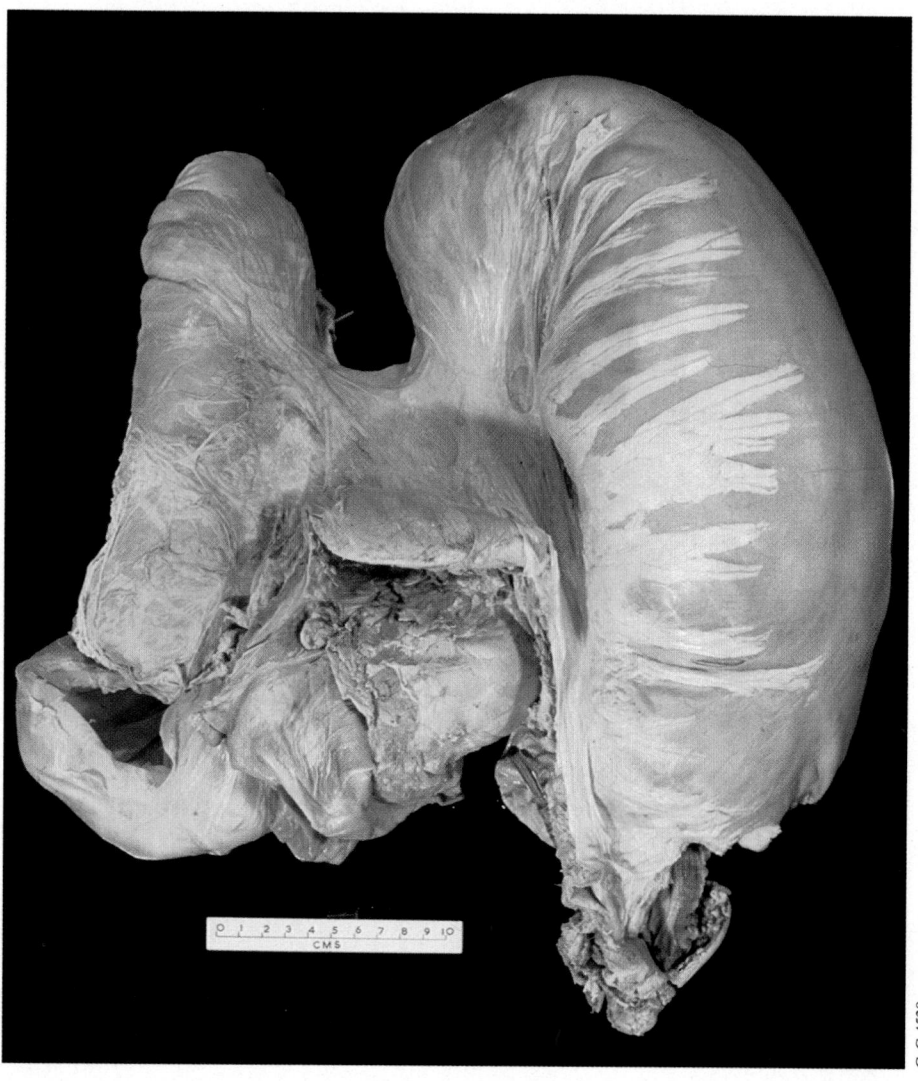

1 From a male aged 9 years the subject of persistent constipation with recurrent obstruction since infancy. The abdomen had become increasingly distended and sigmoidostomy having been performed for 'acute obstruction' he died on the second day after operation. In the specimen illustrated the anal canal and rectum have been laid open and are of normal calibre and development. The sigmoid colon is enormously dilated and occupies the greater portion of the abdominal cavity and on the left side reaches the hypochondrium. The rest of the large bowel and the small intestine are displaced to the right. Recent histological examination of a biopsy from the rectum confirmed the diagnosis. This specimen was donated to the Museum in 1902 and reference in the notes is made to the idiopathic dilatation of the sigmoid colon. Note is made of the enormous dilatation of the pelvic colon while the rectum and anus are regarded as relatively normal.

The disease was originally described by Hirschsprung in 1888 and was regarded as an idiopathic dilatation of the colon probably of neural origin. It was not until 1920 that it was realised that the abnormality lay in the small contracted segment of the rectum below the evident paralysed gut. Here the absence of ganglion cells was recognised.

Patients can be divided into three groups depending on the length of the bowel affected:

        60% – rectum and pelvic colon
        30% – rectum and distal rectum only.
        10% – total colonic involvement.

2

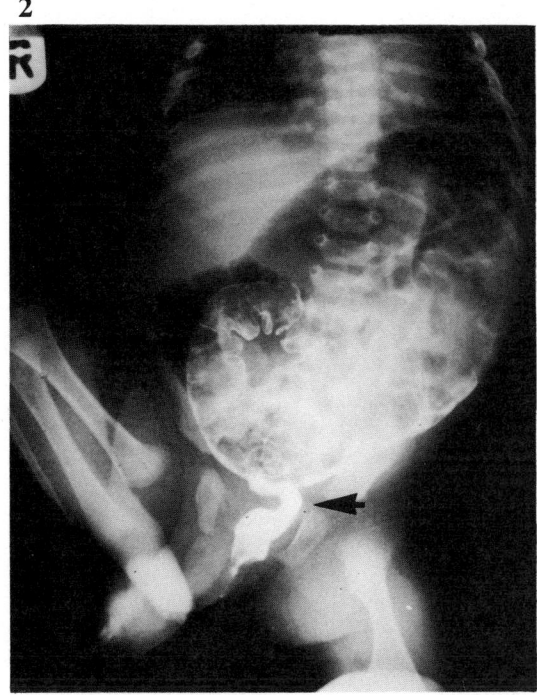

G.C.X.990

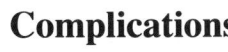

G.C.X.990

2 Barium enema in a neonate with Hirschsprung's disease showing a narrowed aganglionic segment. The proximal normal colon is grossly dilated.

2a Typical appearance at operation showing dilated normal colon proximal to a narrowed aganglionic segment. A biopsy has been taken from the aganglionic zone.

Complications

Enterocolitis is a potentially lethal complication of Hirschsprung's disease associated with distension and diarrhoea. Mortality is in the range 30 to 50% and is highest in the first months of life and in those patients with total colonic disease. Distension of normal bowel leads to mucosal ischaemia and perforation.

Radiologically the picture is similar to that seen in ulcerative colitis. Decompression of the distended bowel is life saving.

3

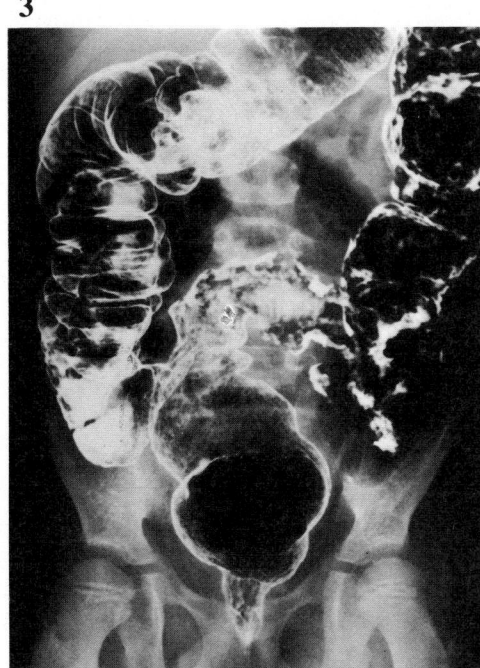

G.C.X.989

3 Barium enema in a 7-year-old boy presenting with enterocolitis. The aganglionic segment involved rectum and distal pelvic colon.

251

Microscopic features

Histological examination of distal narrowed bowel will demonstrate the absence of ganglion cells in association with abnormal nerve fibres. There is a cone shaped transitional zone between the distal aganglionic and proximal dilated bowel, across which there is a gradual return to normal histology.

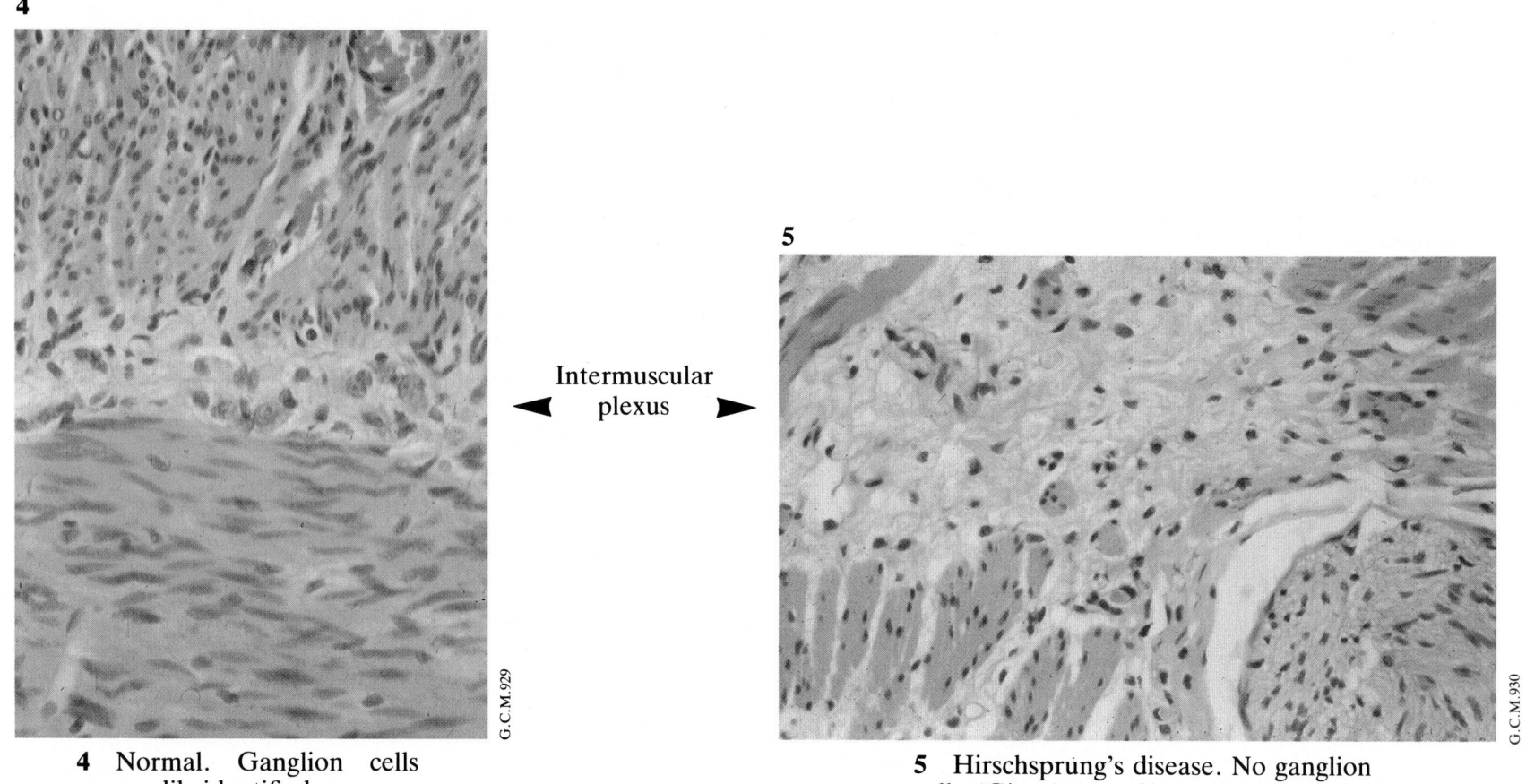

4

Intermuscular plexus

5

G.C.M.929

G.C.M.930

4 Normal. Ganglion cells are readily identified. *(H&E ×300)*

5 Hirschsprung's disease. No ganglion cells. 'Giant' nerve fibres. *(H&E ×300)*

There is a transitional zone between the totally aganglionic and normal colon. At this point the calibre of the bowel changes and ganglion cells begin to appear.

There may be difficulty in interpreting histology in the distal rectum at the level of the internal sphincter and 3 to 4cm proximally, especially in the young and premature infant. In this 'grey area' ganglia may normally be absent or few in numbers, but there is an increase in cholinergic fibres in the mucosa, in both muscularis mucosae and lamina propria.

Full thickness bowel biopsies are hazardous.

Histochemical assay of biopsies in Hirschsprung's disease has shown the presence of large quantities of the enzyme acetylcholinesterase. The demonstration of an increased number and size of the cholinergic nerve fibres in the muscularis mucosae and lamina propria by acetylcholinesterase staining is now an accepted diagnostic technique. Mucosal biopsies are adequate for this staining method.

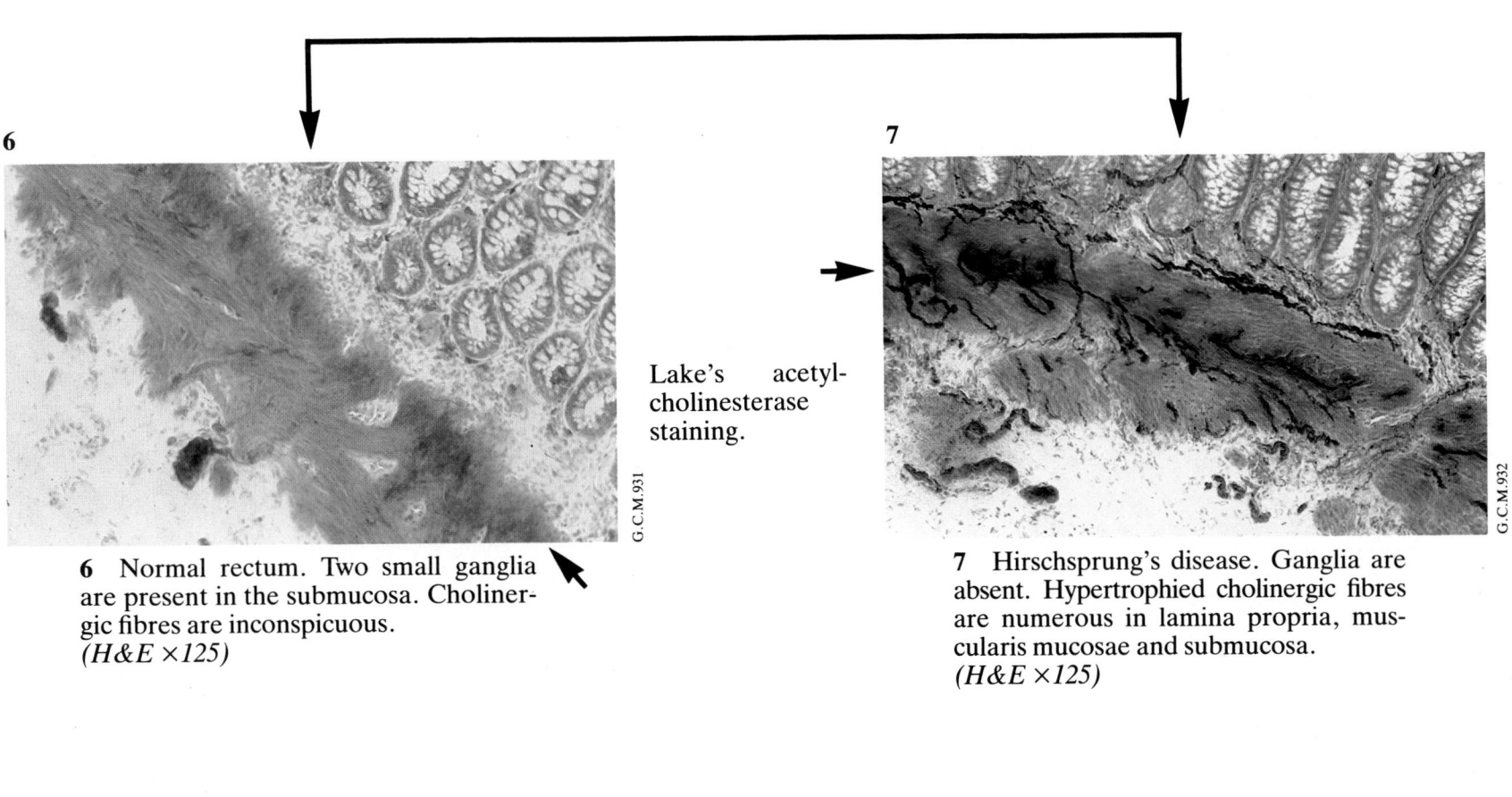

Lake's acetyl-cholinesterase staining.

6   Normal rectum. Two small ganglia are present in the submucosa. Cholinergic fibres are inconspicuous. *(H&E ×125)*

7   Hirschsprung's disease. Ganglia are absent. Hypertrophied cholinergic fibres are numerous in lamina propria, muscularis mucosae and submucosa. *(H&E ×125)*

The internal sphincter in Hirschsprung's disease is abnormal in that the relaxation reflex associated with rectal dilatation is absent. The manometric measurement of this response can be used as an aid to diagnosis.

Chagas' disease

A similar picture to Hirschsprung's disease is seen in chronic Chagas' disease with megacolon and megarectum. There is a quantitive reduction in ganglion cells. The oesophagus may also be affected. Ganglion cells are thought to be destroyed by a neurotoxic agent liberated from the breakdown of pseudocysts and leishmania forms of Trypanosoma Cruzi. Chagas' disease is seen in South and Central America.

W.G. Scobie

The persistent use of anthraquinone and other purgatives is alleged to damage the myenteric plexus of the colon and the condition presents in adults with years of purgative abuse, melanosis coli and the features of adult megacolon and severe constipation. The right colon is principally affected, there is axonal degeneration in the myenteric plexus and the mucosa and muscularis mucosae are flattened or atrophic. There is an eventual failure of gut motility.

Following the long-standing constipation these cases frequently develop melanosis coli.

Melanosis coli

Pigmentation of the colon may be minimal and detected only microscopically or may be of such intensity as to blacken the mucosa. The condition appears to arise either from the use of drugs of the anthracine group or due to degenerative changes in the mucous membrane of unknown cause. The pigment lies in macrophages in the mucous membrane. It is not related to the development of malignant melanomas and the condition appears to be reversible.

1

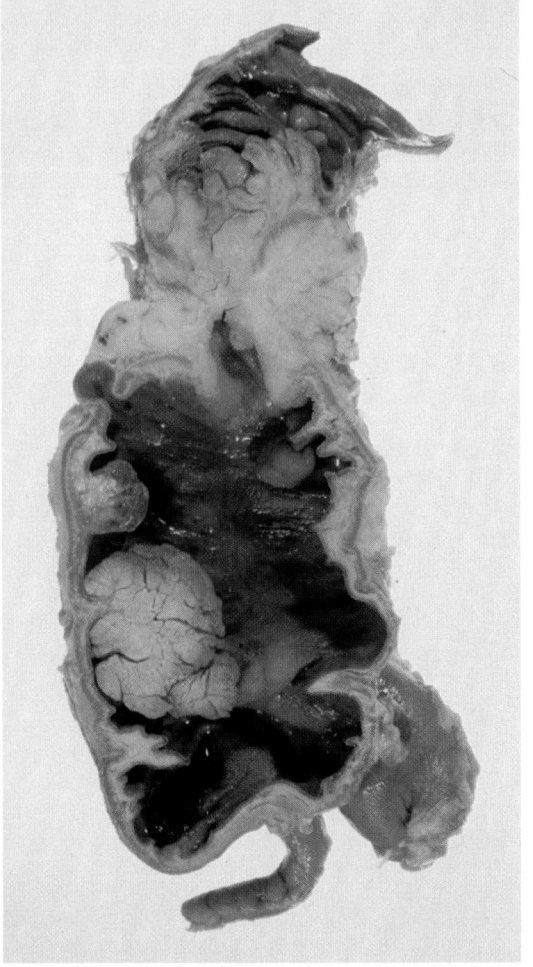

G.C.14672

2

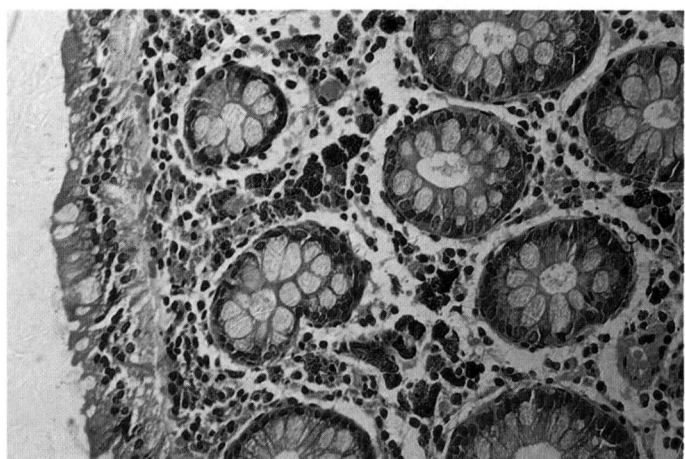

G.C.M.947

2 Colon – Melanosis coli. Brown pigment has accumulated in the lamina propria particularly in its upper layers. *(H&E ×250)*

1 A specimen demonstrating melanosis associated with a carcinoma of the hepatic flexure which is causing a degree of obstruction resulting in dilatation of the caecum and ascending colon. This specimen had the added interest that it demonstrates a separate pedunculated neoplasm in the caecum of glandular structure and projecting as a mass into the lumen of the gut.

A number of lesions of unknown or differing aetiology and in which an inflammatory component is present, occur in the lower small intestine and colon. These principally affect the mucosa but are differentiated from the specific infective colitides. It is convenient to consider these together and draw special attention to the distinctive features by which they can be differentiated. These lesions are:

1   Idiopathic ulcerative colitis
2   Necrotising enterocolitis
3   Crohn's disease of the colon
4   Diverticular disease (see Section 15 BX)
5   Ischaemic colitis (see Section 15 OA)

Idiopathic ulcerative colitis

An ulcerative lesion of the colonic mucosa occurring in younger persons. The disease often runs a prolonged intermittent course with alternating periods of activity and relative quiescence. Of special significance is the development of carcinoma in long-standing cases.

In older records the differentiation of ulcerative colitis and Crohn's disease was confused. The clinical, radiological and morphological features of these two diseases have now been identified and differentiated but in a proportion of cases the characteristics of the two diseases are intermixed. Occasionally typical Crohn's disease has been observed in the small intestine while the large intestine presents the features of ulcerative colitis. Alternatively the features of both diseases are apparent in the same specimen of the colon. These findings often suggest a relationship between Crohn's disease and ulcerative colitis, but most cases will in the long run prove to be Crohn's disease.

The aetiology of ulcerative colitis is unknown. Many investigations have been undertaken but have failed to reveal any specific factor which can be regarded as causative. The disease does not appear to be attributable primarily to infection but a secondary infection, once mucosal damage has occurred, plays an important rôle in the clinical and pathological manifestations. There is also no evidence that enzyme action on the mucosa is a primary cause of the disease.

The modern view is that the disease is attributable to an auto-immune disturbance, the primary effects of which are manifest in vascular and muscular disturbance.

Immunological studies have demonstrated the presence of antibodies to mucosal or organismal antigens.

Age incidence – Most common between 30 and 40 years but cases in early childhood have been reported. The sex incidence is approximately equal. It is uncommon in non-Caucasians. A high incidence has been described in Jews.

The condition affects the mucosa of the rectum and colon, often the first indications being a proctitis or proctocolitis affecting the left colon. Thereafter, in the absence of treatment, the spread of the inflammation is usually proximal, till the rectum and colon in their entirety are affected.

In many instances the colon is involved totally when the patient is first seen and in a few instances the systemic effects of the inflammatory process are extreme. Then the local features of tenesmus with diarrhoea or the passage of blood, mucus and pus from the bowel become of less importance than the spread of infection through the damaged wall of the bowel to cause a bacteraemia.

When the disease is extensive loss of muscle tone occurs with dilatation (the so-called toxic dilatation of the colon).

In long standing disease the colon becomes narrowed and forms a conduit. Through this fluid faeces passes rapidly giving rise to frequent defaecation and sometimes incontinence.

Microscopic features

In the early stages of the disease, the mucosa is infiltrated by lymphocytes and plasma cells and in very active inflammation there may be evidence of extravasated red blood corpuscles as well. Endoscopy shows a mucosa which is pink with oedema, or granular if there has been attempted repair.

1

G.C.M.853

1 Rectum – Mild colitis. The mucin in the surface epithelial cells is partly depleted. The number of plasma cells in the lamina propria is increased. *(H&E ×250)*

2

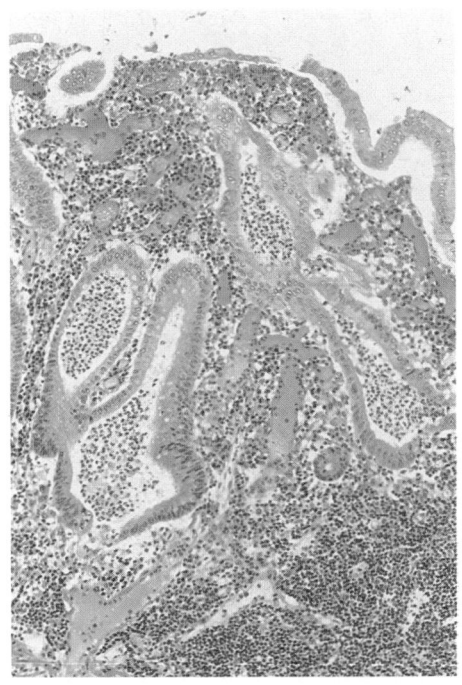

G.C.M.854

2 Colon – Severe active colitis. The mucosa is congested and heavily infiltrated by plasma cells and other inflammatory cells. The epithelial mucin is depleted, the glands are distorted and contain crypt abscesses. A thin layer of epithelium covers a recent erosion. *(H&E ×100)*

Idiopathic ulcerative colitis *(Continued)*

Examination of the more extensively damaged colonic specimen shows that there are areas where the mucosa is eventually lost and other areas of repair. If both ulceration and repair have occurred, islands of regenerative tissue will be seen as the so-called pseudopolypi, more correctly termed the inflammatory polyps of ulcerative colitis.

3

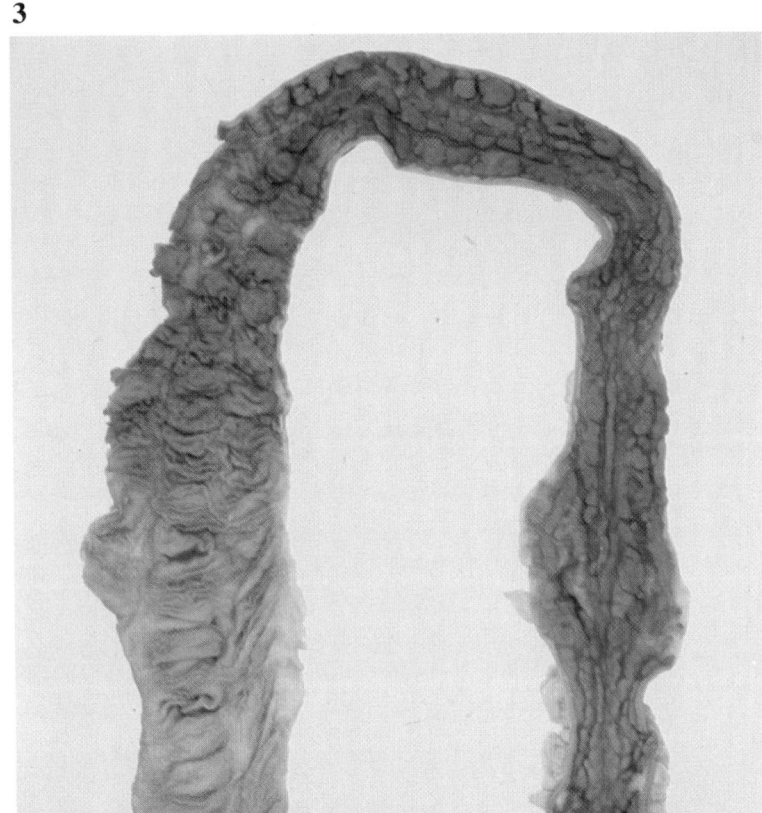

G.C.14482

3a

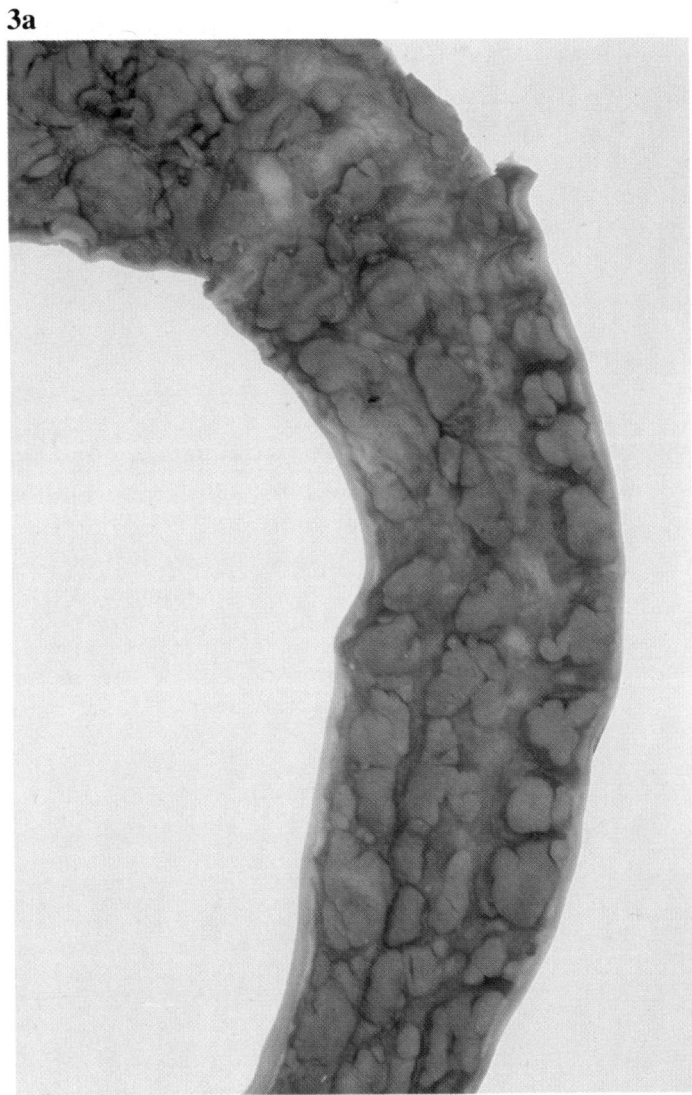

3 From a female aged 35 years. Eight months history of diarrhoea with severe rectal haemorrhage and abdominal pain. Admitted during a severe exacerbation. She was treated by parenteral cortisone. She died suddenly from a massive pulmonary embolus three weeks after colectomy. This is a diffuse ulcerative colitis. Specimen represents the whole length of the colon from the caecum to the sigmoid. Active disease commences close to the hepatic flexure and involves the whole transverse and descending colon. The mucosa is inflamed, oedematous and furrowed with numerous areas of ulceration. The oedematous mucosa has a pseudopolypoidal arrangement in many parts. The vertical furrowing is most prominent in the descending and pelvic colon.

3a Enlarged view of mucosa, splenic flexure and proximal descending colon.

4

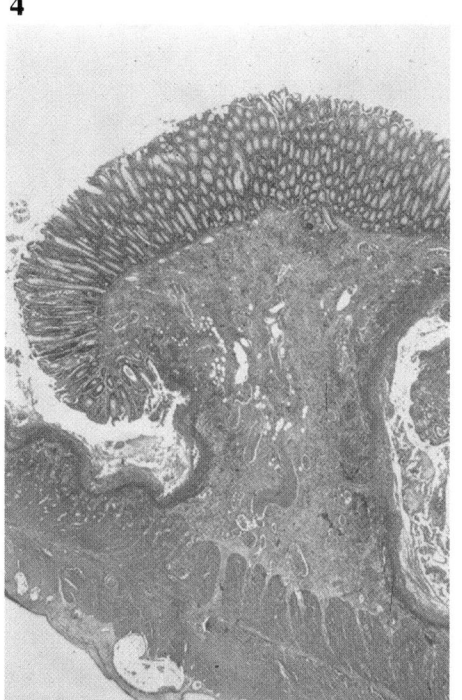

4 Colon – Ulcerative colitis. Inflammatory polyp (pseudopolyp). A surviving portion of mucosa has been drawn out in a polypoid fashion. Its epithelium is hyperplastic and its submucosa thickened by inflammation and fibrosis. To each side of it, ulceration extends to inner muscularis. *(H&E ×12.5)*

5

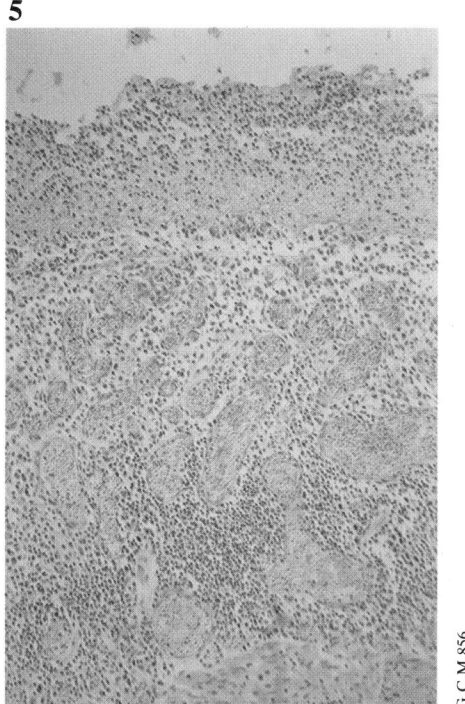

5 Ulcerative colitis. The base of this deep ulcer is formed by inflamed granulation tissue covered by inflammatory exudate. Note the extreme vascularity of the granulation tissue. *(H&E ×100)*

6

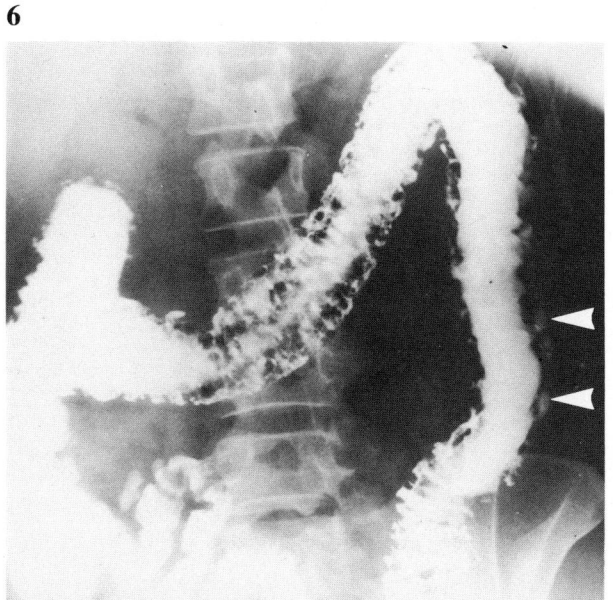

6 From a female aged 49 years. Bloody diarrhoea for many years. Barium enema showed ulcerative colitis with collar-stud abscess and pseudopolyposis. The normal haustration is missing.

7

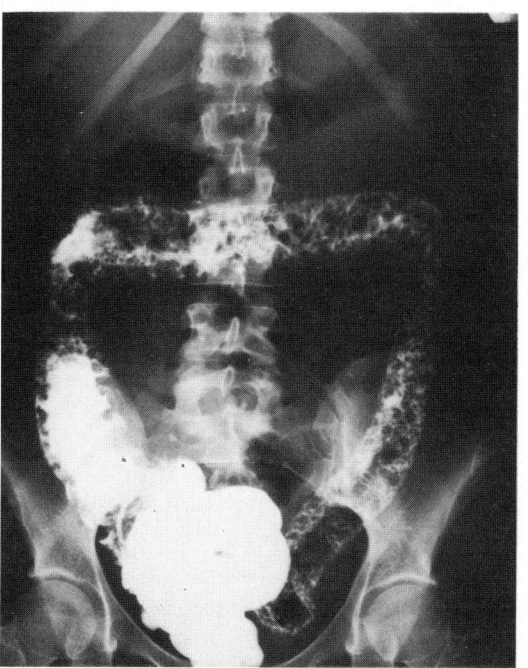

7 From a female aged 28 years. Eight months severe blood-stained diarrhoea. Treated with steroids.

Barium enema shows ulcerative colitis with gross pseudopolyposis due to lymphoid and epithelial hyperplasia between the ulcerated areas of mucosa.

Idiopathic ulcerative colitis *(Continued)*

Toxic dilatation

Myonecrosis is seen microscopically in colon affected by toxic dilatation. Perforation may occur. The muscle is thin and its fibres stretched apart at this stage. The mortality attached to this phase of the disease is 40%. The cause of death is faecal peritonitis. Operative specimens show that many patients have had minor incidents limited by adhesion of the colon to the parietes.

9 From a female aged 25 years with severe bloody diarrhoea due to ulcerative colitis. Barium enema is incomplete because of the extreme contractility of the left half of the colon. The radiograph shows toxic dilatation of the transverse colon which contains large pseudopolyps.

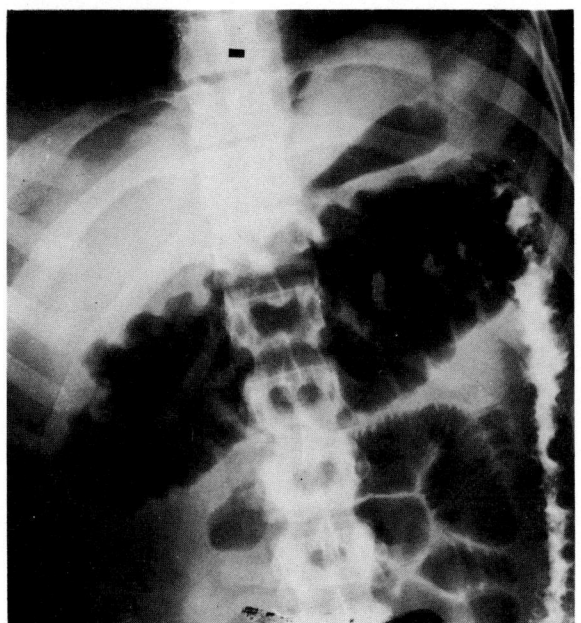

G.C.X.464

Dilatation with distal obstruction

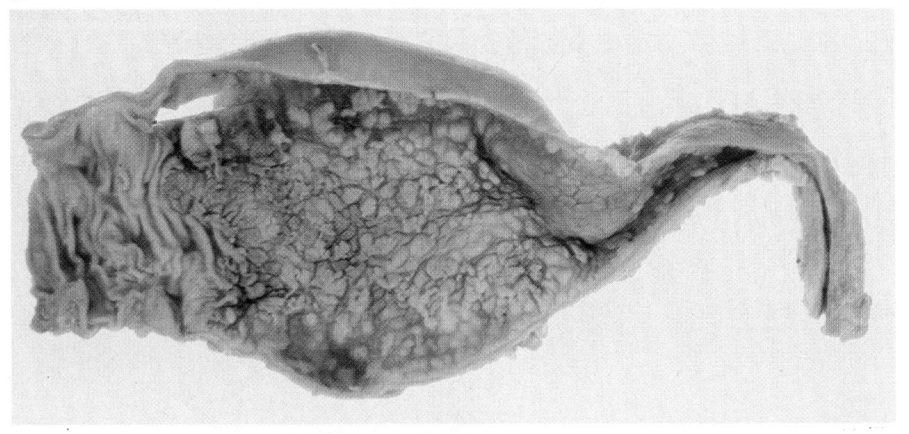

G.C.14631

8 From a female aged 37 years. Ulcerative colitis had been present for 6 years. Controlled by steroid therapy. She had, however, developed faecal stasis and at operation a telemetering capsule swallowed 3 months previously was found in the caecum.

The specimen illustrates dilatation of the transverse colon with the pattern of pseudopolyposis and narrowing of the descending colon associated with hypertrophy and contraction of the muscularis. This combination of proximal dilatation and distal contraction with spasm is recognised in a few cases of ulcerative colitis and may lead to faecal stasis.

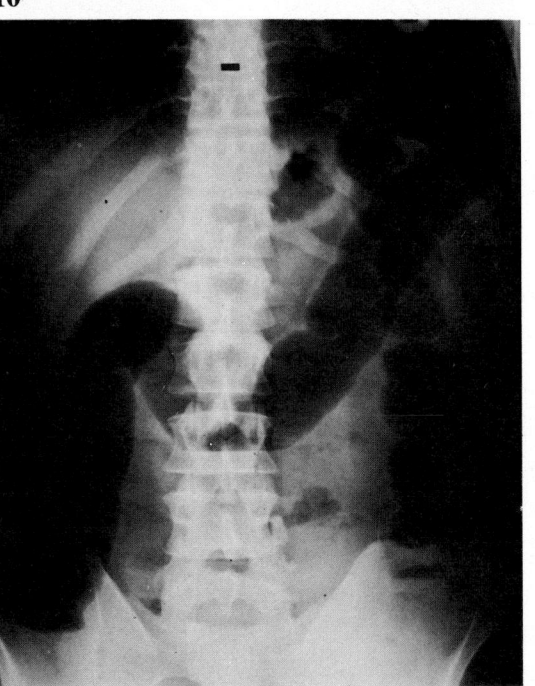

G.C.X.462

10 From a male aged 39 years who suffered from diarrhoea for several years due to ulcerative colitis.

A plain radiograph of the abdomen shows lack of haustration in the ascending and transverse colon with fluid levels in the caecum and lower descending colon. The smooth calibre of the colon is diagnostic of ulcerative colitis and the fluid levels reflect the water content of the bowel.

Complications

Healed lesion

Many patients with ulcerative colitis may have systemic complications. These are:

1 Pyoderma gangrenosum which characterically affects the skin of the lower limbs, chiefly in patches of superficial haemorrhagic necrosis which heal as the general state improves with treatment.
2 Arthropathies – This may affect any joint but a common lesion is that of the sacroiliac joint. The joints usually show a synovitis with effusion.
3 Iridocyclitis – This often indicates an acute relapse after periods of chronic activity of the disease. It responds well if the patient is brought into re-mission.

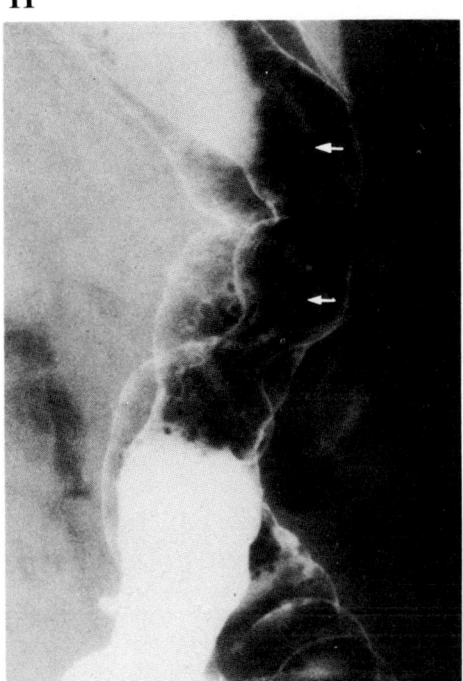

11

11 From a female. Barium enema showed involvement of the sigmoid, lower descending and the distal half of the transverse colon.

Enlargement of the splenic flexure area showing mucosal tags typical of healed ulcerative colitis.

Other complications

As in Crohn's disease a pericholangitis may occur. This is usually associated with long-standing disease with gross shrinkage of the colon.

In long-standing disease renal calculi may develop.

Idiopathic ulcerative colitis *(Continued)*

Carcinoma

The development of carcinomatous change is a recognised sequel of ulcerative colitis and occurs in 5% of cases. This is 10 times the estimated incidence of colonic cancer in the general population. It tends to affect:

1 Those in whom the ulcerative colitis has existed for 10 years or more (50%).
2 Those with total involvement of the colon.
3 Those of the younger age group in whom the ulcerative colitis may have been detected during adolescence.

The malignancy is often multifocal. The lesions may be flat and inconspicuous or clearly evident. As the wall of the bowel is invaded there is stricture formation – an important distinctive feature. The tumour grows rapidly with early metastases to the lymph nodes.

Histologically the tumour is frequently of an infiltrating colloid type and shows a high grade of malignancy.

In cases with carcinoma other areas in the colon will frequently show marked epithelial dysplasia including areas of carcinoma *in situ*.

12

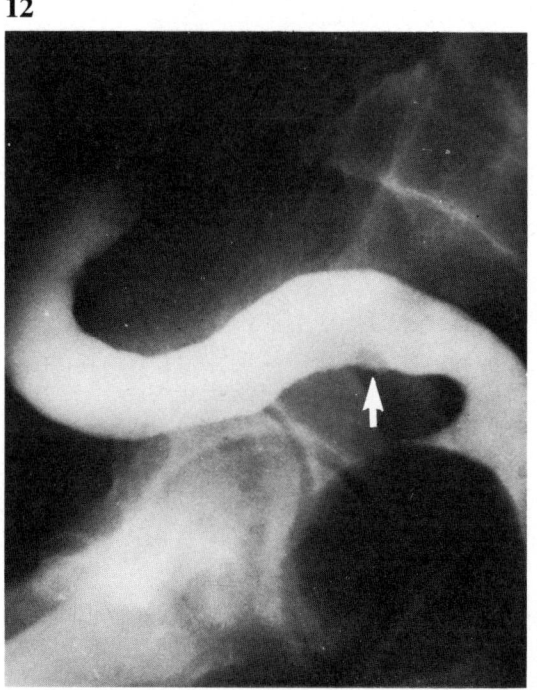

13

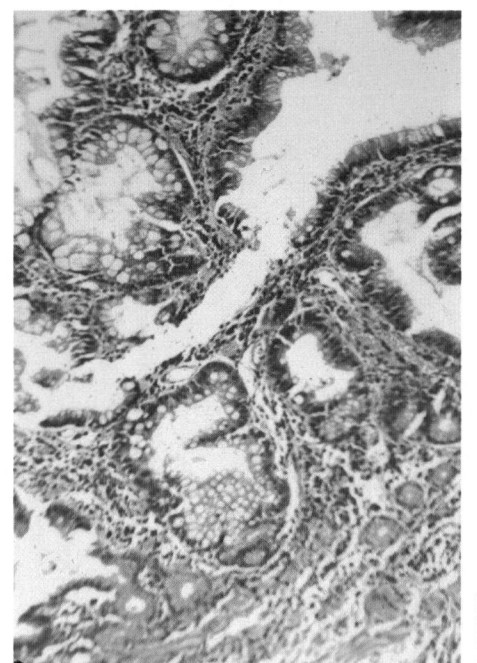

12 From a male aged 56 years. A 10 year history of ulcerative colitis.

Barium enema shows a narrow, smooth, contracted rectum and sigmoid colon with negative filling defect on the anterior wall of the lower sigmoid colon. Sigmoidoscopy and biopsy confirmed that this was due to carcinoma superimposed on ulcerative colitis which is a recognised complication.

13 Chronic ulcerative colitis – dysplasia.

The epithelium is polypoid, hyperchromatic and dysplastic – a premalignant change. *(H&E ×100)*

The disease has frequently metastasised before the diagnosis is established and carries a very grave prognosis in all cases.

Illustrative case

From a female aged 48 years who had suffered from ulcerative colitis for 20 years. Total colectomy was carried out. The specimen demonstrates three distinct areas of carcinoma. In two of these the carcinoma shows as a well marked stricture formation (14).

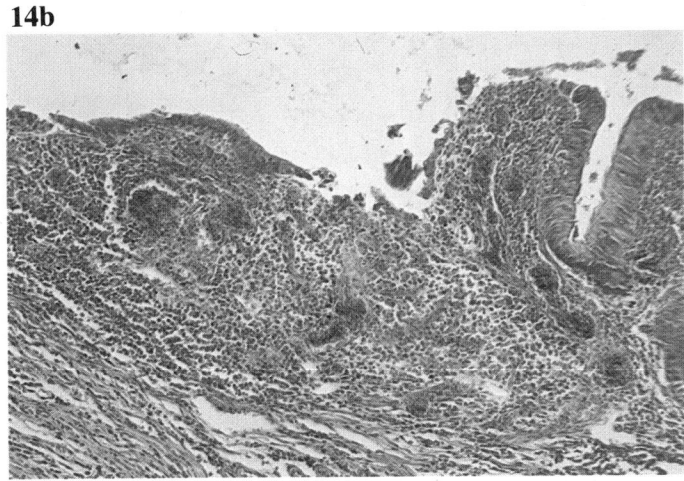

14b Field 2. Margin of re-epithelialising ulcer showing surface carcinoma. *(H&E ×100)*

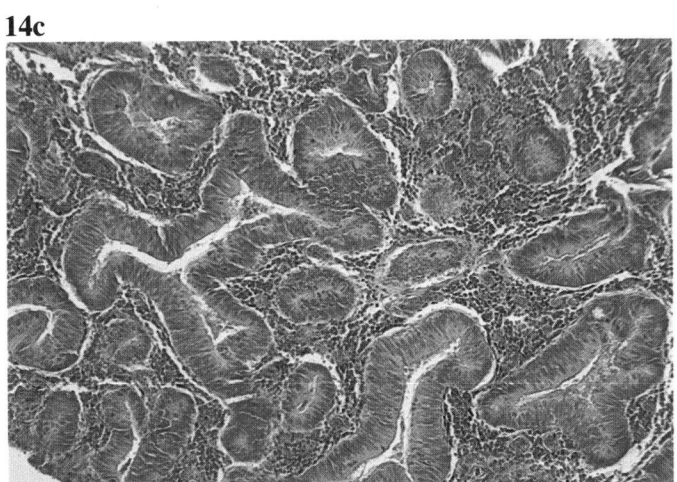

14c Field 2a. Well differentiated adenocarcinoma in area contiguous with field 2. *(H&E ×100)*

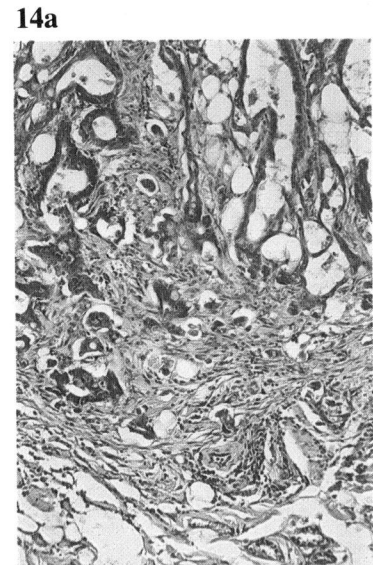

14a Field 1. Moderately differentiated mucin-secreting adenocarcinoma invades the colon as far as outer muscularis. *(H&E ×100)*

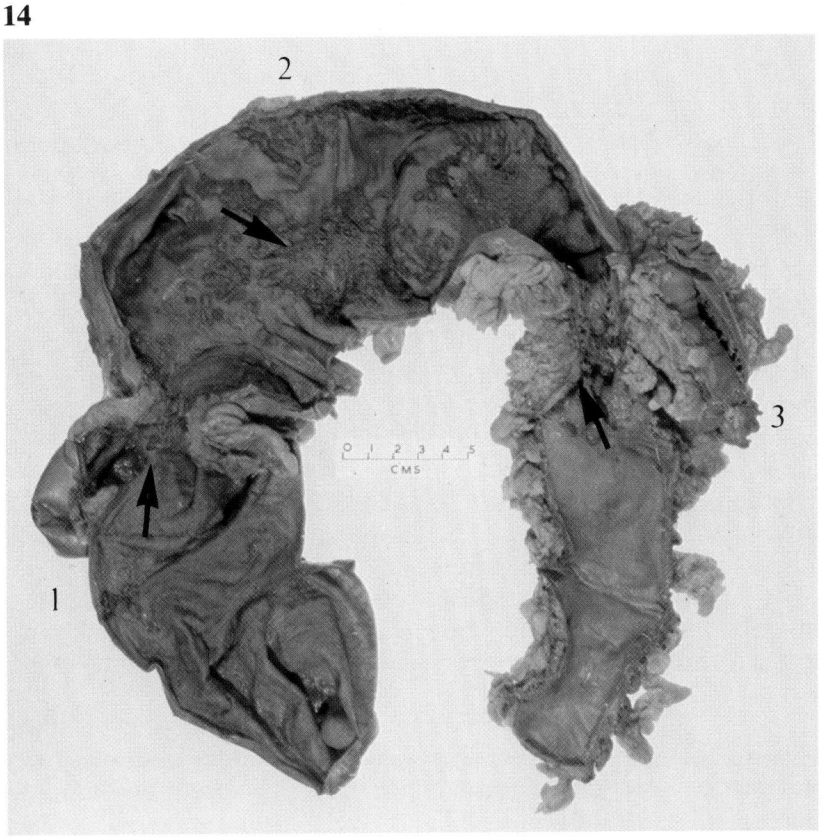

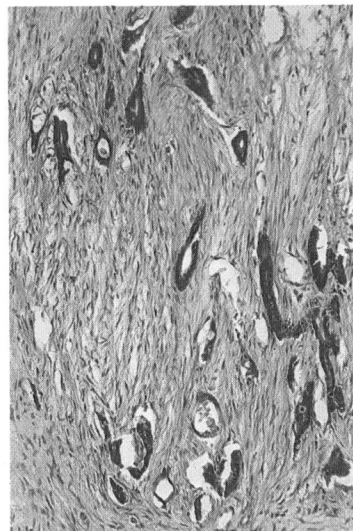

14d Field 3. Less well differentiated tumour infiltrating and provoking fibrosis. *(H&E ×80)*

A.N. Smith

263

Acute necrotising enterocolitis

This form of enterocolitis was first recognised as a dread complication of abdominal surgery. Typically, a few days after operation the onset of diarrhoea was rapidly followed by a state of dehydration, peripheral circulatory failure and a high mortality.

Aetiology and pathogenesis

The condition is of debatable pathogenesis and in the pre-antibiotic era it happened most often after partial gastrectomy or operation for carcinoma of the colon. It could also follow intestinal obstruction or even extra-abdominal operation. The condition became more prevalent after the introduction of antiobiotics especially when used as pre-operative prophylaxis. In a number of cases the disease complicated such medical conditions as myocardial infarction or other cardiovascular disorders, and more recently, cardiovascular operations associated with bypass.

The essential lesion may be intestinal anoxia caused either by occlusion of minute mucosal vessels by thrombi or by spasm, or when circulatory deficiency occurs from hypotension. The condition therefore should be compared with ischaemic colitis in which the vascular insufficiency involves larger vessels (see Section 15 OA).

In recent years the occurrence of necrotising enterocolitis in infancy has been reported with increasing frequency. In particular it has been noted in very premature babies many of whom have been treated in intensive care. It has also become evident that the lesion is more frequent in bottle-fed babies.

Pathology

In the most rapidly fatal cases virtually the whole of the alimentary tract may be involved, but in others only the colon or less often some other part of the alimentary tract shows the characteristic mucosal necrosis.

In fulminant cases the small intestine is usually most severely affected. The bowel wall is oedematous and the serosa dull. The small bowel may contain two or more litres of thin fluid and there may be a small amount of blood-stained transudate in the peritoneal cavity. The surface of the mucosa is devitalised and is covered by a thin 'membrane' of grey or bile-stained inflammatory exudate which is easily detached to float free in the fluid contents of the bowel.

Although the necrosis is extensive it affects only the mucosa, particularly the surface layers. The 'membrane' is composed of fibrin heavily infiltrated by inflammatory cells. The mucosal capillaries and venules may contain thrombi but arteries and arterioles are not affected.

When the disease is mainly confined to the colon but is severe the patient may be left with chronic disease and ulceration and/or stricture formation. A rare complication is perforation.

15

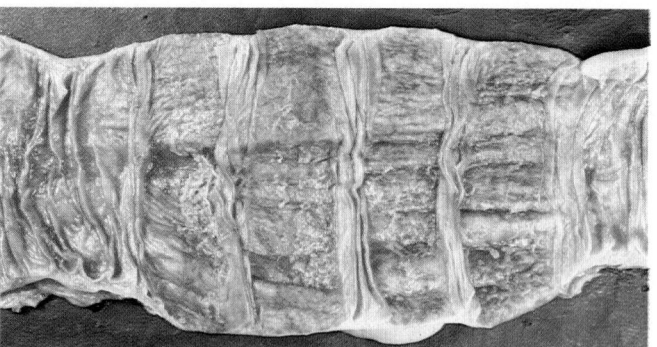

G.C.P.228

15 From an elderly female who developed necrotising enterocolitis following operative relief of an intestinal obstruction.

A portion of dilated small intestine showing inflammatory oedema. Its congested mucosa is partly covered by pseudomembranes of devitalised epithelium and inflammatory exudate.

Pseudomembranous colitis

This is a less catastrophic condition of similar aetiology in which colonic mucosal damage results in formation of 'pseudomembranes'. It sometimes follows the administration of antibiotics both therapeutic and prophylatic, and is then believed to result from an overgrowth of faecal micro-organisms which are relatively resistant to the antibiotic in question. Staphylococci and clostridia have been implicated in this way. In recent years the production of cytopathic toxins by *C. difficile* has been recognised as a possible cause of colitis following antibiotics. Lincomycin and Clindamycin with its powerful action against faecal anaerobes may be responsible for an unduly high proportion of the attacks. The severity of the disease varies to some extent with the severity of the underlying clinical condition.

Pathology

Numerous discrete, raised, yellow plaques varying in size up to 2cm in diameter may be found scattered over the mucosa like paint splashes. In the most severe cases they may coalesce.

16

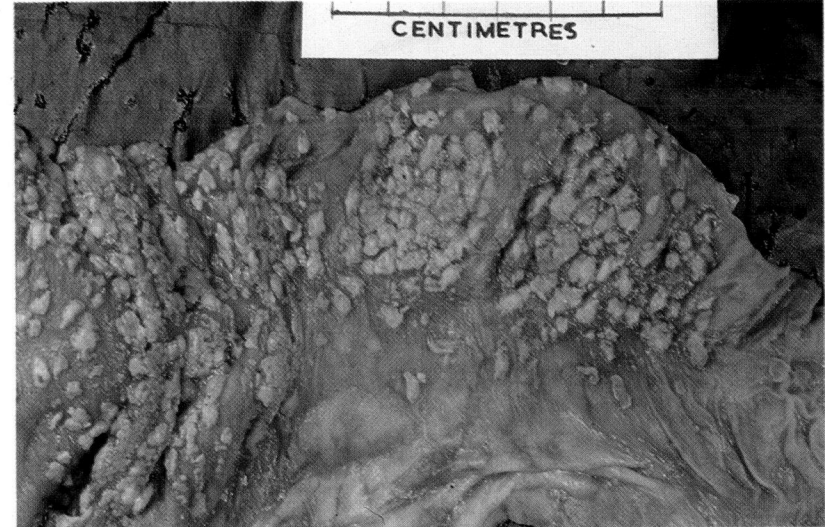

G.C.P.227

16 From a female aged 69 years who died of cardio-respiratory failure resulting from chronic bronchitis and emphysema and pulmonary fibrosis. She had experienced abdominal pain with some diarrhoea for one week before death.

At autopsy the transverse colon was found to be severely inflamed with some inflammatory exudate on its peritoneal surface, and pseudomembranes on the mucosa.

The illustration shows the mid portion of the transverse colon. The yellow colour of the raised pseudomembranous patches contrasts with that of the congested surrounding mucosa.

17

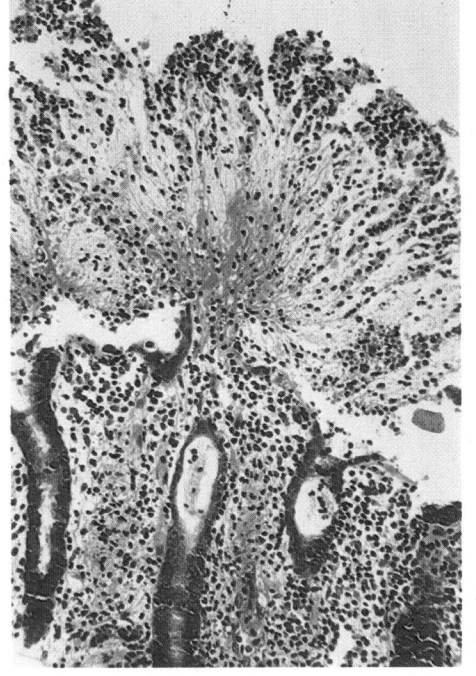

G.C.M.982

17 Mushroom-like aggregates of inflammatory exudate, fibrin and mucin form the 'paint-splashes' seen on the colonic mucosa. (*H&E ×162.5*)

On microscopic examination the severity of the lesions varies considerably. Often only the most superficial layers of the mucosa are involved. Uncommonly the whole depth of the mucosa is affected and the appearance is then difficult to distinguish from that of ischaemic colitis. The most characteristic histological abnormalities are seen in foci of moderate severity. Here small groups of glands are distended by mucin and polymorphs which erupt on the surface giving a mushroom-shaped cap of admixed mucin, fibrin and polymorphs – the bile-stained 'pseudomembrane'. The adjoining mucosa is relatively normal.

N. Maclean

265

Crohn's disease

This is a chronic disease of unknown aetiology in which an inflammatory type of reaction occurs with granuloma formation. This, however, may be a secondary phenomenon. The disease may affect any part of the gastrointestinal tract but predominantly the terminal ileum.

Historical

Though originally described by Dalziel in 1913 the disease is named after Crohn and his associates who described its distinctive features in 1932. His original description was of lesions in the terminal ileum but later it was shown that similar lesions could occur elsewhere in the ileum, jejunum and the colon. It is now possible to differentiate Crohn's disease from ulcerative colitis and tuberculosis (See Figs 18 and 19 opposite). When the disease occurred in the ileocaecal region earlier observers had regarded it as a form of hyperplastic tuberculosis but from which it was appreciated that the tubercle bacillus could not be recovered.

Epidemiology

Crohn's disease is most common in Western Europe and parts of the United States of America and is rare in Africa and South America. There has been a marked increase in the incidence of the disease since 1930. The apparent increase in Crohn's disease of the colon may be due to more accurate diagnosis whereby it is distinguished from ulcerative colitis. Crohn's disease is commoner in Jews than in other ethnic groups.

Incidence

Crohn's disease affects males and females approximately equally. The disease can occur in any age group but is rare below 6 years. It has a bimodal distribution, the main peak occurring between 15 and 30 years and a smaller secondary peak between 55 and 60 years. The second peak comprises mainly women with colonic disease.

The similarity of the naked eye appearances of Crohn's disease and ileocaecal tuberculosis are demonstrated in the accompanying illustrations:

18

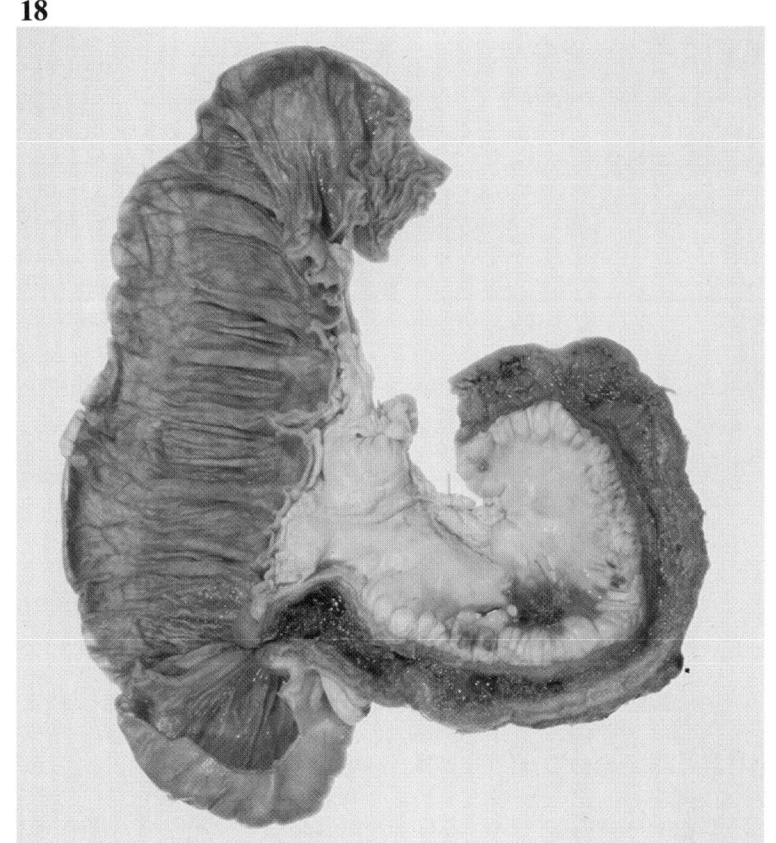

G.C.13228

18   From a female aged 21 years. The patient had a 6 month history of right iliac fossa pain associated with an anal fissure. Occasional attacks of pyrexia. Right hemicolectomy was carried out.

The pathological changes are present only in the terminal ileal loop with involvement of the ileocaecal valve. There is gross ulceration with marked thickening of the mucosa and of the muscularis. There has been haemorrhage into the lumen of the gut. The serosa of the terminal ileum shows many fine adhesions and considerable subserous haemorrhage has occurred. The haemorrhage may well have been due to manipulation at operation. These changes in the wall of the gut have made the terminal loop rigid, producing the typical 'hose pipe' stricture. The mesenteric lymph nodes are enlarged and prominent.

Microscopically the picture is that of the chronic stage of Crohn's disease.

19

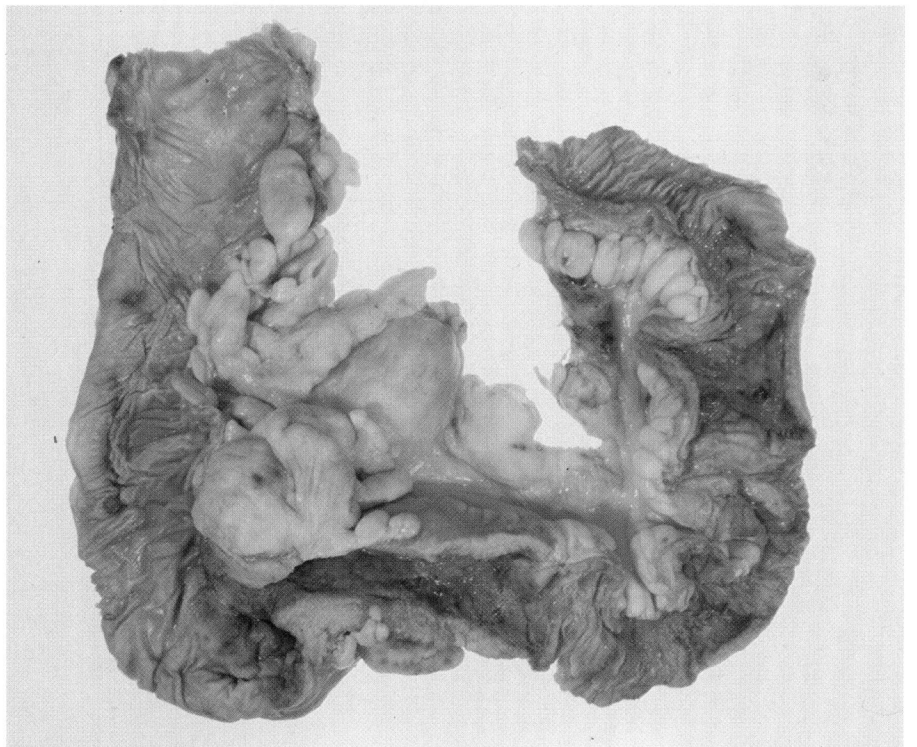

G.C.12225

19   From a female aged 73 years admitted to hospital as an 'acute appendicitis'. Right hemicolectomy was performed.

Externally the pathological features are limited to the terminal ileum close to the ileocaecal valve. The affected segment is congested and covered with shaggy adhesions. The mesentery appears to be thickened. The intestine has been opened to demonstrate the mucosa which is the site of several ulcers. These are most marked close to the ileocaecal valve. Typically the floor of each ulcer is congested and nodular.

The outstanding feature in this specimen is that both in the subserosa and in the mucosa there are numerous small tubercles and histologically this is a clear case of tuberculosis of the intestine.

These two specimens can be differentiated essentially by the presence of tubercles in one and not in the other. The other changes in the mucosa, muscularis and serosa are almost identical.

Crohn's disease (*Continued*)

Aetiology

This remains unknown but the following hypotheses have been advanced:

a   Infection – animal transmission studies using extracts of homogenised Crohn's disease tissue have been shown to induce epithelioid granuloma when injected into rodents. The characteristics of the filtrate that can induce lesions suggests either a virus or a cell-wall-deficient bacterium. However, other workers have failed to reproduce these findings.

b   Cellular immune deficiencies have been observed but whether these abnormalities are primary or secondary is undetermined.

c   The rising incidence of Crohn's disease recently has led to speculation about food additives and other dietary factors. Low fibre diets and increased consumption of refined carbohydrates have been implicated.

There is an increased risk in the siblings of patients with the disease. Furthermore relatives of patients with Crohn's disease have a greater frequency of ulcerative colitis and vice versa, suggesting an inherited predisposition to inflammatory bowel disease.

Macroscopic appearances

Irrespective of the segment of gut affected the appearances are similar, any differences being due to anatomical variation and the stage of the disease. The lesions may be solitary but when more than one segment is affected, the intervening bowel is normal (skip lesion).

In the early acute stage of the disease the lesion, usually in the terminal ileum, appears as an erythematous oedematous zone fading rapidly into normal bowel. The associated mesentery is thickened and the regional lymph nodes enlarged and fleshy. The mucous membrane is ulcerated, the ulcers varying in size from small aphthoid ulcers to large serpiginous ulcers.

20

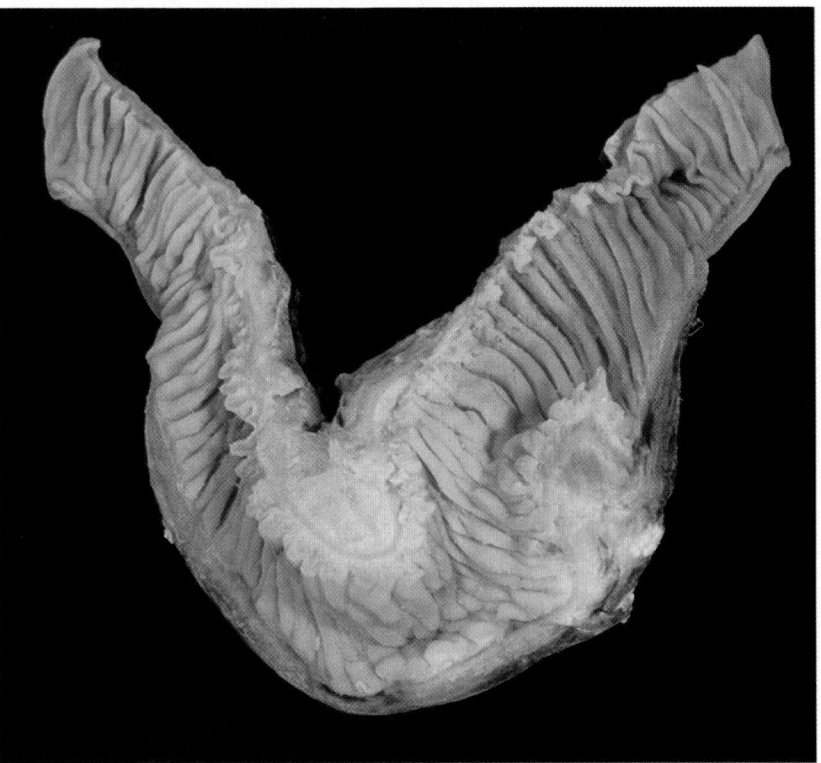

G.C. 14314

20   From a male aged 62 years. During admission for another condition a swelling was noted in the left iliac fossa. This appeared to subside but 4 months later he was again admitted to hospital and developed evidence of intestinal obstruction. A laparotomy was carried out when an inflammatory lesion of the small intestine adherent to the bladder and pelvic colon was discovered. This was resected.

The resected segment of ileum shows the presence of a localised lesion characterised by gross thickening of the muscle and subserosa but without ulceration of the mucosa.

Microscopic examination showed widespread hyalinisation and 'fibrosis' affecting the submucosa and subserosa with hypertrophy of muscle layers. Lymphatic dilatation was prominent and there were numerous foci of lymphocytes; no giant cells were present and there were no signs of neoplasm. These features were consistent with Crohn's disease.

Strictures often develop and the affected segment of bowel has a thickened rigid wall – the so-called 'hose pipe' stricture. The serosa loses its normal lustre, becoming paler, but the serosal blood vessels may become prominent and reticular.

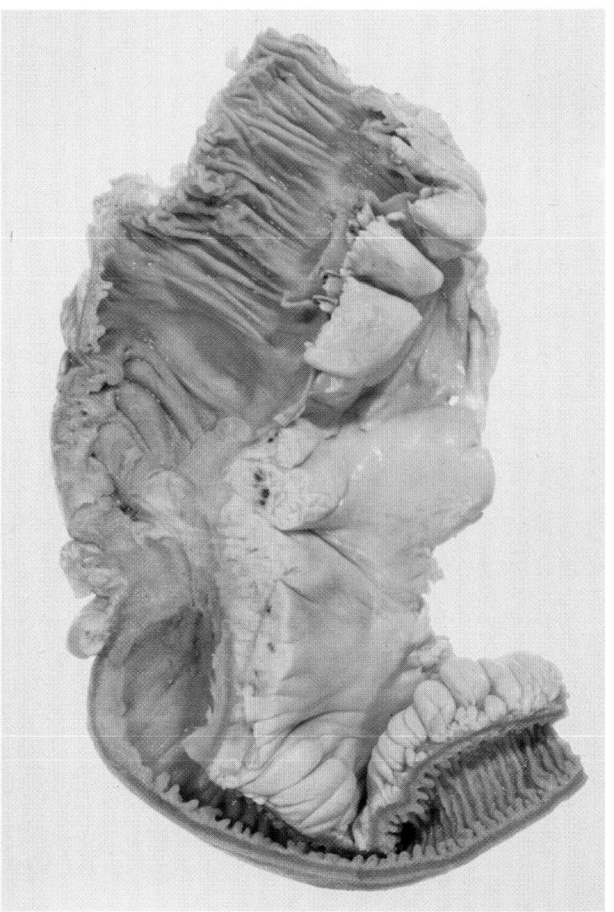

G.C.11413

22 From a male aged 50 years with a 10 year history of abdominal colic frequently located in the right iliac fossa and lower abdomen. Bowel habit was normal. The patient noted that occasionally after meals there was a feeling of fullness in the upper abdomen associated with exaggerated borborygmi after which the fullness disappeared.

X-ray demonstrated a persistent deformity with filling defects in the caecum and spasticity, irritability and narrowing of the terminal ileum. A right hemicolectomy was performed.

The specimen shows congestion of the terminal ileum and caecum. On section there is a mass of fibrous tissue at the ileocaecal junction with almost complete obliteration of the lumen of the gut. The terminal ileum shows muscular dilatation and hypertrophy. The mucosa of the last 5 cm of the ileum just proximal to the stenosed area shows ulceration and superficial necrosis. Note that the affected segment of gut is strictly limited and elsewhere the mucosa is normal. The mesentery of the ileum is markedly thickened with enlarged lymph nodes into some of which there has been localised haemorrhage.

Microscopically the main changes are those of long-standing inflammation with gross oedema and fibrosis.

21

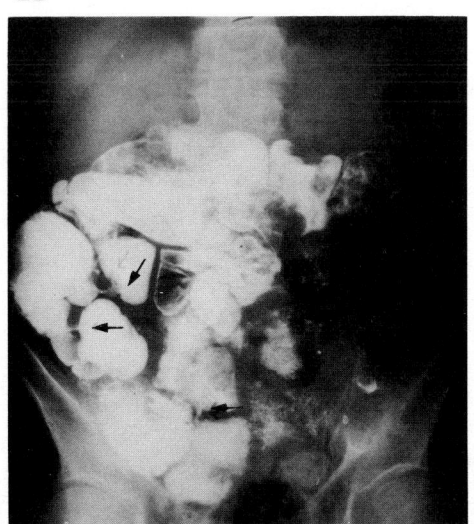

G.C.X.1003

21 From a male patient aged 64 years. Barium meal demonstrating multiple strictures of the jejunum associated with Crohn's disease.

Crohn's disease *(Continued)*

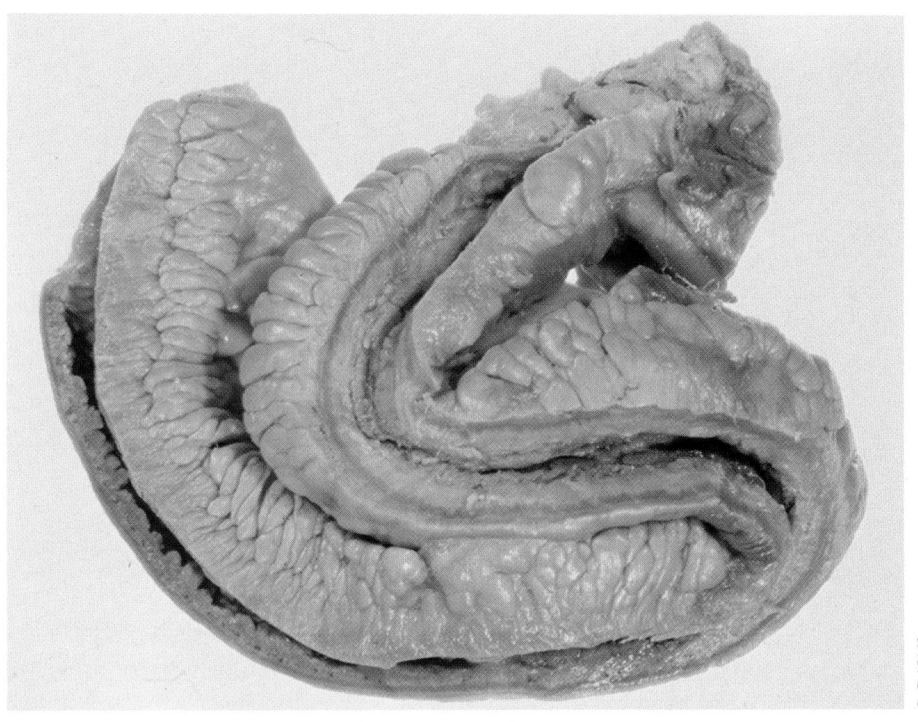

23 Loop of ileum in which the coils appear to have become matted together and show the gross evidence of Crohn's disease. The bowel wall is grossly thickened and the mucosa shows ulceration and haemorrhage. The major changes are in the submucosa and muscularis. There has been marked narrowing of the lumen of the gut over a long segment and obstruction must have occurred. This is the deformity described as a 'hose pipe' stricture.

G.C.15169

24

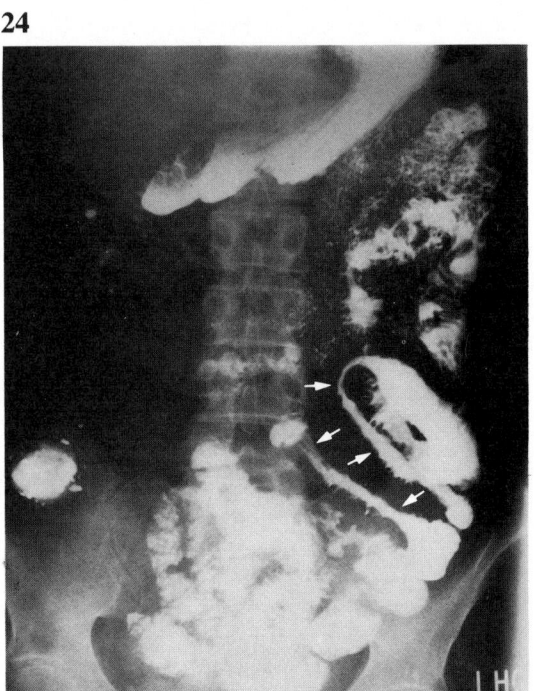

G.C.X.895

25

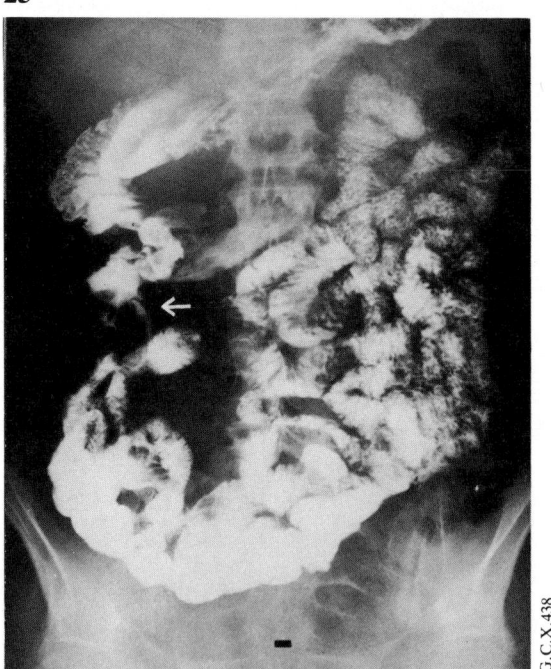

G.C.X.438

24 From a female who suffered from abdominal pain and diarrhoea for several years.

Barium follow-through shows typical involvement of a segment of lower jejunum associated with stricture formation and obstruction.

25 From an adult female.

A known case of regional enteritis treated by ileo-transverse colonic anastomosis and right hemi-colectomy. Barium-follow through shows a recurrence in the terminal 10 to 15 cm of the anastomosed ileum with ulceration and stricture formation.

The diagnostic 'cobblestone' appearance of the mucosa is present in less than a quarter of all cases. This appearance is due to intercommunicating fissures surrounding islands of inflamed oedematous mucosa.

26

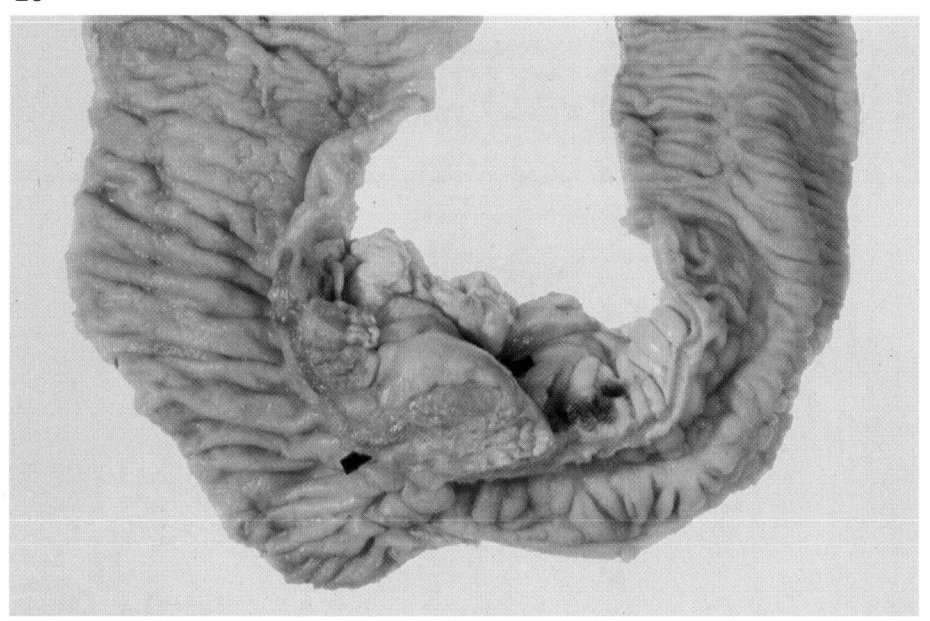

G.C.15051

26 The illustration is of the terminal ileum showing the changes of Crohn's disease. The bowel wall is thickened. Note the marked oedema of the mucosa which is raised and gives an early cobblestone pattern. A perforation is present which is possibly due to a deep fissure at this site (indicated by a black rod).

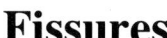

27

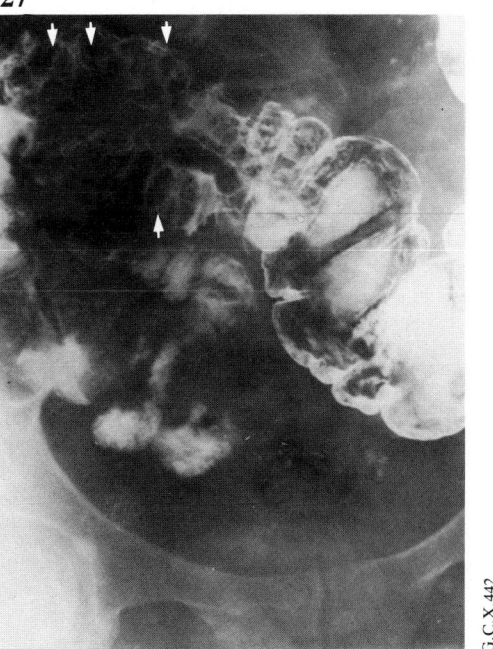

G.C.X.442

27 From an adult female showing recurrent Crohn's disease after right hemicolectomy and ileo-transverse anastomosis .

Note the 'cobblestone' appearance of the mucosa of the ileum.

Fissures

Fissures allow infection to penetrate transmurally the wall of the intestine leading to the formation of adhesions or internal fistulae. The most common fistulae are between adherent loops of small intestine: fistulae to colon, vagina and bladder are less common.

Abscess formation may occur and rarely free perforation. Cutaneous fistulae may follow bowel resection.

28 From a female aged 54 years. There was a history of abdominal pain over a period of 3 weeks prior to admission. Following a short phase of vomiting and general distress she was found to have evident features of peritonitis. Marked rectal tenderness on the left side.

At operation there was free fluid in the peritoneum and the affected loop of intestine was adherent to the bladder (1). A loop of intestine 35 cm long showing a diffuse inflammatory change with loss of peritoneal sheen and the presence of adhesions. A perforation is present in the wall of the gut at the site where intramural haemorrhage has occurred (2). Small areas of haemorrhage into the wall of the bowel have occurred at other points (3). There was a general thickening over the affected segment of the gut but the rest of the intestine showed no change and the appearances were therefore compatible with the diagnosis of Crohn's disease.

28

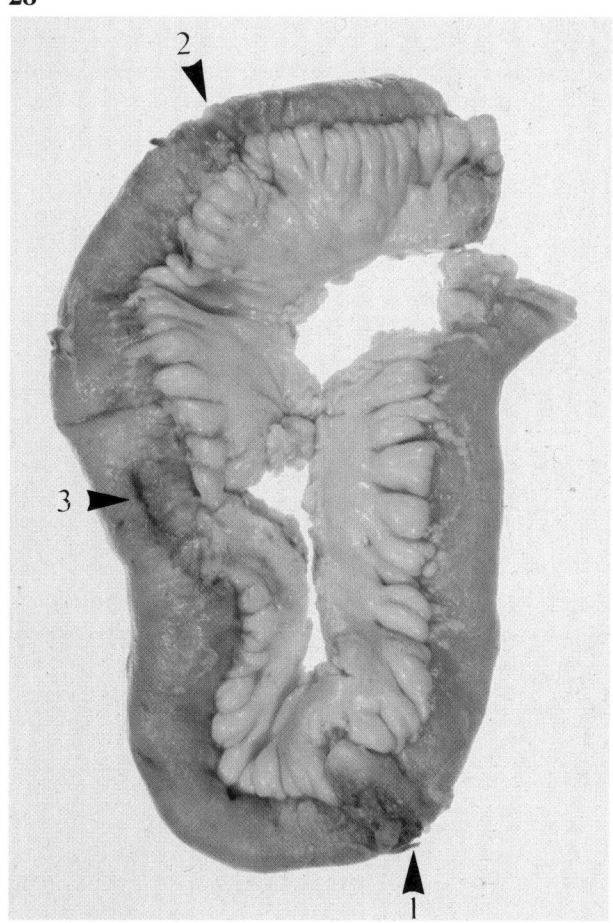

G.C.11497

Crohn's disease *(Continued)*

Relative incidence of Crohn's disease of small and large intestine.

There is considerable variation between series and the prevalence of Crohn's colitis may be under-estimated by misclassification of some cases as ulcerative colitis. Referral patterns in different centres may vary causing apparent atypical distribution.

Small bowel only	21–66%	average 40%
Small and large bowel	30–58%	average 39%
Large bowel only	16–27%	average 19%
Other (stomach, duodenum and rectum)	0–5%	average 2%

Colon

Pathological changes in Crohn's disease of the colon are similar to those described in the small intestine. Both colon and small intestine may be affected together; indeed, an ileal lesion with involvement of all or part of the right colon is one of the commonest distributions.

The disease presents in two forms:

1 The predominantly submucosal lesion spreading ultimately through the wall as a pan-colitis. Lymph nodes may be affected though less than in small bowel lesions.

2 Discontinuous or segmental 'skip' lesions.

As in the small intestine minimal aphthoid ulcers may be found or grosser granulomatous nodules sometimes referred to as 'sarcoid'.

Internal fistulae may result comparable to those noted previously. Dilatation of the colon and carcinomatous change do occur but much less frequently than in idiopathic ulcerative colitis.

29

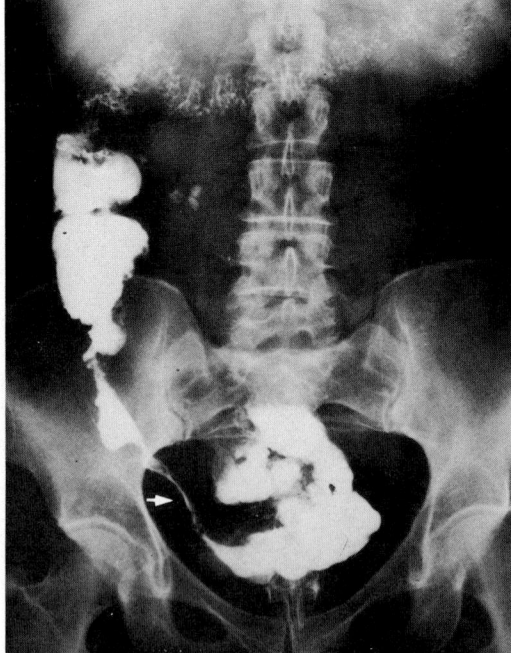

29 From a female aged 45 years. The classical picture of Crohn's disease. The terminal 20 cm of ileum shows irregular narrowing, the caecum is drawn up and the terminal ileum and ascending colon are in one line – the typical 'string' sign is present.

G.C.X.433

30

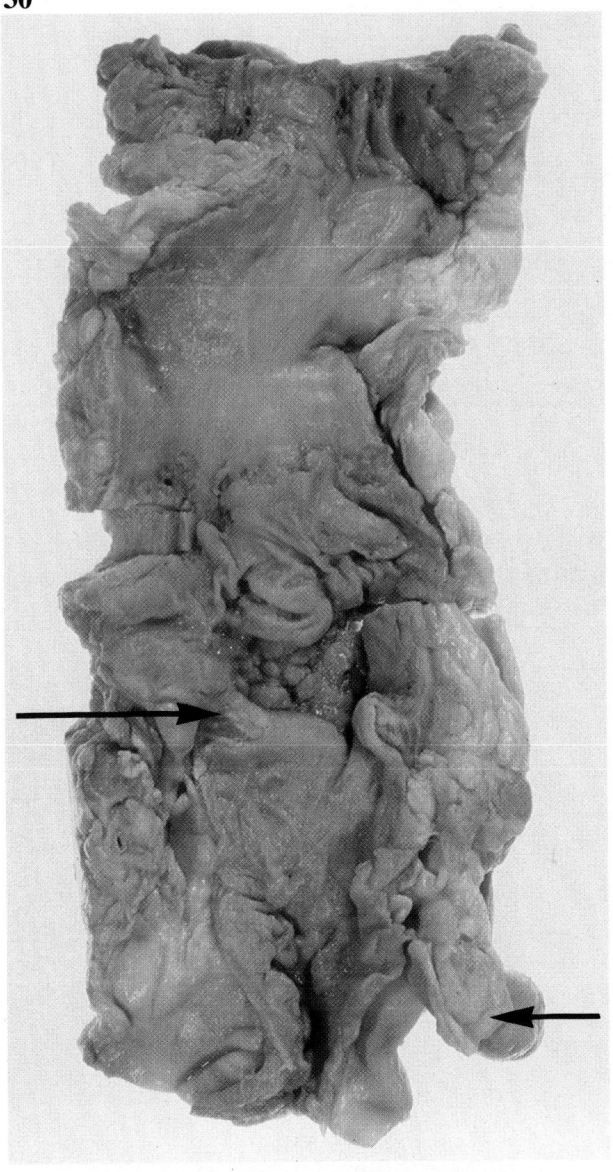

Ileocaecal
junction

Appendix

G.C.7618

30 From a female aged 49 years. History of vomiting and marked loss of weight for 18 months. This is an older specimen in the collection (1930) and at operation was regarded as tuberculosis rather than a carcinoma of the caecum. It was only at later re-examination of the specimen the diagnosis of Crohn's disease was recognised.

An irregular ulcer has destroyed part of the caecal mucosa. The edge of the ulcer is slightly raised and in places undermined. Irregular islets of mucous membrane are present on the floor of the ulcer. The mucosa in the immediate neighbourhood is puckered. Distal to the ulcerated area a considerable portion of the mucosa is smooth and has a cicatricial appearance. The appendix was stiff, thickened, kinked and adherent. The retrocaecal fat is abundant.

Note how the ileum has been drawn up and the ileocaecal angle straightened out.

31

G.C.X.434

31 From a female aged 40 years. Diarrhoea for several years. Barium enema shows extensive involvement of the colon due to Crohn's disease. The radiograph shows shortening of the colon, loss of the normal haustration and multiple pseudopolyposis due to mucosal hypertrophy. The terminal ileum is also involved and the disease is more severe in the right half of the colon than the left half of the colon. Both these features help to differentiate the condition from ulcerative colitis.

Crohn's disease (Continued)

Colon (Continued)

32

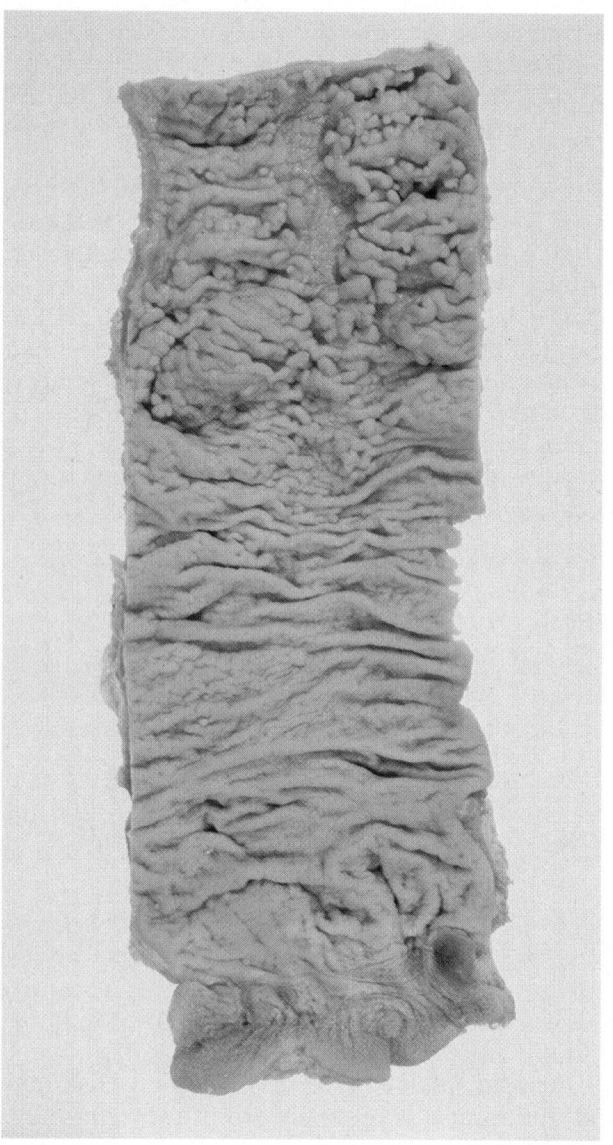

G.C.14663

32 The pelvic colon shows several large sessile polypoid masses, suggesting areas of mucosal oedema but without evidence of ulceration. Some deep crevasse formation is present running transversely. In the rectum at the lower end of the specimen there is marked mucosal change with polyp formation and ulceration. This surrounds the whole gut. The picture conforms to the diagnosis of Crohn's disease which had been established histologically.

33

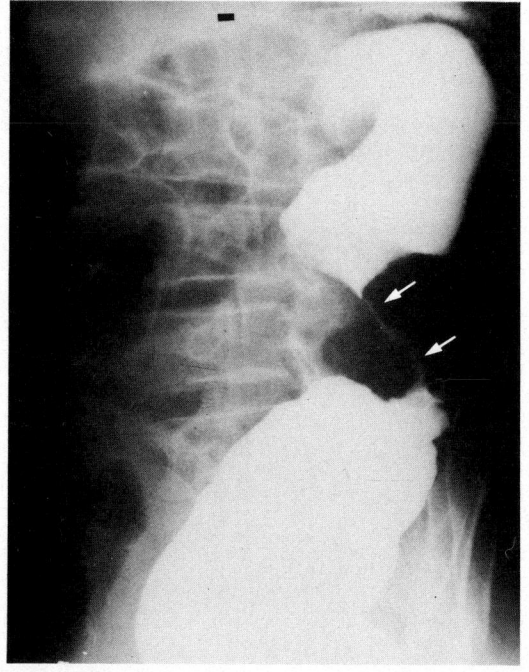

G.C.X.417

33 From a patient with known Crohn's disease of the terminal ileum.

Barium enema shows the stricture of the pelvic colon. This is a second or 'skip' lesion. The stricture has tapered ends, indicating its inflammatory nature.

Rectum

The disease may be confined to the rectum alone or may be associated with colonic or ileal disease. The main features are diffuse ulceration with or without areas of normal mucosa, short strictures or a thickened rigid bowel.

Anal/perianal

Perianal lesions may present in a variety of forms:
a   Skin lesions – maceration and superficial erosions are common. Occasionally deep ulceration and sub-cutaneous abscess formation occurs. Skin tags (oede-matous perianal skin) are very common.
b   Anal canal lesions – fissures, often multiple, always painless, rarely midline.
c   Ulceration – may be cavitating deeply into sphincter muscles. Stenosis with induration is a sequel to long-standing fissures or indolent ulceration.
d   Fistulae – low fistulae-in-ano and low rectovaginal fistulae are usually the result of abscess extension. High fistulae result from deep penetrating ulcers of the rectum giving rise to ischiorectal abscesses.

Perianal disease where the colon is chiefly affected presents as a fissure or fistula. Biopsy at this site gives a diagnosis. These features are of great importance since perianal disease can sometimes be the first clinical manifestation, often preceding intestinal disease by years.

34

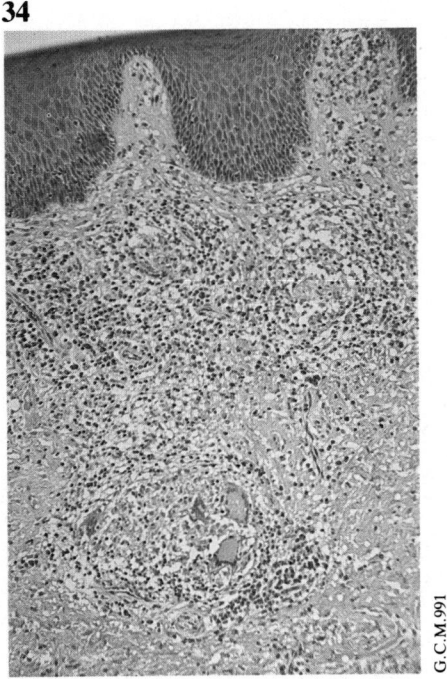

34 Anus – Crohn's disease. Non-caseating granulomas have formed in the anal wall. The deepest contains several giant cells. *(H&E ×100)*

Incidence

The reported incidence of anal/perianal disease varies widely probably related to the care taken in searching for the lesions. Approximately 3 patients out of 4 with Crohn's disease either of the small or large intestine will also have anal/perianal lesions.

Crohn's disease has been described in a variety of other sites including mouth, oesophagus.

Stomach

Usually affects the distal half of the stomach and may simulate linitis plastica. The mucosa shows a cobble-stone appearance. The diagnosis is usually established only by histological examination, the clinical features in the absence of small bowel disease being impossible to distinguish from infiltrating carcinoma.

Crohn's disease *(Continued)*

Microscopic features

General pattern

Typically a transmural inflammation of the whole thickness of the bowel wall. Focal collections of chronic inflammatory cells, mainly lymphocytes, are scattered throughout the layers of the bowel wall. Submucosal oedema is marked. Lymphangiectasia and neuromatous hyperplasia are non-specific features. Vascular changes may be inflammatory or degenerative. The mucosa shows ulceration, fissuring and crypt abscess formation.

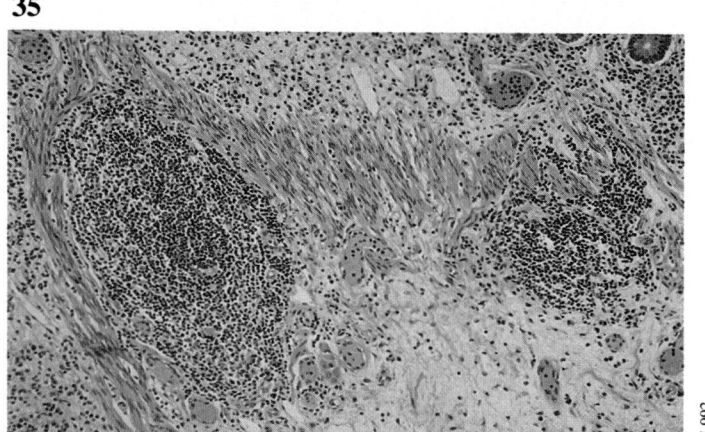

35 Ileum – Crohn's disease has caused oedema and lymphoid hyperplasia in the muscularis. *(H&E ×100)*

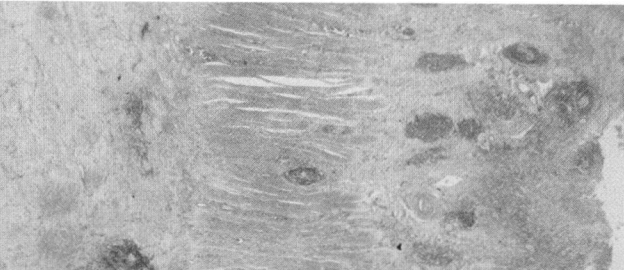

36 Ileum – Crohn's disease has caused mucosal ulceration and inflammation of the full thickness of the bowel wall. Lymphoid hyperplasia is marked. *(H&E ×15)*

Fissures

Fissures are almost pathognomonic of Crohn's disease. The penetrating knife-like clefts, sometimes branching, and lined by granulation tissue, pass deeply into the bowel wall and are the basis of internal fistula formation.

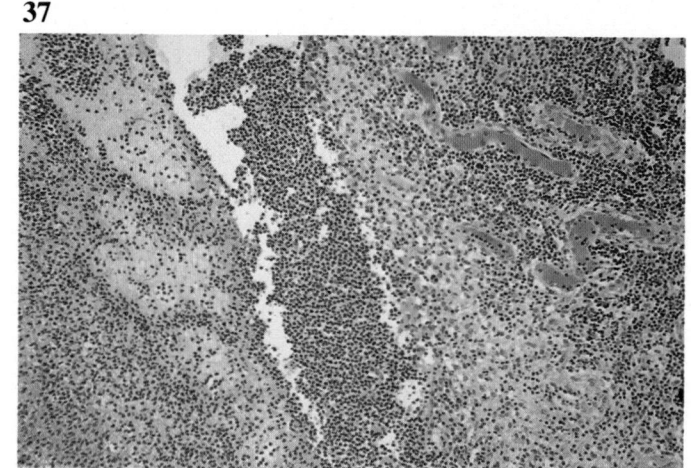

37 Ileum – Crohn's disease. A fissure lined by non-specific granulation tissue penetrates deeply into the bowel wall. *(H&E ×100)*

38

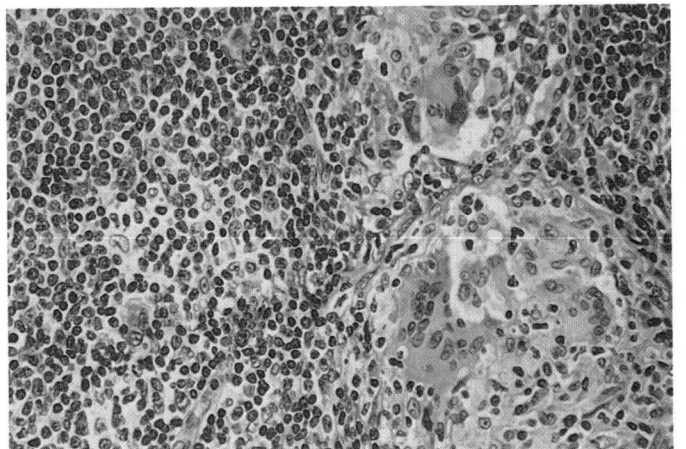

38 Lymph nodes – Crohn's disease. In addition to hyperplasia the lymph nodes associated with a segment of bowel affected by Crohn's disease may also show giant-cell follicles. *(H&E ×312.5)*

Granulomas

The presence of granuloma is one of the most valuable diagnostic features of Crohn's disease, being present in 50 to 70% of all cases. The granulomas are composed of epithelioid cells and often giant cells of the Langhan's type. The numbers vary from a few easily missed granulomas to large numbers. Granulomas are also found in the regional lymph nodes in 25 to 38% of cases.

39

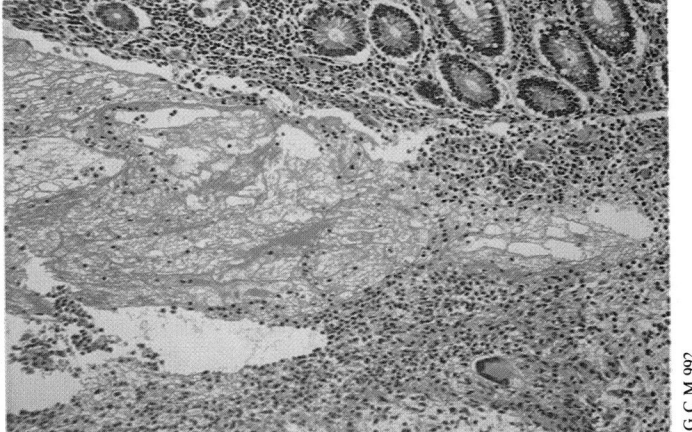

39 Ileum – Crohn's disease. The mucosa is undermined at the margin of an ulcer and a multinucleated giant cell can be seen in the granulation tissue. *(H&E ×125)*

40

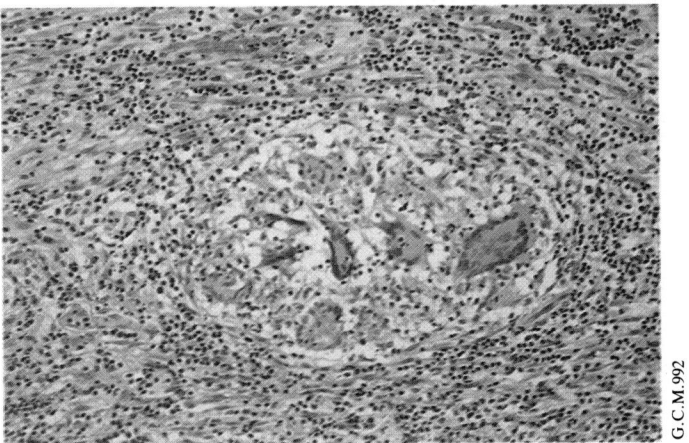

40 Ileum – Crohn's disease showing a non-caseating, giant-cell granulomatous follicle. *(H&E ×150)*

In the later stages of the disease ulceration is absent and the mucosa shows patchy atrophy with fibrosis of the muscularis mucosae. The oedema and inflammatory infiltrate are replaced by an excess of fibrous tissue in all layers. The granulomas undergo hyalinisation but without calcification.

Crohn's disease *(Continued)*

In Crohn's disease a number of factors lead to malabsorption:
1   Direct mucosal damage leading to a reduced surface area for absorption.
2   Mucosal damage causing a reduced bile salt reabsorption and a reduction in the entero-hepatic circulation.
3   Bacterial colonisation following stasis giving in effect the blind loop syndrome.
4   Fistulae.
5   Lymphangiectasia.
6   Problems due to surgical resection which may have had to be extensive or multiple.

Extra intestinal manifestations

Many apparent systemic effects have been regarded as attributable to Crohn's disease. These include:
1   Arthritis.
2   Ankylosing spondylitis.
3   Erythema nodosum.
4   Pyoderma gangrenosum.
5   Iritis.
6   Uveitis.
7   Stomatitis.
8   Hydronephrosis; renal calculi (usually oxalate).
9   Biliary calculi.
10 Hepatic dysfunction is common and usually minor, but hepatitis, pericholangitis and cirrhosis can occur.
11 Osteoporosis which is attributable to the malabsorption may develop.
12 Amyloidosis has been reported as a late complication.

These manifestations have been described as occurring prior to the recognition of intestinal Crohn's disease. In established cases systemic disturbance is usually regarded as an index of the activity of the intestinal lesion.

Carcinoma

Recent studies have shown an increased incidence of both small bowel and colonic adenocarcinoma in patients with Crohn's disease. The associated cancers tend to occur in the distal small bowel in areas involved by the disease and in surgically by-passed loops. There is also some evidence that pancreatic cancer may be increased in patients with Crohn's disease.

Mortality

The death rate is approximately twice that expected from an age and sex matched control population.

J. Anderson

Ulceration of the colon occurs in uraemia and it is convenient to consider this lesion and contrast it with the other ulcerative conditions of the intestine.

Uraemic colitis

In advanced uraemic disease the mucosa of the colon and rectum is subject to damage. This is partly due to circulating toxins but also to submucosal haemorrhages. The damaged mucosa is liable to be invaded by organisms from the lumen of the gut with the development of ulceration. Microscopic examination confirms these findings.

41a

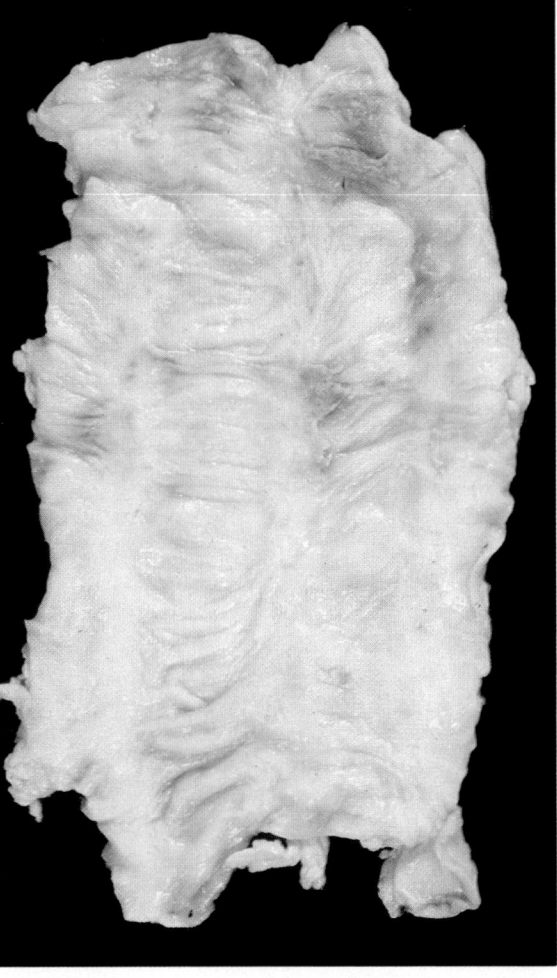

41 From a male aged 54 years. The patient was admitted to hospital with the clinical evidence of failing renal function. His blood pressure was elevated. There were retinal changes. His blood urea was elevated.

While in hospital he developed lower abdominal colic, diarrhoea and the passage of blood per rectum. An exploratory laparotomy was carried out but revealed only an inflammatory reaction of the right colon. Following operation there was a rapid fatal increase in renal failure.

41

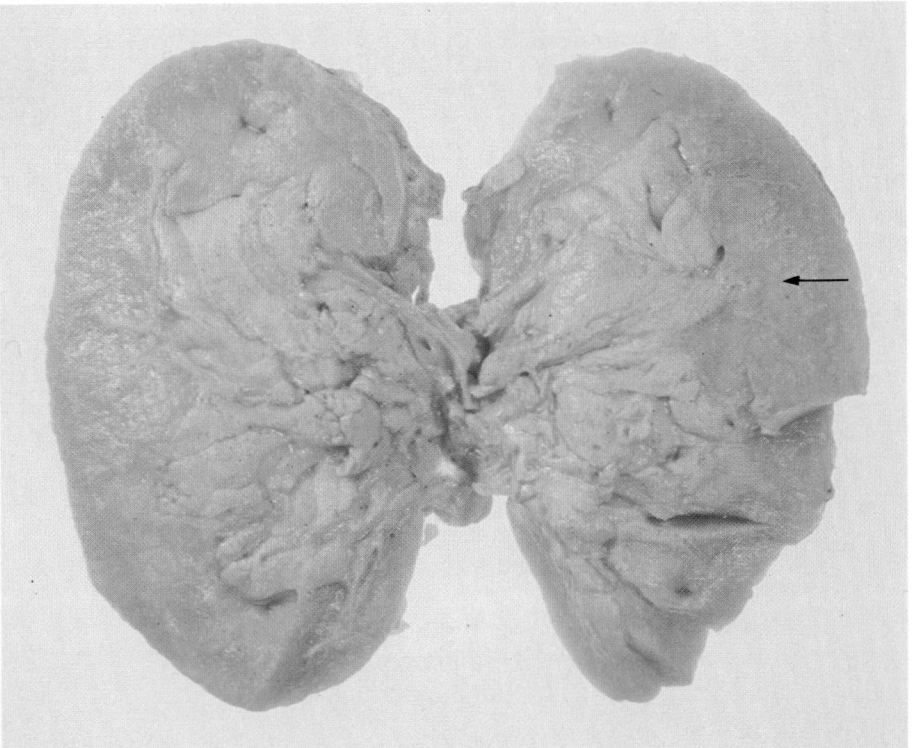

The specimen of kidney demonstrates marked reduction in cortical bulk and marked yellow pigmentation of tubules, presumably due to lipoid accumulation. The cortex was paler than normal and the appearance is that of an advanced degree of chronic nephritis.

41a The caecum and ascending colon showed marked ulceration which involved approximately two-thirds of the mucosa of the caecum. The ulcers were shallow and were covered by a yellow-grey exudate. The gross ulceration continued for some distance into the ascending colon. From that point onwards to just beyond the splenic flexure the mucosa was generally congested and there was a line of ulceration along each taenia coli similar to that in the caecum. No ulceration was present in the pelvic colon or rectum. The illustration is of a segment of colon.

Tuberculosis of the intestine, the abdominal nodes and the peritoneum was formerly common in the United Kingdom. The incidence has been greatly reduced by the pasteurisation of milk, eradication of tuberculous infected milk herds, and the introduction of childhood immunisation. The disease remains common in many parts of the world, especially the Indian subcontinent where 1% of hospital admissions are due to this condition.

Routes of infection

Primary tuberculosis of the gastrointestinal tract is due to the ingestion of M tuberculosis bovis carried in infected milk. The bovine bacillus penetrates the intestinal mucosa without causing structural damage and reaches submucous lymphoid tissue and the mesenteric lymph nodes. These changes correspond to the Ghon focus in the lungs.

In persons already sensitised by previous exposure, ingestion of the bacilli may lead to a localised ulceration of the intestine. Secondary tuberculosis of the gastrointestinal tract is caused by M tuberculosis hominis and occurs in persons suffering from pulmonary tuberculosis. It is usually spread by direct invasion of the alimentary tract from swallowing infected sputum. Rarely the spread to the intestinal tract is haematogenous. The abdominal cavity may become infected from the female genital tract.

Site of lesion

Oesophagus:	Rare, often associated with a bronchial fistula.
Stomach:	Uncommon, due to rapid transit, lack of lymphatic tissue, low pH; antrum most often affected.
Duodenum:	Uncommon.
Ileum:	Most frequently affected portion of the gastrointestinal tract – often with caecal involvement. Lesions may be single or multiple.
Colon:	Tuberculous colitis is rare and occurs in two forms – hypertrophic and ulcerative. It may progress to fistula or stricture formations and may be associated with skip lesions.
Ano-rectal:	Four types described – ulcerative (most common), varicose, lupoid and miliary.

Pathology

Three types of lesion have been described: (a) ulcerative, (b) sclerotic and (c) hypertrophic.

Ulcerative

1 This is most common in persons with active pulmonary tuberculosis and often a terminal event. The length of involved intestine is variable. The lesions are usually found in the ileum, corresponding to the normal sites of lymphoid tissue (Peyer's patches). They may be due directly to the action of the tubercle bacillus on the mucosa or to an ulcerative hypersensitivity within the lymphoid follicles of the submucosa. The ulcers are oval and lie transversely. Subperitoneal miliary tubercles may be seen and the draining lymph nodes are usually enlarged.

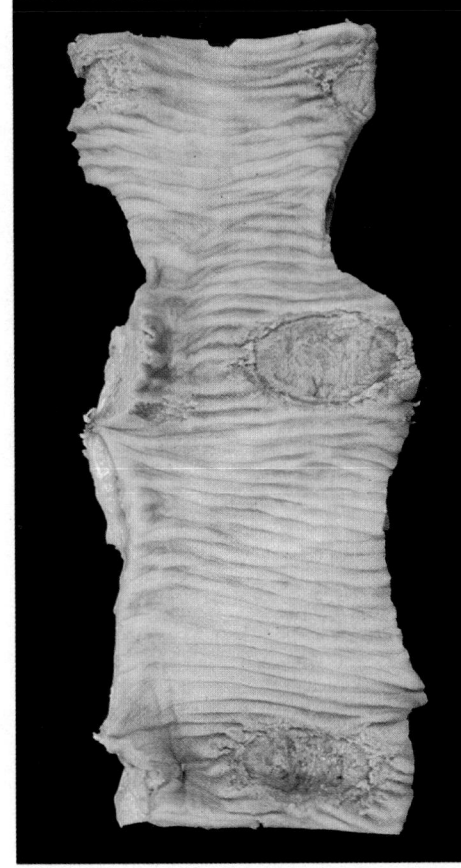

G.C.2513

Sclerotic

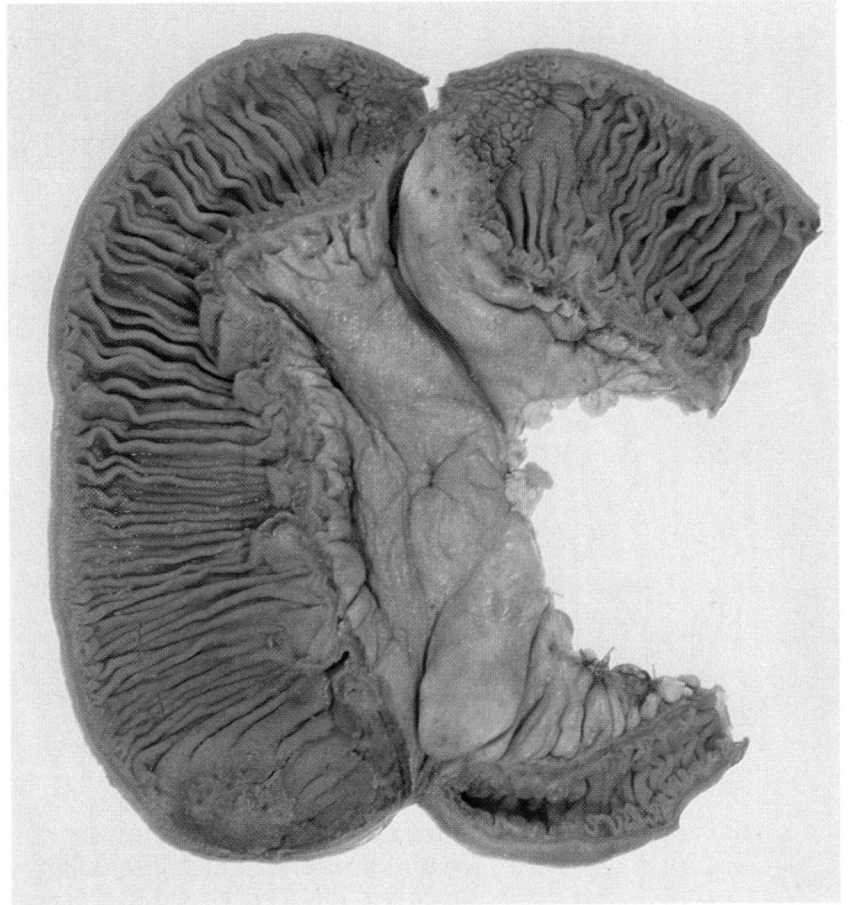

G.C.13147

2 Following the healing of an ulcerative lesion sclerosis occurs causing stenosis of the bowel lumen.

The illustration demonstrates such a lesion.

From the internal aspect the gross stricture formation can be observed. Proximally and between the strictures the bowel is distended and there is some hypertrophy of the muscle wall. On both sides of each of the strictures the mucosa shows a granular ulceration. Externally the peritoneal coat in the vicinity of the strictures was covered with tubercles.

Hypertrophic

3 This usually occurs in the ileocaecal region. The typical lesion is a bulky swelling involving ileum, caecum and ascending colon. Following contraction of fibrous tissue, the ileum is drawn upwards with obliteration of the ileocaecal angle; the caecum and ascending colon are shortened, the ileocaecal valve distorted and the appendix is contracted and may not be identifiable. The mucosa shows a variable degree of ulceration and sometimes a polypoid formation. The gut lumen is narrowed and tortuous and this may result in obstruction. Adhesions can develop and fistulae may occur. Caseation is usually not observed although small minute caseous tubercles in the serosa may be seen. These may be few or numerous.

Hypertrophic tuberculosis may simulate Crohn's disease, carcinoma or amoeboma.

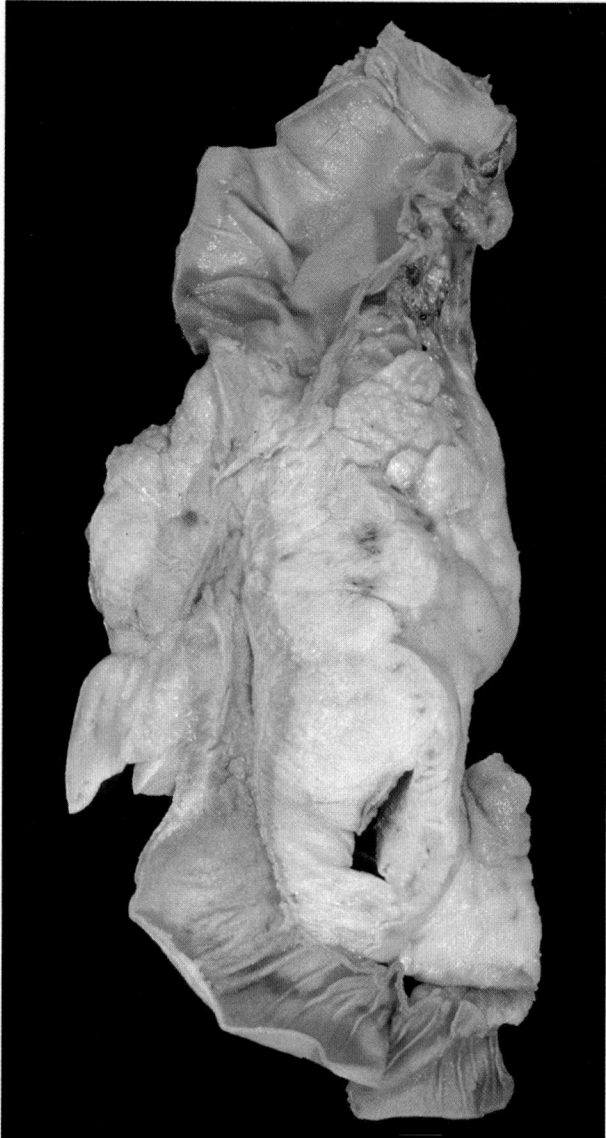

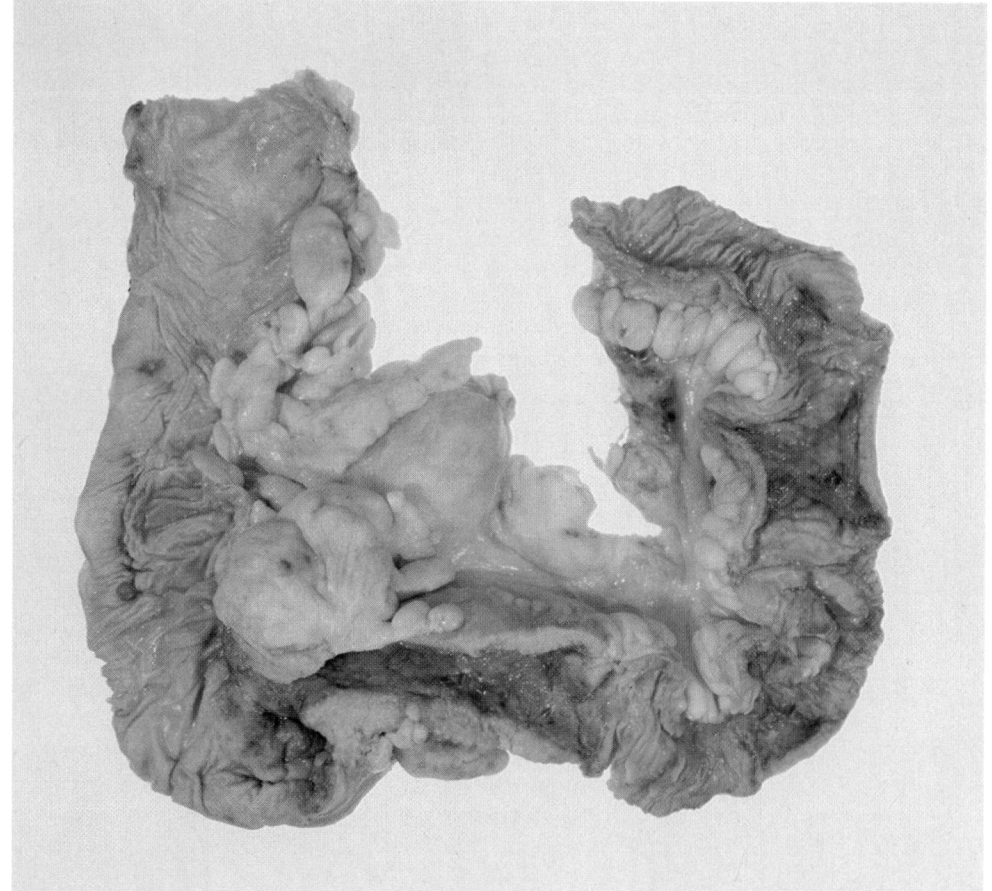

4 Prior to the identification of Crohn's disease in 1930 as a separate entity, this lesion was generally confused with tuberculosis and regarded as a varient characterised by the absence of caseation and failure to identify the causal organism. This point is noted in Section 15 E where one of the specimens illustrated had originally been diagnosed as tuberculosis. This specimen of proven tuberculosis has been previously shown in contrast with typical Crohn's disease (see Section 15 E **19** and **30**).

Microscopic features

Tubercle formation, caseation, ulceration and fibrosis, the cardinal diagnostic features of tuberculosis are frequently seen but are not invariable. Caseation necrosis may be absent and therefore the histological appearance, being atypical, presents diagnostic difficulties. Identification of the tubercle bacillus is rarely achieved. Differentiation between ileocaecal tuberculosis and Crohn's disease may be impossible and in this situation emphasis is laid on the presence of tuberculous lesions in other parts of the body especially the lungs.

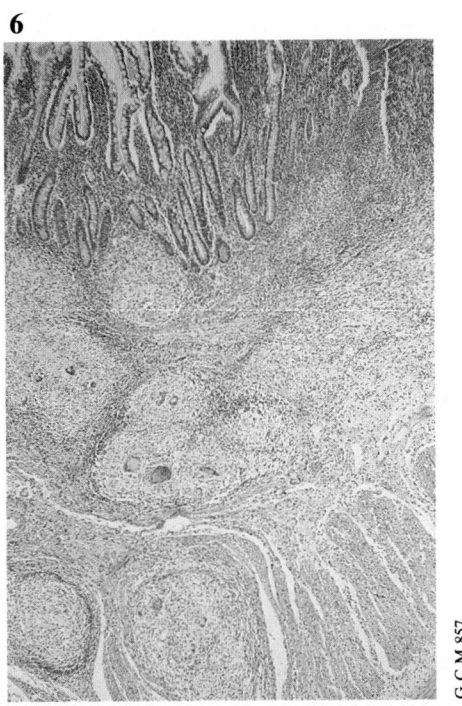

6

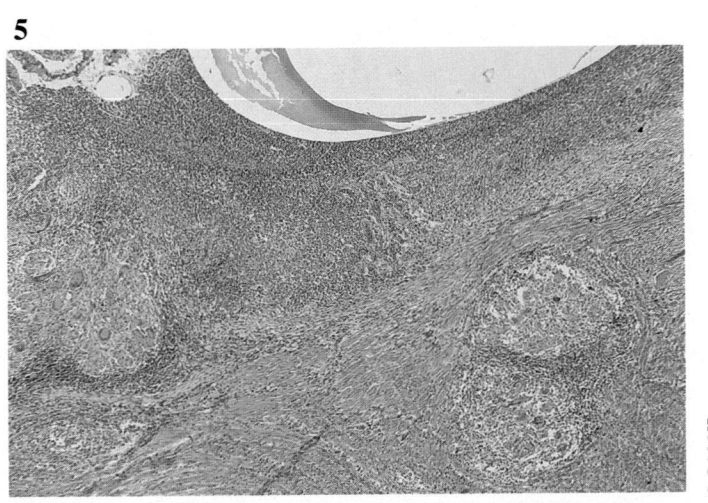

5

5 Ileum – Tuberculosis. Part of a tuberculous ulcer lined by granulation tissue. Giant cell follicles are present in the submucosa and muscularis. *(H&E ×37.5)*

6 Ileum – Tuberculosis. There are tubercles in the mucosa, submucosa and muscularis. *(H&E ×37.5)*

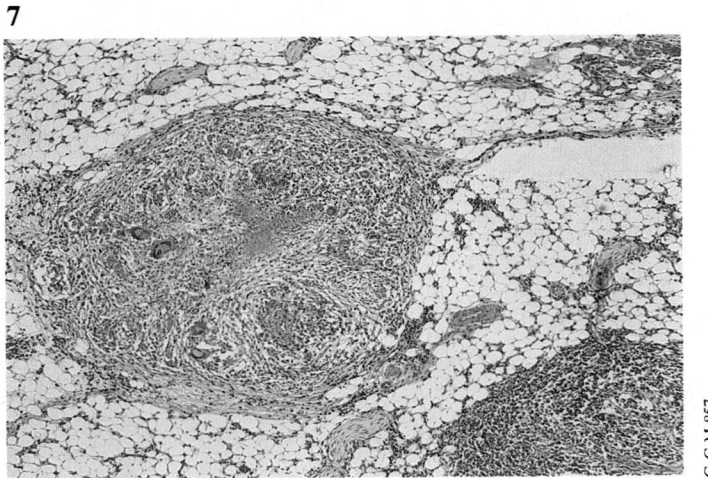

7

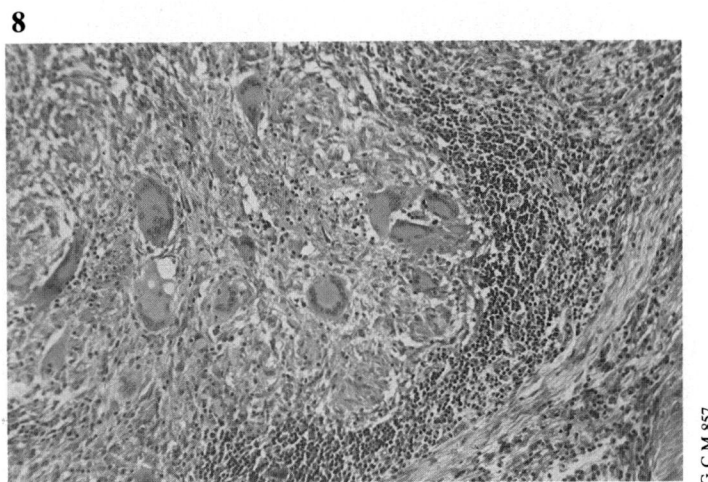

8

7 Ileum – Tuberculosis. Same case. A mesenteric tubercle with giant cell follicles shows slight central caseation. *(H&E ×125)*

8 Ileum – Tuberculosis. A submucosal tubercle composed of epithelioid cells and multinucleated giant cells surrounded by lymphocytes. *(H&E ×125)*

Abdominal lymph nodes

Tuberculous disease of abdominal lymph nodes is a common lesion and was formerly particularly prevalent in Scotland. It is still common in some countries.

The disease is most common in childhood and young adult life.

9 The usual mode of infection is by spread of the tubercle bacillus from a tuberculous ulcer located in the lower ileum and the infecting organism is of the bovine type derived from infected milk. However, the portal of entry may not be identifiable.

The affected lymph nodes are usually located in the mesentery especially in the right iliac fossa.

9

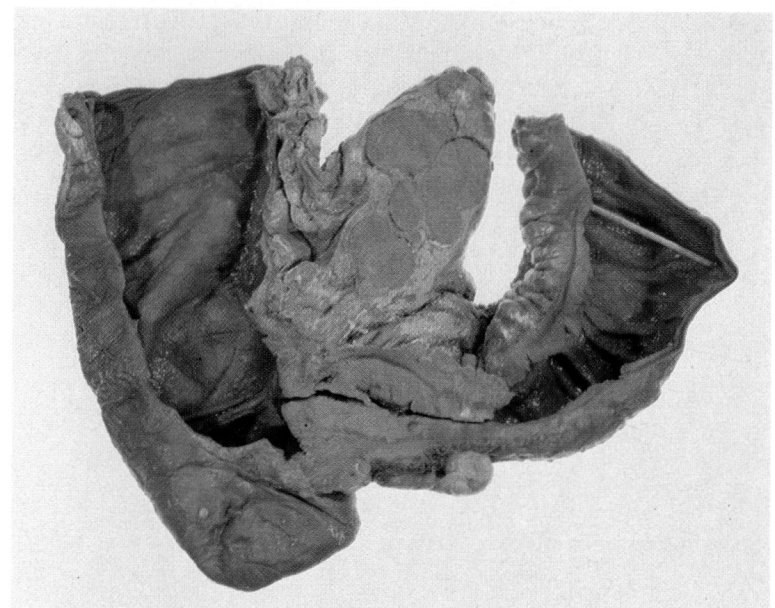

The lesions may proceed to caseation but many heal by a process of fibrosis and calcification. The extent of nodal involvement varies. Solitary nodes or a group of nodes presenting as a matted mass are commonly found. Rarely a widespread involvement is observed, in which event the possibility of a haematogenous origin may be considered.

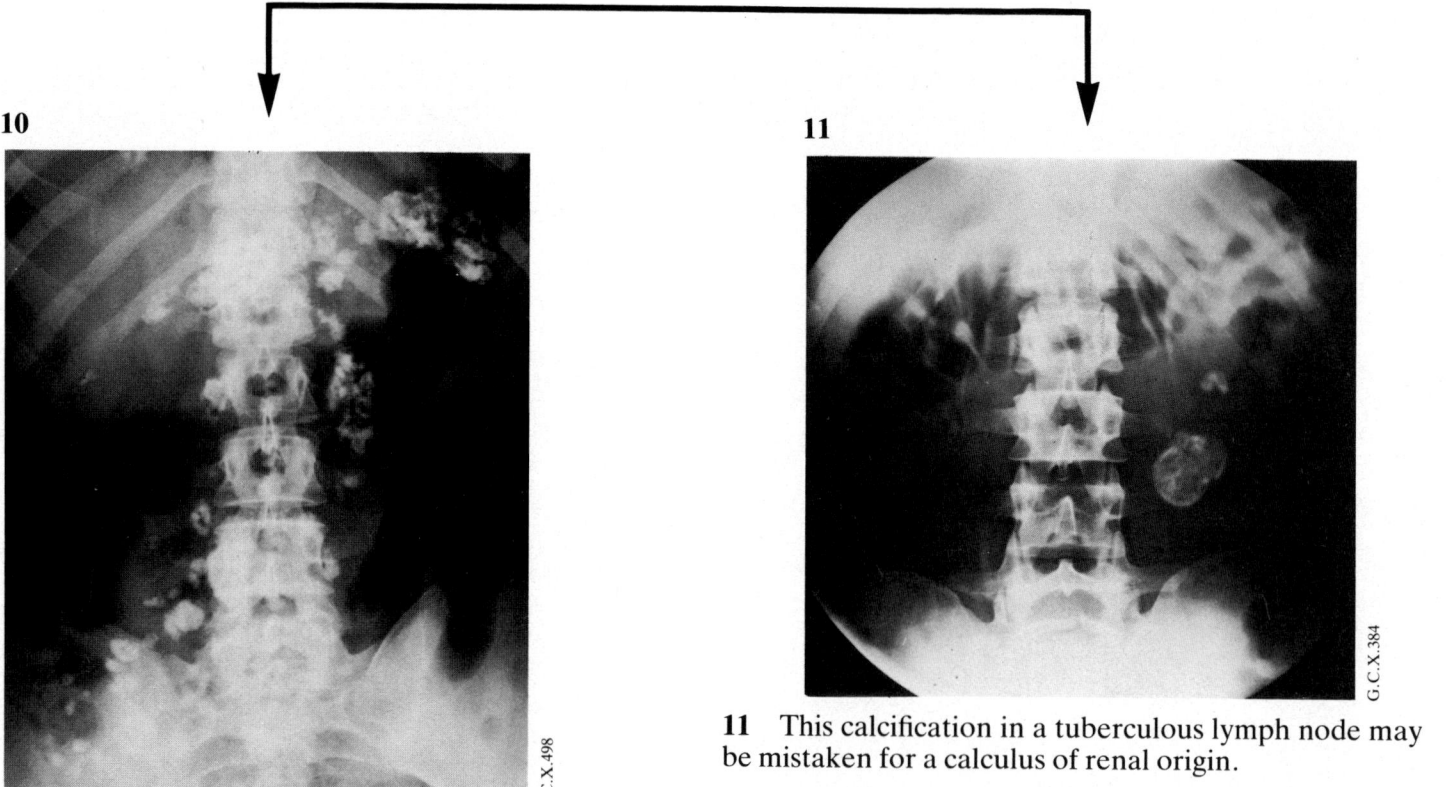

10

10 Diffuse calcified mesenteric nodes.

11

11 This calcification in a tuberculous lymph node may be mistaken for a calculus of renal origin.

284

Occasionally a tuberculous lymph node may increase with liquefaction and the formation of a localised abscess. Rupture of such a lymph node into the peritoneal cavity leads to a localised or diffuse peritonitis.

The node may become adherent to adjacent coils of intestine causing kinking or obstruction.

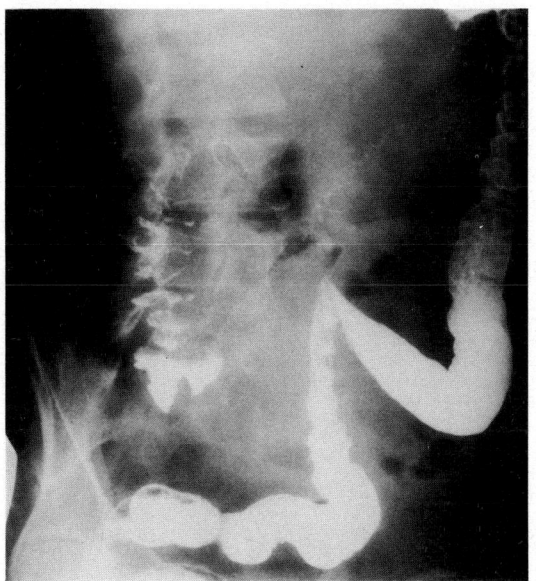

12 Example of adhesion from a mesenteric tuberculous node becoming attached to the pelvic colon which is drawn upwards with resulting deformity.

Peritoneum – tuberculosis

Tuberculous peritonitis is a lesion rarely seen in the United Kingdom today. It has been eradicated by the rising standards of living and nutrition; the elimination of infected milk, the introduction of immunisation and the control of tuberculous lesions when discovered by modern drug therapy.

The clinical description of the lesions, when found, is based upon older observations.

Tuberculous peritonitis may occur at any age but is most frequently observed during childhood or adolescence. It is most commonly the result of extension of disease from a local focus in the intestine or a mesenteric lymph node. It may also be derived as a complication of tuberculosis of the Fallopian tubes. Rarely the condition results from haematogenous spread from an extra-abdominal focus.

The disease may run an acute course usually with involvement of the whole peritoneal cavity and with marked effusion. More often it runs a chronic course and tends to be more localised. A third variant of the disease is a localised cystic lesion.

Acute tuberculous peritonitis

This is an acute illness associated with marked cachexia which carried a high mortality prior to the introduction of modern therapy.

The whole peritoneal cavity is involved and the characteristic feature is the multiplicity of small tubercles over the whole peritoneal surface. There is usually a serous effusion containing many lymphocytes, but it may be difficult to identify tubercle bacilli microscopically although animal inoculation demonstrates the organisms. Splenic enlargement is common.

Occasionally the effusion is purulent and this is found most frequently in young females. The peritoneum is thickened and the effusion gelatinous and commonly greenish in colour.

Chronic tuberculous peritonitis

The course of the disease may be slower and chronic. It may present in a variety of ways according to the dominant reaction.
1   There is marked peritoneal effusion.
2   The characteristic feature is the formation of adhesions and minimal outpouring of peritoneal fluid.
3   The disease may form a localised 'cyst'.

Ascitic

The disease here runs a more chronic course and the peritoneal lesions vary in size from discrete miliary tubercles to conglomerate masses. The effusion may be considerable, is clear and yellowish in colour and, as in the acute form, it may be difficult to identify the causal organism. In boys a patent processus vaginalis allows fluid to distend the scrotum.

Dry

13   A form of the disease is also recognised in which the effusion is more limited but in which there is much matting of the tissues due to many adhesions. The affected tissues form irregular masses and the omentum often presents as an irregular cylindrical swelling. Areas of caseation can be identified. The parietal peritoneum is thickened. In this form of tuberculous disease fistula formation is common and because of the manner in which the intestinal loops are bound together intestinal obstruction frequently occurs. The illustration is of such a tuberculous mass which has been sectioned.

13

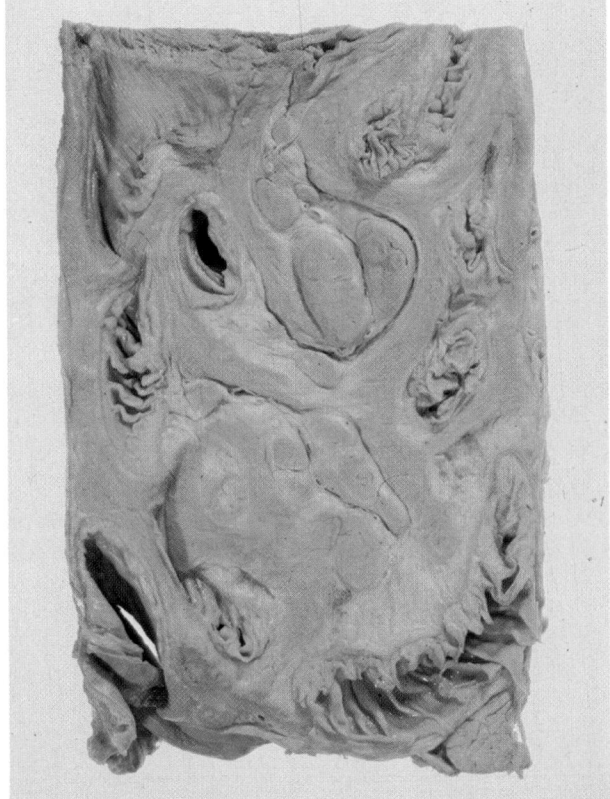

G.C.2989

14

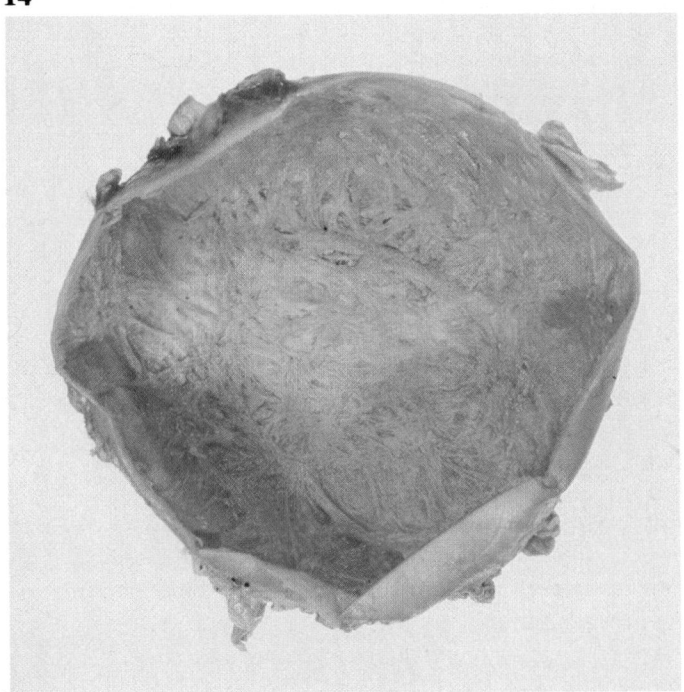

G.C.5986

Encysted

14   The disease has become limited by adhesion formation and presents as a localised cystic mass. It is frequently pelvic in position and clinically may simulate an ovarian cyst.

J. Anderson

The cause of actinomycosis is an anaerobic strepto-thrix, *Actinomyces israeli*, which is present as a commensal in the human mouth. Given a portal of entry such as a wound in the skin, a recent extraction socket or a carious tooth in the mouth or some break of the mucous membrane in the ileo-caecal region, the organism enters the submucosa and is followed by secondary infection to form the characteristic pyogenic granuloma. The resulting inflammatory mass is 'woody' hard and consists of a honeycomb of fibrous tissue and multiple abscess cavities in which lies the pus containing the diagnostic 'sulphur granules'.

Actinomycosis does not spread by lymphatics but involves tissues adjacent to the site of the primary infection by direct spread. From the mouth it spreads to involve salivary glands, bone and the tissues of the face and neck and in the ileo-caecal region the peritoneal cavity and the abdominal wall. When the disease occurs in the ileo-caecal region it forms initially a hard swelling which simulates tuberculosis or neoplasia or a chronic appendicular abscess. In both sites the skin is penetrated by multiple sinuses which discharge the characteristic pus and heal, only for new tracks to form and point. Actinomycosis may also occur in the lungs where it may spread to the chest wall without infecting the pleural cavity and has to be distinguished from pyogenic or tuberculous osteomyelitis of a rib.

Amoebiasis

An endemic protozoan disease in tropical countries caused by the entamoeba histolytica. The disease is transmitted by the passage of ova in the faeces of affected persons and from this source food and vegetables are contaminated. Ova in encysted form are ingested with contaminated food. After ingestion the cysts reach the large intestine and there invade the bowel wall.

Carriers may or may not have experienced a previous attack of the disease.

The initial lesion is a small elevated yellowish mass in the mucosa which breaks down to form a transverse ulcer with ragged undermined edges. The base of the ulcer is covered by yellow slough and the surrounding mucosa shows a zone of hyperaemia. The extent of the disease varies. Ulcers are most frequently found in the caecum and rectum. Diffuse colitis is the most dangerous form of the disease, the ulceration becoming confluent leaving islands of hyperaemic mucosa amongst large areas of necrosis.

1

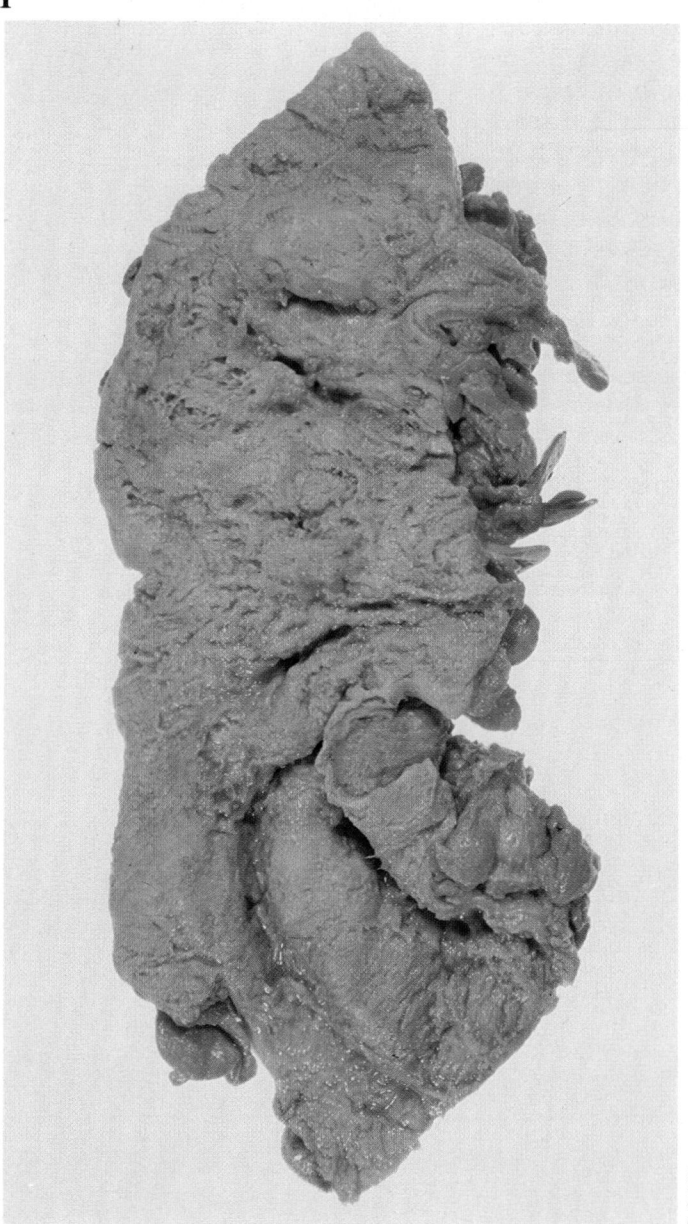

G.C.4421

1 From an adult. The colon is thickened. The mucosa is wholly involved. There are numerous irregular ulcers extending more-or-less completely through and in places undermining the mucosa which forms a shaggy necrotic surface. Amoebae histolyticae are present in the ulcerated areas.

In all cases the diagnosis is established by the identification of the entamoeba histolytica.

Caecum – Amoeboma

Occasionally a chronic form of the disease develops characterised by a local swelling – the so-called amoeboma. This can develop months or years after the original infection and clinically may simulate carcinoma, hypertrophic tuberculosis or a diverticular or appendicular mass.

An amoeboma arises as the result of a secondary infection. There is tissue necrosis with a surrounding wall of fibrous tissue. The contents of this granulomatous lesion vary in consistence and the peritoneum overlying the swelling is congested.

2

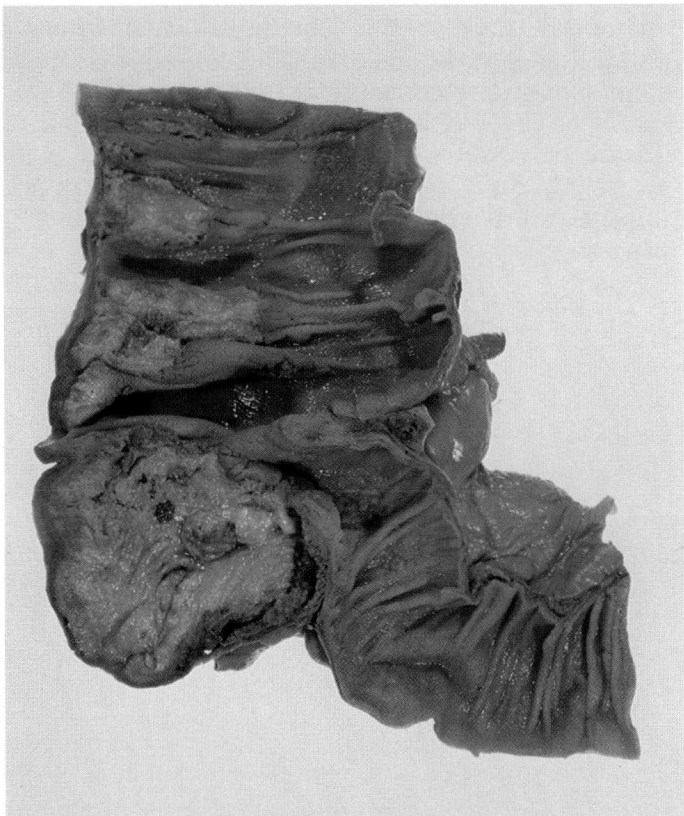

G.C.10664

2 From a Chinese male aged 40 years who gave a history of 14 days abdominal pain chiefly colicky in nature and associated with some general malaise and slight fever. On local examination a tender palpable mass was present in the right iliac fossa. The stools did not show amoebae. There was no history given of 'dysentery'. The condition was observed for 48 hours and as the tenderness appeared to be increasing laparotomy was carried out. At operation the caecum was found to be congested, the walls thickened and rigid, and there were no obvious enlarged lymph nodes. A provisional diagnosis of tuberculosis of the caecum was made and the right colon resected. The patient died 2 days later.

Operative intervention in the presence of entamoeba histolytica is a dangerous procedure precipitating spread of the parasite.

3

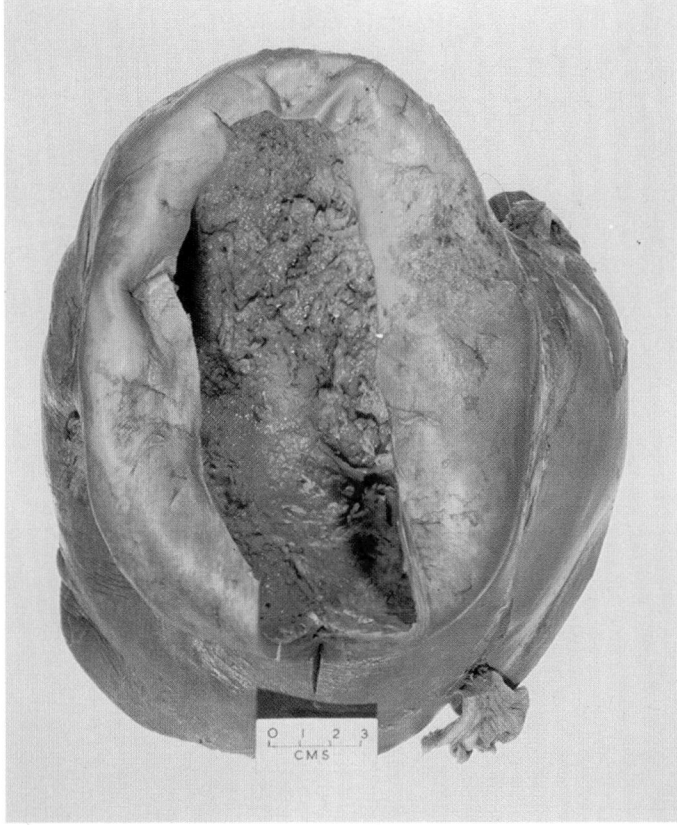

G.C.8210

3 The most serious complication is invasion of the portal venous system with subsequent metastatic amoebic liver abscesses or amoebic hepatitis. Rupture of an abscess will spread the disease to the peritoneal cavity, pleural cavity or into the lung substance. A chronic abscess may become encapsulated with fibrous tissue and eventually undergo calcification. Rare complications include perforation of the colon and massive necrosis (see Section 16/1 E).

Schistosomiasis (bilharziasis)

Three species of schistosoma occur in man, *Schistosoma mansoni* (Africa and South America), *Schistosoma haematobium* (Africa) and *Schistosoma japonicum* (Far East). *Schistosoma mansoni* and *Schistosoma japonicum* involve the intestine, particularly the left colon and rectum, and *Schistosoma haematobium* involves the bladder.

Infection occurs in agricultural workers wading in waters infested with the larval form of the parasite (cercaria) which have been released from the appropriate snail intermediate host. The cercariae penetrate the skin, enter the circulation through the lymphatics and after extensive migration settle in the veins of the portal system (*Schistosoma mansoni* and *japonicum*) or bladder (*Schistosoma haematobium*). There the male and female worms lie in copula and the ova are deposited in the terminal venules. The ova have a spine which serves both as an anchor while they develop and later to assist their passage into the lumen. An intense granulomatous inflammatory reaction occurs in the submucosa of the colon and rectum, and with ulceration in the bladder epithelium. The initial changes are those of acute proctitis and colitis and in the bladder of acute ulcerative cystitis.

Later the condition becomes chronic with polypi, fibrosis and stricture formation and in the bladder wall calcification. Parasites may also spread via the portal vein to the liver leading to an inflammatory reaction in the portal triads and to fibrosis which obstructs the portal flow into the liver with the consequent development of portal hypertension (see Section 16/1 O). It has been held that the development of malignant disease may follow long-standing schistosomiasis as in ulcerative colitis, but the precise nature of the relationship has not been established. There is no doubt that schistosomiasis is a precancerous condition in the bladder.

4

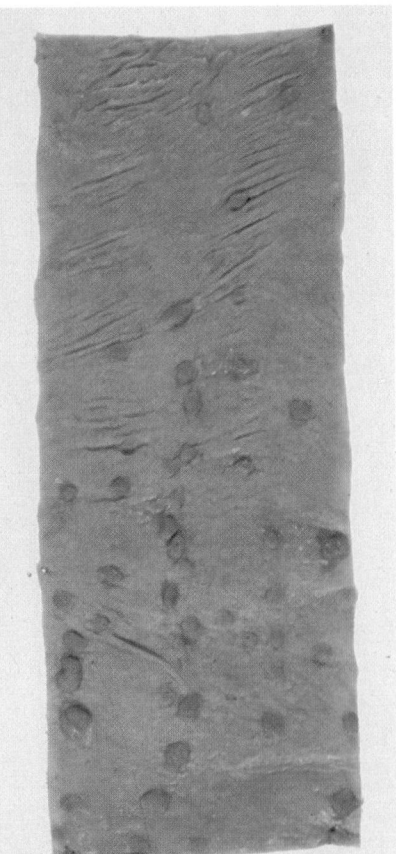

G.C.5168

4 From an Egyptian patient. Colon showing multiple discrete, brownish, nodules some of which have a warty appearance on the surface. Some ova have become calcified.

5

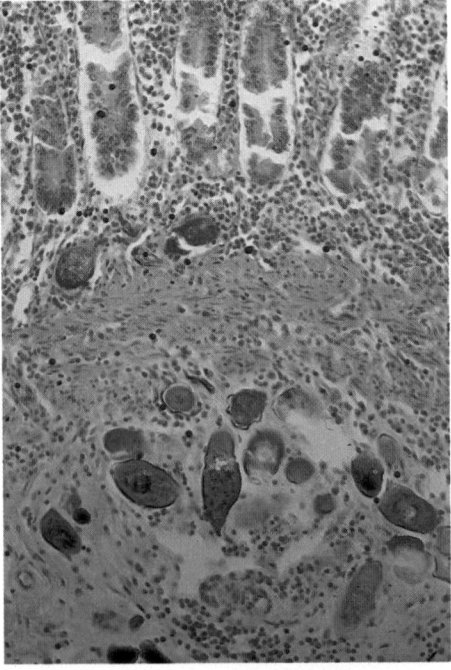

G.C.M.1004

5 Colon – Schistosomiasis. In this section of inflamed colonic wall schistosoma ova can be seen in deeper mucosa and particularly in submucosa. *(H&E ×150)*

Ascariasis

Infestation of the intestinal tract by ascaris lumbricoides is common in tropical countries.

Life cycle – After ingestion the young larvae leave the egg, penetrate the mucosa of the intestine, enter the blood stream and eventually become arrested in the alveoli of the lung. The larvae further develop and enter the bronchi and trachea after which they are swallowed and reach the jejunum where they become attached as adult worms. In its adult form the ascaris is cylindrical in shape, pointed at both ends and some 15 to 35 cm in length. It is white in colour.

The worm attaches itself to the mucosa of the small intestine, especially the jejunum. When numerous they lie in masses which may occlude the lumen and cause some degree of obstruction. Ascaris *in situ* may be demonstrated radiologically after a barium meal. Frequently the degree of infestation is severe especially in childhood and the patient often is pot-bellied. A degree of anaemia is common since the parasites feed on blood sucked from the mucosa and the anaemia is usually associated with an eosinophilia, especially in the early stages when there is pulmonary invasion.

While the chief habitat is in the jejunum the parasites frequently migrate.

1 They may ascend through the stomach into the oesophagus and may be vomited: or they may be aspirated into the respiratory tract and cause pneumonia. A worm has been recorded as ascending the Eustachian tube.
2 The worms may enter the common bile and pancreatic ducts leading to obstructive jaundice.
3 Worms may pass downwards and may cause appendicitis or be voided in the faeces. The passage of worms occasions an intense irritation.

The eggs of the worm are discharged in the faeces. This is a source of a fresh round of infection and affords a means of diagnosing the condition.

For details of the nature and life cycle of the parasites text books of tropical diseases should be consulted.

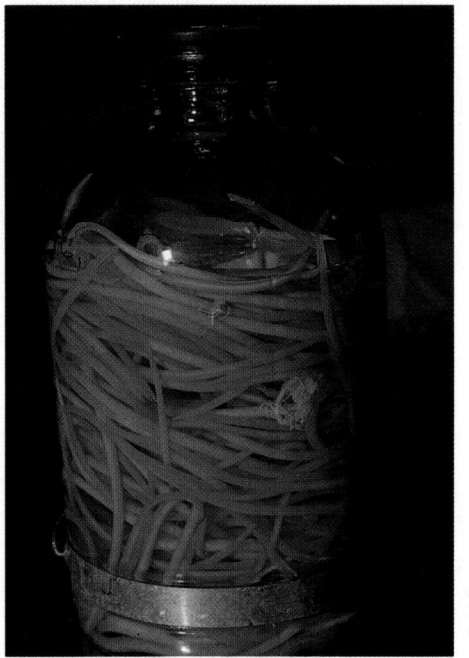

6 Ascaris lumbricoides passed per rectum.

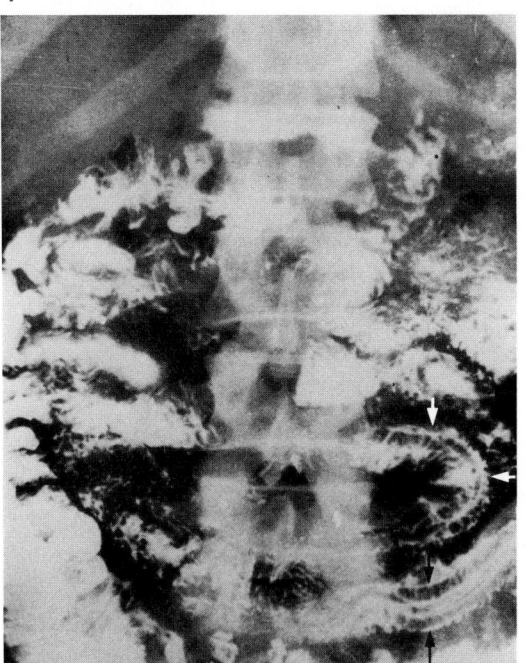

7 Radiograph demonstrating ascariasis.

Two factors predispose to the formation of faecoliths.
1 The presence of a nidus. This may be indigestable vegetable material including fruit stones or a gallstone which has reached the intestine and about which layers of new material are laid down.
2 Stasis. It is rare for stasis of the contents within the lumen of the gut to be such as to permit the formation of a calculus. Only in cases of most severe constipation persisting over a prolonged period are faecoliths formed. This may occur in patients suffering from mental disease and in Hirschsprung's disease.

The majority of faecoliths are found in diverticula or pouches of the intestine where faecal material may remain for long periods. The most common example is the appendix. Intestinal pouches in which calculi may form have usually resulted from adhesions.

Faecoliths may be single and ovoid but if multiple are faceted. They are dark in colour and on section show a laminated structure and the deposition of calcium salts. The essential risks of these faecoliths are ulceration and intestinal obstruction. Gallstone ileus is the classical example of obstruction.

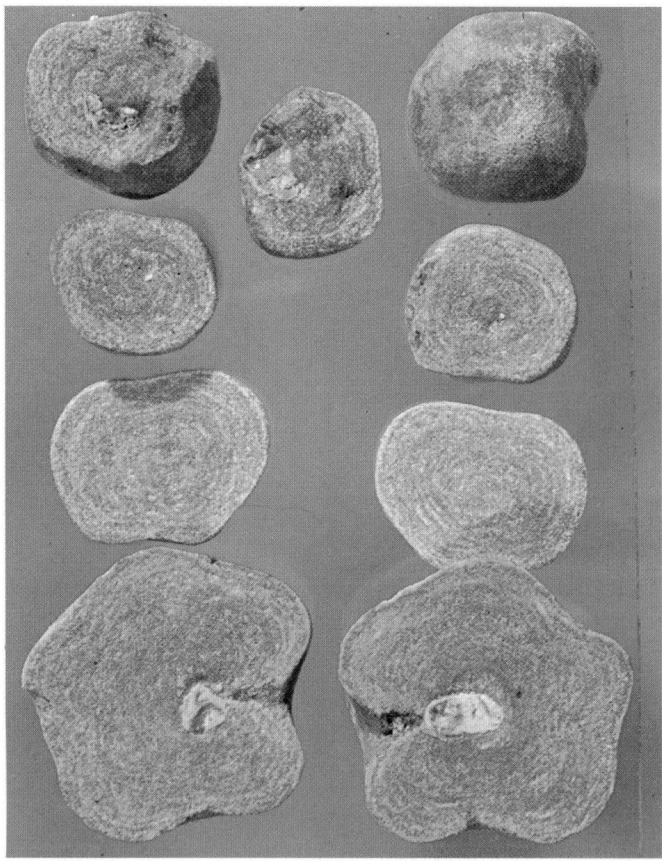

G.C.1458

1 From a male aged 9 years who died of abdominal tuberculosis.

The faecoliths were removed post mortem from the transverse colon.

The faecoliths are irregular, spherical, not faceted, light yellow in colour and on section appear to be arranged in ill-defined laminae.

2 and **2a** From a female aged 77 years. There was a history of an abdominal operation 30 years previously but for what condition and the details of the operation no information is available.

The patient was admitted to hospital with the presenting feature of a mass in the right iliac fossa provisionally diagnosed as an appendicular abscess.

Radiological examination showed the presence of four large stones, each of which had a slightly translucent centre – considered to be vesical calculi. Cystoscopic examination showed this to be incorrect.

At operation the calculi were found to lie in convoluted, dilated and adherent loops of terminal ileum and associated with this was a carcinoma of the ileo-caecal junction. A right hemicolectomy was carried out. The patient survived for two years.

The illustration shows the adherent dilated loops of the ileum which are some 25 to 30cm proximal to the ileo-caecal valve. The loops appear almost to have formed three separate cystic compartments in the lowermost of which lie the four faceted calculi. At the ileo-caecal junction there is an ulcerating carcinoma with necrotic base and the ulcer surrounds the whole circumference of the bowel. Histologically the tumour was a well differentiated glandular carcinoma. Examination of the wall of the distended ileum showed marked inflammatory cell infiltration and oedema.

2

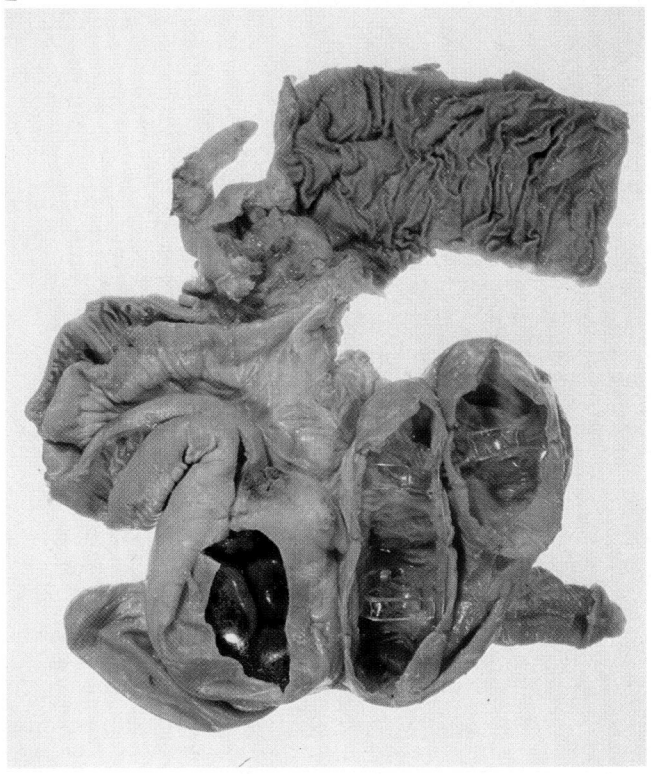

G.C.13894

2a

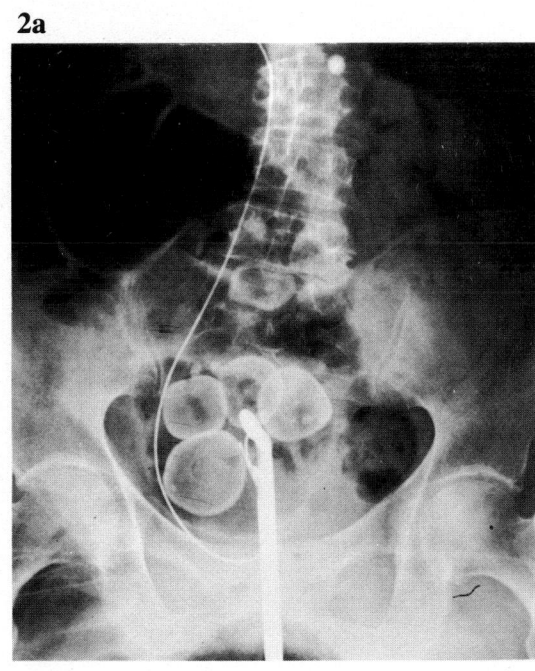

Stercoral ulceration

Localised ulceration may occur as the result of prolonged pressure on the mucosa by abnormally hard scybalous masses. The condition is particularly liable to be present in elderly patients and it has been suggested that an ischaemic factor is frequently present and partially causal. The ulcers may be single or more commonly multiple and occur in any part of the colon but are most frequent in the left colon, and rectum. There is full thickness mucosal loss. The edges are irregular and surrounding death of tissues may be observed. Perforation may occur.

Blood supply

1

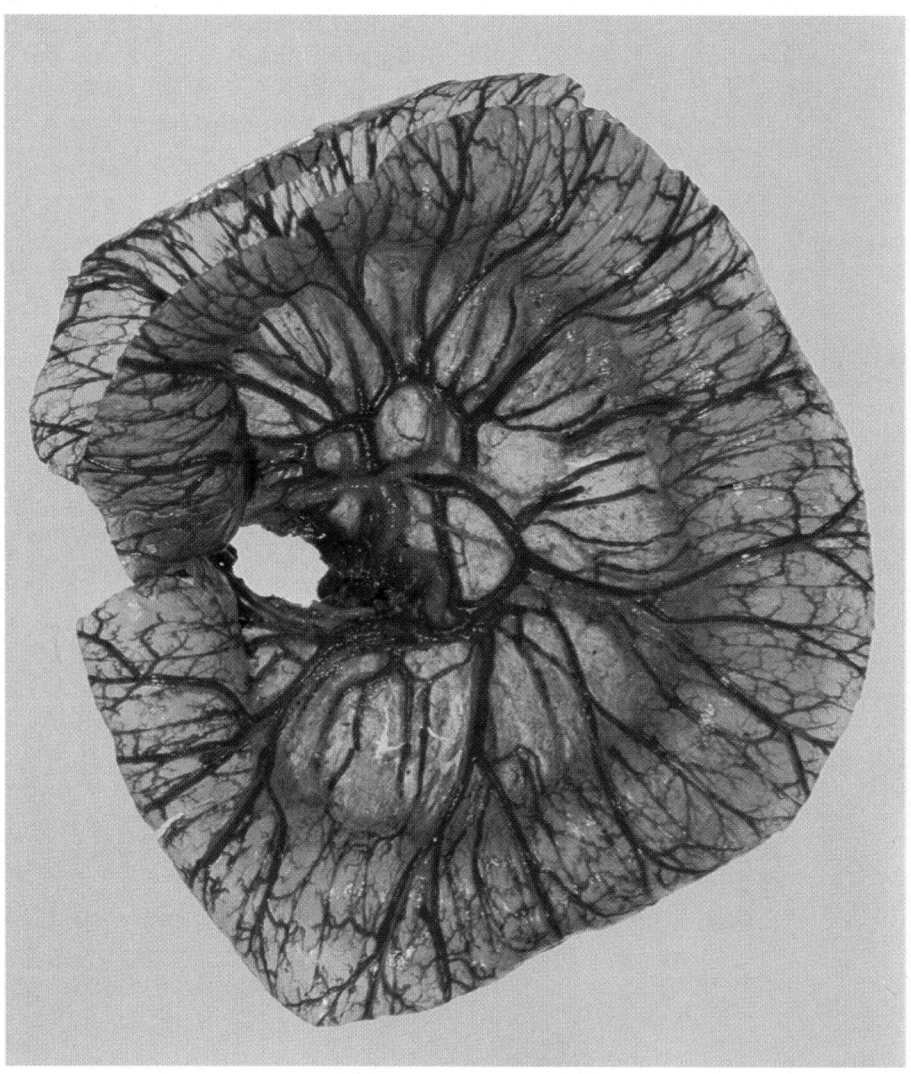

The blood supply of the stomach and intestine follows a general pattern. The branches of the main arteries form a series of anastomosing arcades. In relation to the small intestine more peripheral (secondary) arcades are present.

From the arcades straight vessels pass directly to the intestinal wall. These, after running for a variable distance beneath the peritoneum, penetrate the muscle coat to reach the submucosa. Variations of this general pattern occur in relation to the stomach, different parts of the small intestine and the colon.

1 The illustration is of an injection specimen demonstrating the blood supply of the intestine and prepared by Sir Charles Bell. This item was part of the original collection from the Great Windmill Street School of Anatomy, London, 1823.

The three principal arteries of the alimentary tract correspond to the embryological areas, i.e. foregut – coeliac axis; midgut – superior mesenteric artery (SMA); hindgut – inferior mesenteric artery (IMA).

2

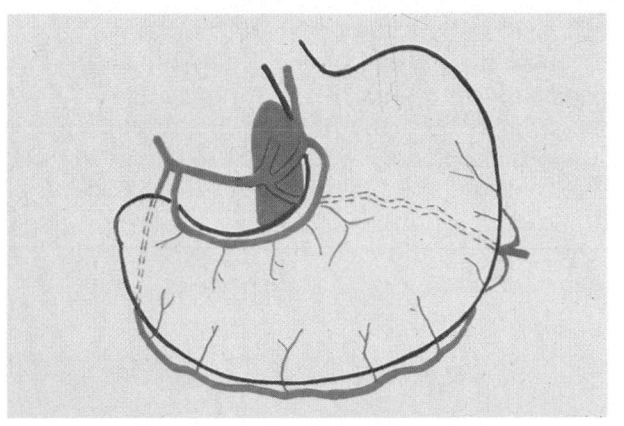

2 The coeliac axis supplies the lower oesophagus, stomach, duodenum, liver, spleen, pancreas and gall bladder. There is a rich collateral supply with the phrenic, oesophageal and lower intercostal arteries and with the SMA via the pancreatic arcades. At the extreme fundus of the stomach the blood supply is only just adequate and this segment is therefore most at risk of infarction.

3

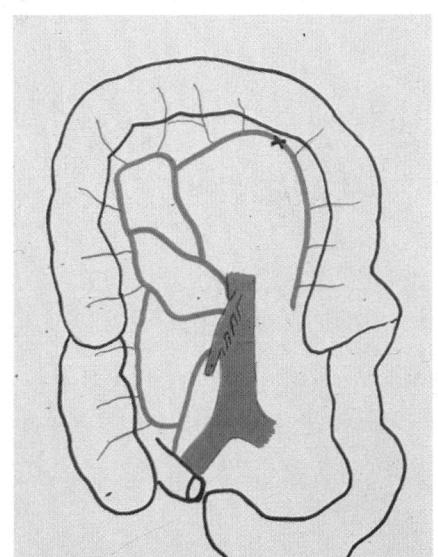

3 The SMA supplies the small intestine and proximal half of the colon. The intestinal arteries come from its left side and form a series of arcades increasing in number and complexity towards the ileum. It is from the most peripheral of these arcades that the straight arteries, as noted, pass to the gut and, after running subserosally for variable distances, penetrate the muscle coat to end in the submucosal plexus. Single arterioles then pass to each villus. From the right side of the SMA three main colonic vessels end by forming the marginal artery from which the vasa recta and vasa brevia pass to the colon.

4

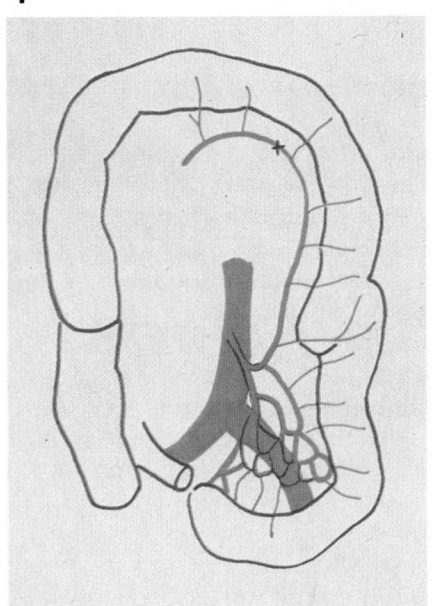

4 The IMA divides into two or three branches, the left colic usually reaching the splenic flexure where it should anastomose with the middle colic artery but the continuity may be broken at this point.

The sigmoid branches anastomose to a variable degree with each other before the vasa enter the colon. The blood supply of the rectum comes from the terminal branches of the IMA supplemented by the middle and inferior haemorrhoidal arteries from the internal iliac system.

Caused by arterial obstruction

Insufficiency of the blood supply to the intestine may result from aortic occlusion or mesenteric arterial occlusion.

Two-thirds of the population over the age of 55 years have partial or occasionally total occlusion of the SMA as shown by post mortem and radiological studies. This is due to atherosclerosis and is usually asymptomatic.

Acute occlusion follows embolus or thrombosis superimposed on atherosclerosis. The unique importance of mesenteric embolism is that if diagnosed early it is curable. Comparable lesions occur much less commonly in the IMA but ligation of this artery during lower abdominal aortic surgery may lead to colonic ischaemia.

5

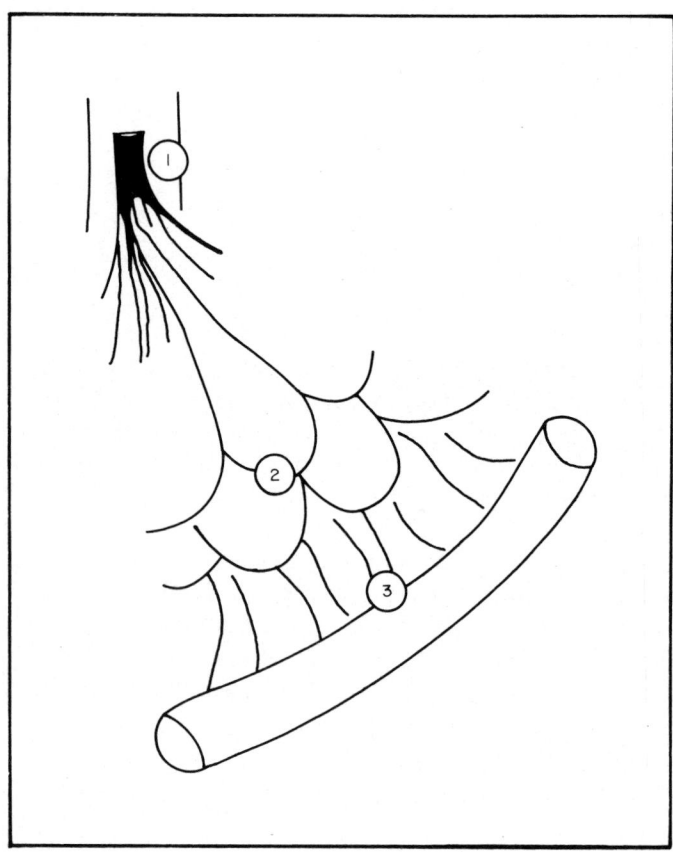

5 Because of the anatomical arrangement:
1 Acute occlusion of the SMA at its origin usually leads to widespread infarction.
2 Acute occlusion of the arcades is not usually associated with damage to the bowel because of the free anastomosis.
3 Acute occlusion of the small straight branches may result in localised necrosis.

Caused by venous thrombosis

Extensive venous thrombosis can cause intestinal infarction. Venous gangrene differs slightly from arterial gangrene in that mucosal necrosis so frequently seen with arterial lesions is uncommon. Venous gangrene mainly affects the submucosa and muscle and loss of the mucosa is a secondary process.

Venous occlusion is usually secondary to peritoneal sepsis, portal hypertension or blood dyscrasia.

Caused by other factors

'Non-occlusive' infarction without structural vascular change is considered by many to be numerically more frequent than embolus or thrombosis and may be caused by:
1 Diminished mesenteric blood flow:
   – congestive cardiac failure
   – trauma
   – shock
2 Haemoconcentration – trauma
                        – severe burns
                        – septicaemia
                        – anaphylaxis
3 Mucosal invasion by virulent *Clostridia* –
   releasing a powerful enterotoxin
   inducing intense mucosal vasoconstriction.

The bowel wall becomes intensely congested, deep plum coloured and oedematous, loses its peristalsis and becomes necrotic and permeable, permitting the escape of intestinal contents into the peritoneal cavity. Considerable controversy still exists regarding the relative importance of toxic absorption and fluid depletion as the main cause of death in this condition.

Massive infarction – main trunk

6

Thrombus has formed on an atherosclerotic patch occluding the SMA and partly obstructing the orifice of the coeliac axis. The renal vessels are not involved. In the mounted specimen the upper element has been rotated so that the superior end of the aorta is shown below.

The mesenteric vessels show diffuse thrombosis involving the arcades.

A segment of ileum has undergone complete infarction and is dark blue.

6 The specimen was obtained from a female patient with multiple thrombosis including the hepatic artery and superior mesenteric arteries. The specimen is mounted to show the effects of superior mesenteric thrombosis.

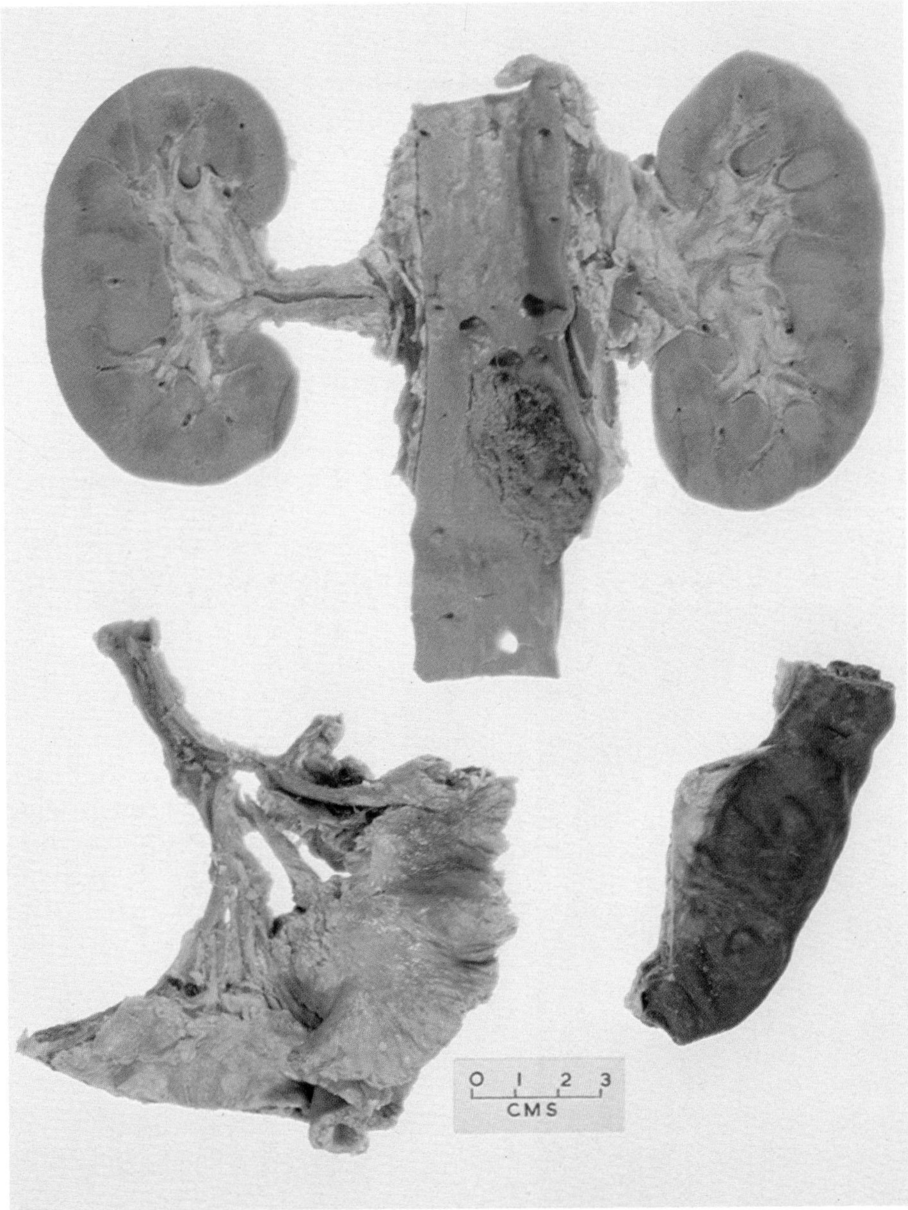

Acute occlusion of arcade arteries

Occlusion of a branch artery forming part of the arcade system does not usually lead to infarction since the collateral circulation is free.

More commonly, where a relatively small segment of gut is affected, the long term result is the formation of a fibrous stricture.

From a male aged 59 years who had a suprapubic prostatectomy. A week later he developed intestinal obstruction. An exploratory laparotomy was performed but no abnormality was found. Eight days later the patient developed a small intestinal fistula and further exploration of the abdomen revealed a limited necrotic segment of small intestine. A fatal peritonitis ensued.

This is a case in which the initial vascular insufficiency caused only circumscribed infarction which, however, continued to extend so that after eight days gross bowel necrosis was present and a major mesenteric vessel showed thrombosis.

7

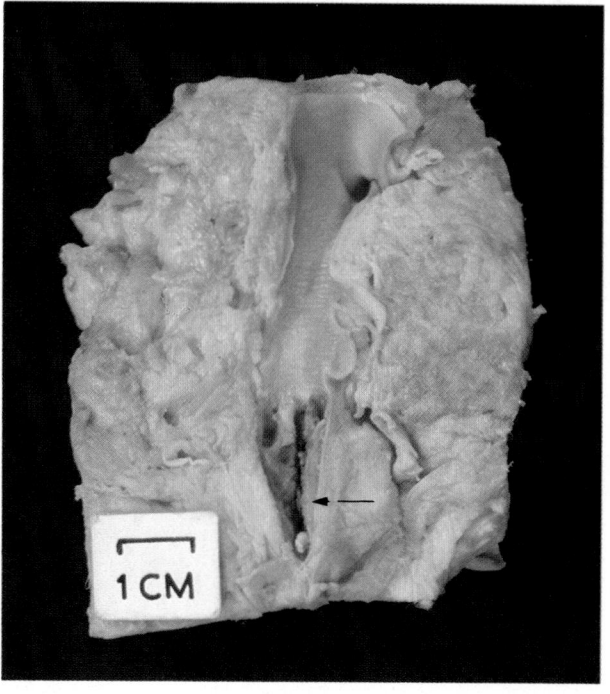

1 CM

G.C.14466

7 Segment of mesentery with a corresponding segment of the superior mesenteric artery which has been opened and demonstrates thrombosis within the lumen of the vessel.

Continued opposite page. ➡

8

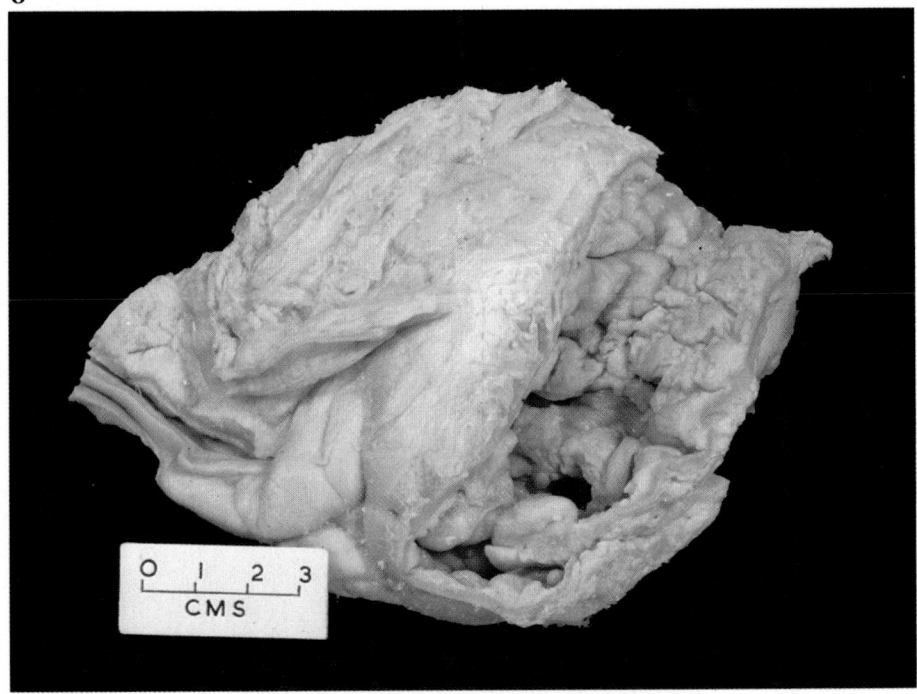

8 Section of ascending colon. There is no evident change of colour suggesting congestion but the bowel, which has been opened up, shows massive oedema with a pseudopolyp formation.

9

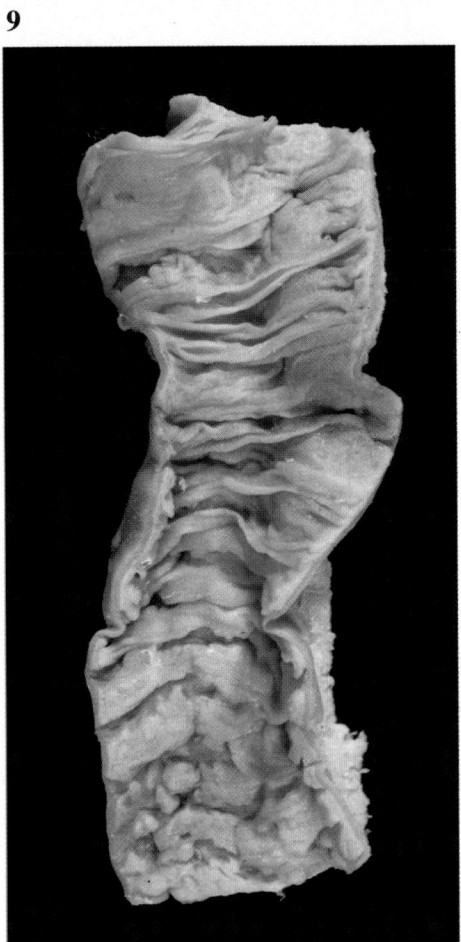

10

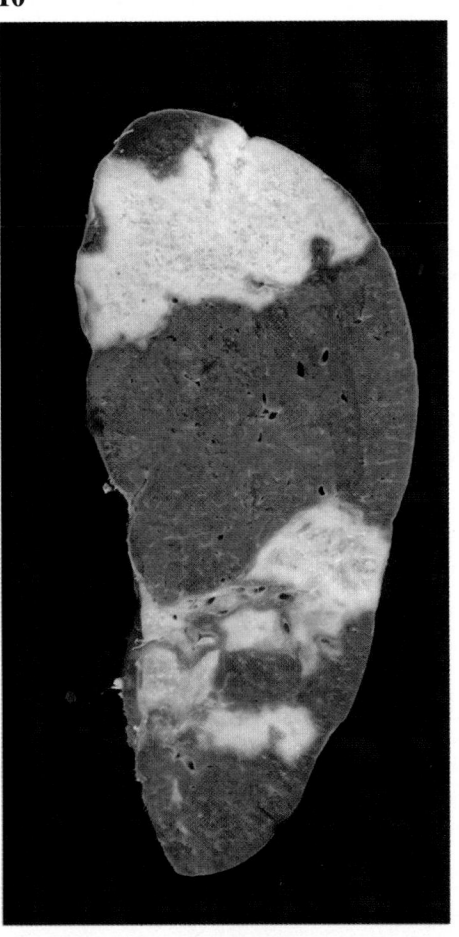

9 Segment of ileum shows comparatively little change and is of normal colour but the mucosa is oedematous and there is some loss of the normal folds.

10 The spleen shows several areas of complete infarction. There has been occlusion of 'end-arteries'. The contrast between this and the lesions in the gut is explained by the differences in the circulation. In the gut anastomosing vessels are present. In the spleen the end-arteries are occluded.

Acute occlusion of the terminal arteries

Occlusion of the terminal straight arteries may result from:
- Mesenteric haematomas following blunt abdominal trauma.
- Minute emboli of thrombus or cholesterol from ulcerated atheromatous patches.
- Inflammatory disease of the vessels of the gut wall.
- Radiation injury.

The lesions may be multiple or single and the length of the bowel involved varies. The arterioles of the villi are peculiarly susceptible to vascular insufficiency leading to mucosal death. This allows organisms to reach the submucosa. The resulting ulceration varies in extent and depth according to the degree and severity of the infection. When the condition resolves fibrosis of the submucosa and muscularis causes stricture formation.

Potassium stricture

The iatrogenic lesion known as the 'potassium stricture' results from high concentrations of potassium salts applied to the intestinal mucosa causing local ischaemia, thrombosis and ulceration. Perforation may occur but the lesion usually heals resulting in a fibrous stricture. Pre-existing intestinal ischaemia enhances this effect.

11

11 Small intestine: potassium ulceration. The ulcer is covered by inflammatory exudate and blood (left). Granulation tissue is present in the full depth of the mucosa. *(H&E ×50)*

Polyarteritis nodosa

12

12 In this case of polyarteritis nodosa several patches of bile-stained necrotic mucosa were present in the colon at necropsy.

13

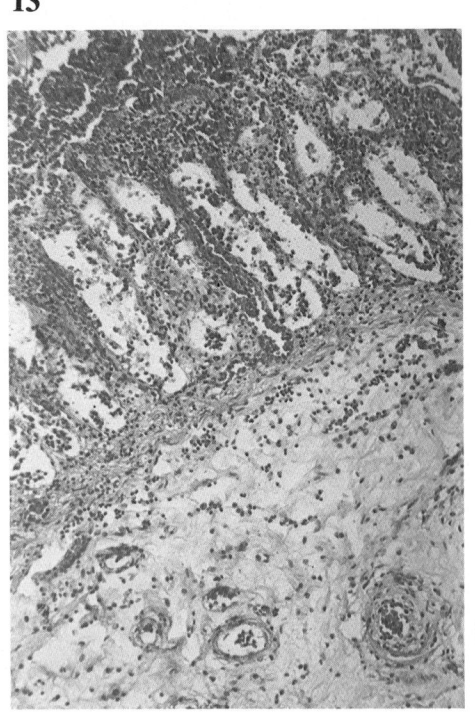

13 Microscopically the devitalised mucosa is infiltrated by inflammatory cells. In the oedematous submucosa the wall of a small artery is thickened by fibrosis. *(H&E ×125)*

Ischaemic colitis

14

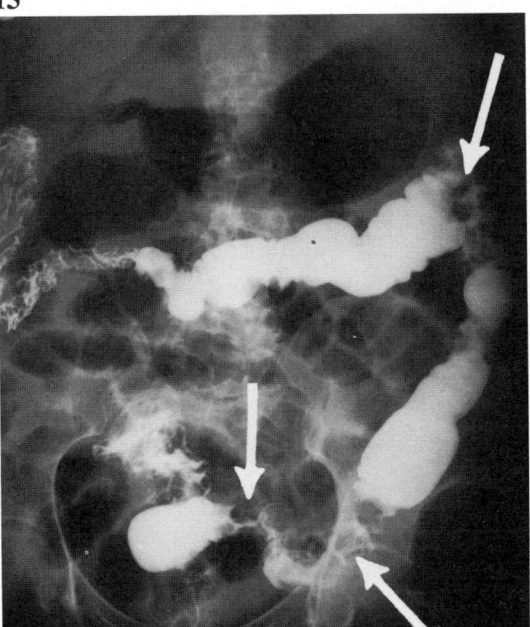

G.C.14327

15

G.C.X.643

15 Barium enema showing two segments of ischaemic colitis located at the splenic flexure and in the sigmoid colon. The typical thumb print filling defects are indicated by arrows.

Ischaemic colitis may follow operation but commonly arises in a setting of a non-surgical condition. Predisposing factors include mesenteric atheroma, respiratory insufficiency and anaemia.

Precipitating factors may be hypotension due to myocardial infarction or endotoxic shock, or splanchnic vasoconstriction due to cardiac failure or digitalis intoxication.

The part of the bowel with the most precarious blood supply, the splenic flexure and upper descending colon, usually suffers most. At this site there is a tenuous and variable anastomosis between branches of the middle colic artery and the left colic artery and the usually continuous system of arterial arcades may be deficient. The affected portion of the colon is intensely congested and haemorrhage may occur into its mucosa and lumen.

Mucosal necrosis and submucosal inflammation of a patchy nature with intervening areas of unaffected mucosa follow. These areas are usually oedematous and give rise to the 'thumb printing' seen on barium enema (as illustrated).

16

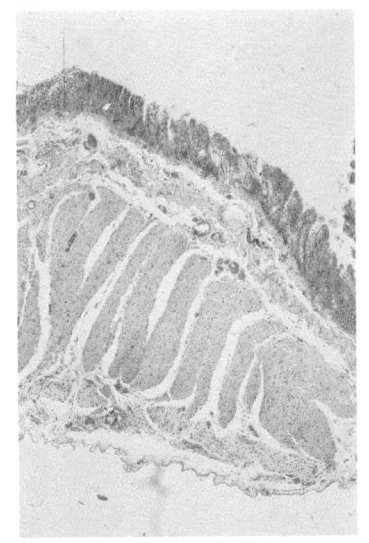

G.C.M.950

17

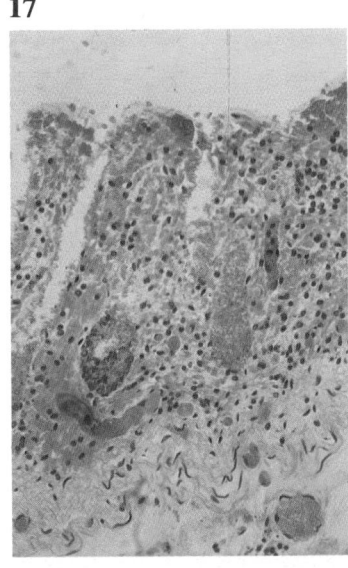

G.C.M.950

16 Necrosis is extensive in the mucosa but does not involve other parts of the wall. *(H&E ×32)*

17 Red necrotic substance replaces the normal stromal tissues. Only blue nuclear debris survives in the colonic glands. *(H&E ×200)*

The later development of a stricture is difficult to forecast on initial clinical presentation. Ischaemic proctitis can occur and may be confused with other types of rectal inflammation.

Irradiation

The intestinal wall is readily damaged by irradiation. Although the stomach and small bowel are more sensitive to X-rays the colon is more often damaged especially after pelvic irradiation for bladder and uterine cancer. Intestinal complications may occur at any time from shortly after treatment to many years later.

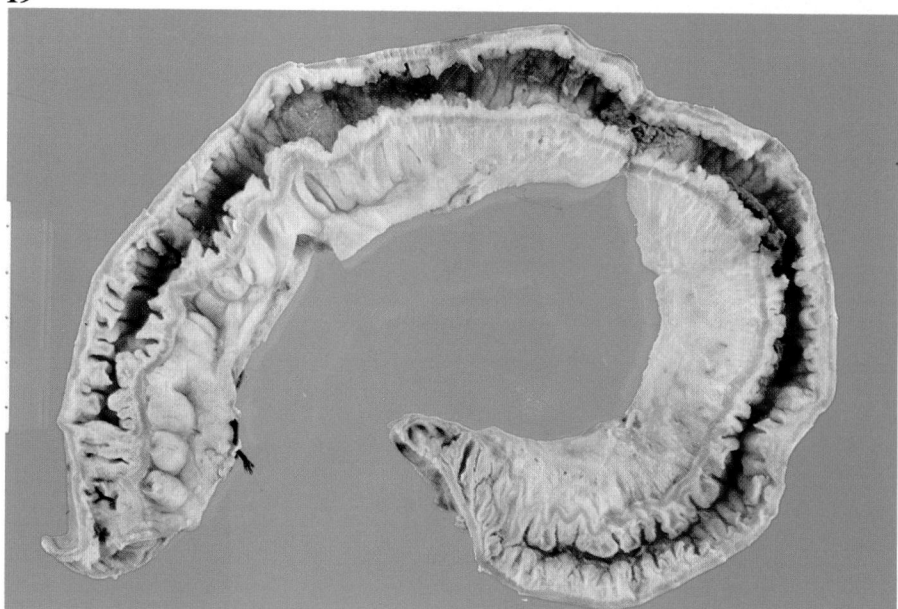

G.C.P.212

19 Thickened rigid ileum with narrowed lumen following radiotherapy for carcinoma of the bladder.

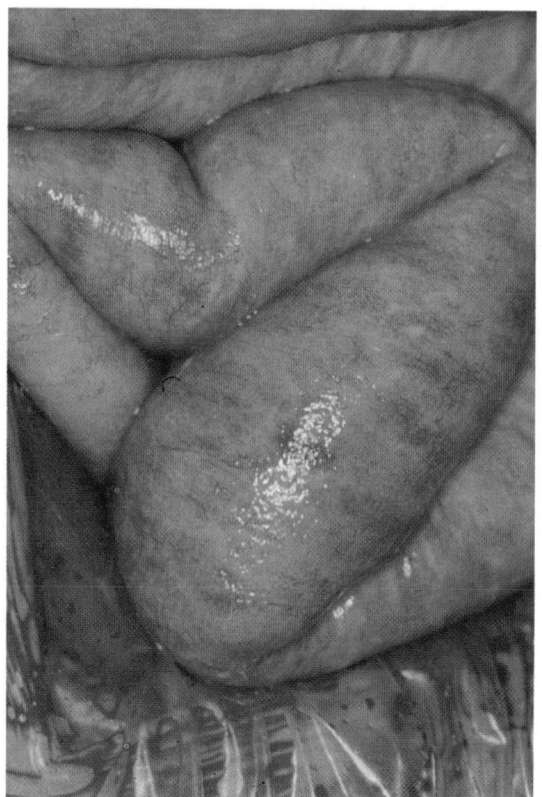

G.C.P.211

18 Illustration of appearances at operation showing pale small bowel due to thickening of the serosa.

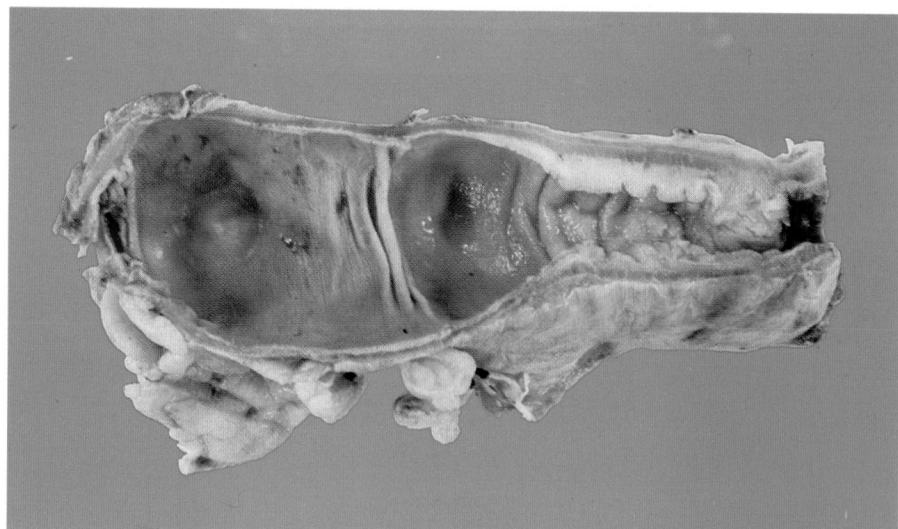

G.C.P.213

20 A 3.5 cm stricture in sigmoid colon with marked submucosal fibrosis following external and intracavity radiation for carcinoma of the cervix.

Early effects

Small intestinal biopsies in the immediate post irradiation period show loss of villi and severe damage to the crypt epithelium. Complications at this stage include focal necrosis of the whole bowel wall with perforation and fistula formation. This ulcerative phase is followed by regeneration which shows flattened, thickened villi on convoluted ridges. Adhesions to adjacent loops form. Similar changes occur in the colon. The arteries and arterioles show endarteritis obliterans, and there is proliferation of bizarre fibroblasts.

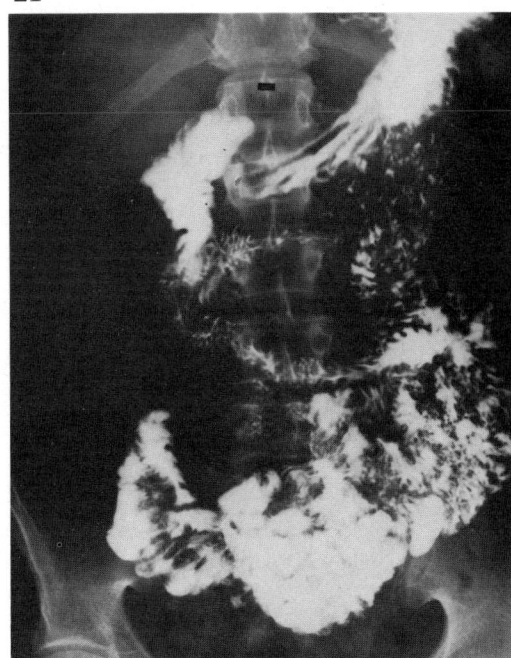

21 From an adult male who had received radiotherapy for a seminoma of the testis and later developed diarrhoea with passage of mucus.

Radiologically the small intestine exhibits hypermotility and abnormality of pattern.

Late effects

Progressive submucosal and subserosal fibrosis in the small intestine leads to malabsorption and subacute obstruction with eventual stricture formation. In the colon and rectum the mucosa appears granular and haemorrhagic and may show areas of ulceration. Fistulae and stricture formation may occur.

Histological examination reveals partial loss of the mucous membrane with chronic inflammation of the surviving mucosa. There is marked submucosal fibrosis and endarteritis obliterans of the arteries and arterioles. Bizarre fibroblasts and macrophages are seen. Carcinoma of the rectum has been reported following pelvic irradiation but causal relationship is uncertain.

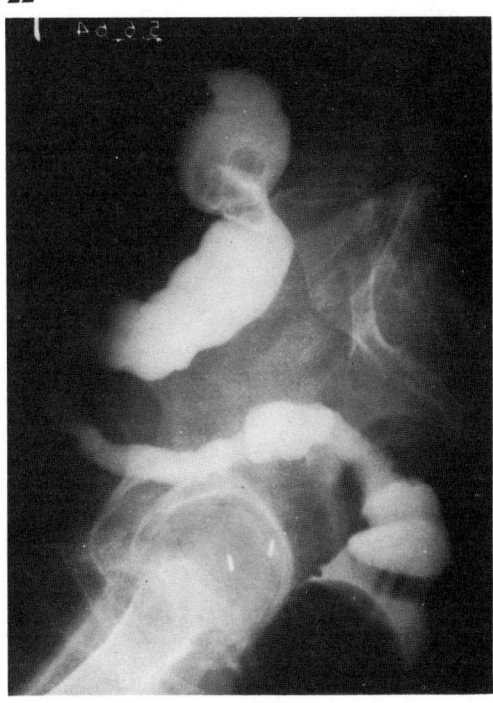

22 From a female aged 64 years. Treated by radiotherapy for advanced carcinoma of the cervix. Subsequent development of chronic diarrhoea.

Radiologically there is irregular stenosis of the sigmoid colon regarded as post radiation colitis.

J. Anderson

Pneumatosis cystoides intestinalis

Gas cysts are found most frequently in the small intestine. In the large intestine they most commonly occur about the region of the splenic flexure and left colon. The cysts present singly or as clusters, are thin walled, do not communicate and are readily punctured. The cysts may be sessile or pedunculated.

The cysts are located principally in the mucosal and submucosal layers but also occur beneath the serosa. It is now recognised that the condition has a pronounced association with airway obstruction or emphysema of the lungs. It is believed that air escaping from the alveoli and bronchi, especially if there are bullae, passes into the mediastinum. It tracks downwards into the retroperitoneal tissue and then into the mesentery to reach the gut along the line of lymphatic or vascular channels. Gas cysts may form at any point in this pathway or in the bowel wall.

Another theory is that gas-forming organisms have penetrated into the submucosa following an inflammatory process. Here colonisation by the organisms leads to the formation of gas cysts. This is followed by an elevation of breath hydrogen and methane. Many of the patients have been on steroids which may have facilitated transfer through the mucosa.

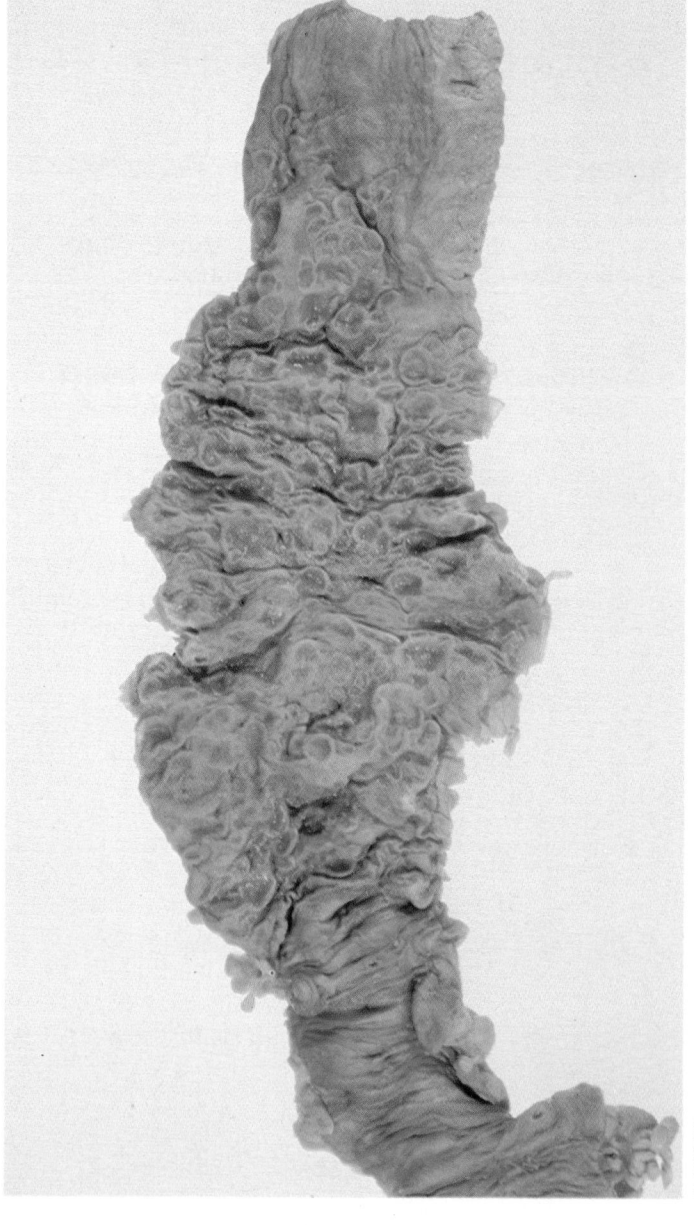

1 From a male aged 79 years. The patient suddenly became restless and confused 24 hours before admission and had frequent calls to stool which subsequently became uncontrollable. The stools were black in colour containing streaks of red blood. He was markedly shocked and the clinical picture suggested intestinal haemorrhage. He died shortly after admission from acute peripheral circulatory failure.

At post mortem examination there was a considerable sanguinous peritoneal exudate. The pelvic mesocolon showed a circular defect through which some 3.5 metres of small bowel had herniated. This had undergone torsion and showed partial gangrene. In the pelvic colon a segment some 30 cm long showed thickening and when opened demonstrated mucosal gas cysts.

The affected segment of bowel is sharply demarcated from the other normal parts above and below.

G.C.1347z

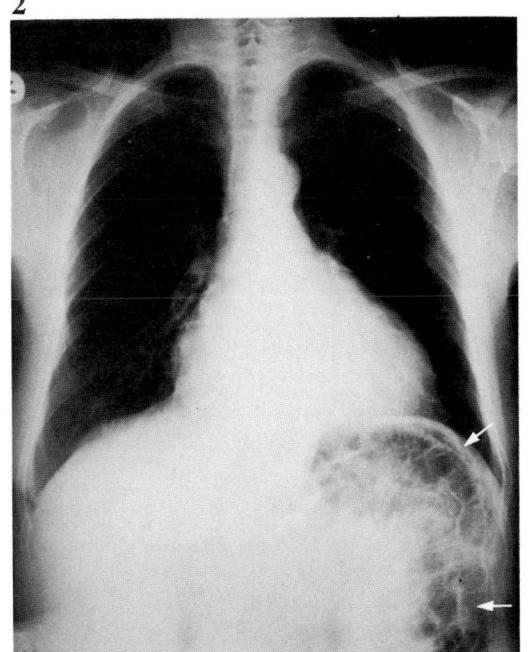

2 This X-ray demonstrates the presence of multiple gas filled cysts in the large intestine involving the splenic flexure and descending colon.

The cysts may cause partial intestinal obstruction.

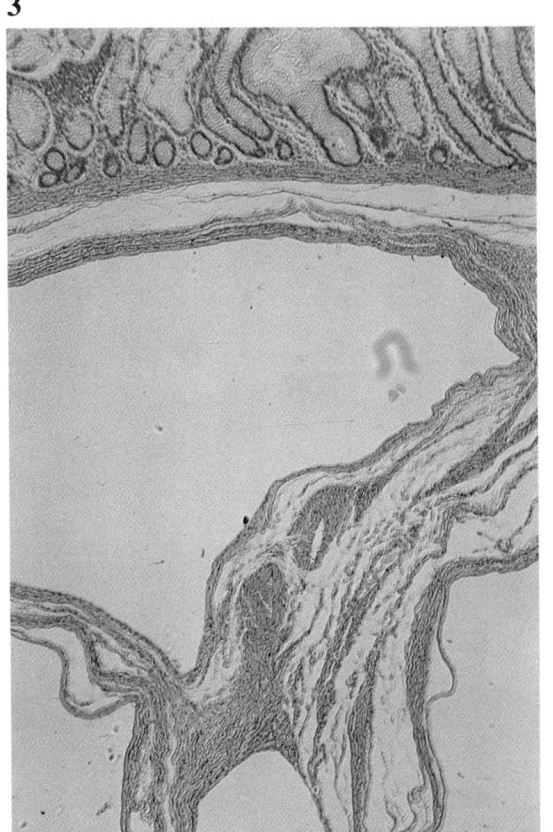

3 *Pneumatosis coli.* Several gas cysts can be seen beneath the mucosa. *(H&E ×48)*

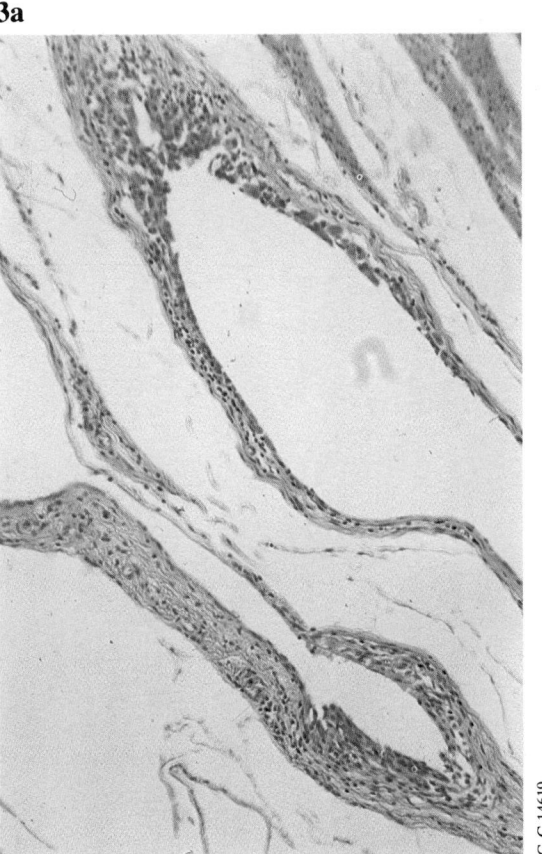

3a *Pneumatosis coli.* Multinucleated cells with eosinophilic cytoplasm may line the cysts. *(H&E ×120)*

Colitis cystica profunda

This lesion is characterised by intramural mucous cysts associated with hypertrophy of the muscularis mucosae. The abnormality is located in the lower colon and rectum and may be seen either as a single polypoid mass or affect a considerable area of the bowel mucosa presenting as a plaque.

The condition has been ascribed to pre-existing inflammation with ulceration, the mucosal response including a downgrowth of the mucus-secreting cells along granulation tracts. This forms the origin of the submucous lakes.

Comparable changes have been observed in ulcerative colitis.

The patients present with mucoid discharge, partial prolapse of the rectum or the passage of blood per rectum. It is associated with lower abdominal colic. Sigmoidoscopy shows a proliferative mucosa with elevated rounded cysts.

Alternatively, there may be an elevated polypoidal plaque or a densely sclerosed ulcer, often with a vessel exposed in the base.

The condition is highly recurrent if locally excised.

Because of the three different naked eye appearances of the lesion and in spite of the same pathology and probably aetiology, three names have been applied:

1 Colitis cystica profunda.
2 Inverted hamartomatous polyp.
3 Solitary rectal ulcer.

4

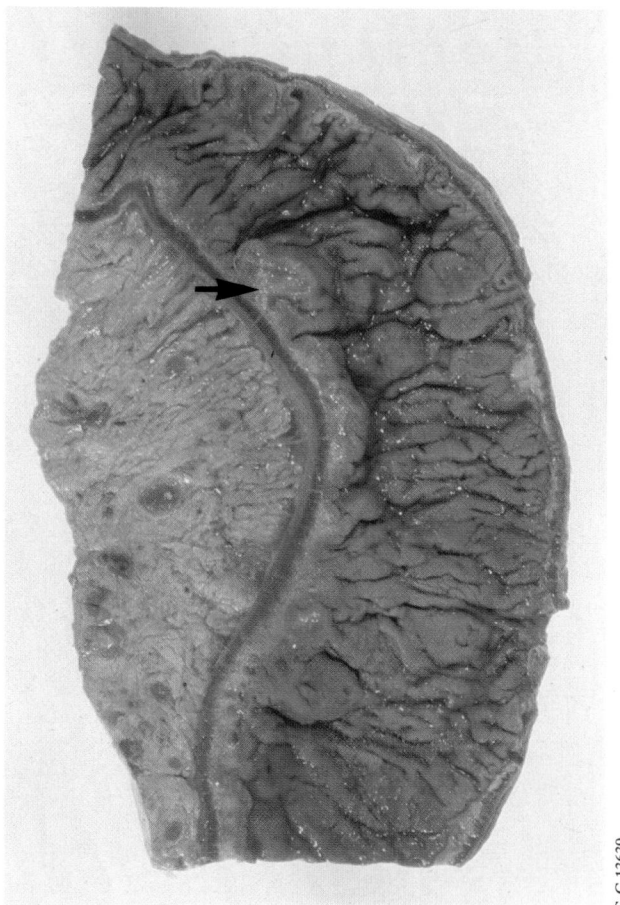

G.C.13639

4 From a male aged 43 years with a six month history of abdominal colic associated with diarrhoea. There was evidence of malnutrition including atrophic glossitis, oedema of the ankles, diffuse follicular keratosis and hyperkeratosis of legs. Marked anaemia and hypoproteinaemia. Achlorhydria. There was passage of blood and mucus with the faeces. Radiology demonstrated a stenosing lesion of the pelvic colon. The appearances suggested a mucous carcinoma and a resection was carried out.

The specimen consists of the distal pelvic colon and rectum. Diffuse thickening of all layers of the bowel wall and of the pelvic mesocolon. The mucosa of the pelvic colon and upper rectum was irregularly thickened and raised into numerous folds and bosses by submucosal mucoid cysts. Small ulcers were associated with several of the larger cysts. From some of the cysts mucus could be expressed into the lumen. The muscularis was thickened and the fibres were separated by oedema.

5

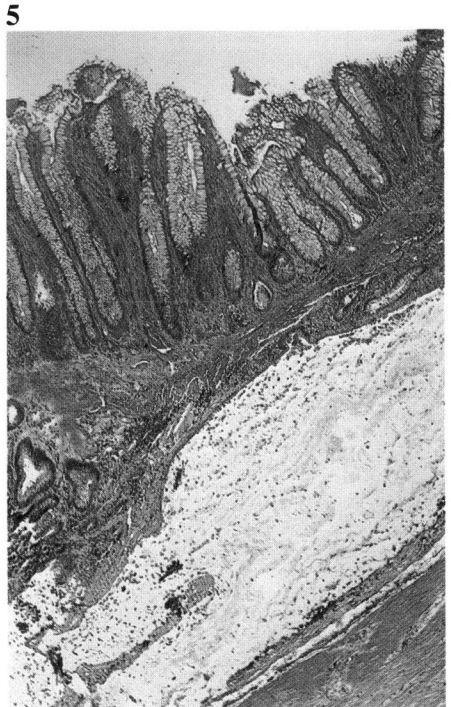

G.C.13639

5 Colitis cystica profunda showing a submucous cyst filled by mucin. Most of the epithelial lining of the cyst has been shed and only one small segment lying below the muscularis mucosae can be seen. *(H&E ×40)*

6

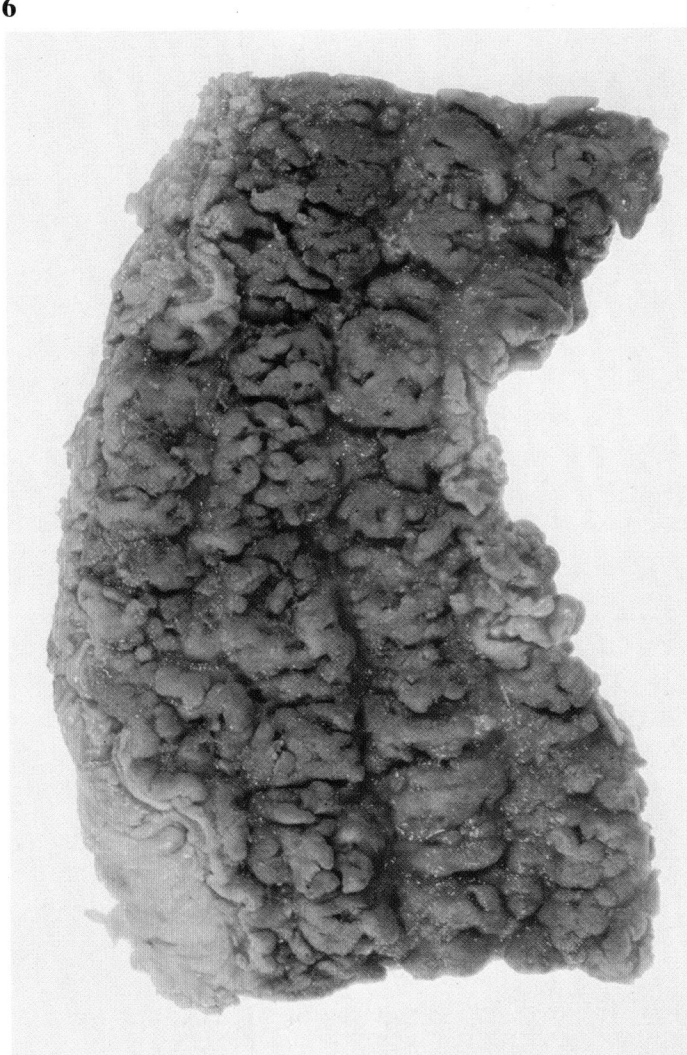

G.C.13693

6 From a female aged 24 years. Three week history of diarrhoea with blood and mucus. A comparable attack had occurred four months previously.

Sigmoidoscopy suggested ulcerative colitis. The condition did not respond to medical treatment and an ileostomy was performed, followed on a later occasion by a removal of the colon.

At operation many adhesions were present and the bowel showed severe inflammation. The patient died three months after the operation.

The specimen consists of the pelvic colon. Congestion and ulceration are present. There are ulcers varying in size, many being large and confluent. The intervening mucosa is thickened, granular, friable, polypoid in places and raised into numerous folds. Microscopically the muscularis appears thickened and shows widespread and intense inflammation in addition to the presence of epithelial lined cysts. The lymphoid follicles show abscess formation. The ulcerated areas show evidence of healing with regenerating epithelium extending deep to the muscularis mucosae.

The submucosal cysts are confined to the pelvic colon and vary in size. There is continuity between the mucus secreting surface epithelium and the deeply placed cysts below the muscularis. The appearances can be interpreted as those of chronic ulcerative colitis with reparative changes which have resulted in post-inflammatory polyposis and cyst formation (colitis cystica profunda).

A.N. Smith

Mesoblastic tumours

Tumours arising from connective tissue elements occur in all parts of the alimentary tract including the oesophagus, stomach, small intestine and colon, although the site incidence of each tumour type varies. These tumours are relatively rare and usually both benign and malignant forms are described. Many are slow growing and cause few symptoms.

In all varieties of alimentary tract tumours where growth is rapid or the tumour projects into the lumen of the gut, complications occur. These include intussusception, obstruction, ulceration with haemorrhage, infection and necrosis (following vascular insufficiency caused by stretching or torsion of pedicle). Perforation and malabsorption are other complications. Occasionally there has been spontaneous extrusion of the tumour.

For convenience and to avoid repetition the mesoblastic tumours, irrespective of site, are considered together in this section.

Lipoma

Incidence

These are rare tumours with an incidence of 0.5% (post mortem series). Sex incidence equal.

Site incidence

Stomach	12%	Lipoma of the oesophagus has
Small intestine	36%	been described but is very
Large intestine	52%	rare.

In the small intestine the ileum is the commonest site and in the colon the most frequent sites are the caecum and ascending colon.

Pathology

These tumours may arise either in the submucosa or in the serosal fat. The former are more common. They present as a lobulated soft pale yellow mass and may be difficult to feel through the bowel wall. They are usually solitary but multiple and diffuse forms have been described (see Section 19 T).

1

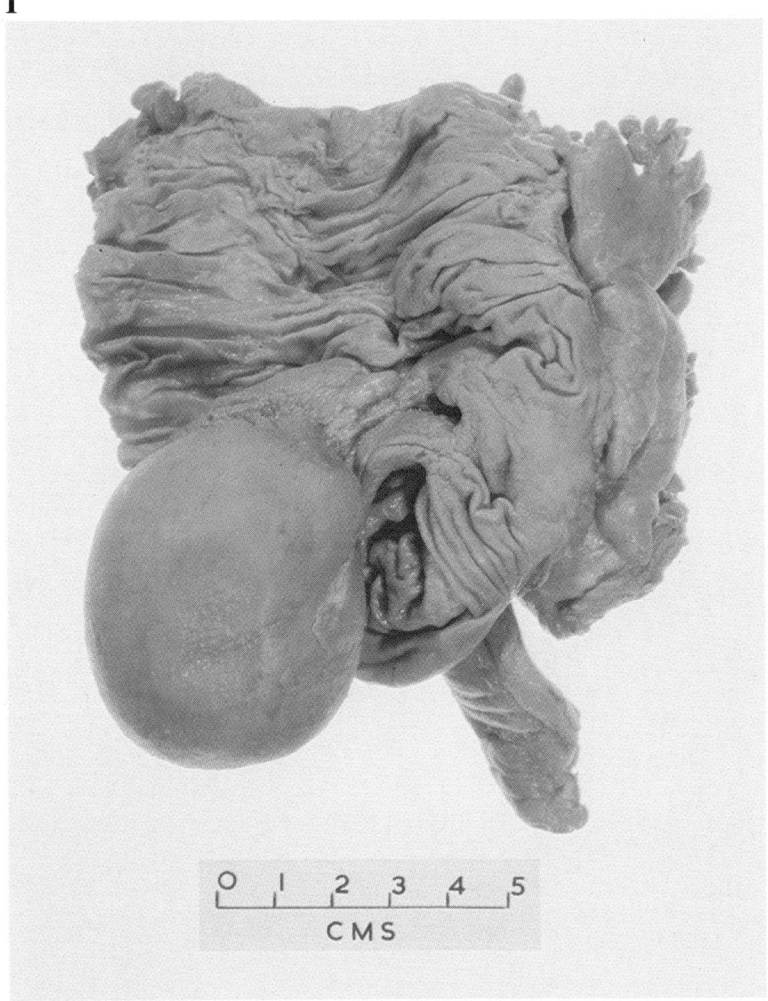

O 1 2 3 4 5
C M S

G.C.8064

1 From a middle-aged female suffering from intestinal obstruction of short duration. The tumour is globular and attached to the bowel by a comparatively narrow pedicle inferior to and at some distance from the openings of the ileum and vermiform appendix. It projects into the lumen of the gut. Microscopic examination showed a lipoma of submucous origin covered by the muscularis mucosae and intestinal epithelium. There was some inflammatory cell infiltration and exudate in the mucosa.

Histology

The tumours consist of mature fat cells and the overlying mucosa may show atrophy due to pressure. The muscularis is not involved but may show stretching and atrophy.

Leiomyoma

Morgagni (1761) quoted a case which was most probably a leiomyoma. Foerster (1858) recorded the first definite case.

Incidence

It is impossible to estimate accurately since many are symptomless and found incidentally either at laparotomy or at post mortem. The estimated incidence is approximately 20% of all benign small bowel tumours.

Estimated Site Incidence

Oesophagus	Rare
Stomach	55 – 65%
Duodenum	5%
Small intestine	20%
Colon and rectum	10%

2

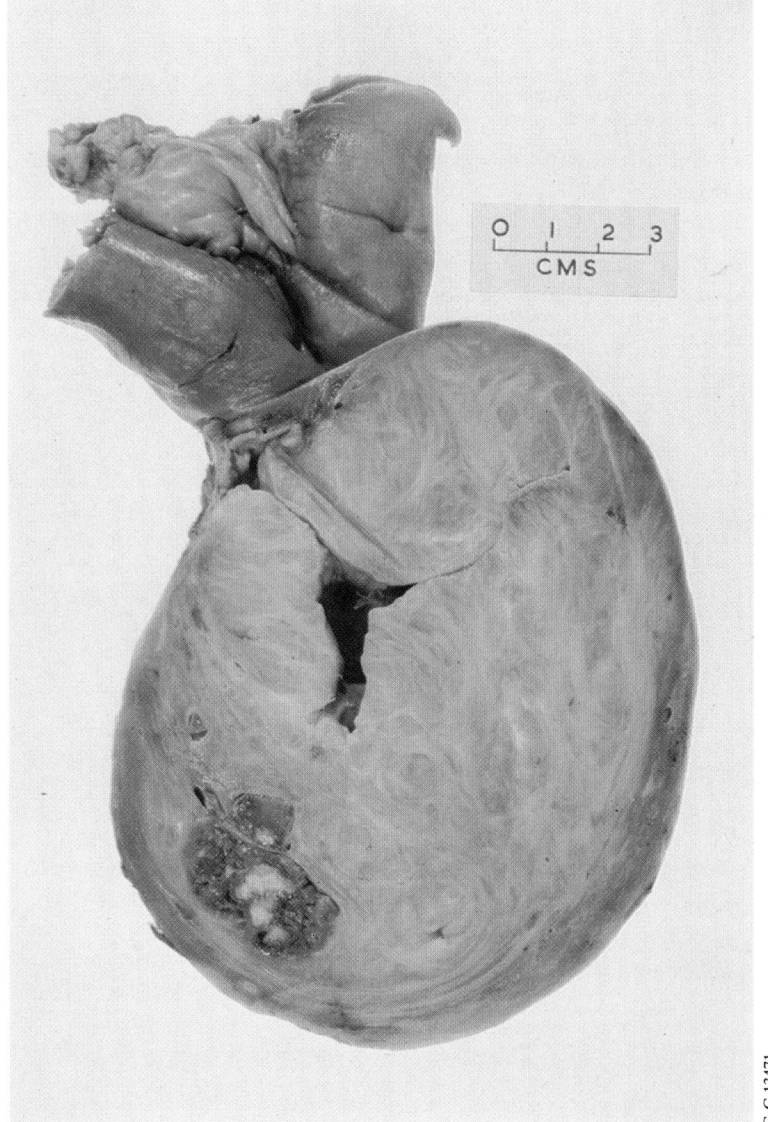

G.C.1347I

2 Jejunum – Leiomyoma. From a female aged 71 years. Six month history of loss of weight and appetite. Palpable tumour below the umbilicus and descending into the pelvis. The tumour measured 14 × 10 cm. The histological picture was regarded as benign. This is a subserous leiomyoma showing the characteristic features which are detailed in the text.

Pathology

These tumours arise in the muscle coat of the gut – very rarely from the muscularis mucosae. Initially growth may be described as mural but later the tumour becomes either submucosal or subserosal. 'Dumb-bell' tumours with masses under the serosa as well as the mucosa are recorded. Rarely they produce diffuse or constricting lesions.

The tumours illustrated demonstrate the typical well defined mass, round or lobulated. They are relatively avascular although large vessels may lie on the surface. Central necrosis with cavity formation and the development of a fistulous tract leading to the mucosal surface is well demonstrated. The cut surface is pinkish white and whorled. Calcification, cyst formation and occasionally perforation can occur.

The tumours of the submucosal group are associated with ulceration of the mucosa and haemorrhage. Bleeding is episodic but sometimes fatal. These tumours may cause obstruction but more frequently intussusception. Subserosal tumours tend to be bulkier, sometimes with a narrow attachment to the gut.

The two specimens shown are so similar that they illustrate the difficulty of differentiation between benign and malignant leiomyomas (see **2** and **3**).

3

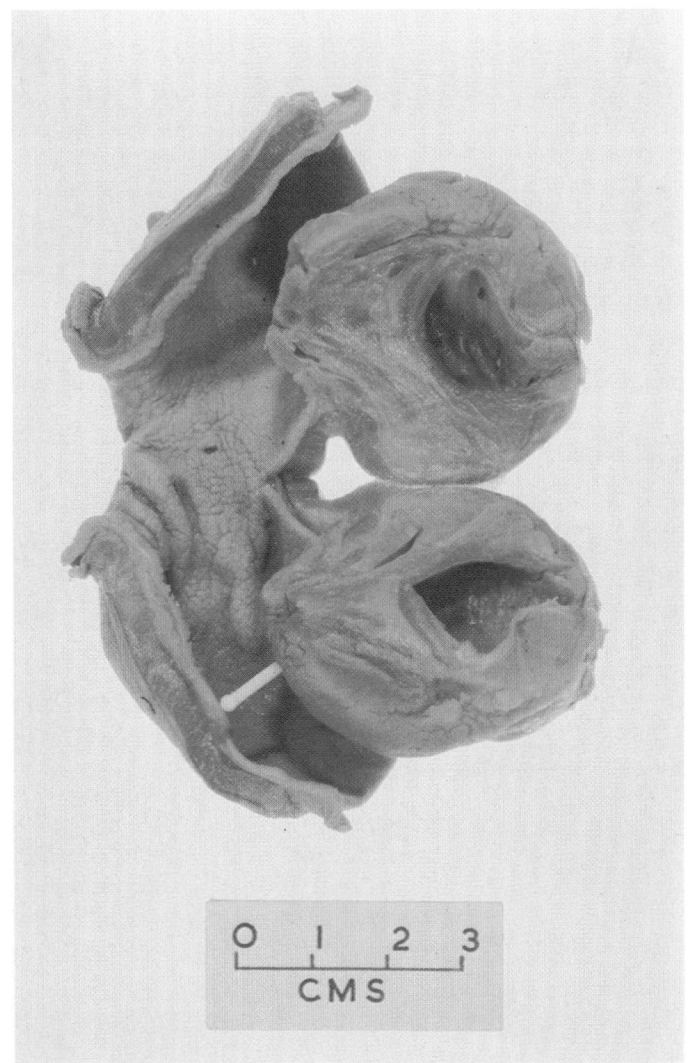

3 Pylorus – Leiomyosarcoma. From a female aged 53 years. Two year history of anaemia, anorexia and latterly vomiting. She had two attacks of haematemesis and blood was present in the stools. Histological examination showed evidence of malignancy. The tumour measured 4 × 3.5 cm.

G.C. 6669

311

Leiomyoma *(Continued)*

Histology

Composed of bundles of smooth muscle cells more or less whorled and interspersed with a scanty stroma. The nuclei may have a characteristic palisade pattern which may simulate that of a neurilemmoma or neurofibroma. It is difficult to differentiate benign from malignant lesions. The two most important features which help to distinguish benign from malignant lesions are the number of mitoses and the size of the lesion. Increased cellularity, pleomorphism and giant cells may be found but usually indicate degeneration rather than malignancy. The tumour cells at the periphery interdigitate with the normal muscle cells of the bowel wall and closely simulate the appearance of an infiltrating tumour. This is not regarded as diagnostic of malignancy. Excluding purely mural tumours 30 to 50% will metastasise usually to the liver. Lymph node metastases are rare.

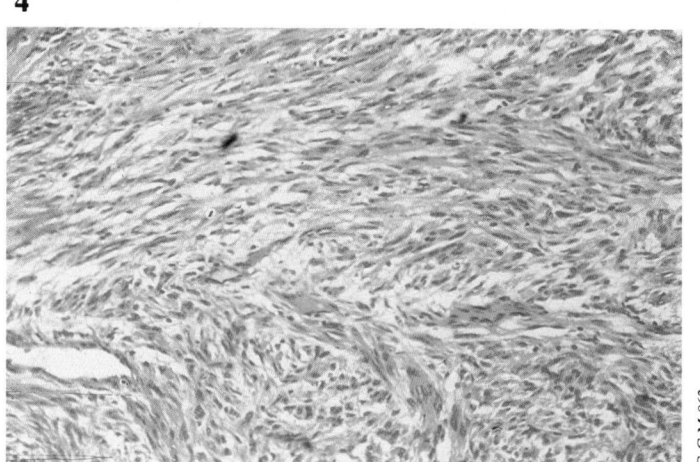

4 Well differentiated leiomyoma of jejunum. *(H&E ×100)*

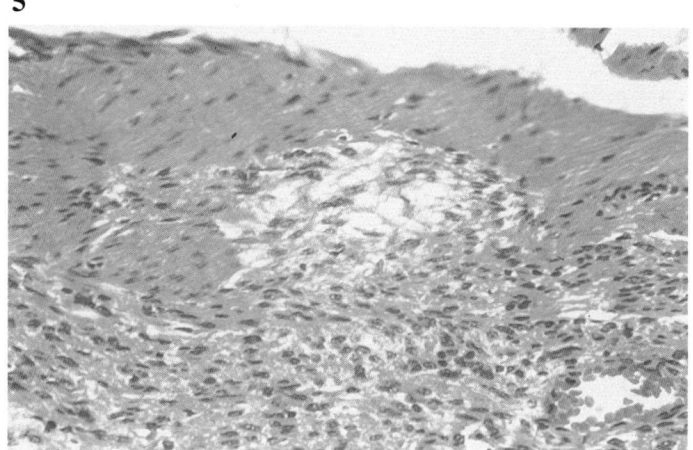

5 Leiomyoma showing interdigitation of peripheral cells with normal smooth muscle. *(H&E ×312.5)*

Complications

The major complications are obstruction, strangulation, intussusception and perforation.

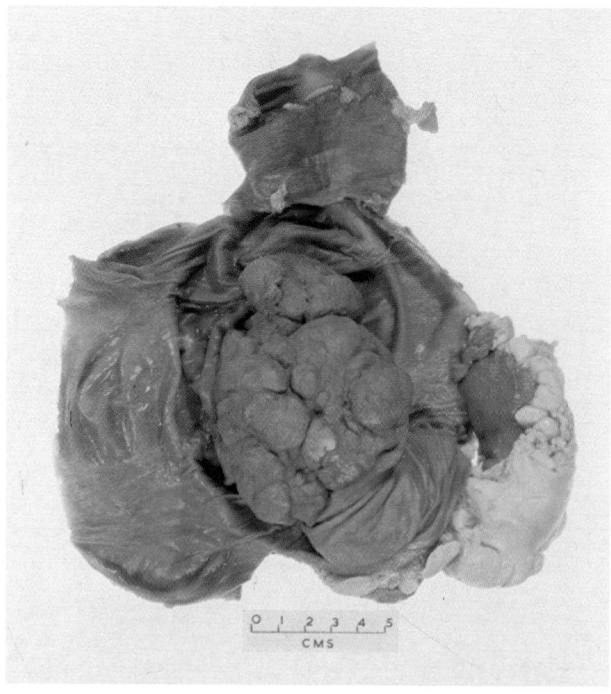

6 From a male aged 63 years. A large ileocolic intussusception induced by the presence of a myofibrosarcoma of the ileum. Histologically pleomorphism and the presence of giant cells was noted. Malignancy was confirmed by the presence of numerous mitoses.

Radiology

Radiological examination frequently demonstrates the rounded shadow of the tumour but in barium series the contrast medium may be seen extending from the lumen of the affected segment into the central necrotic area of the neoplasm.

7

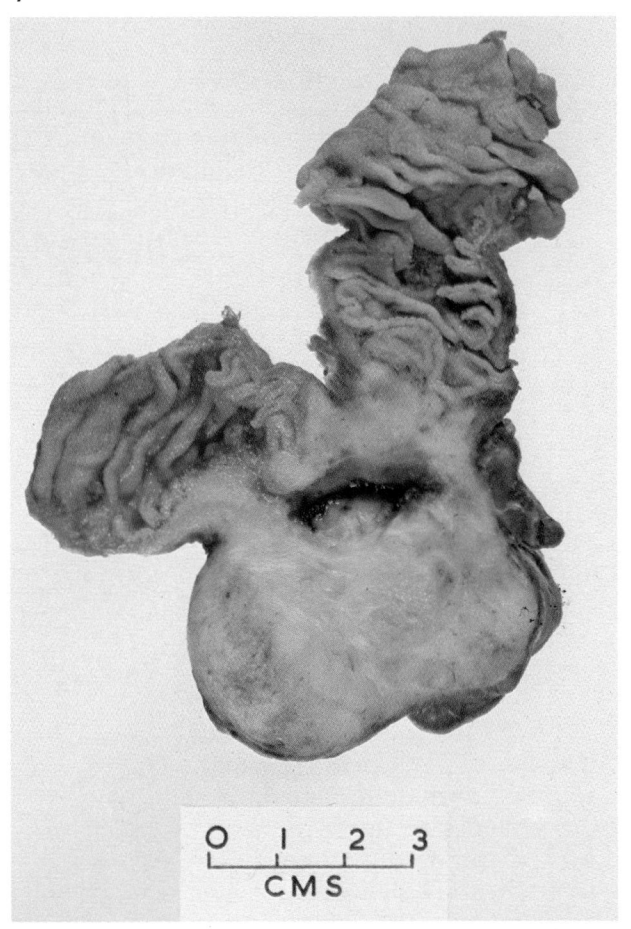

7a

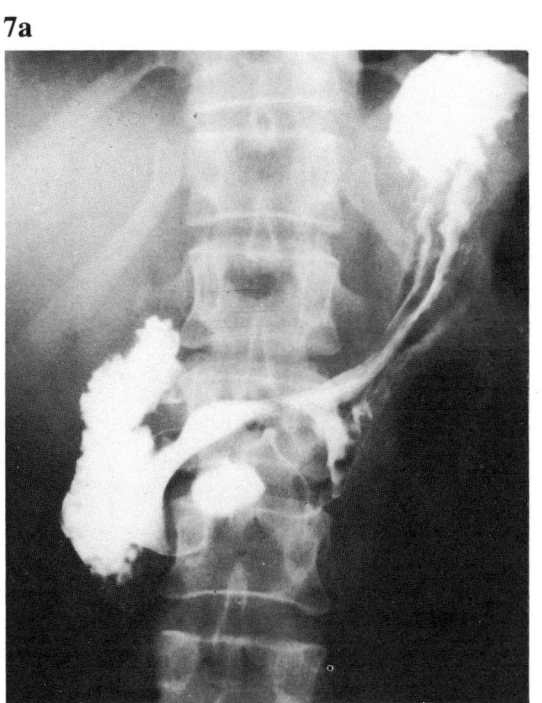

7 and **7a**   From a male aged 55 years. Short history of dyspepsia associated with vomiting, loss of weight and anorexia. Blood was present in the stools. Palpable swelling right hypochondrium. The tumour was mobile and associated with visible peristalsis. The X-ray shows a barium crater leading into the centre of the tumour. The tumour was removed surgically and measured 5 × 4.5 cm.

Nerve sheath tumours

These tumours were first described by Verocay in 1910 and called 'neurinoma'. Subsequent investigation showed that two tumour types occurred – the neurofibroma and the neurilemmoma respectively. To the latter the name 'Schwannoma' has also been applied.

Incidence

Neural tumours are very rare. They are more frequently found in the stomach than the intestine and the incidence appears to be higher in females. The precise location of the tumour may be (a) submucous; (b) subserous or (c) mural, derived from Auerbach's plexus between the circular and longitudinal muscle coats.

Pathology

Neurofibroma

Typically neurofibromas are small and solitary but may be multiple. Intestinal neurofibromas also occur in generalised neurofibromatosis (Von Reckling-hausen's disease). The tumours are rounded, oval and firm. The cut surface is pink in colour and shows fasciculation.

Neurilemmoma

The neurilemmomas are usually larger, rounded and lobulated. In the presence of central degenerative changes which are common, the tumour is comparatively soft. The cut surface may be pale or a pinkish-yellow colour and will show degenerative cysts containing reddish fluid.

Neurofibromas are frequently regarded as hamartomatous in nature. The Schwannoma, however, is considered to be a true neoplasm.

Also found in relation to nerves are occasional small nodules which represent a non-neoplastic hyperplasia sometimes attributed to preceding trauma. These are small and multiple. A very rare tumour occasionally found in the intestinal wall is a ganglioneuroma.

8

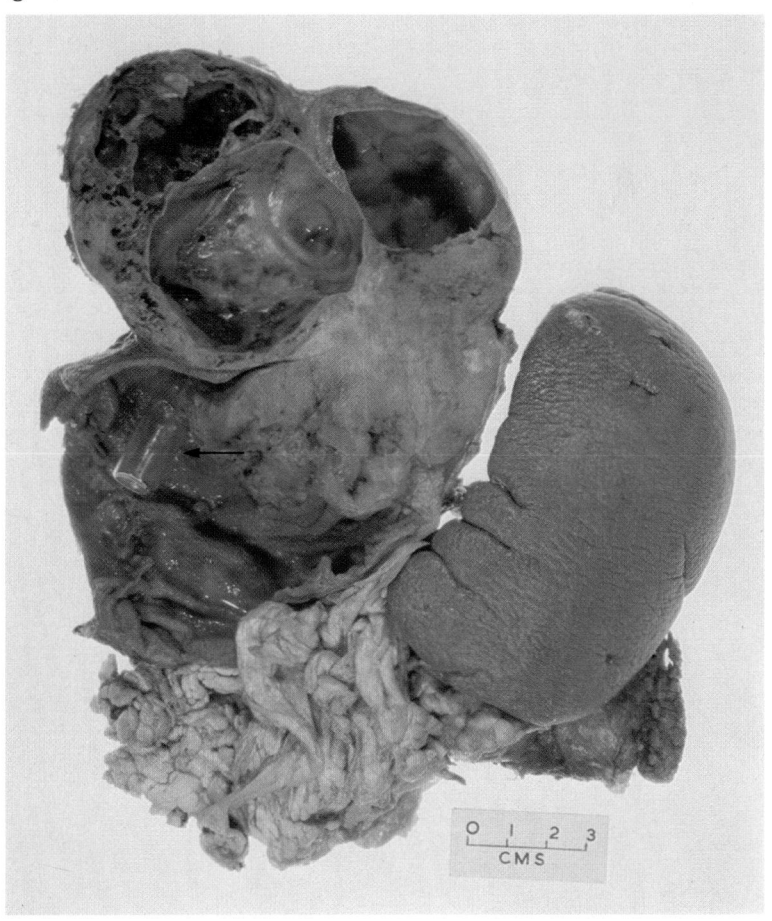

G.C.10510

8 From a male aged 51 years. Seven year history of abdominal discomfort and flatulence. The tumour involves the fundus of the stomach. A glass rod indicates the gastro-oesophageal orifice. Note the presence of an ulcerating mass projecting into the lumen and the presence of cystic spaces due to degeneration. Histologically the tumour is a neurilemmoma. (See Figure **12**, page 316.)

9 From an elderly female patient with a history of dyspepsia for six months. Radiological examination disclosed lesions in both the oesophagus and the stomach. Total gastrectomy was performed. Oesophageal lesion – a typical ulcerative squamous carcinoma of the lower oesophagus with considerable penetration. Histological examination confirms this diagnosis. Gastric lesion – an ovoid tumour projecting into the lumen of the distal part of the stomach measuring 7 × 4.5 × 4.5 cm. The tumour has not invaded either the serosa or mucosa. The cut surface of the tumour was friable and mottled by recent haemorrhage. Histologically the tumour is a neurilemmoma showing degenerative changes but no mitoses are present.

9

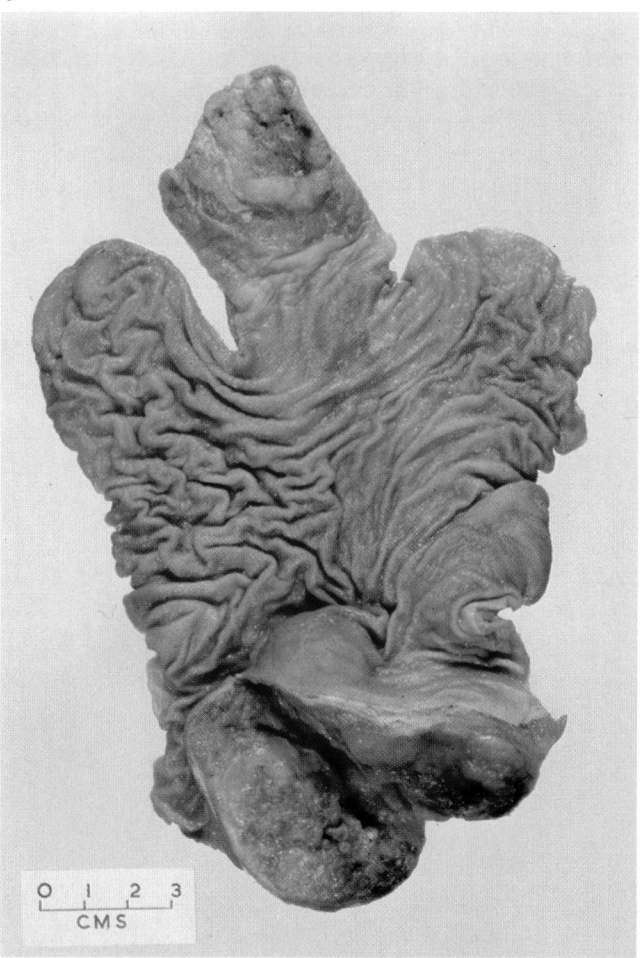

G.C.14649

Nerve sheath tumours *(Continued)*

Histology

Neurofibroma

10 The tumour is comparatively acellular and composed of undulating bundles of fibres with long thin nuclei. Nerve fibres may be observed between the bundles. *(H&E ×100)*

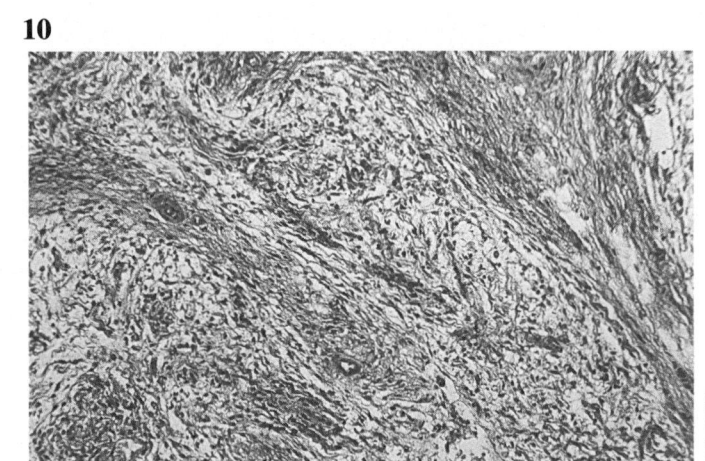

Neurilemmoma

Neurilemmomas are composed of two main types of tissue in varying proportions.

Type 'A' is fibrillary with long, slender, wire-like fibres, straight or undulating with a tendency to palisading of the cell nuclei.

Type 'B' is reticular with no structural pattern. It shows microcysts and areas with a mucinous appearance. In the absence of these characteristics differentiation from leiomyomatous tumours can be difficult. The tumours are essentially benign and slow growing.

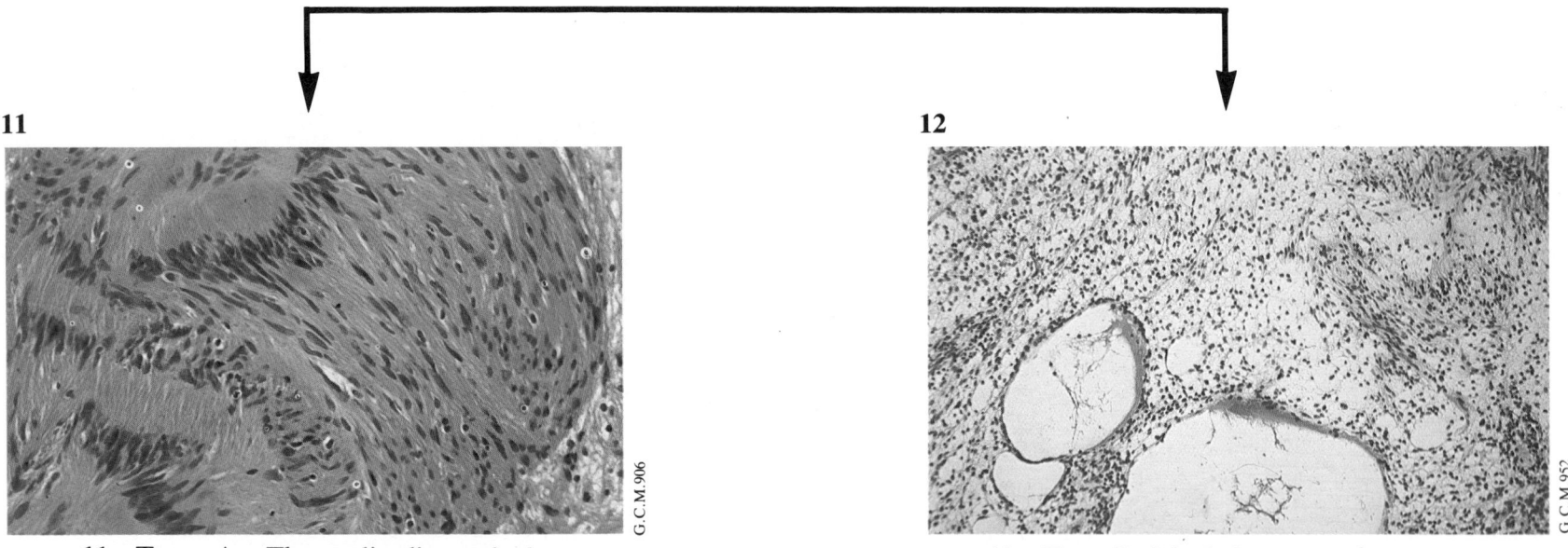

11 Type A. The palisading of the nuclei is well shown. *(H&E ×250)*

12 Type B. Much looser oedematous tissue with small cysts. *(H&E ×100)*

Fibroma

Fibromas and myxomas have been described but are rare findings and are comparable to lipomas in their presentation and complications. They may be single or multiple. Many supposed examples of fibromas on careful histological examination prove to be tumours of other types, e.g. leiomyomas, with an unusually large fibrous component.

Site incidence

Stomach	Less than 1%
Duodenum	5%
Jejunum	15%
Ileum	60 – 70%

The differentiation of a true fibroma from a neurofibroma is often extremely difficult and cannot be based upon the study of a single section since the picture varies throughout the tumour.

13

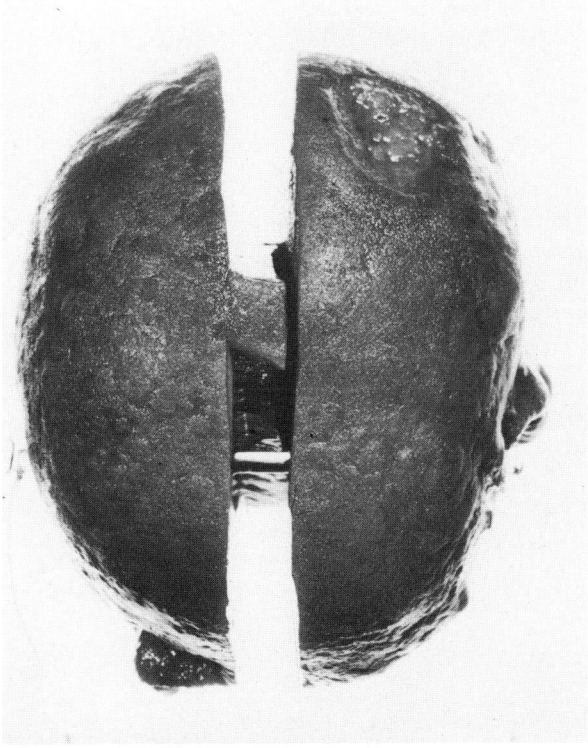

G.C.6450

13 Operative specimen removed from an adult. The tumour which measured 5 × 4 × 2.5 cm, is oval and smooth on the surface except at one portion where there is a small area of ulceration. Two large wedges of tissue have been removed for histological examination. It appears to have originated in the cellular tissue of the muscle coat. Histologically it presented the appearance of a cellular fibroma. There was some degree of pleomorphism suggesting cellular activity and possibly early malignant change.

Lymphoma

This is a complex group of tumours of lymphoid origin and may affect virtually any organ of the body. They are discussed in detail in a later section.

Incidence

Lymphoma of the alimentary tract is comparatively uncommon in the United Kingdom but the incidence is higher in the Middle East especially in the valley of the Nile. These neoplasms show a slight male preponderance (2:1). They are more common in patients over 40 years of age but similar lesions are found in children during the first decade.

Site incidence

Any part of the alimentary tract may be involved. The majority of the tumours are found in the stomach, small intestine and colon, with the ileum the commonest site.

A definite association exists between gluten-sensitive enteropathy (coeliac disease) and idiopathic steatorrhoea and malignant lymphoma. Irradiation may also predispose to lymphoma.

14

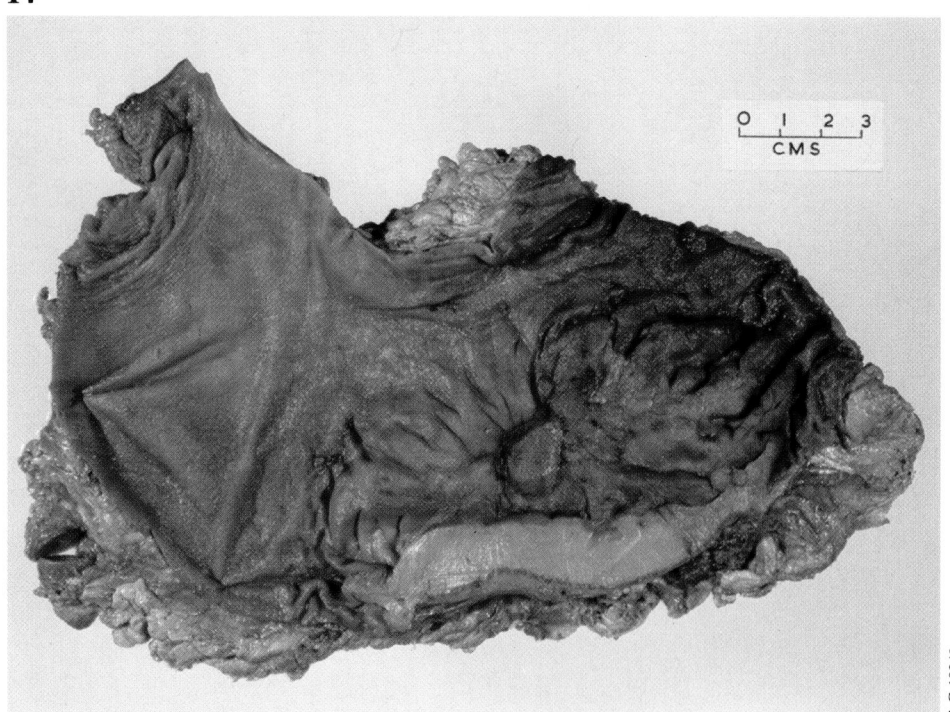

G.C.10249

14 From a female aged 43 years. Two years debility. Six weeks prior to admission transient severe melaena. Three week history of epigastric discomfort. Gastrectomy performed. Symptom-free 2 years 6 months later. The cut surface shows thickening of 1.5cm over a distance of 11cm along the greater curvature due to the growth of pale, structureless tissue chiefly located in the submucous layer. The mucosa shows ulceration.

Pathology

The initial lesion is sited in the mucosa but the main proliferation of tumour cells is seen in the submucosa. This may give rise to a bulky polypoidal lesion which may initiate intussusception. Alternatively the tumour may spread submucosally giving rise to an annular constricting lesion producing obstruction. Initially the overlying mucosa is intact but ulceration soon follows. Central necrosis may occur in the large bulky tumours giving rise to apparent dilatation of the lumen, a condition described sometimes as aneurysmal. Perforation may occur. These tumours may be multiple.

15

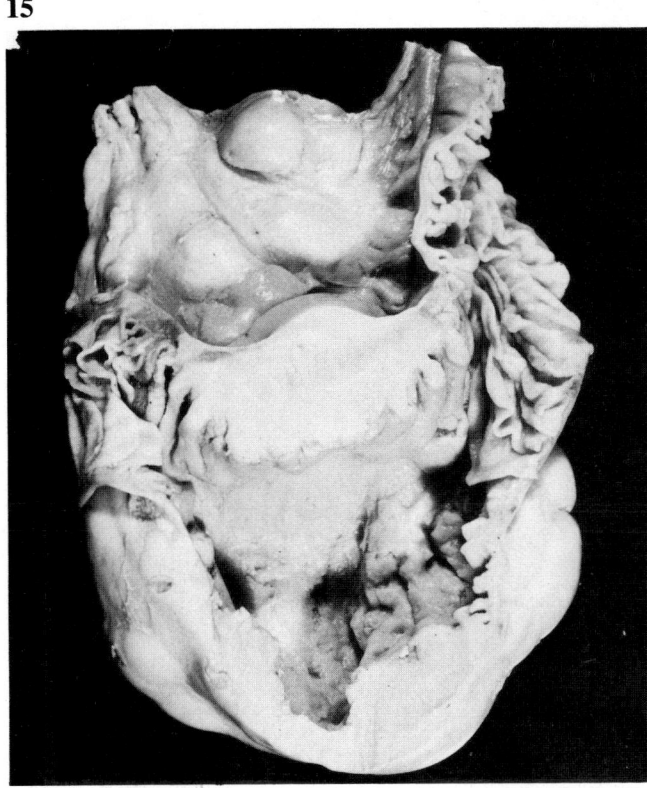

15 An older specimen from the Museum collection presenting the classical appearance of the 'aneurysmal' lymphosarcoma.

Two variants have been described:
(a) multiple lymphomatous polyposis – where multiple small tumours project into the lumen.
(b) diffuse involvement of the intestinal tract by malignant cells without polyp formation (Mediterranean lymphoma) may be:
  1 Associated with severe malabsorption and ∝ chain disease.
  2 Linked with Waldenstrom's macroglobulinaemia.

The serosa is usually intact and the cut surface is homogeneous, fleshy and greyish white in colour. It is softer in consistence than a carcinoma and is often described as 'rubbery'.

16

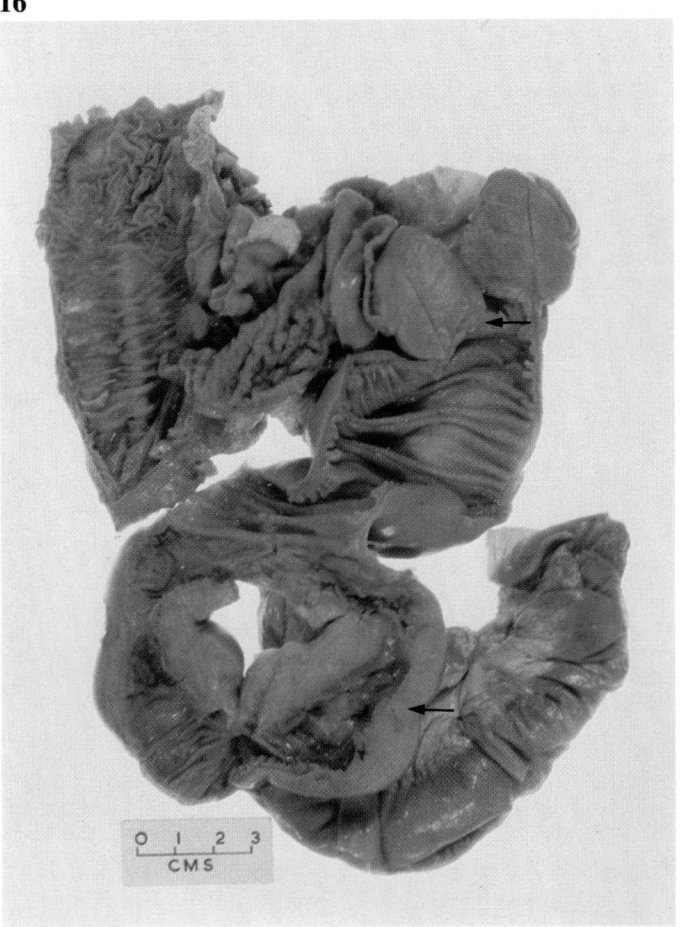

16 From a male aged 6 years. This is an example of multiple lymphoma of the intestine. Note that one of the lesions measuring 3.5 × 3cm presents as a mass protruding into the lumen of the gut (polypoid form), while the other lesion, 6 × 1.5cm in diameter, is of more tubular character with ulceration of the mucosal surface.

Lymphoma *(Continued)*

Hodgkin's lymphoma

18

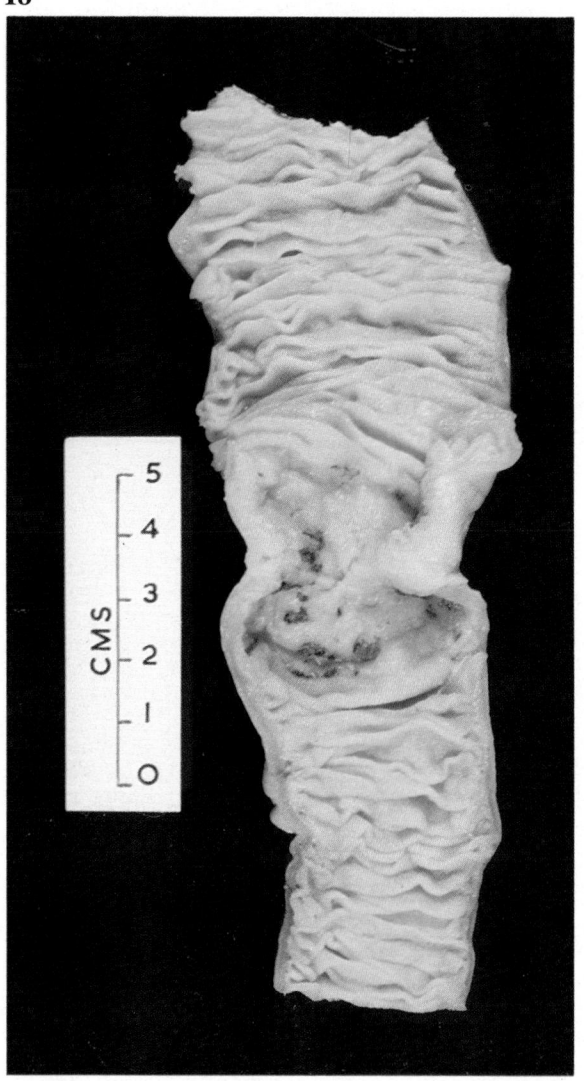

G.C.14686

18 From a patient suffering from Hodgkin's lymphoma in whom a jejunal lesion was discovered at post mortem. Externally there is an area of constriction but without change in the overlying serosa. On section a circular ulcerative lesion measuring 4 × 4cm is present encircling the wall with raised everted edges. The mucosa in the rest of the preparation shows no evidence of ulceration. The appearances are those of a typical malignant ulcer and where the edges of the lesion have been sectioned the tumour is homogeneous and fleshy, situated chiefly in the submucosa and without serosal involvement. There is a degree of infiltration and destruction of the muscularis.

Multiple lymphomatous polyposis

17 Case report. From a male aged 42 years. Vague abdominal pain with tumefaction of the abdomen for 15 months. Sigmoidoscopy revealed a polypoid tumour. Histology established the diagnosis of reticulosis. Later an exploratory laparotomy demonstrated that the whole length of the small intestine, the caecum and the ascending colon were studded with masses, the caecum being most grossly affected. The lymph nodes of the mesentery were enlarged, one close to the caecum being the size of a clenched fist. There were numerous sites of intussusception in the ileum which could be reduced but recurred. The appendix was removed for examination. The lesion responded rapidly to radiotherapy and four and half years later the patient was well and had returned to work.

17

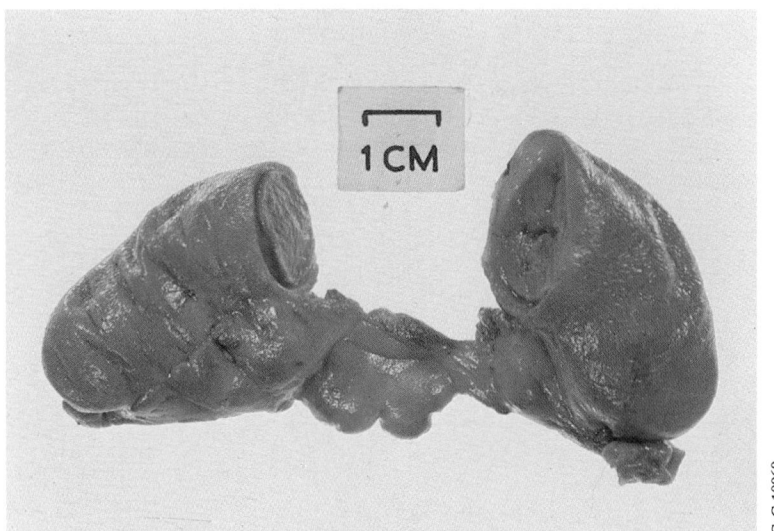

1 CM

G.C.10969

The appendix has been sectioned transversely to demonstrate that the wall of the organ is normal in structure but the lumen is completely occupied by a homogeneous fleshy mass.

Histology

These tumours are composed of sheets and aggregates of neoplastic lymphoid cells. Classification into Hodgkin's lymphoma or non-Hodgkin's (further subdivided into groups according to cell type and degree of differentiation) can be difficult. Involvement of regional nodes does not necessarily worsen the prognosis.

Patients with tumours composed predominantly of small lymphocytic cells or having a pronounced follicular pattern generally do best. Large cell tumours tend to do badly.

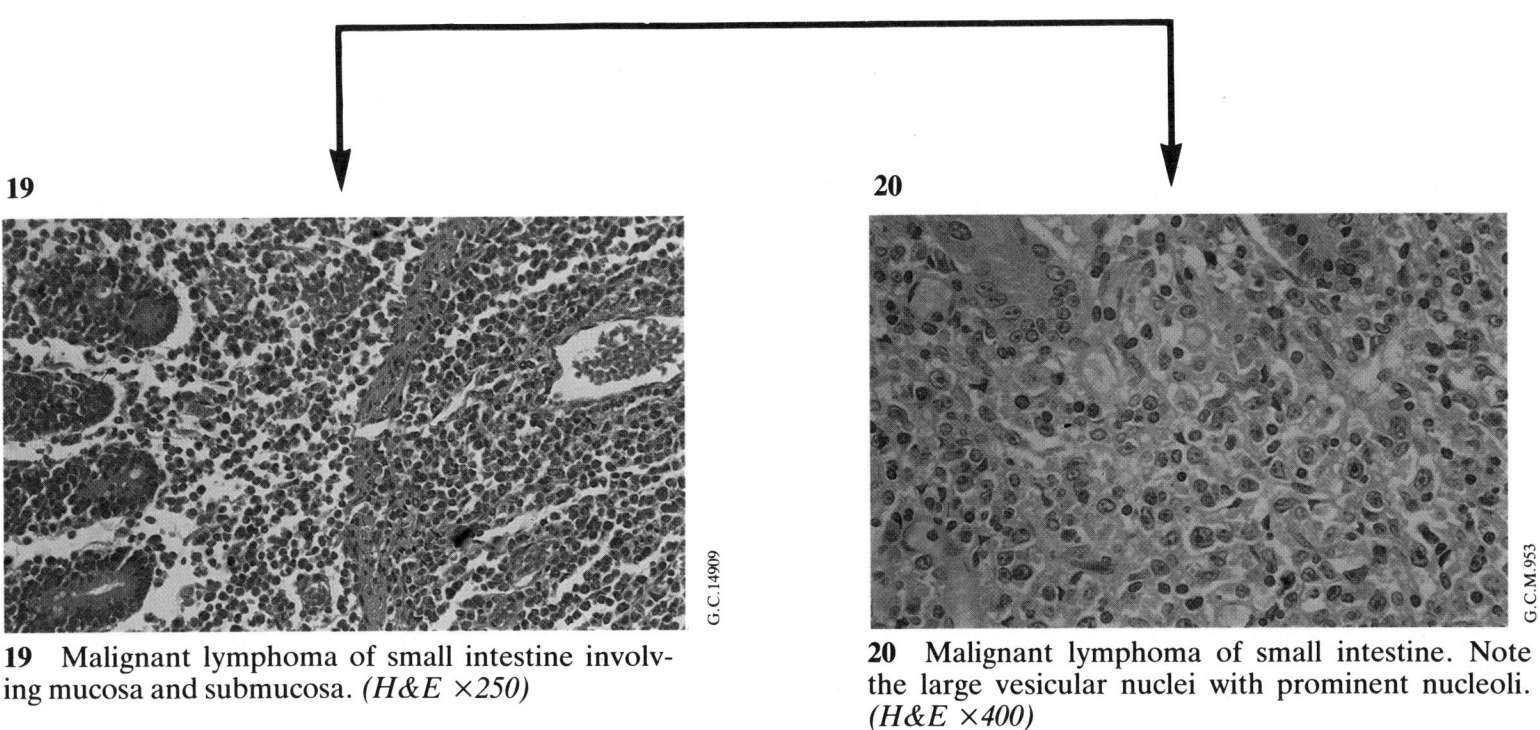

19 Malignant lymphoma of small intestine involving mucosa and submucosa. *(H&E ×250)*

20 Malignant lymphoma of small intestine. Note the large vesicular nuclei with prominent nucleoli. *(H&E ×400)*

Generalised lymphoma

Involvement of the gastrointestinal tract may be found in 15% of patients with malignant generalised lymphoma. These lesions are usually small, infiltrative and often multiple and rarely confused with primary gastrointestinal lymphoma.

Benign lymphoid hyperplasia

Benign lymphoid hyperplasia may occur anywhere in the gastrointestinal tract. The gross appearance may simulate neoplasia but distinction can usually be achieved by a study of the histological appearances.

Haemangioma

These tumours may be confined to the intestine or be associated with comparable lesions in other parts of the body. Both simple and malignant forms of the tumour occur.

Incidence

Account for approximately 0.3% of all gastrointestinal tumours and show a male preponderance of 2:1.

Site incidence

The large majority of the tumours are to be found in the small intestine (45%) and the colon (30%). Lesions in other sites are rarer.

21

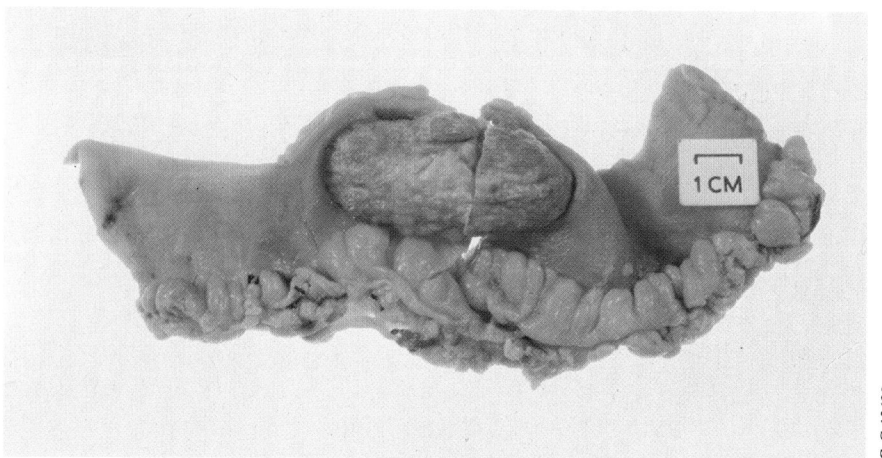

22

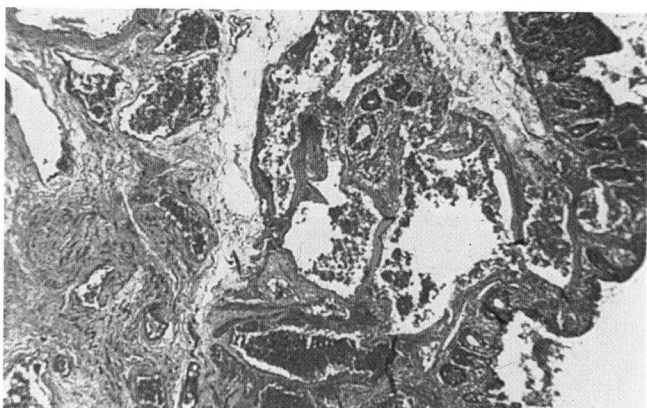

21 Female aged 66 years. Ten year history of recurrent intestinal colic. Finally admitted with acute intestinal obstruction. A localised haemangioma measuring 4.5 × 2.5 cm was found in the ileum, 125 cm proximal to the ileocaecal junction.

22 A section of the tumour showing mucosa and submucosa. Cavernous vascular spaces in the submucosa extended deeper into the bowel wall. *(H&E ×40)*

Pathology

The term 'angioma' is commonly applied both to congenital abnormalities and true neoplasms of vascular origin since the structure of these frequently cannot be differentiated. The congenital anomalies are in the nature of hamartomas the growth of which continues only during the period of normal development of the tissue from which it arises.

Haemangiomas present three patterns of growth:
(a)   Diffuse infiltrating cavernous haemangioma – usually single but apparently infiltrating the gut wall – cause haemorrhage or obstruction.
(b)   Circumscribed cavernous haemangioma – usually a single, polypoidal lesion projecting into the lumen – associated with haemorrhage, obstruction or intussusception.
(c)   Simple capillary haemangioma – single or multiple occurring in younger age groups.

23

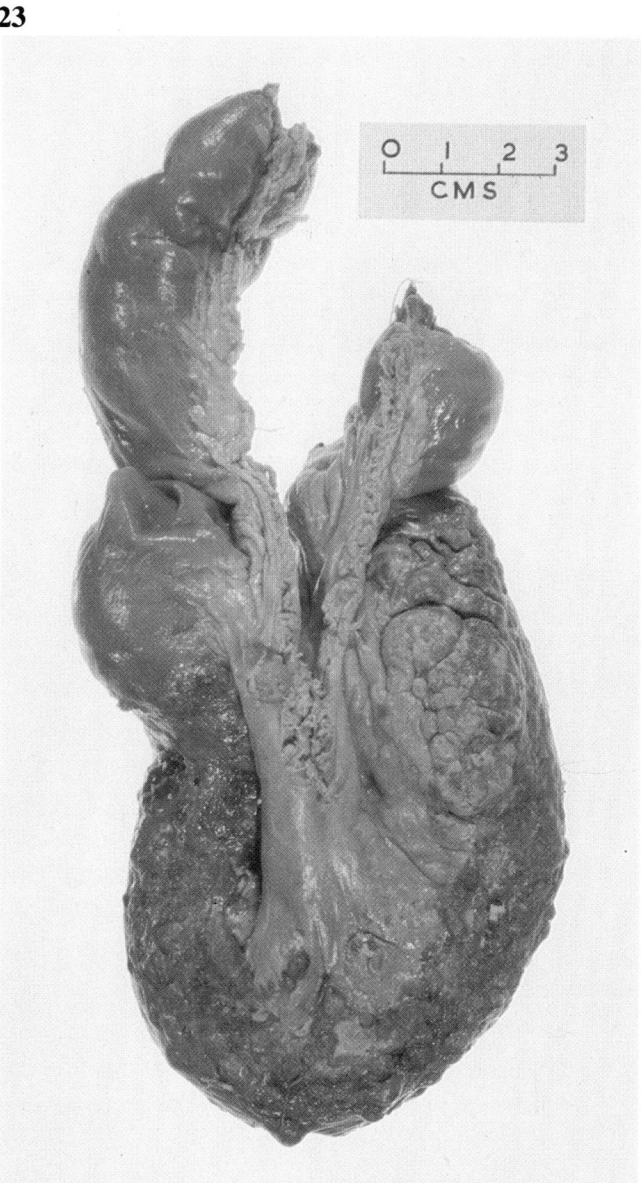

23   Male aged 10 years. Five year history of recurrent abdominal colic and general ill health with anaemia. The diagnosis was only established when he was admitted on the last occasion for acute obstruction and a palpable mass was present in the lower abdomen. At operation a loop of jejunum approximately 20cm in length with a cavernous haemangioma was found to be the site of the volvulus. The child died nine days later and at post mortem a further area of telangiectasis was disclosed in the jejunum.

Haemangioma *(Continued)*

Haemangiomas fall into three groups according to their gross nature:
- A   Diffuse – infiltrative or expansive
- B   Multiple
- C   Single or circumscribed

Lesions of groups A and B are most probably hamartomatous malformations. Lesions in group C may be true tumours. These tumours may also be grouped according to their histological structure:
- (a) capillary
- (b) mixed capillary – cavernous
- (c) cavernous

Simple capillary haemangiomas may be single or multiple submucous lesions. Microscopically composed of closely packed, small blood vessels with marked proliferation of endothelium with minimal stroma. The endothelial proliferation may obliterate the lumen. Haemangiomas in group A (Diffuse) or group C (Single) are usually cavernous in character. Microscopically such lesions consist of large blood spaces with single or multiple layers of lining endothelial cells with scanty supporting connective tissue.

Hereditary haemorrhagic telangiectasia

(Rendu–Osler–Weber syndrome)

Gastrointestinal lesions develop early in adult life. The lesions are multiple, may be nodular and are found either in the submucous or subserous zones. Cutaneous lesions and multiple small haemangiomas of the nasal and oral mucosa are a constant feature and appear in childhood. The condition is familial, inherited as a Mendelian dominant. Histologically the lesions resemble small cavernous haemangiomas

Multiple telangiectasis

This condition is essentially a localised dilatation of arterio-venous anastomoses in the submucosa and subserosa. There is frequently involvement of other viscera. It is not certain whether this represents dilatation of existing vessels or a genuine hamartoma.

Malignancy

Malignant vascular tumours are rare and represent 10 to 15% of the true neoplastic angiomatous group.

Angiosarcoma

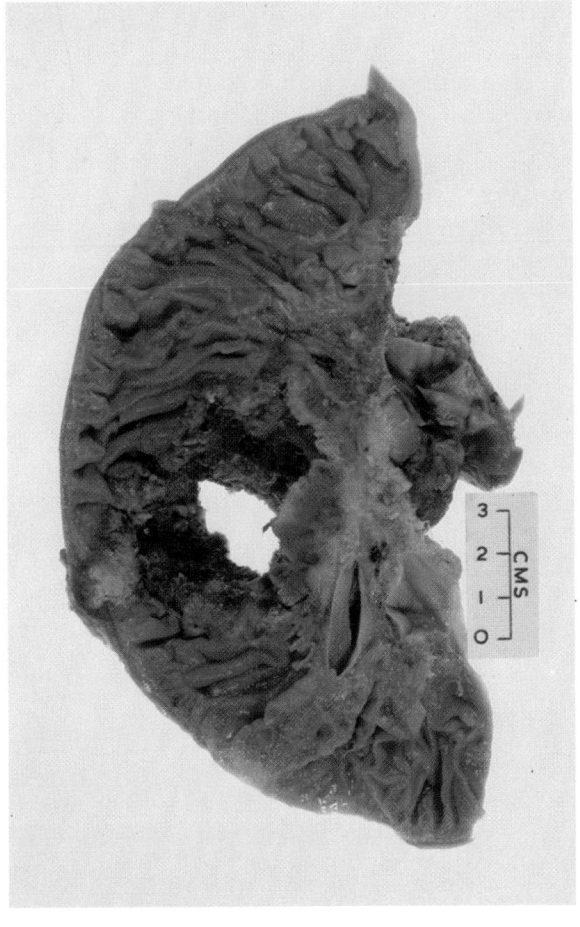

G.C.14636

This is a unique specimen from which several lessons can be learned.

The patient was a middle aged male who for six weeks had had subcostal pain which had moved downwards in the abdomen two weeks prior to admission to hospital. He had suffered from diarrhoea. A mass was palpable in the abdomen. At operation a perforated tumour of the upper jejunum which was adherent to the colon, was found and was resected. The vascularity of the tumour and its infiltration suggested the diagnosis of angiosarcoma.

The operative specimen consists of the resected jejunum and attached colon.

Histological examination at first appeared to confirm the diagnosis of angiosarcoma but further study revealed the presence of trophoblastic derivatives thus indicating that the tumour was in fact a choriocarcinoma.

There was no evidence on clinical examination of any testicular neoplasm. At operation there was no evidence of any retroperitoneal tumour which would suggest a neoplasm originating in an undescended testis.

The occurrence of testicular tissue 'rests' in the retroperitoneal space has been described as the possible origin of testicular teratomatous tumours comparable to tumours of the undescended testis. Testicular tumours have also been known to undergo a regression whilst their metastases progressed. The origin of some of these very rare abdominal visceral tumours, however, is apparently inexplicable. Interesting examples of the co-existence of a trophoblastic tumour and a carcinoma have been reported in the stomach.

24a

G.C.14636

24a Small intestine – A malignant vascular tumour invades the mucosa and submucosa. *(H&E ×100)*

24b

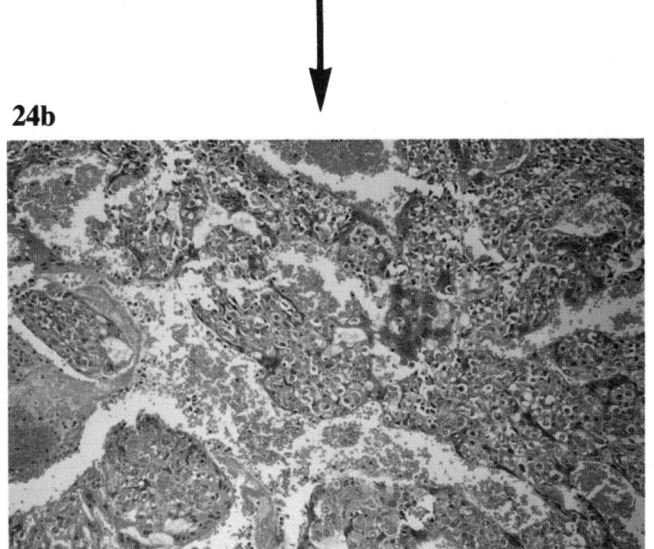

G.C.14636

24b Same case. Part of the tumour shows syncytial cells and cells of Langhans' layer – diagnostic of chorionic carcinoma. *(H&E ×100)*

J. Anderson

325

A primarily non-neoplastic tumour-like malformation of tissue development characterised by a mixture of tissues indigenous to that part, presenting at birth or in the post-natal period. Hamartomas can undergo neoplastic change.

Peutz–Jeghers syndrome

This familial anomaly is characterised by the presence of intestinal polyps and pigmentation of the lips and oral mucosa. It was first described by Peutz in 1921 and by Jeghers in 1944.

Incidence

This is a rare disease showing an equal sex incidence and transmitted as a Mendelian dominant in 55% of recorded cases.

1

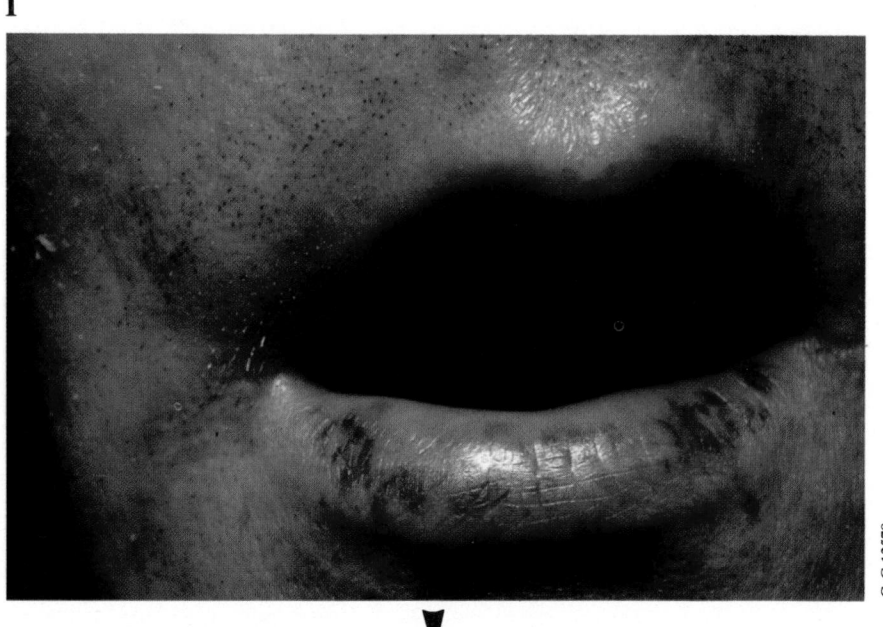

G.C.12578

Pigmentation

Round, bluish lesions due to melanin deposition are present in the circumoral skin especially the lower lip and in the buccal mucosa but the tongue is not usually affected. Comparable pigmentation occurs in the toes and fingers.

1 From a male aged 36 years with a 7 week history of abdominal colic and vomiting. Barium meal showed duodenal ulcer. Settled on gastric diet and drugs, but had persistent melaena, and symptoms recurred. Because of the marked pigmentation about the lips a diagnosis of Peutz–Jeghers syndrome was given. At operation an intussusception of the small intestine was discovered and resected.

The illustration on the opposite page (**1a**, page 327) demonstrates the affected segment and detached from the specimen is the large polyp which was responsible for the intussusception. Mucosal haemorrhage and devitalisation resulted and two shallow mucosal ulcers can be seen. The patient subsequently developed a carcinoma of the maxillary antrum.

Intestinal lesion

1a The intestinal polyps may be single or multiple. These may affect any part of the alimentary tract but are most commonly located in the jejunum. They vary in size and usually appear later than the pigmentation. The polyps show a coarse lobulation, resembling adenomas but histologically the essential feature is a branching core of smooth muscle covered by normal epithelium and lamina propria.

There is a marked tendency to haemorrhage and intussusception.

1a

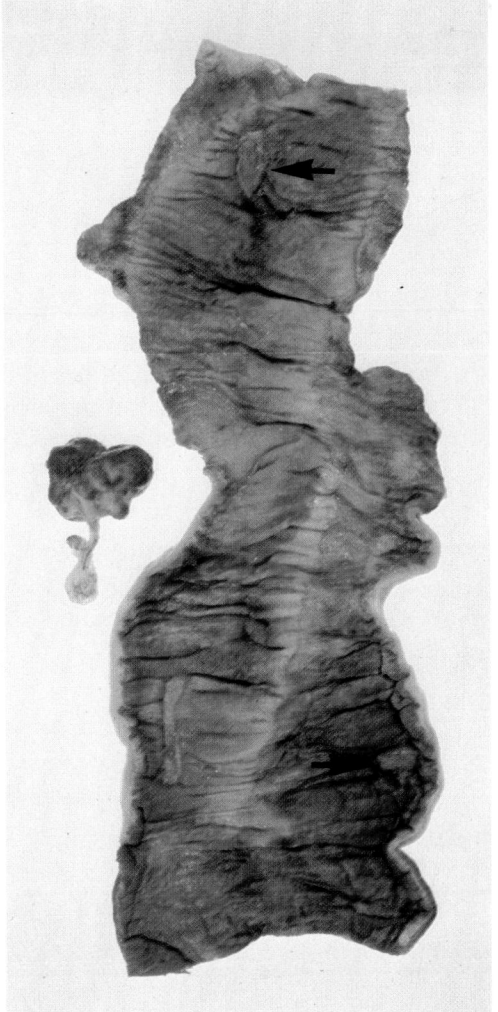

G.C.12578

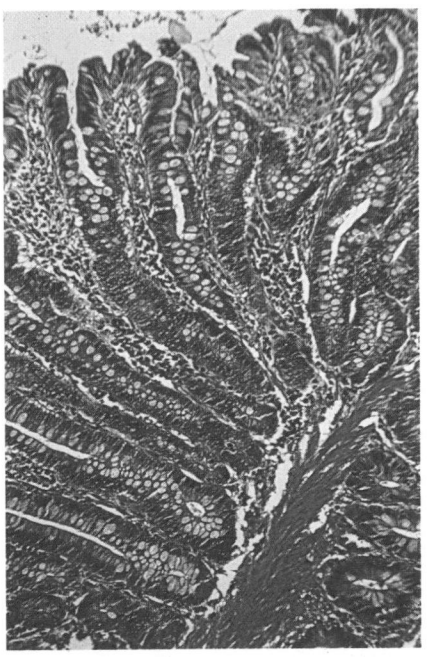

G.C.M.864

2 Jejunal polyp from a child with Peutz–Jeghers syndrome. There is an overgrowth of mucosal epithelium set regularly on an arborisation of the lamina propria and muscularis mucosae. *(H&E ×112.5)*

Complications

Carcinomatous change occurs occasionally in these polyps but the risk is not great.

Cronkhite – Canada syndrome

A rare lesion characterised by gastrointestinal polyposis combined with alopecia, hyperpigmentation, nail atrophy and excess protein loss from the gut. Stomach and colon more regularly involved than small intestine.

J. Anderson

327

Benign

Benign epithelial tumours occur in both the small and large intestine but are much less frequent in the former. They usually present as polyps and may be single or multiple. The statistical studies of incidence, sex, site, etc., are drawn from larger series of cases and refer essentially to the lesions occurring in the colon and rectum.

Incidence

In the general population (post mortem series) the incidence of simple papillomatous and adenomatous tumours is 4 to 10% where there is no carcinoma of the intestine present. The incidence rises to a 70% association when cancer is present.

Site

Site distribution

Adenomas and papillomas of the small intestine are rare. They do occur in the duodenum and the jejunum but the majority of reported cases are located in the ileum.

These lesions, however, occur frequently in the colon and the site distribution is shown.

Adenoma – Figures on outer (lateral) border

Papilloma – Figures on inner (medial) border

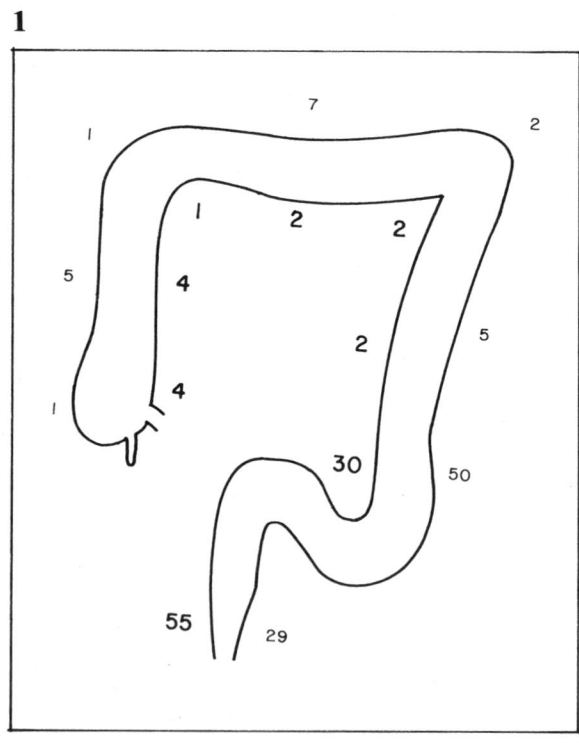

1 Distribution shown as approximate percentages.

Two forms of simple epithelial tumours are described:

Tubulo-adenoma

Tubulo-adenoma – structurally characterised by the presence of closely approximated tubules lined by columnar epithelial cells. The tumour, which is generally small, may be single or multiple and initially sessile (68%). The margins may be difficult to define. The surface of the tumour is smooth but may show lobulation due to the presence of clefts. Surface ulceration may occur. When the tumour becomes pedunculated the base of the pedicle may be wide and the short stalk covered by normal mucosa or the pedicle may be of considerable length.

This is the most common form of benign tumour of colon. A large proportion are found in the sigmoid colon and they are slightly more common in men than women. Rectal bleeding occurs and intussusception may develop.

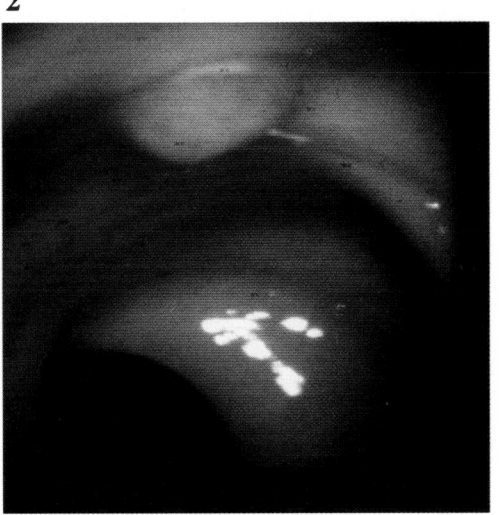

2 A sessile tubulo-adenoma showing characteristic darker colour than the surrounding mucosa.

Villous adenoma

Villous adenoma (papilloma) – structurally consists of closely approximated villi covered by a single layer of columnar epithelium presenting as finger-like fronds on a broad base. The lesion is usually soft and sessile (90%) with shaggy, papilliferous surface and well defined edges. These tumours are generally single and of considerable size. They are darker in colour than surrounding mucosa. The tumour is believed to have a greater tendency to malignant change than other adenomas of the colon and recurrence after excision is frequent.

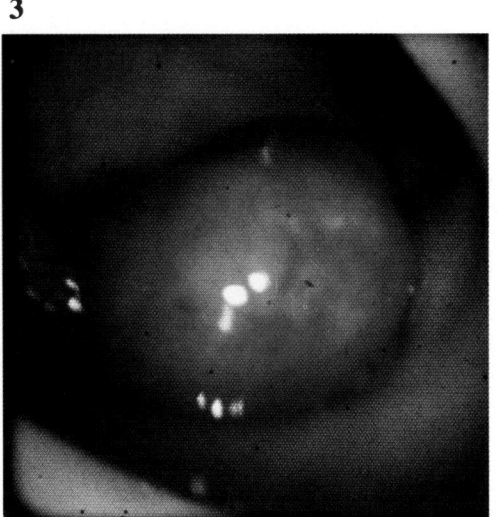

3 The vascular red appearance of this villous adenoma and the copious mucus production are typical features.

4

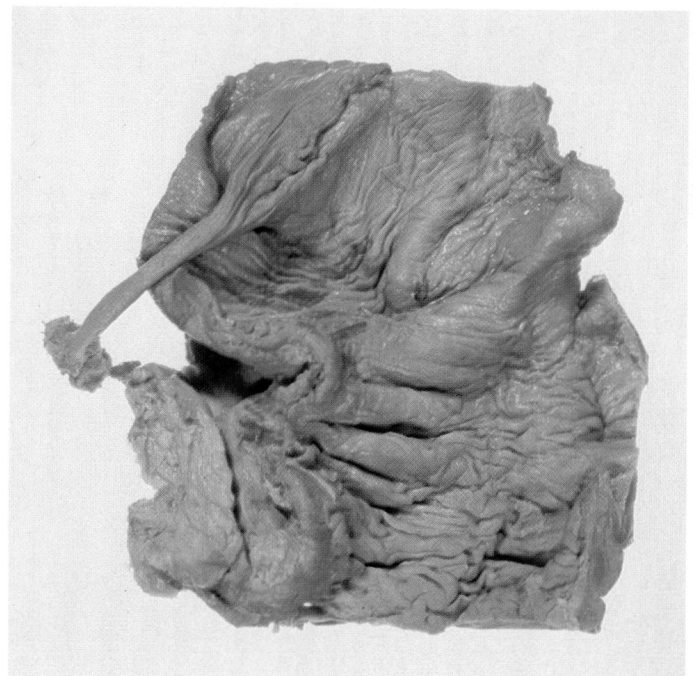

G.C.2764

4 From an adult male. A pedunculated tumour which protruded from the anal canal. The tumour is ovoid and warty and is connected by a smooth rounded pedicle 50mm long to the ampulla of the rectum. Histologically the tumour is a simple adenoma.

5

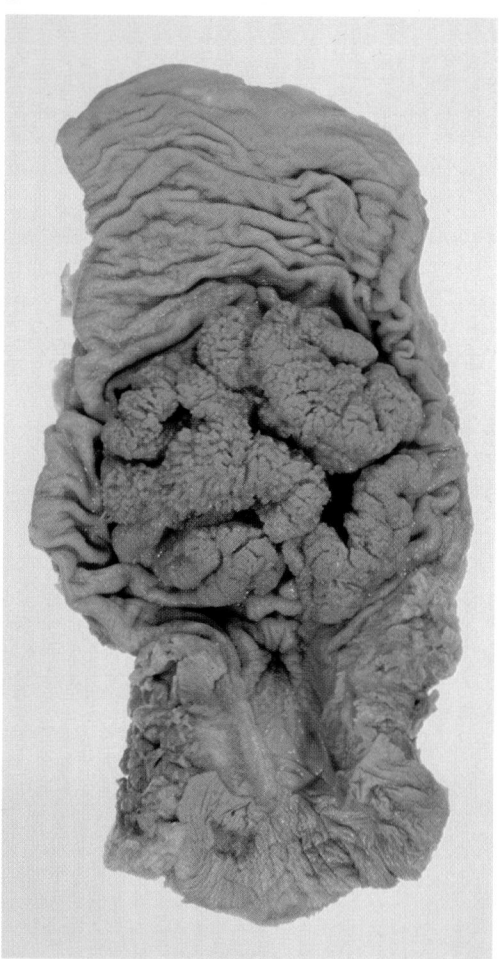

G.C.10080

5 From a female aged 65 years who had suffered from 'diarrhoea' for five months with discharge of watery fluid from the rectum. There had been some loss of weight. This is a soft tumour projecting into the lumen of the gut and possessing a short pedicle. Its surface is lobulated or gyrate and presents small superficial ulcerations. Microscopically the tumour is a papillary adenoma.

6

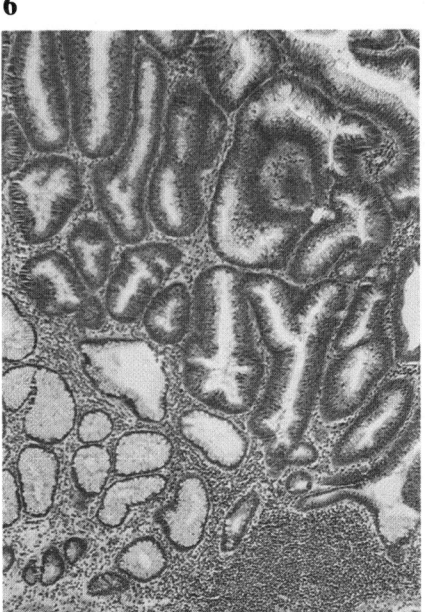

G.C.M.976

6 Part of a single tubulopapillary adenoma (adenopapilloma). The darker epithelium of the actively growing part of the tumour contrasts with that of the more normal glands below. *(H&E ×50)*

Special feature

Larger adenomas (> 1 cm), especially if sessile and/or associated with apical ulceration, should be regarded with suspicion. Malignant change may occur (*vide infra*) and histological examination is required.

7

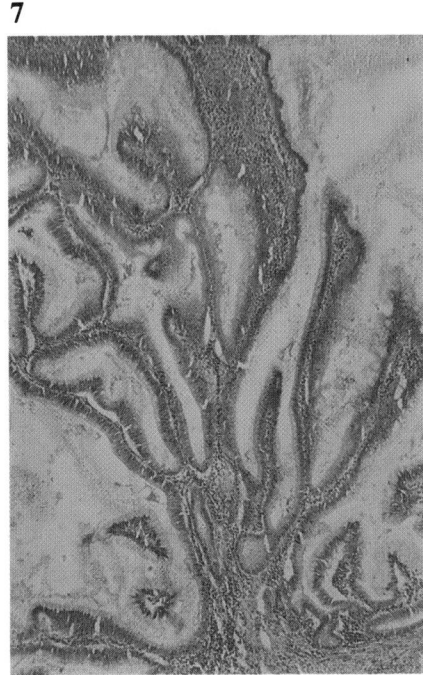

G.C.14678

7 Villous papilloma. The delicate papillary branches of this tumour are covered with columnar epithelium secreting mucin. *(H&E ×50)*

In adenomas arising in the small intestine the gross and microscopic features are similar to those of colonic tumours. Malignant change occurs in a significant proportion of these tumours.

Hamartomatous lesions frequently presenting as polypoid masses may be confused macroscopically with adenomatous lesions. The histological picture, however, is distinctive. Such lesions are found in the Peutz–Jeghers syndrome (see Section 15Ta).

Potassium-secreting papilloma

This is a comparatively rare lesion. The relationship of a simple papillomatous colonic tumour with a related marked disturbance of water and salt balance was first recognised in 1954. The papilloma is usually located in the distal colon or rectum, with marked mucus secretion, and occurs in patients in late adult life. Both sexes are equally affected.

In the fresh specimen the surface is covered by mucus and compression of the mass leads to extrusion of more mucus. Histologically the tumour does not differ structurally from the villous papilloma already described but there is a very marked dominance of the mucus-secreting elements.

Electrolyte loss

There is an excessive secretion of mucus from these tumours and this is rich in potassium. Typical figures demonstrate the loss of water and salt:

	Water	Sodium	Potassium
Normal daily faecal loss	100–200 ml	2–5 mmol	10–15 mmol
Villous	Greatly increased	103–158 mmol	15–80 mmol

From tumours low in the colon or rectum excessive secretion may be intermittent or continuous and is due to the very large secreting area of the tumour. A contributory factor is that in lesions located low in the colon, in contradistinction to those occurring in the proximal colon, reabsorption does not occur. As the result of fluid loss and differential electrolyte loss a condition of hypovolaemia develops associated with hypokalaemia, hyponatraemia and hypochloraemia. There is consequently disturbance of renal function and the development of oliguria, azotaemia and acidosis.

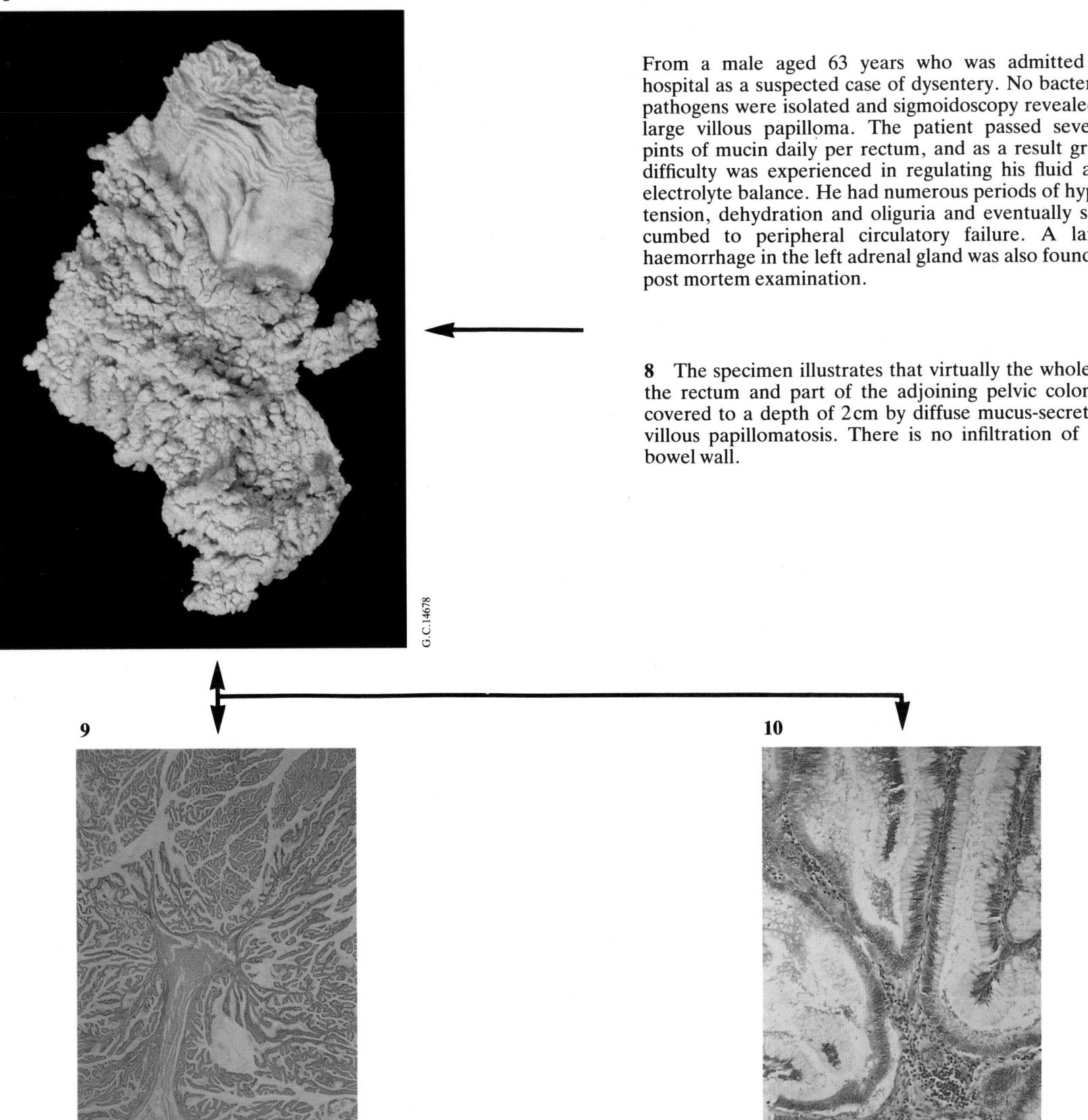

G.C.14678

From a male aged 63 years who was admitted to hospital as a suspected case of dysentery. No bacterial pathogens were isolated and sigmoidoscopy revealed a large villous papilloma. The patient passed several pints of mucin daily per rectum, and as a result great difficulty was experienced in regulating his fluid and electrolyte balance. He had numerous periods of hypotension, dehydration and oliguria and eventually succumbed to peripheral circulatory failure. A large haemorrhage in the left adrenal gland was also found at post mortem examination.

8 The specimen illustrates that virtually the whole of the rectum and part of the adjoining pelvic colon is covered to a depth of 2 cm by diffuse mucus-secreting villous papillomatosis. There is no infiltration of the bowel wall.

9 Part of the base of the tumour. It consists of a complex of slender branching epithelial fronds set upon delicate stroma. *(H&E ×10)*

10 The tall columnar epithelium secretes copious mucus. Although there is no sign of malignancy in this tumour, villous papillomas are prone to undergo carcinomatous change. *(H&E ×125)*

Adenomas – malignant change

The presence of adenomatous polyps indicates an abnormal state of the mucosa which renders it liable to tumour formation which may be simple initially but has a malignant potential.

The finding that an adenoma or a papilloma is present in the gut raises three questions for both the clinician and the pathologist:

1 Is this a solitary lesion?
2 Has it undergone malignant change?
3 Is it associated with another possibly malignant lesion?

Pre-malignant change

On histological examination a significant finding may be areas of dedifferentiation recognised by:

1 Atypical arrangement of cells
2 Deeper staining of nuclei
3 Frequency of mitosis

but without evidence of invasion indicative of malignant change.

Malignant transition

When these changes are more marked and the transition to malignancy is occurring the term 'polyp cancer sequence' is employed and three stages of this process are described:

1 *In situ* change   2 Invasive spread   3 Frank carcinoma

11
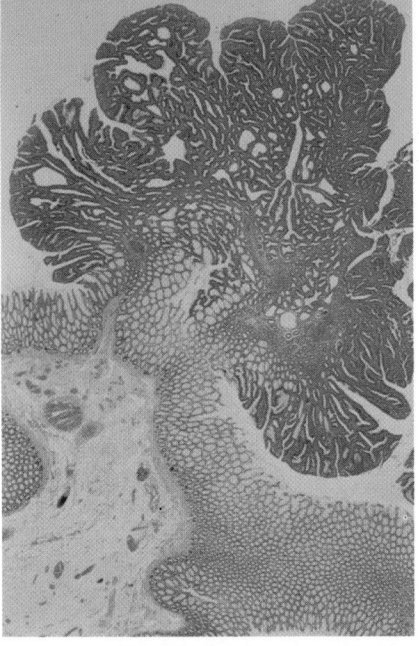
G.C.M.867

12
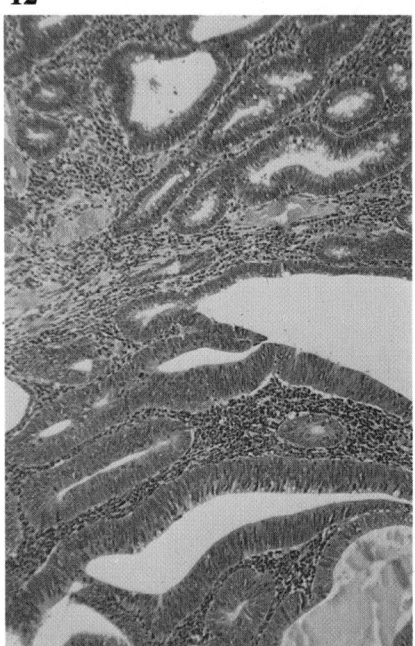
G.C.M.867

13
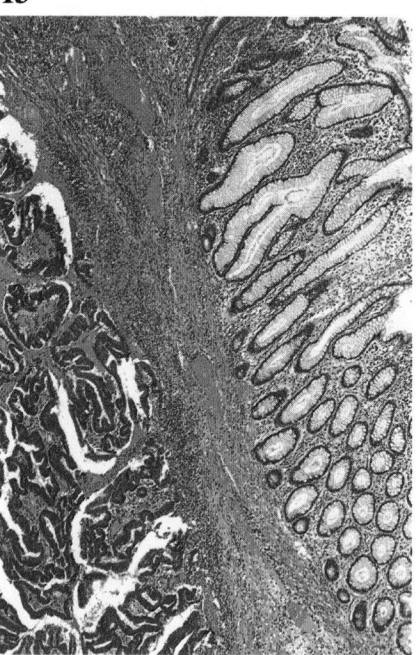
G.C.M.977

11 A well-differentiated papilloma. In part of the tumour (top right) the glands are crowded together and their lumina are inconspicuous. *(H&E ×10)*

12 A higher-power view of the suspicious area. Below, malignancy has supervened and the carcinoma cells are large, hyperchromatic and multilayered. *(H&E ×100)*

13 Invasive carcinoma. The normal mucosa at the edge of a colonic carcinoma is undermined by infiltrating tumour. *(H&E ×40)*

Frequency of malignant change

2.5% of adenomas subsequently become malignant.
30% of villous papillomas subsequently become malignant.

Removal of a polyp is followed by recurrence in 40% of cases or by a carcinoma in 12 to 15% of cases.

The presence of polyps proximal or distal to a carcinoma is very frequent as noted.

14a

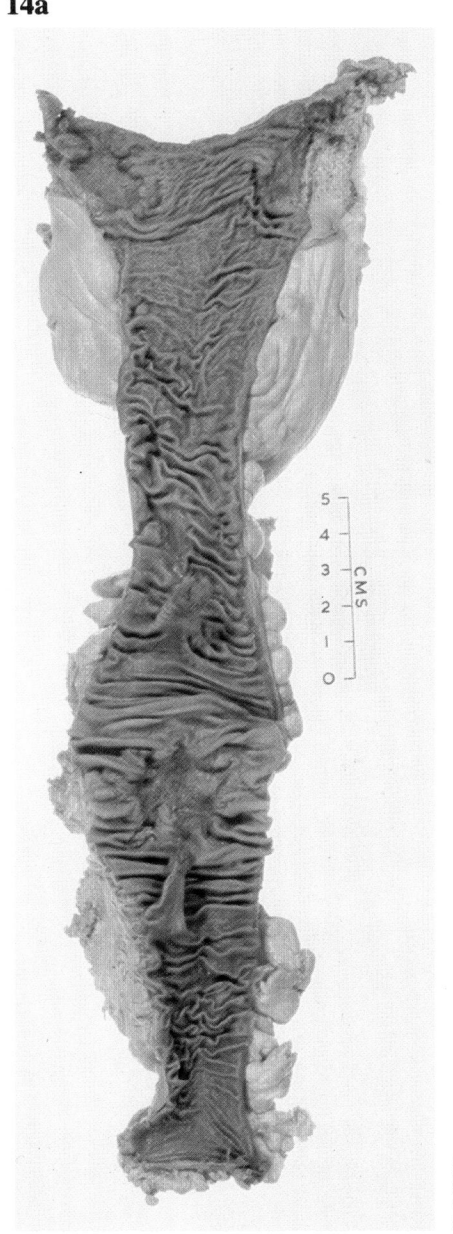

G.C.10198

14a and **14b** From a male aged 67 years. Two month history of irregularity of bowel action. At operation a carcinoma was found in the rectal ampulla. A second carcinoma was found in the sigmoid colon.

14b

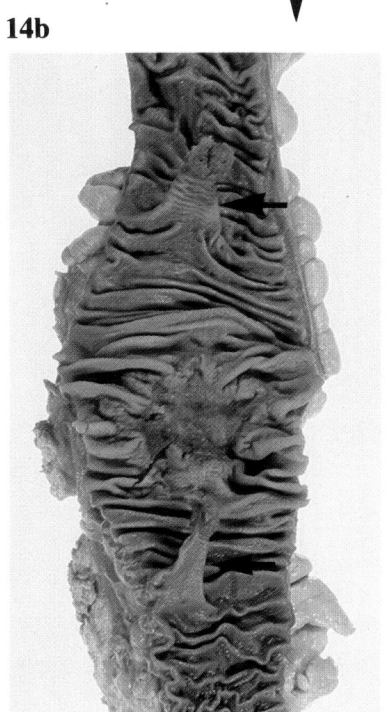

On examination of the specimen of the rectum two pedunculated adenomas (indicated by arrows) were found above and below the carcinoma. See enlarged illustration (**14b**).

Following the removal of a carcinoma of the colon or rectum the subsequent development of a carcinoma in another part of the residual colon and apparently from an independent adenoma is common.

Familial adenomatous polyposis

Although this condition has been known for over a century and the risk of subsequent malignant change recognised, it was not until 50 years ago that Dukes demonstrated that it was a disease transmitted as a Mendelian dominant.

The characteristic feature of the disease is that there are numerous adenomatous polyps from the caecum to the rectum. These appear in the colon after puberty but they have been reported to occur in childhood. Malignancy develops with 100% certainty usually after the age of 25 years with a peak incidence at 40 years. In a majority of cases other members of the family will be or have been affected. New cases are probably the result of mutation. Both sexes are equally affected.

Family tree demonstrating the incidence of polyposis

The disease was first discovered in the eldest brother and the other members of the family were accordingly examined. Two younger brothers were found to be affected. The other brother and a sister were free from the disease. There is no knowledge of the cause of the death of the father who died at the age of 55 years. The mother was alive and well.

1st brother
35 years old. Minor rectal bleeding. Condition discovered on sigmoidoscopy.

2nd brother
31 years old. Three fibrous polyps found in the anal canal. Not regarded as multiple papillomas. Repeated examination surveillance organised.

3rd brother
23 years old. No clinical features but on examination the diagnosis of multiple polyposis was established. Proctocolectomy.

4th brother
20 years old. Asymptomatic. No polyps found.

Sister
Her precise age is not known. Asymptomatic. No polyps found.

Specimens from these patients are in the Museum collection.

G.C.1347

Nodules of hyperplastic tissue first appear and later become fully formed adenomas. They are diffusely scattered throughout the whole length of the colon but are most numerous in the sigmoid and the rectum. Very rarely the small intestine may be affected and this is observed in a younger age group. The number of tumours is always large. The tumours vary in size but are generally small. The individual tumours are comparable in all respects to the solitary adenomas described previously.

15

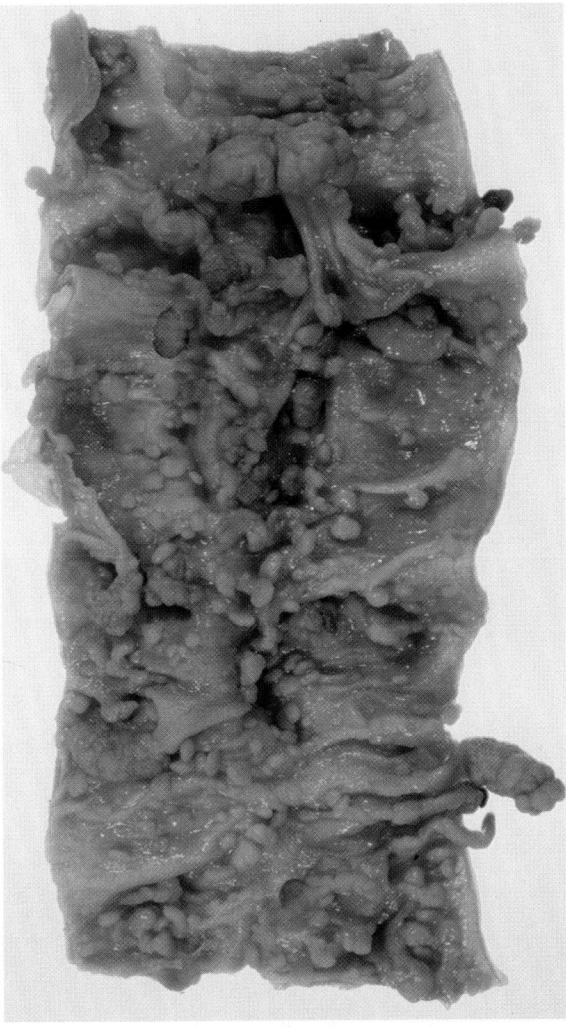

15 Segment of gut on the mucosal surface of which are innumerable polyps. Some of these possess relatively long pedicles, others are sessile and a few show ulceration. Some show submucous haemorrhages due to trauma. There is no evidence of typical malignant ulceration or infiltration.

16

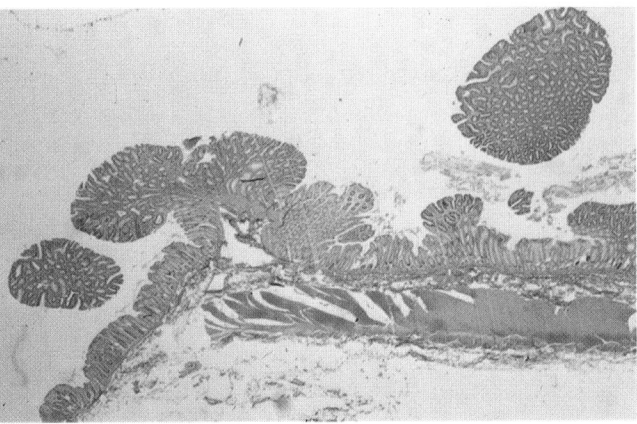

16 From a case of multiple polyposis. Sessile and pedunculated polyps are numerous in the section of colon shown above. *(H&E ×10)*

16a

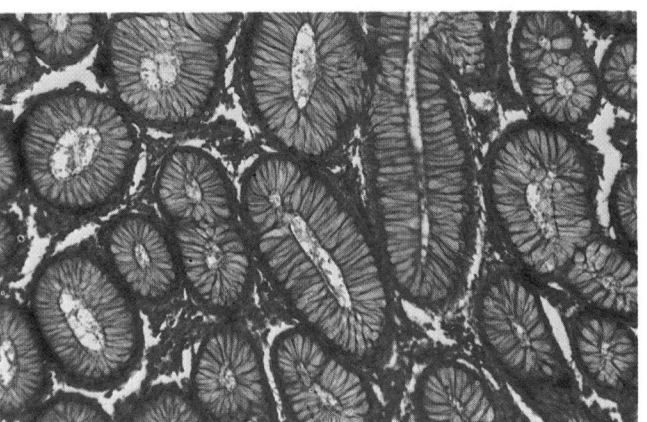

16a Part of a simple polyp from another case of familial polyposis. It is composed of tubules and acini lined by a single layer of very regular tall columnar, mucin-secreting epithelium. There is no suggestion of malignancy in this polyp. *(H&E ×125)*

Familial polyposis with malignancy

Malignancy is frequently multifocal initially appearing at the tips of the polyps, never in the intervening normal mucosa. Early spread to lymph nodes occurs. The tendency to early malignant change makes prophylactic colectomy essential as soon as the diagnosis is made.

17a

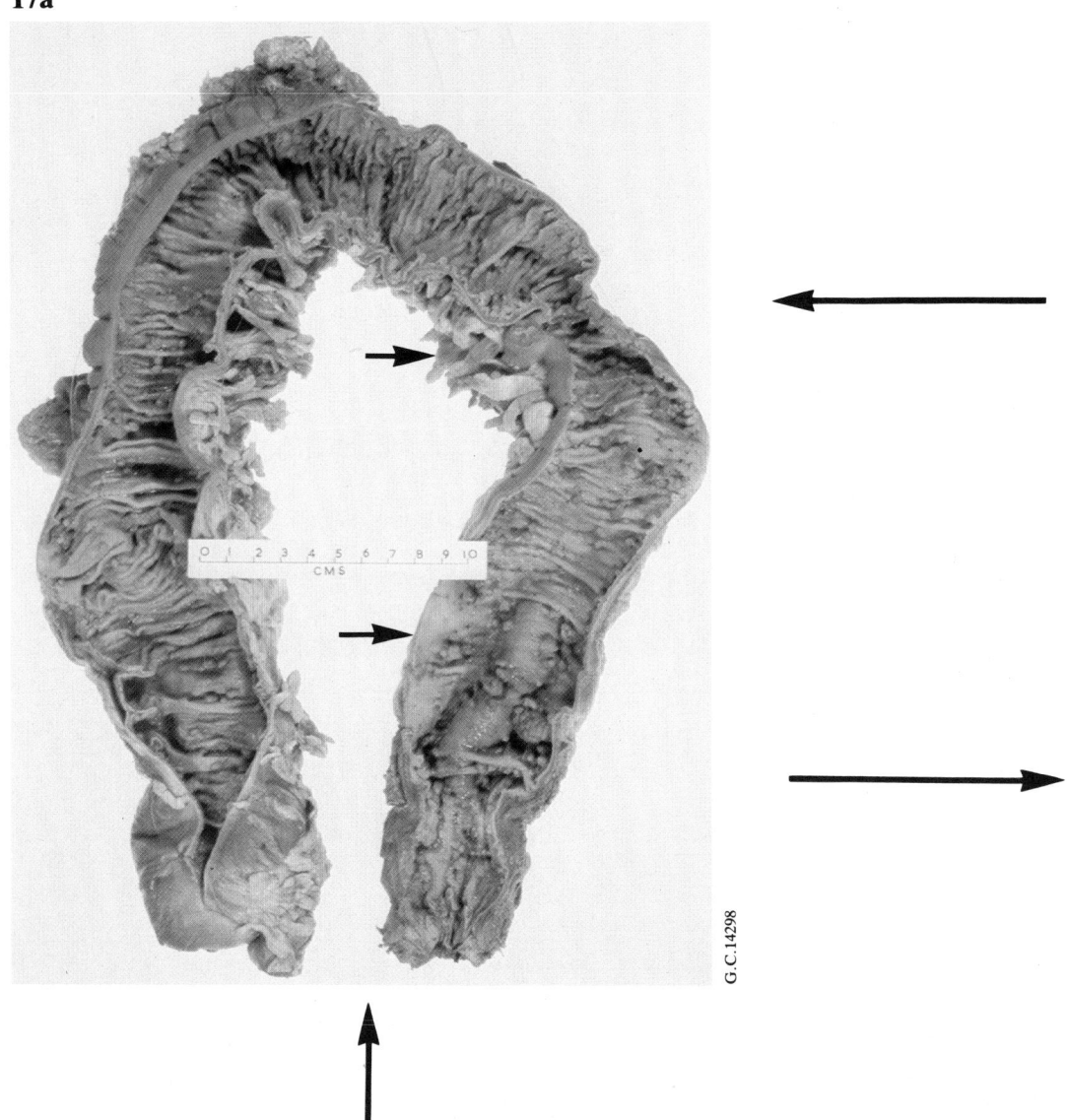

G.C.14298

17a From a female aged 37 years. Two year history of diarrhoea with the presence of blood in the stools. Endoscopy revealed multiple polyposis.

The patient had a sister also the victim of polyposis on whom a colectomy had been performed. The patient has two children aged 7 and 11 years who presently show no evidence of the disease and who are to be kept under review.

17b

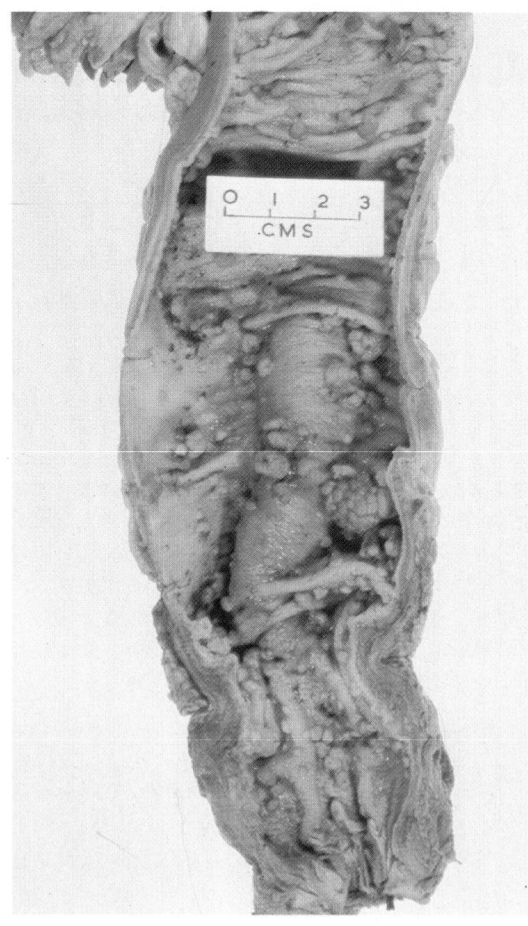

17b The specimen shows multiple polyps in the colon. These commence in the caecum where the polyps are few in number but increase distally. There are two points of overt malignancy, one close to the splenic flexure and a second in the pelvic colon (arrows). The lesion in the pelvic colon has been enlarged to show detail.

17c

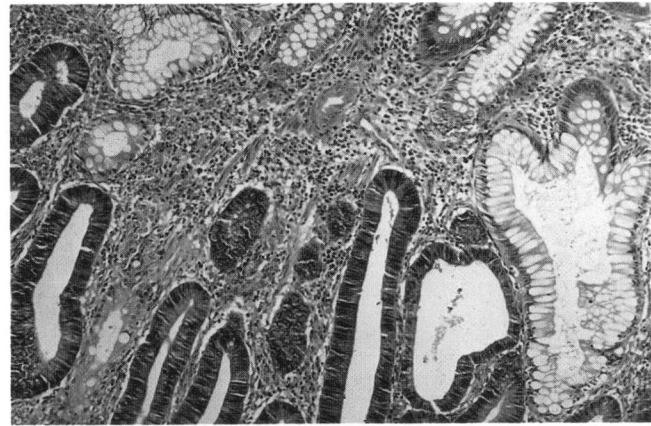

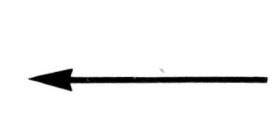

G.C.M.865

17c A 1cm polyp from a patient with familial polyposis. The main part of the polyp was composed of regular mucus-secreting glands. The focus of dark-staining glands indicates that malignant change has occurred. *(H&E ×100)*

Sixty per cent of patients presenting as familial polyposis on detailed examination will already show carcinomatous change. The age incidence at which carcinoma develops in these patients will be 20 years earlier (40 years of age) than patients suffering from carcinoma without polyposis. The average age of death, 40 to 45 years, is likewise 20 years earlier than in patients who have cancer without polyposis.

Gardner's syndrome

This is a rare hereditary condition characterised by familial polyposis, usually of the colon, accompanied by soft tissue tumours and osteomas. It is transmitted as an autosomal dominant.

Colonic polyps appear by the second or third decade and small bowel polyps rarely occur. The polyps undergo malignant change. The first signs may be dental abnormalities and/or osteomas of the mandible, maxilla or sphenoid.

Patients show a tendency to develop fibromas in incisional scars and mesenteric fibrosis after abdominal surgery.

Tumours may develop in the second part of the duodenum and may also occur in the thyroid, adrenal and terminal ileum. Eight per cent of polyposis coli show the features of Gardner's syndrome.

Juvenile polyp

Hamartomatous polyps of the colon and more frequently of the rectum occur in childhood. These lesions may be sessile or pedunculated, solitary or multiple and are liable to prolapse, undergo torsion, or cause haemorrhage.

18

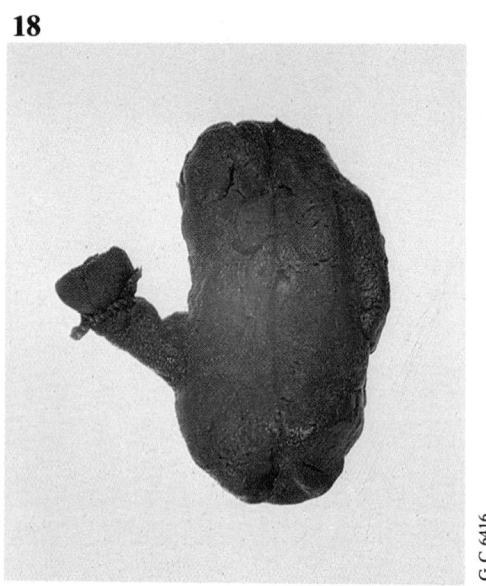

G.C.6416

18 From a male aged 2 years 8 months in whom the occasional projection of a tumour at the anus was not accompanied by bleeding. This is a typical infantile polyp. Note the narrow pedicle by which it had been attached to the bowel wall. The tumour measures 30mm in long diameter. It was removed during a period of extrusion from the anus and there was consequently intense congestion. Microscopic examination showed the polyp covered by a stratified squamous epithelium indicating that it had originated low down in the ano-rectal canal with some subepithelial and perivascular inflammatory cells, a moderate degree of hyperkeratosis, but no evidence of neoplastic tissue. There was no telangiectasis and no vascular thrombosis.

Site distribution

19

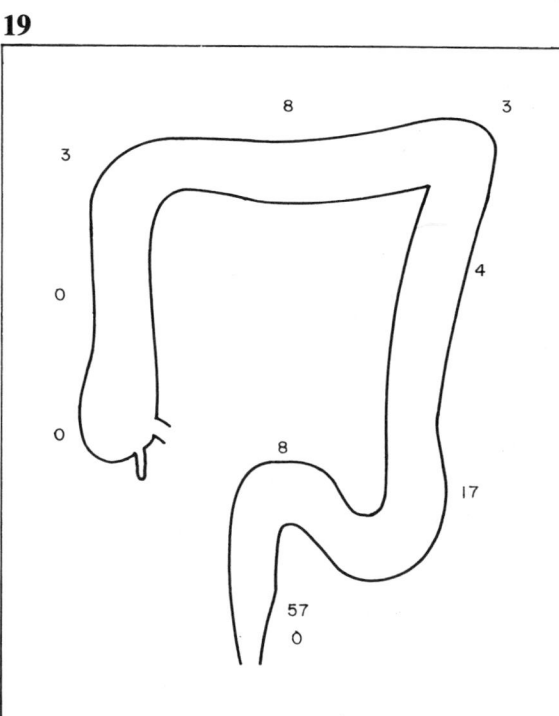

19 Distribution shown as approximate percentages.

These tumours vary in size and structurally the main mass consists of cellular vascular tissue containing small cystic spaces lined by columnar epithelium – mucus-secreting. Marked infiltration with inflammatory cells. The surface of the tumour is covered by mucous membrane but after traumatisation shows ulceration and replacement by granular tissue. The pedicle is covered by normal rectal and colonic mucosa.

20

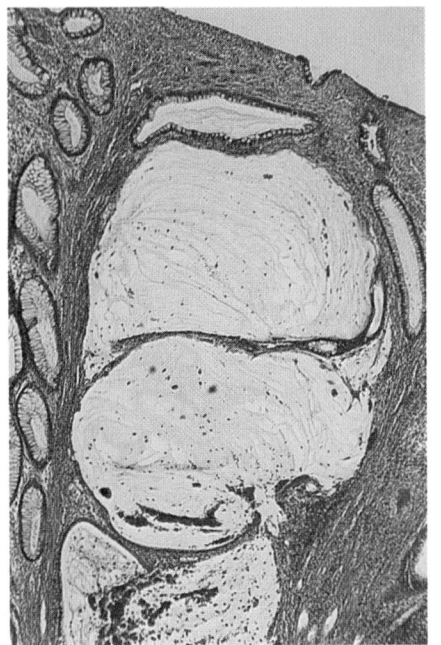

20 Part of a juvenile polyp of rectum showing a microcyst distended with mucus. Some of the surface epithelium has been exfoliated and the stroma is infiltrated by inflammatory cells. *(H&E ×40)*

21

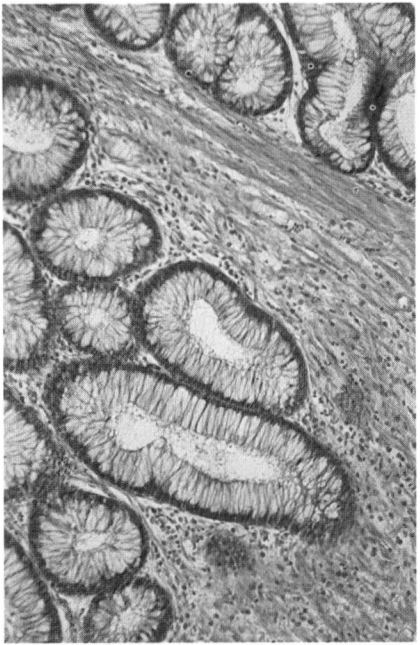

21 The glandular component of the polyp is regular and well differentiated. There is no sign of malignancy. The glands are set in stroma containing both fibrous tissue and smooth muscle. *(H&E ×125)*

Peutz–Jeghers syndrome

In Peutz–Jeghers syndrome polyps may occur in the colon and rectum. This condition has already been described in detail (see Section 15Ta).

Carcinoma

Carcinoma of the intestinal tract is one of the most common and fatal forms of malignant disease. It is convenient to present the main features of these tumours as a single subject while recognising that variation of incidence, complications, clinical features and prognosis occurs according to the precise location of the lesions.

Site incidence

The incidence of tumours of the small intestine is much less than that of the colon and rectum and varies in different reported series between 1 and 9%.

Site distribution

22

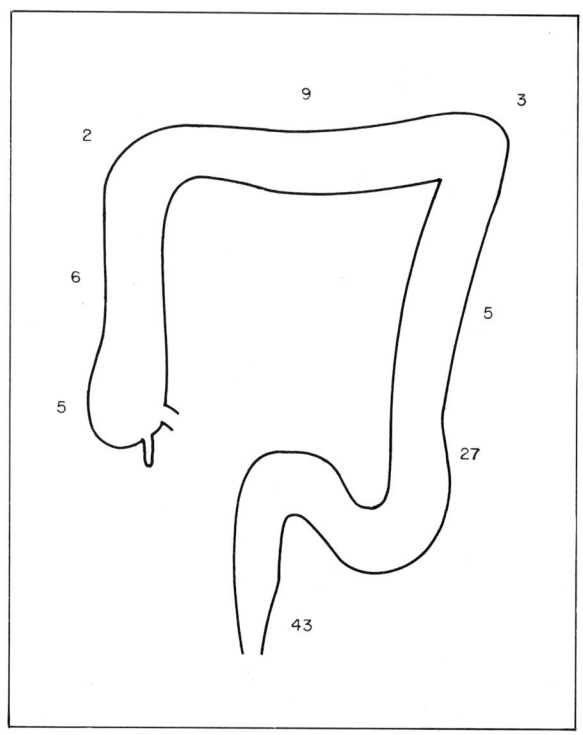

22 Distribution shown as approximate percentages.

Three per cent of cases show the presence of more than one malignant lesion. Where the tumour arises as the sequel to ulcerative colitis the condition is multicentric and numerous foci of disease will be found to show neoplastic change.

The number of deaths annually from carcinoma of the colon and rectum in England and Wales is 15000. The maximum incidence is in the 60 to 70 year age group. There is a slight preponderance of females over males. The number of persons affected by colo-rectal cancer has increased steadily since last century.

The incidence is high in the Western World and low in Africa and Asia. Environmental factors are held to be responsible for the difference as is shown by the fact that American negroes and Japanese born in the USA have a comparable mortality to Americans of European ancestry.

23

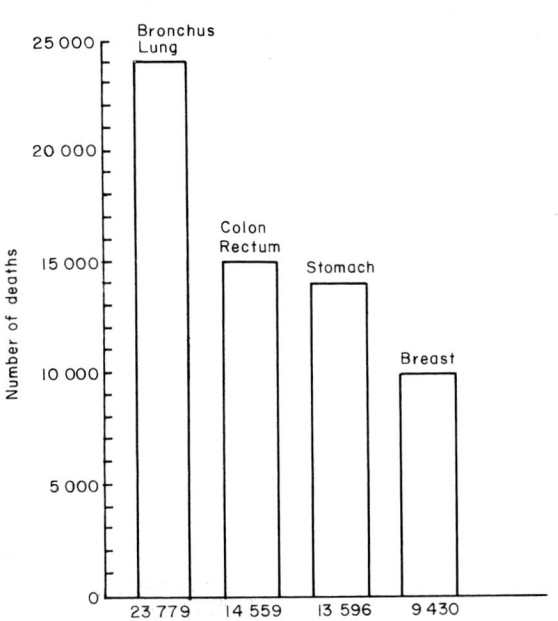

24

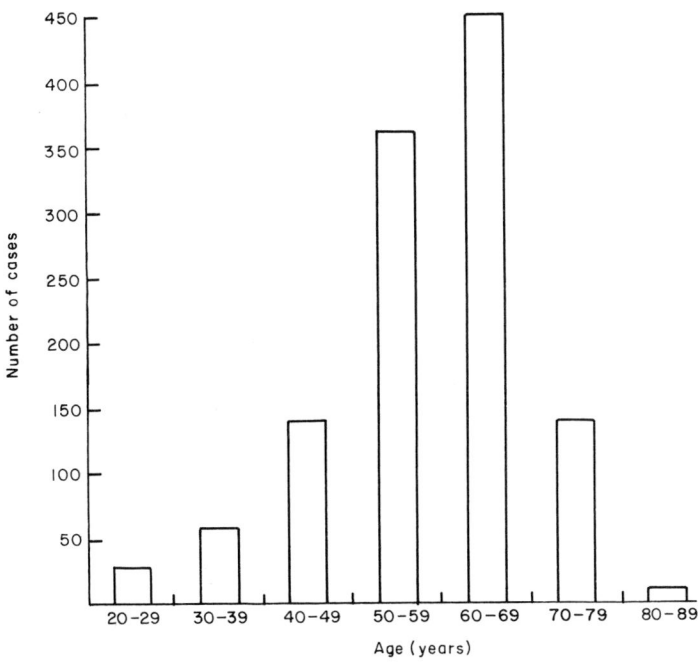

23 Relative annual death rates. Adapted from Goligher.

24 Age incidence.

Perforation

Perforation as a complication of carcinoma occurs in 6 to 7% of patients. The majority result from extension of the neoplasm and the minority (1 in 5) are stercoral ulcers distant from the tumour.

Obstruction

Acute intestinal obstruction occurs as a complication of carcinoma in 15 to 20% of cases. The incidence of obstruction is twice this figure where the tumours are located in the left colon.

Aetiology

The development of a carcinoma in a pre-existing adenoma or papilloma (which may be an isolated condition or associated with a familial predisposition) has already been described.

This may explain the occurrence of carcinoma in several generations in some families. In other instances, however, the same familial pattern may not be associated with the presence of adenomas.

Pre-existing disease

Carcinoma as a sequel to pre-existing ulcerative colitis and less commonly, Crohn's disease is a well recognised complication.

The period from the commencement of the ulcerative colitis to the onset of carcinoma is prolonged – often over 20 years.

Carcinoma is not a sequel to diverticulitis, amoebic dysentery, recurrent dysentery or tuberculosis.

Diet

World wide research has been conducted into the relationship of diet, bowel habits and the incidence of bowel cancer. A modern view is that a protracted intestinal transit allows the conversion of faecal bile acids to carcinogens. Clostridial organisms of the dehydrogenating variety may be particularly important in the reaction and their presence may explain why only certain individuals are susceptible to the development of bowel cancer. Dietary factors may also be important and a high fat intake is said to be found in those affected. Cooking fats at high temperature may result in a splitting of the fats with the production of carcinogens.

Antigen reaction

Especially in carcinomas arising in the colon the presence of CEA (carcino-embryonic antigen) in the serum is of some diagnostic significance but this glycoprotein occurs in a variety of other tumours and there is therefore no specificity. It has been noted that CEA disappears with the apparently successful removal of a colonic tumour but reappears if the neoplasm recurs.

344

Macroscopic features

Macroscopic examination of the gross specimen may be by the study either of thin sections of the tumour or detailed scrutiny of the full specimen.

By the preparation of thin sections of tumours the two basic patterns of the lesions, the proliferative and the invasive are distinguishable as is also the presence of surface ulceration and invasion of deeper tissues.

Proliferative

Invasive

25

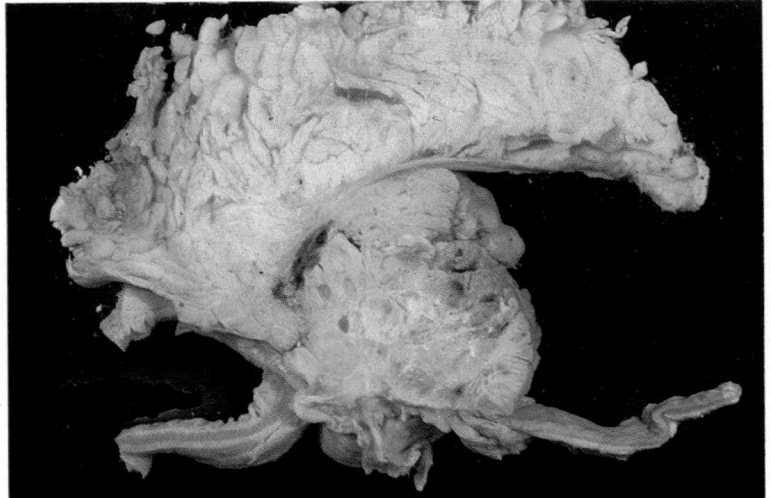

26

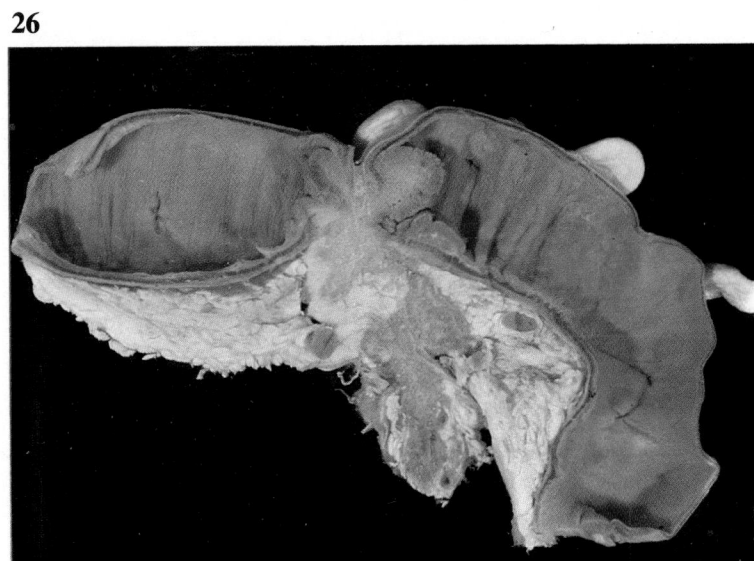

25 From a female aged 68 years. Five months right sided abdominal discomfort. Three months recurrent diarrhoea. This is a proliferative tumour arising at the ileocaecal junction. There is also some degree of stenosis. The ileum is to the left and the caecum to the right.

26 From an adult with acute intestinal obstruction. String carcinoma of the sigmoid colon excised. The tumour had spread deep into the mesocolon.

The appearance of gross lesions as seen in the fresh specimen show great variation depending upon such factors as:
1   The pattern of growth of the tumour – proliferative or invasive.
2   The degree of narrowing of the bowel lumen.
3   The presence or absence of associated infection and the accompanying inflammatory reaction.
4   Other complications.

Examples of these varieties are illustrated on the following pages.

Patterns of tumour growth

Papilliferous carcinoma

A relatively flat tumour which retains a papilliferous or multiple polypoid pattern. The major bulk of the tumour is intraluminal and invasion of the muscle is late. This type of tumour is common in the rectum.

27

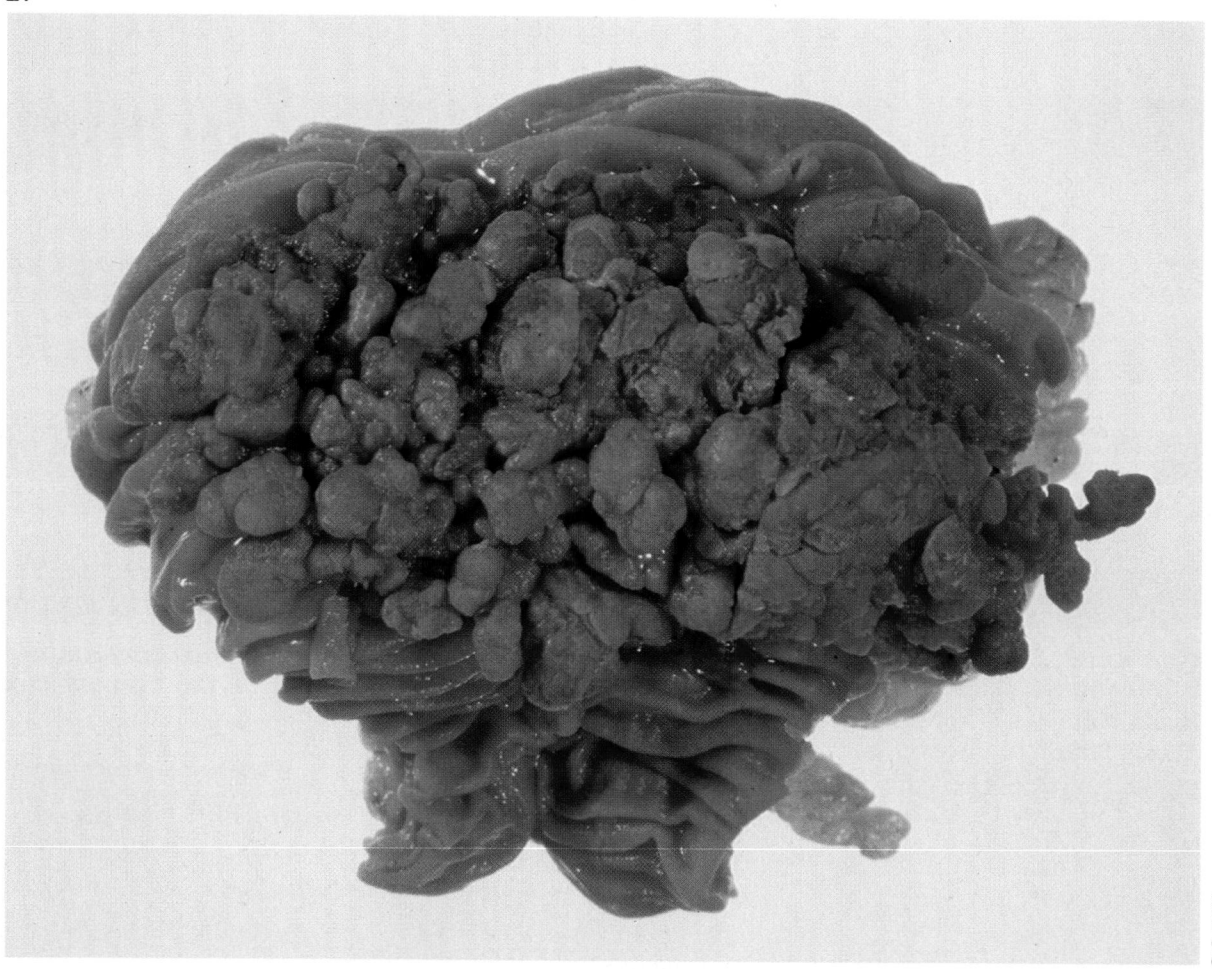

G.C. 10493

27 Sigmoid colon – carcinoma. From a male aged 65 years. Haemorrhoids 3 years. Occasional rectal bleeding and diarrhoea for 2 years.

Polypoid carcinoma

Essentially tumours of lesser malignancy. The bulk of the tumour is within the lumen of the gut. Invasion of the muscle coat is minimal and late and the peritoneum is involved only in the advanced stages. Externally, therefore, the neoplasm is recognised by the presence of the bulky swelling which is defined on palpation. Proximal and distal spread in the bowel wall is relatively limited. This type of tumour is frequently found in the caecum.

28

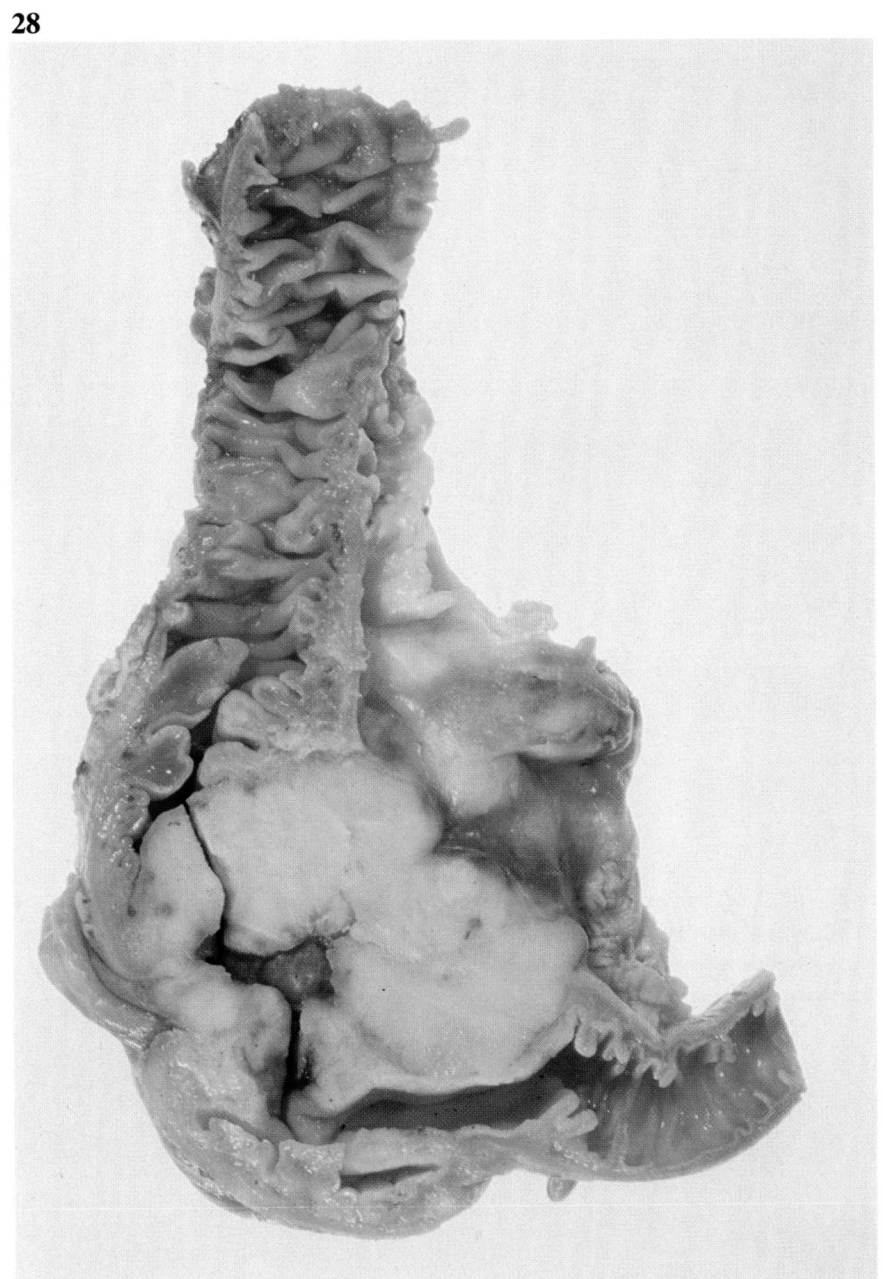

G.C.11929

28 Caecum – late stage of a polypoid carcinoma. From a male aged 78 years. Loss of weight. One month diarrhoea and pyrexia. Mass in right iliac fossa one month.

Carcinomatous ulcer

A malignant ulcer with raised everted edges and a central sloughing base. Tumour growth is relatively slow and complete encirclement of the gut lumen usually takes 6 to 9 months. There is infiltration of the underlying muscle and later the peritoneum is involved, small nodules of tumour being seen. This type of tumour is most frequently found in the rectum and occasionally in the caecum.

29

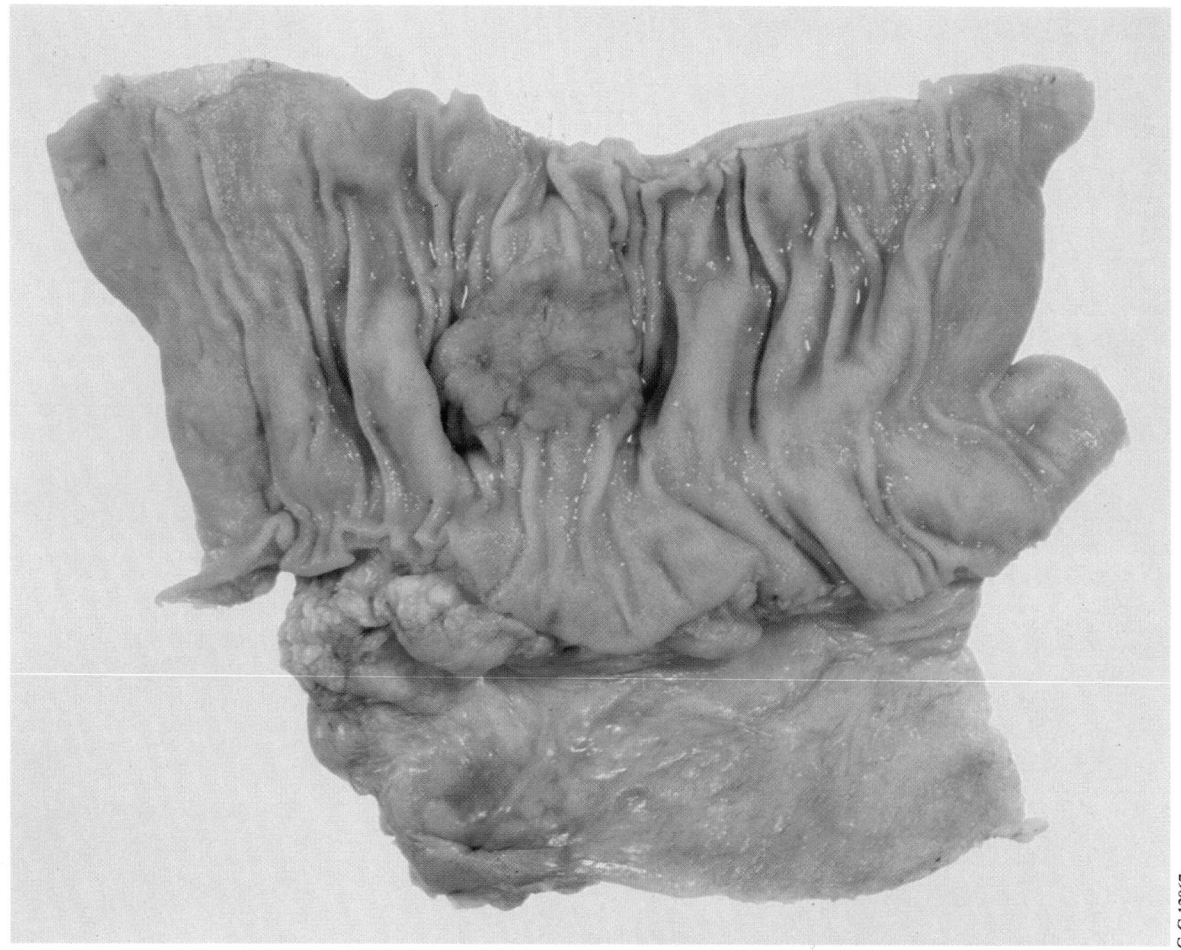

G.C.12067

29 Sigmoid colon – carcinoma. From a female aged 45 years. Passage of blood and mucus 8 months. Radiological examination did not disclose the lesion. At operation lymphatic involvement was discovered.

Stenosing carcinoma – string stricture cancer

The ulcerated area usually remains small but there is marked infiltration of the bowel wall in a circumferential manner. Fibrosis is marked and the lumen of the gut greatly narrowed. The external appearance of this tumour well justifies the name 'string stricture carcinoma' looking exactly as if a ligature had been tied round the gut. This type of tumour is common in the colon and especially characteristic of lesions of the sigmoid colon.

30

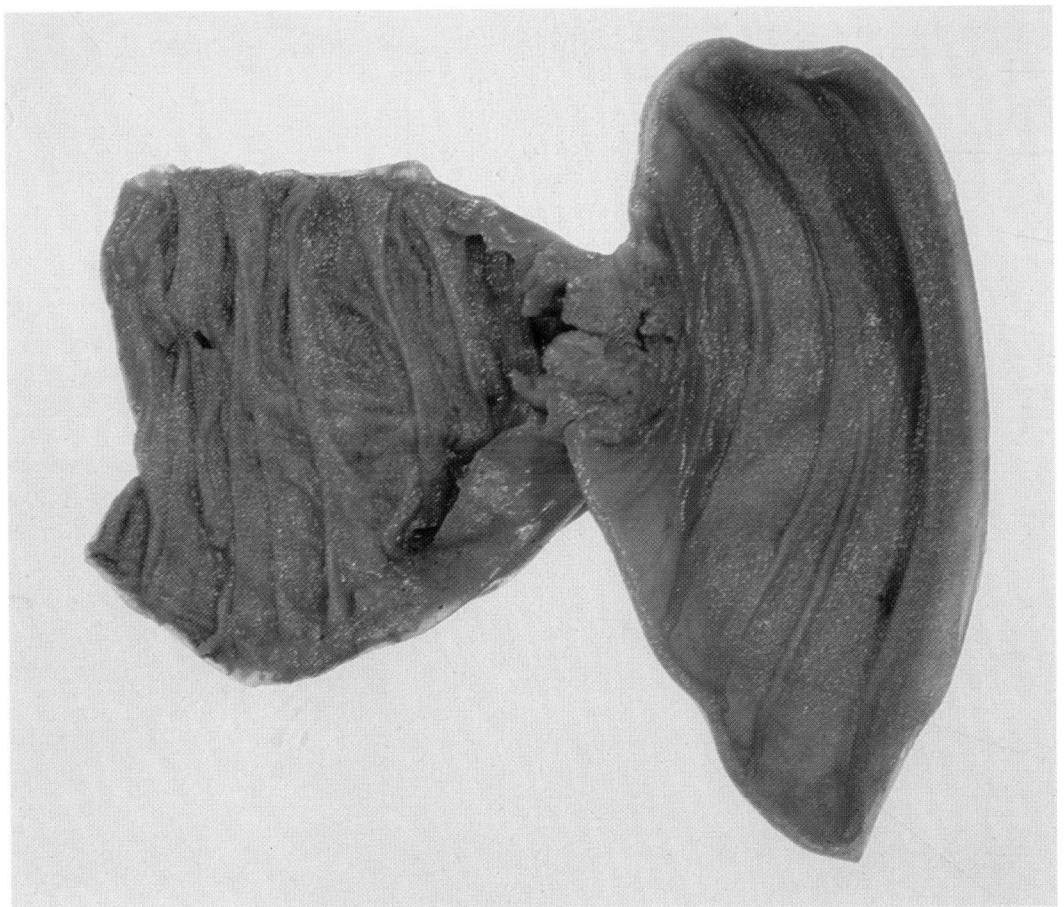

G.C.7388

30 Ileum – carcinomatous stricture with dilation and hypertrophy above the stricture (Rt). From an adult patient who was admitted to hospital as a case of acute intestinal obstruction.

Because the contents of the ileum are fluid, obstruction occurs late and under these circumstances the stricture has to become very marked before acute features develop.

Tubular carcinoma

A rarer form of neoplasm in which ulceration and infiltration have occurred over a length of gut with narrowing of the lumen. This form of carcinoma tends to be seen when malignant change occurs in ulcerative colitis. This lesion occurs most frequently in the distal colon.

31

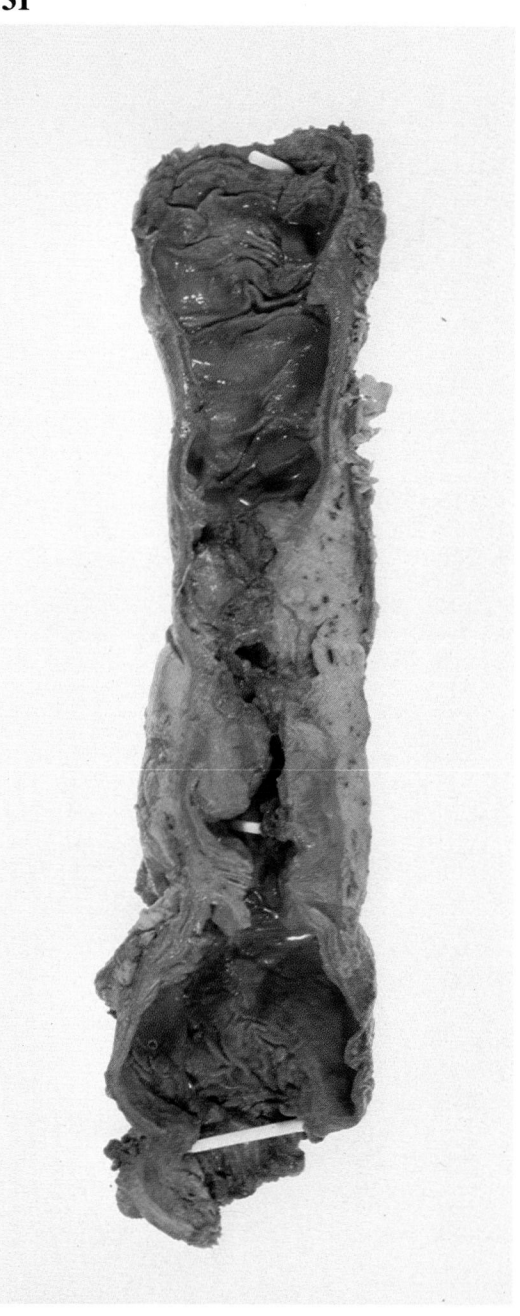

G.C.11222

31 Rectum – carcinoma. From a male aged 67 years. Two years alternating constipation and diarrhoea. Passage of blood and mucus.

Carcinoma of the colon

31a

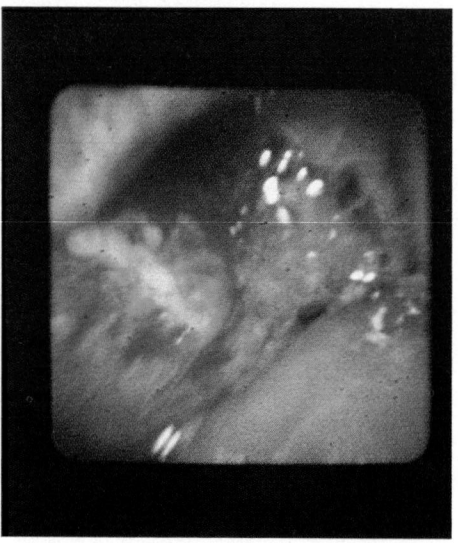

G.C.P.238

31a Endoscopic examination showing a scirrhous carcinoma encircling the lumen of the sigmoid colon with friable surface and excessive amounts of mucus.

Mucoid carcinoma

These tumours are characterised by their gelatinous appearance due to the large mucus content. They are typically bulky tumours of rapid growth. The peritoneum and underlying wall appear oedematous and the cut surface shows the infiltration through the whole thickness of the tumour. Diffuse metastatic peritoneal involvement is common. This type of tumour occurs most frequently in the caecum and rectum.

32

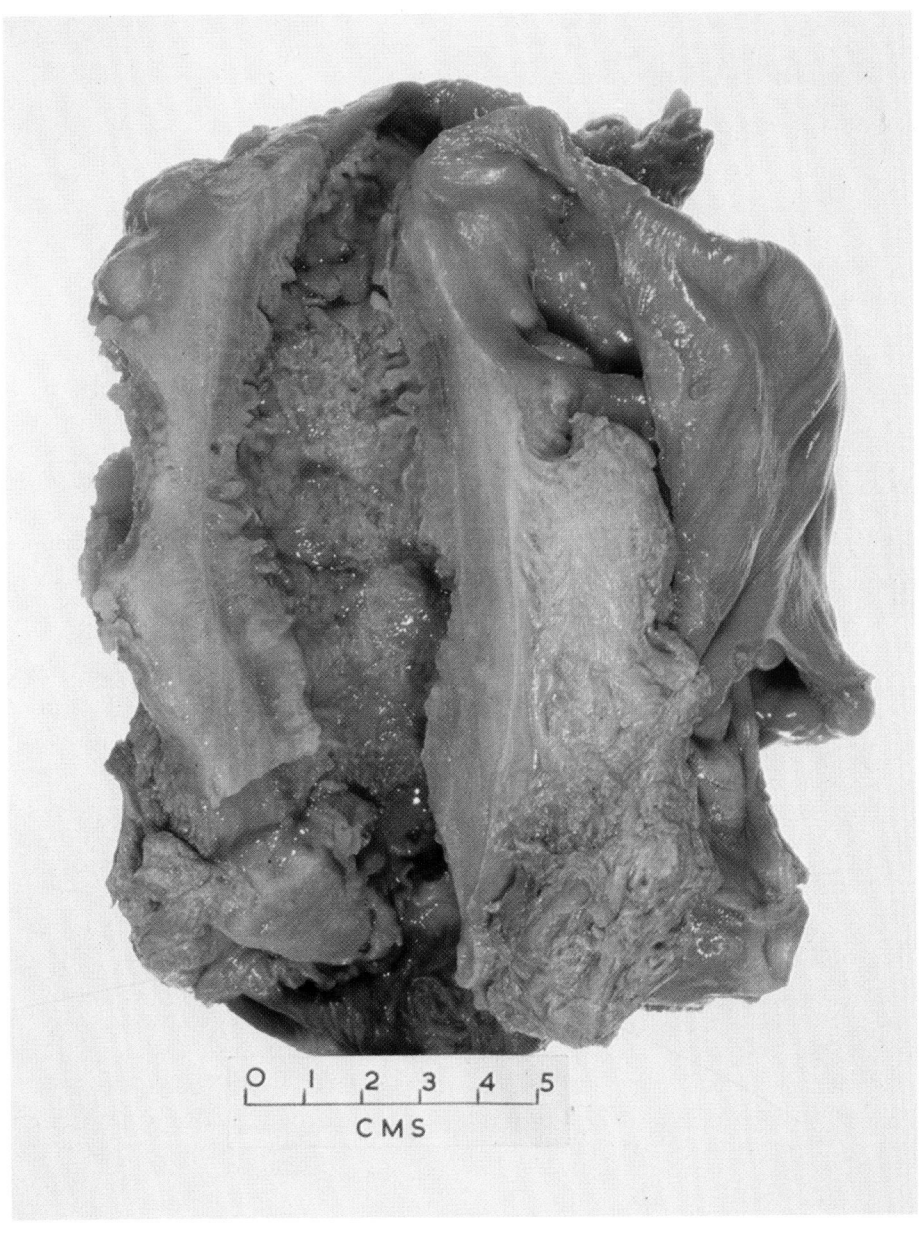

32 Sigmoid colon – carcinoma. From a male aged 56 years. 'Abdominal symptoms' one year.

The view has been expressed that in some instances a colloid carcinoma found in the caecum is a metastatic lesion arising originally in the stomach.

Multiple carcinoma

In the colon it is not uncommon to find that associated with a carcinoma are adenomatous tumours which may be closely related to or widely separated from the malignant lesion. Indeed the carcinoma may have arisen in an adenoma.

The presence of multiple malignant lesions which do not appear to have resulted from spread from one focus is seen in approximately 3 to 5% of cases.

Following apparently successful resection of a carcinoma, malignant disease may arise later in another part of the intestine. This appears to be in many instances a fresh and separate neoplasm. Possibly in both these last two instances the carcinomas may arise in pre-existing adenomas.

33

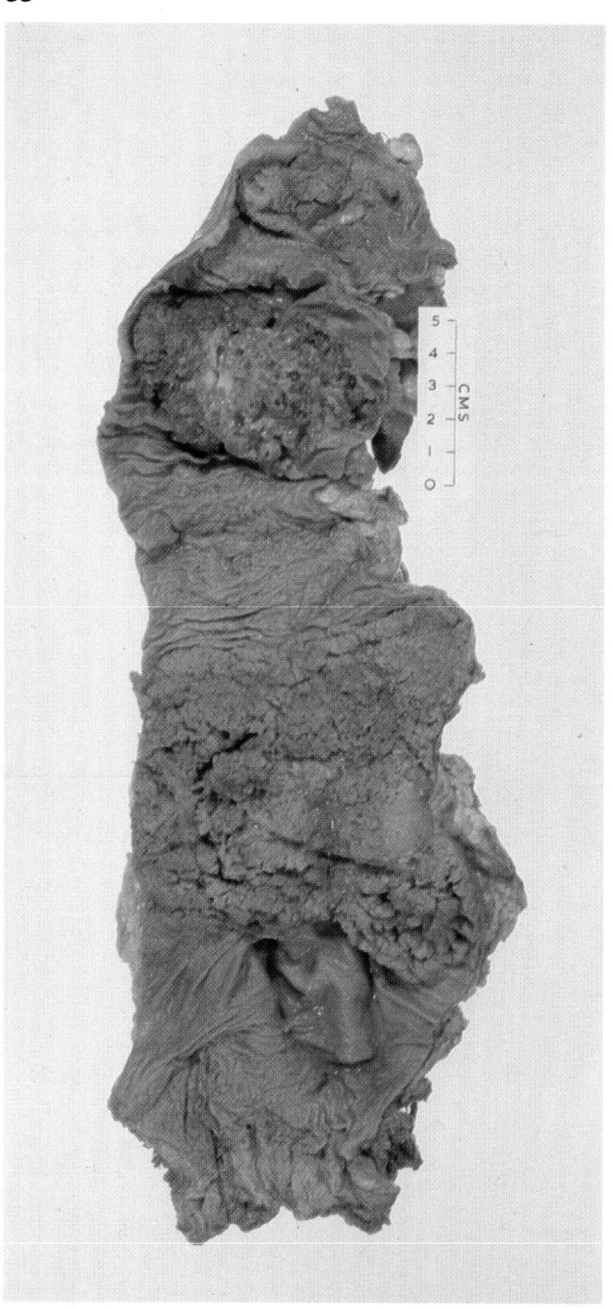

G.C. 10083

33 From a male aged 62 years with a four year history of diarrhoea with the passage of mucus and latterly blood. Rectal examination revealed the presence of a tumour in the ampulla. A barium enema revealed a second tumour at a higher level and at operation a third independent and still higher tumour was discovered.

The lowermost and largest tumour completely encircles the gut and measures 75 mm in the long axis. The second tumour separated from the first by 60 mm is located in the sigmoid colon and is a large, sessile tumour. The third tumour, a small hard sessile tumour is separated from the previous lesion by 35 mm. Histologically all three tumours are papillary carcinomatous lesions with a large mucoid component. There is no evidence of lymphatic dissemination or continuity of tumour growth between the lesions. It is interesting to speculate whether the second and third arose as a result of undetected lymphatic penetration from the rectal growth, or were independent formations.

Diffuse carcinoma

A typical case of ulcerative colitis is shown below in which malignant change has occurred. The incidence of malignant disease as a complication of ulcerative colitis is well recognised and has been described previously. The specimen demonstrates at least three separate malignant foci indicative of the diffuse predilection of the mucosa to undergo neoplastic change, but the number of sites at which malignant change has occurred frequently is dependent upon the number of sections which have been prepared for examination.

34a

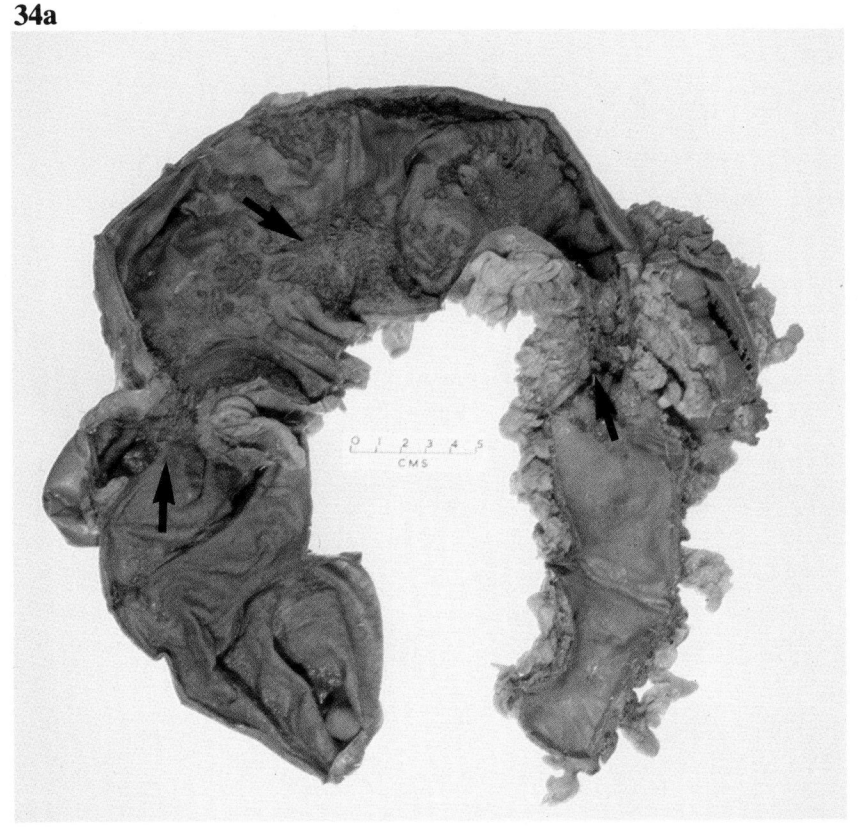

G.C.10976

a Malignant areas indicated by arrows. On the left an ulcerated carcinoma has narrowed the bowel. Note the lesions of ulcerative colitis above.

34b

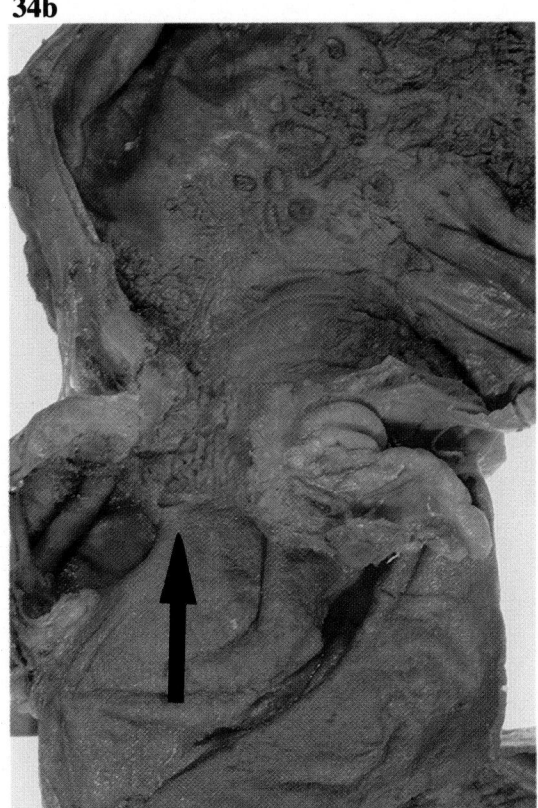

b Enlarged view of ulcerated area.

34 From a female aged 48 years with a 20 year history of ulcerative colitis. Initially the clinical features were most severe – diarrhoea and pain – but latterly were characterised only by looseness of bowel habit. Ileostomy was performed at 44 years of age and total colectomy 4 years later when the presence of carcinomatous lesions was recognised.

Microscopic features

35

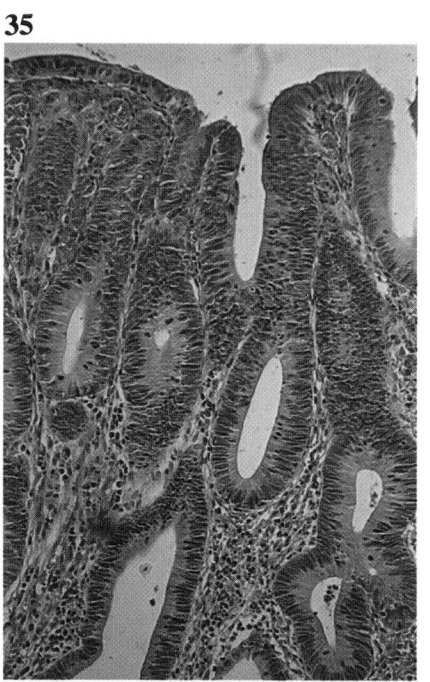

35 Surface portion of a well-differentiated carcinoma of the colon. The tumour cells are regularly arranged in a single layer. *(H&E ×125)*

36

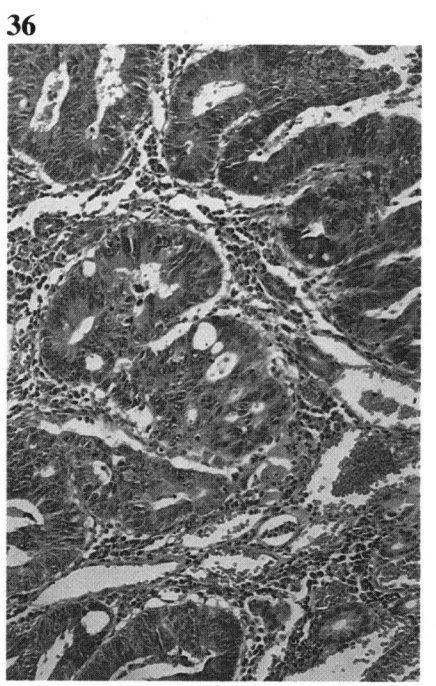

36 A moderately differentiated carcinoma. The tubulo-papillary pattern is still well defined but the arrangement is less regular and the epithelium tends to be heaped up into more than one layer. *(H&E ×125)*

37

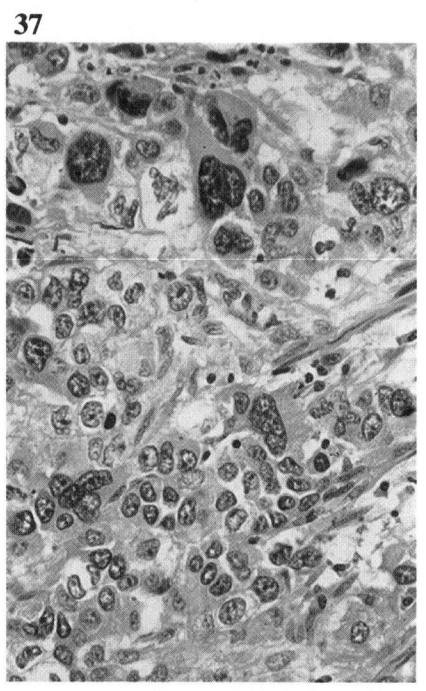

37 Poorly differentiated carcinoma. The glandular pattern has been lost. The cells are pleomorphic and multinucleated tumour giant cells are present. *(H&E ×312.5)*

38

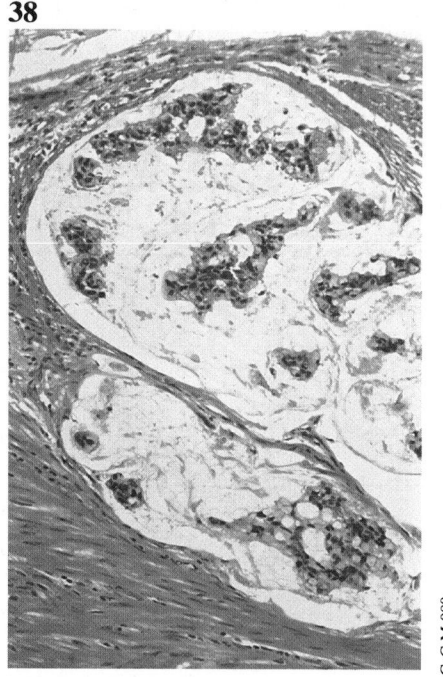

38 Mucoid carcinoma invading muscularis. Groups of tumour cells lie in extracellular mucus. *(H&E ×125)*

The degree of differentiation observed histologically has been used as a system of 'grading' the tumours and is regarded as an index of malignancy:

Grade I   Demonstrating high differentiation,
Grade II   Demonstrating a moderate degree of differentiation,
Grade III   Demonstrating marked dedifferentiation – anaplastic carcinoma.

39   By preparing a montage illustrating the histological features over a complete tumour it is possible to view the point of contact between malignant and normal cells. The contrast between these is clearly discernible.

39

Point of junction of normal and neoplastic mucosae.

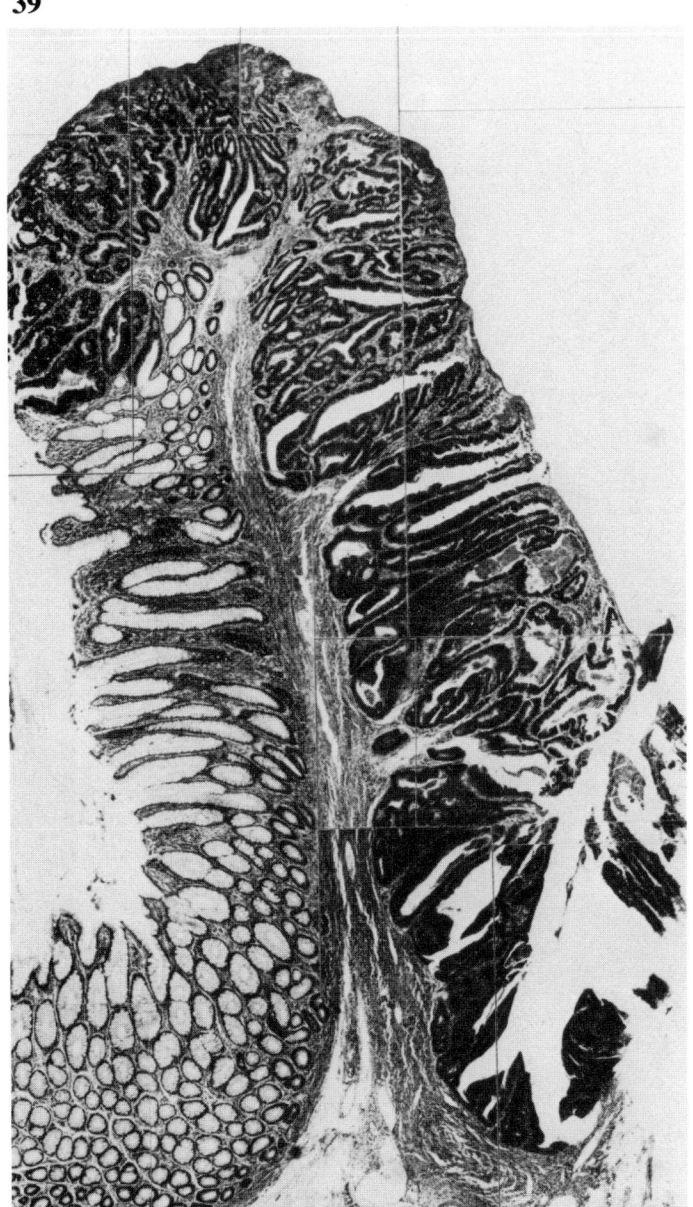

Deeply staining proliferating malignant cells.

Normal mucosa.

G.C.M.981

Whole section study

The study of tumours by the whole section technique has the advantage that it demonstrates on microscopic study the pattern of growth of the neoplasm although detailed cellular structure may be less clearly defined. The particular points to which attention is paid in these whole sections of the intestine are:

1. The pattern of growth – whether proliferative or infiltrative,
2. Whether the muscular coat is invaded or destroyed,
3. Whether the peritoneal coat shows involvement.

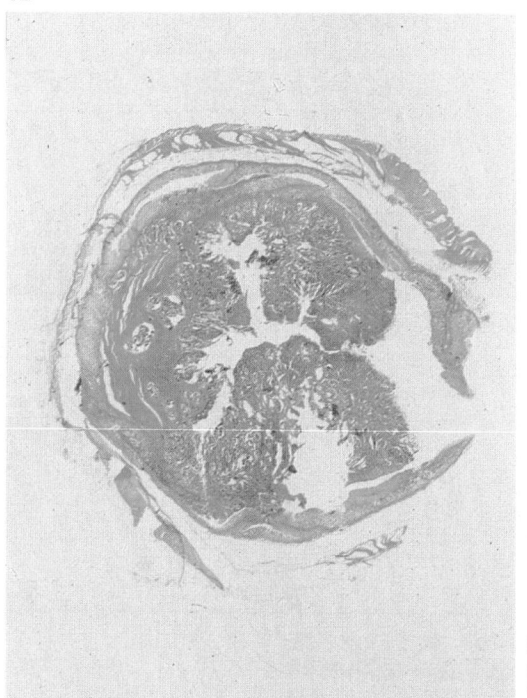

G.C.M.404

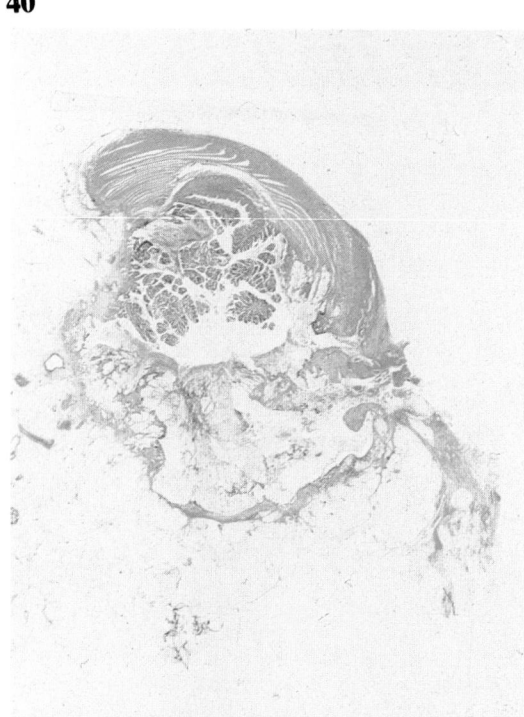

G.C.M.394

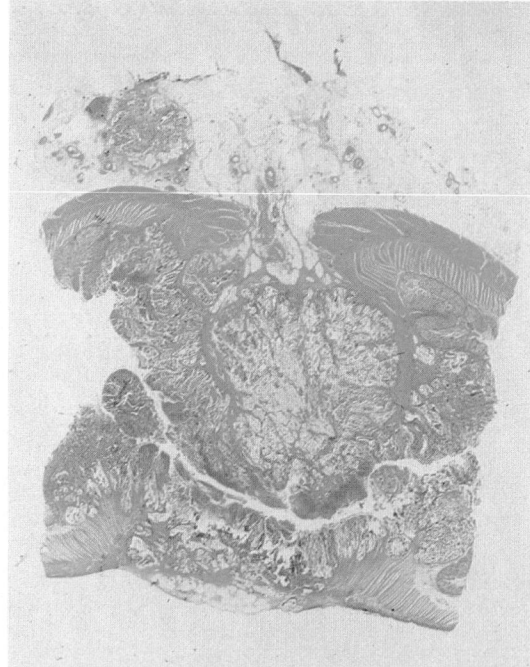

G.C.M.367

41 Adenocarcinoma of a papillary type which is occupying almost the whole of the lumen of the gut. In this transverse section there is invasion of the muscle wall but no evidence of complete penetration and no evidence of involvement of the peritoneal coat.

40 Cross section of a colonic carcinoma showing papillary ingrowth into the lumen at one point and at another place transmural spread of mucoid carcinoma into the mesocolon.

42 This is a longitudinal section of gut with a large bulky tumour which has caused almost complete obstruction. The tumour has invaded and destroyed the muscle coat and appears to have breached the peritoneum, and (top left) invaded lymph node.

Local spread

Local spread of carcinoma is largely determined by the anatomical arrangement of the lymphatic channels. These run circumferentially in the wall of the gut and then directly to the marginal (e.g. epicolic) lymph nodes. There is little lateral connection of lymphatics in the bowel wall and the spread along the gut wall proximally and distally is therefore limited. The primary tumour therefore remains relatively localised.

Malignant ulceration in the colon has a superadded infection which may extend from the lumen leading to the formation of pericolitis with adhesions or abscess formation. Consequently, the affected segment of bowel may become adherent to surrounding organs such as:
1 Stomach
2 Small intestine
3 Bladder and ureters
4 Uterus and vagina

While fixation may be primarily infective in origin, neoplastic involvement may be concomitant or arise later.

43

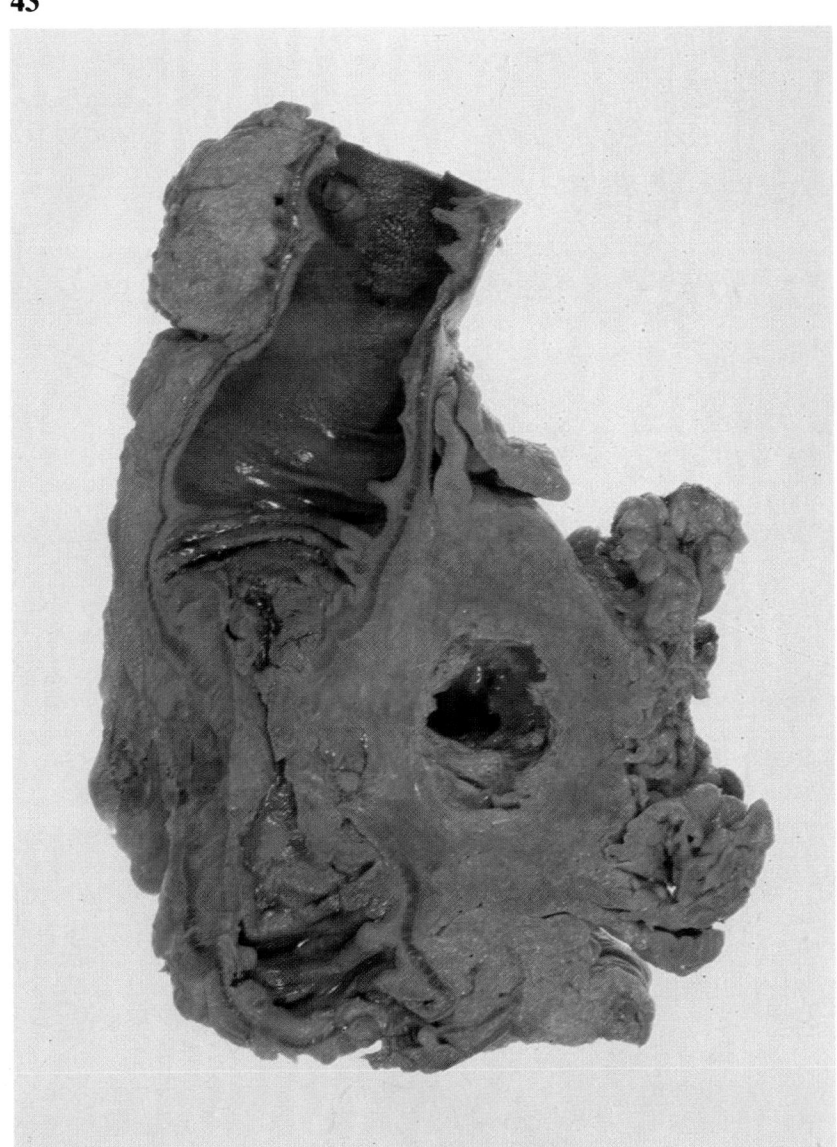

G.C.5315

43 From a female aged 61 years. The tumour involves some 50mm of the colon and almost obliterates its lumen. Proximally and distally the tumour is well defined and between these limits the surface is ulcerated. It has involved the whole thickness of the bowel wall and, having extended into the meso-colon, has consolidated a mass of fat which in its centre is necrotic and cystic.

Local spread *(Continued)*

44

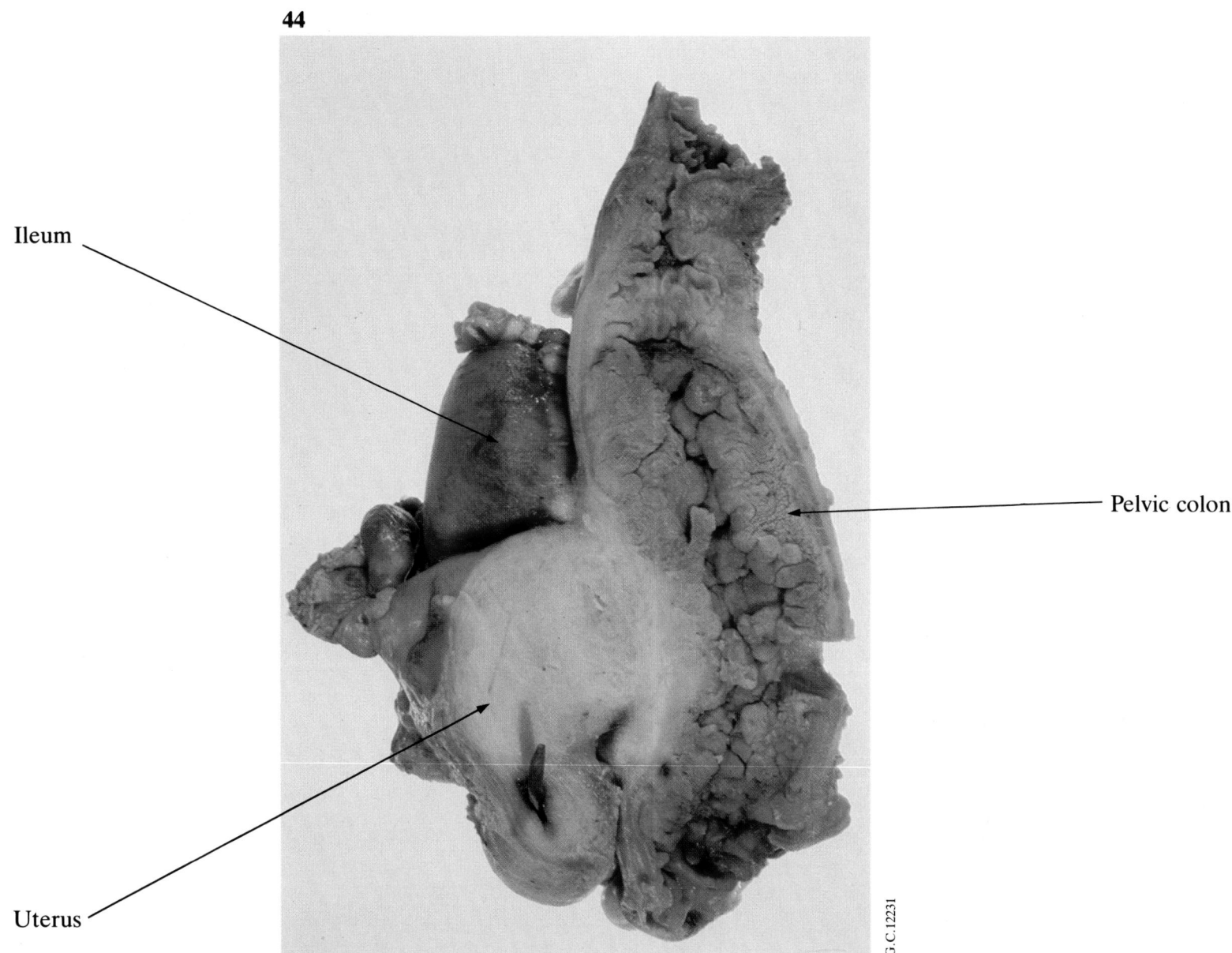

Ileum

Pelvic colon

Uterus

G.C.12231

44 From a female aged 55 years who was admitted to hospital for acute colonic obstruction. An emergency colostomy was performed and followed four weeks later by resection.

The pelvic colon is the site of a diffuse polypoid carcinoma which has penetrated the wall of the gut. The uterus has become adherent to the colon and has been invaded by carcinoma. At this site an abscess has formed consequent upon secondary infection. A loop of ileum is adherent both to the uterus and colon but this is due to the inflammatory reaction and not extension of the malignant disease. A rod indicates the cavity of the uterus.

Histologically the tumour was a characteristic well differentiated glandular carcinoma.

Fistula

By necrosis a fistula eventually is formed between the bowel which is the site of the primary lesion and the other adherent hollow viscera.

45

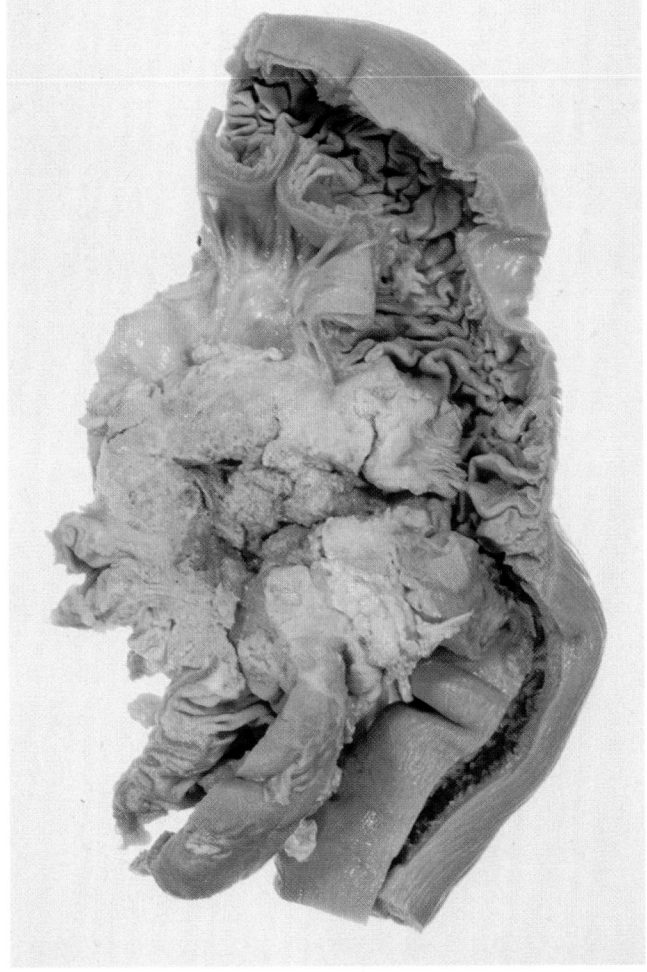

G.C.14028

45 From a male aged 50 years. History of 6 weeks vomiting and diarrhoea.

The specimen demonstrates the transverse colon the wall of which over a considerable length shows an infiltrating ulcerative type of carcinoma. A large mass exists involving the wall of the colon on its mesocolic aspect. It extends into the extra colic tissues forming a globular mass which distant from the colon is attached to a loop of jejunum. The mass has been sectioned and demonstrates a fistulous channel passing from the colon to jejunum.

Histologically the tumour was a mucoid adenocarcinoma.

Varieties of fistulae

1 Jejuno-colic or ileo-colic. Involvement of the small intestine including the duodenum with subsequent fistula formation leads to an acute inflammatory reaction with marked diarrhoea, loss of fluids and rapid malnutrition. General symptoms indicative of toxaemia also occur.

2 Vesico-colic fistula. This occurs in lesions low in the sigmoid colon or rectum with malignant infiltration of the bladder wall. The entry of faecal material into the bladder leads to an acute and marked cystitis associated with pneumaturia. Ascending infection of the kidneys occurs.

3 Utero- or vagino-colic fistula. The result of organisms from the colon reaching the female genital tract causes a marked foul vaginal discharge. There is acute endometritis.

Peritoneal spread

Where the tumour has penetrated all coats of the bowel wall and now involves the serosa, tumour cells becoming detached may lead to diffuse peritoneal involvement. This is usually a late phenomenon except where the tumour is of the mucoid type.

46

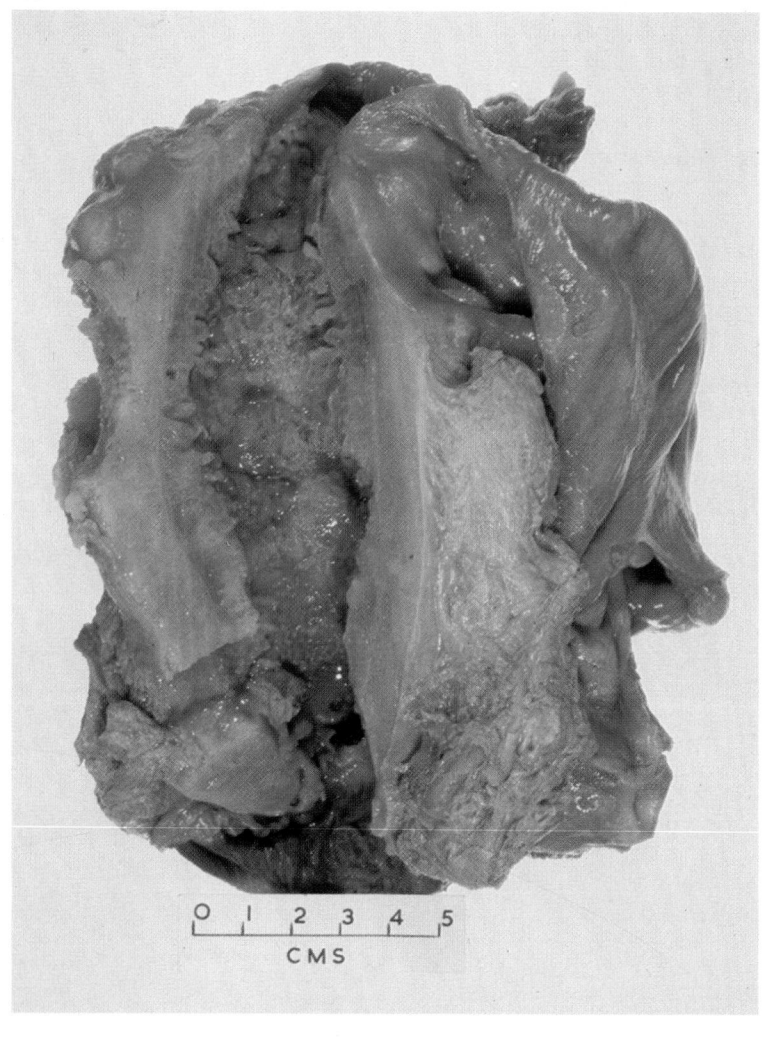

47

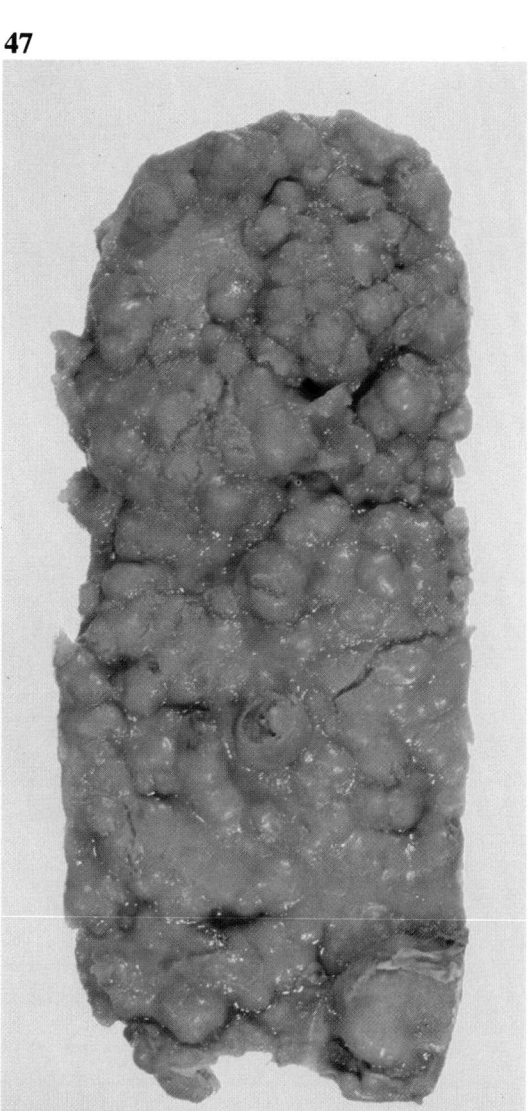

46 and **47**   From a male aged 56 years. Carcinoma of pelvic colon. Symptoms had lasted for over one year.

46   Sigmoid colon. The wall of the bowel is infiltrated with carcinoma, stiff and thick and of a translucent gelatinous appearance. The mucosa is rough and irregular but the calibre is only slightly diminished. Gelatinous carcinomatous nodules project under the peritoneum and in places are attached to the surface. The lymph nodes were similarly involved.

47   Omentum. The greater omentum is thickened to the extent of 40mm in places by carcinomatous infiltration, firm, translucent and gelatinous. The fat for the most part has disappeared. The surfaces of the omentum are irregular and nodular with thin, flocculent, fibrinous deposit. Histologically the tumour was a mucoid carcinoma.

Lymphatic spread

In the bowel wall the lymphatic channels run circumferentially and there is relatively little communication between them in the long axis of the gut. These lymphatics drain into the mesenteric lymphatics and there are frequently lymph nodes at the point of attachment of the mesentery to the gut, e.g. para colic. The lymphatic channels then follow the line of venous drainage (superior and inferior mesenteric veins). Nodes may be found along the veins (intermediate) or close to the point of formation of the portal vein (central). There is variation of the precise lymphatic drainage according to which segment of the intestine is the site of carcinoma.

48   **49**

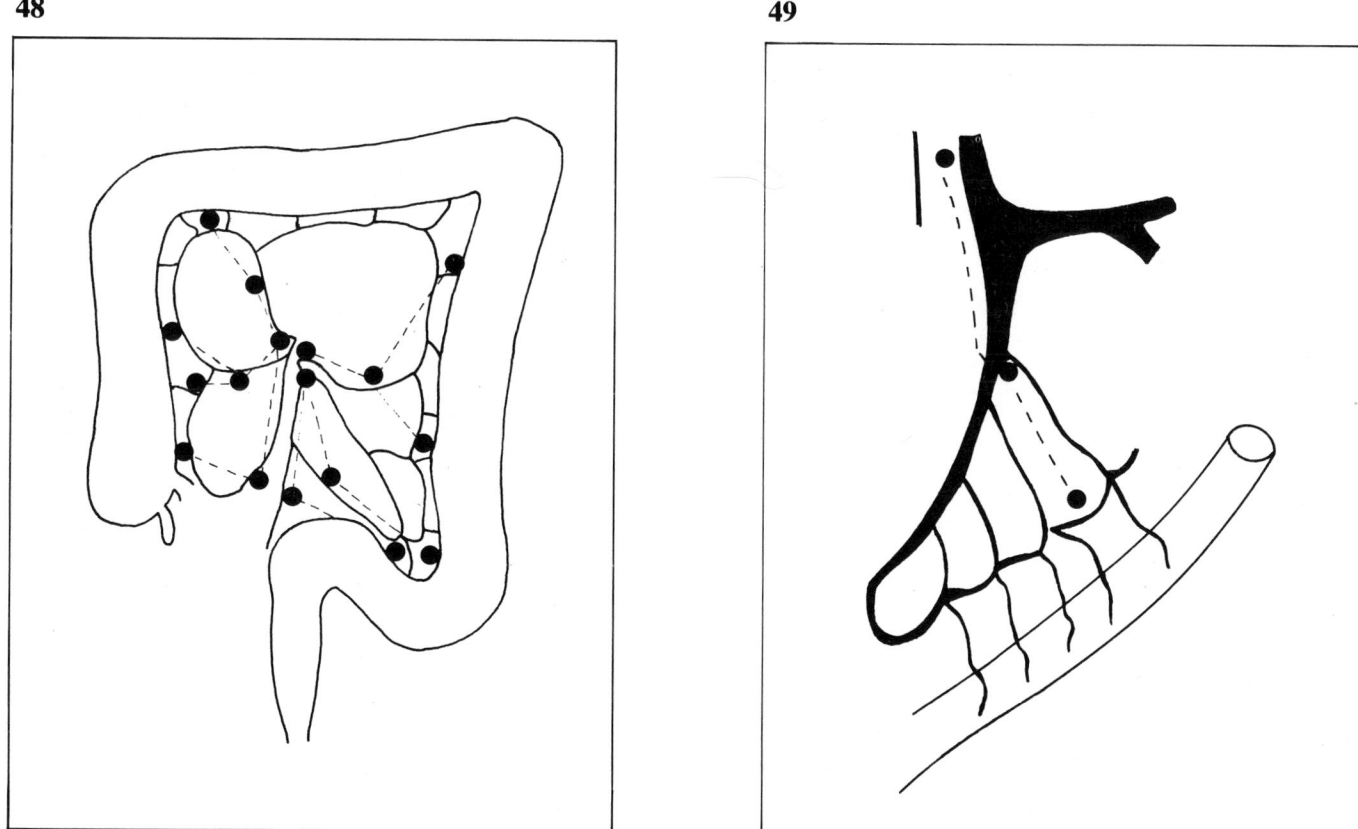

48 and **49**   Lymphatic drainage of colon and small intestine demonstrating the location of the lymph nodes.

Evidence of regional glandular involvement in carcinoma of the colon is a relatively late phenomenon in contrast to the spread of carcinoma in other organs, and usually does not occur before the peritoneal coat has been involved.

In contradistinction carcinoma of the small intestine is associated with early involvement of the lymph nodes.

Lymphatic spread from a carcinoma of the intestine has already occurred in a high percentage of cases at the time of their original operation.

Haematogenous spread

Post mortem studies show 35% of cases to have spread to the liver. In operation series approximately 12% of patients will already have evidence of hepatic metastases. The detection of such metastases pre-operatively is facilitated by the use of ultrasonography, radio-isotope liver scan and aspiration cytology. In spite of such investigations and careful examination of the liver at operation a few patients later develop metastases (occult metastases).

Blood samples from the inferior mesenteric vein taken during operation may show the presence of malignant cells. This finding does not appear to indicate that liver metastases are inevitably present or that the prognosis was thereby adversely affected.

A rare form of spread results from malignant invasion of the cisterna chyli or where there is an overlying carcinoma as for example of the jejunum, leading to invasion of the thoracic duct with entry of the malignant cells into the left brachio-cephalic vein.

Distant metastases occur to the lungs and occasionally to bones.

Implantation

Recurrence of carcinoma after resection is known to occur occasionally at the line of anastomosis and is attributable to the implantation of detached malignant cells present in the lumen of the gut. The incidence is lessened by washouts of the bowel and the preparation of the ends of bowel for anastomosis by cytotoxic agents. An important factor is the avoidance of rough handling of the tumour-bearing area and the early application of occlusion clamps.

Grading

In 1928 C.E. Dukes introduced a method of categorising the extent of the tumour according to the degree of invasiveness as found in operation specimens and showed that this was a useful guide to prognosis.

It is difficult by clinical examination, radiology or endoscopy to make a completely accurate assessment of all cases.

Results of treatment (St. Mark's Hospital series)

Category A

50 Cancer has spread into the tissues of the bowel wall but not beyond the muscle coat. No lymph node metastases. Seen in 15% of operation cases. Prognosis – excellent. Eighty per cent 5 year 'cures'.

Category B

51 Cancer has spread beyond the muscle coat into the pericolic or perirectal tissues in continuity. No regional lymph node metastases. Seen in 35% of operation cases. Prognosis – 60% five year 'cures'.

Category C

52 Direct spread as previously. Lymph nodes involved. Seen in 50% of operation cases. Prognosis – under 30% five year 'cures'.

50

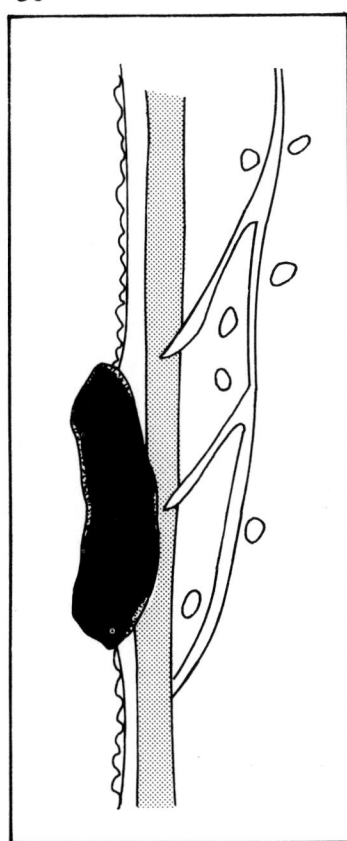

51

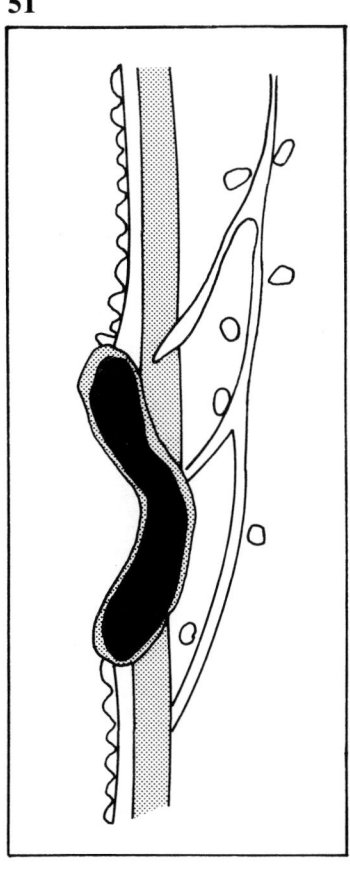

52

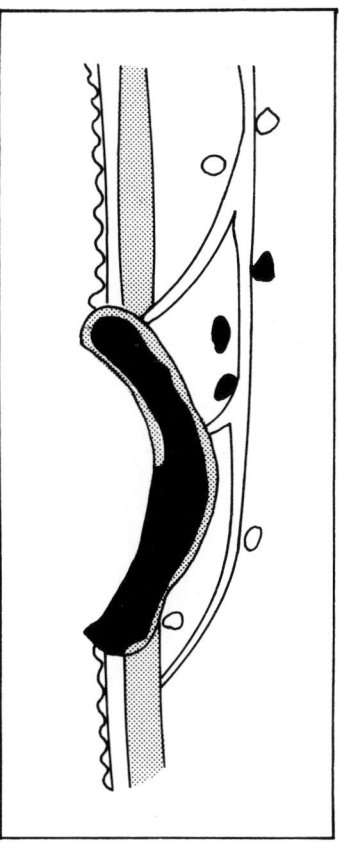

In contrast, the survival figures for an entire region rather than a single hospital reveal that there is a less than 30% crude survival for all patients treated over a five year period.

Complications

Obstruction

Obstruction may result from the filling of the lumen by a bulky tumour or from narrowing of the lumen by a stenosing lesion. Partial obstruction is associated with dilatation of the gut and hypertrophy of the muscle coat proximal to the lesion. Acute obstruction usually supervenes when a scybalous mass becomes impacted especially in an oedematous colon.

Because of the fluid nature of the content in the small intestine and right side of the colon, obstruction is late.

53

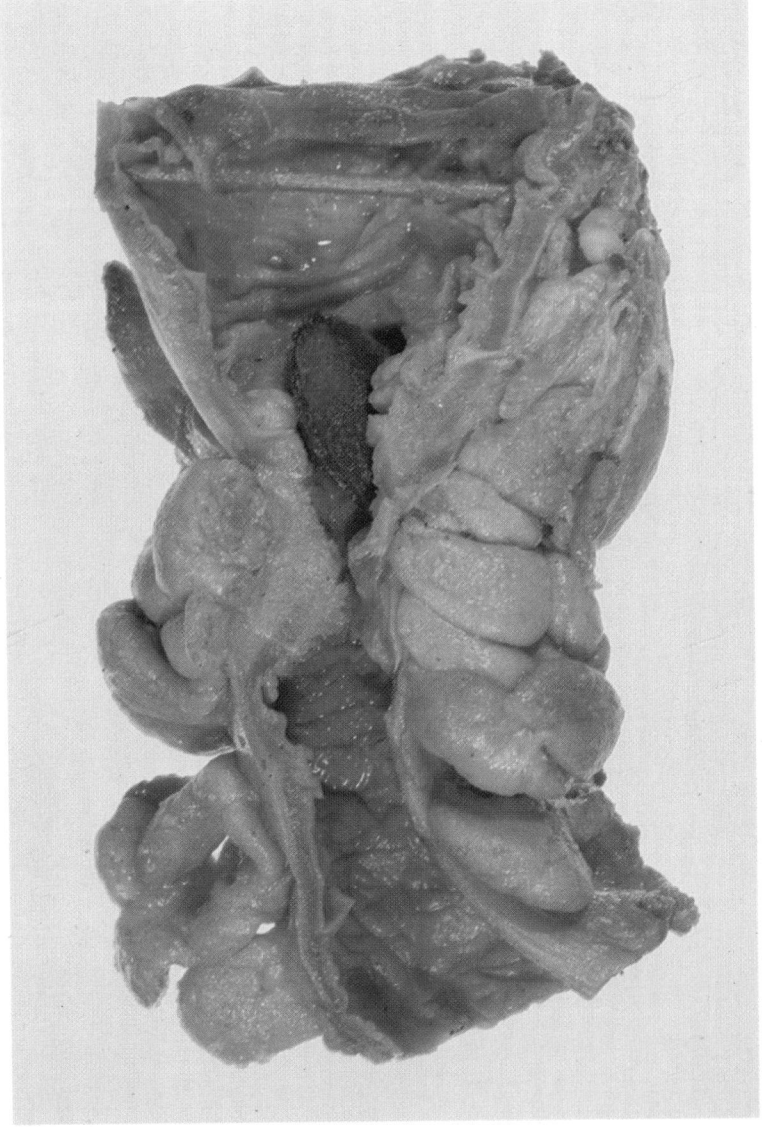

G.C.10037

53 From a female aged 75 years who had suffered loss of appetite and loss of weight for three or four months. Symptoms of subacute obstruction necessitated her admission to hospital for emergency operation. The carcinoma is a small scirrhous, stenosing tumour, and has given rise to a 'string stricture' of the gut. The colon proximal to the tumour is hypertrophied and dilated. A prune stone is impacted in the growth and has clearly been responsible for the development of the acute obstructive symptoms. Microscopically the growth was a moderately differentiated adenocarcinoma.

In the presence of an obstructing carcinoma of the colon, especially in the ascending or transverse segments, if the ileocaecal valve is competent the features of closed loop obstruction are evident. The caecum becomes grossly distended and its anterior wall may show ischaemic necrosis and perforation.

54

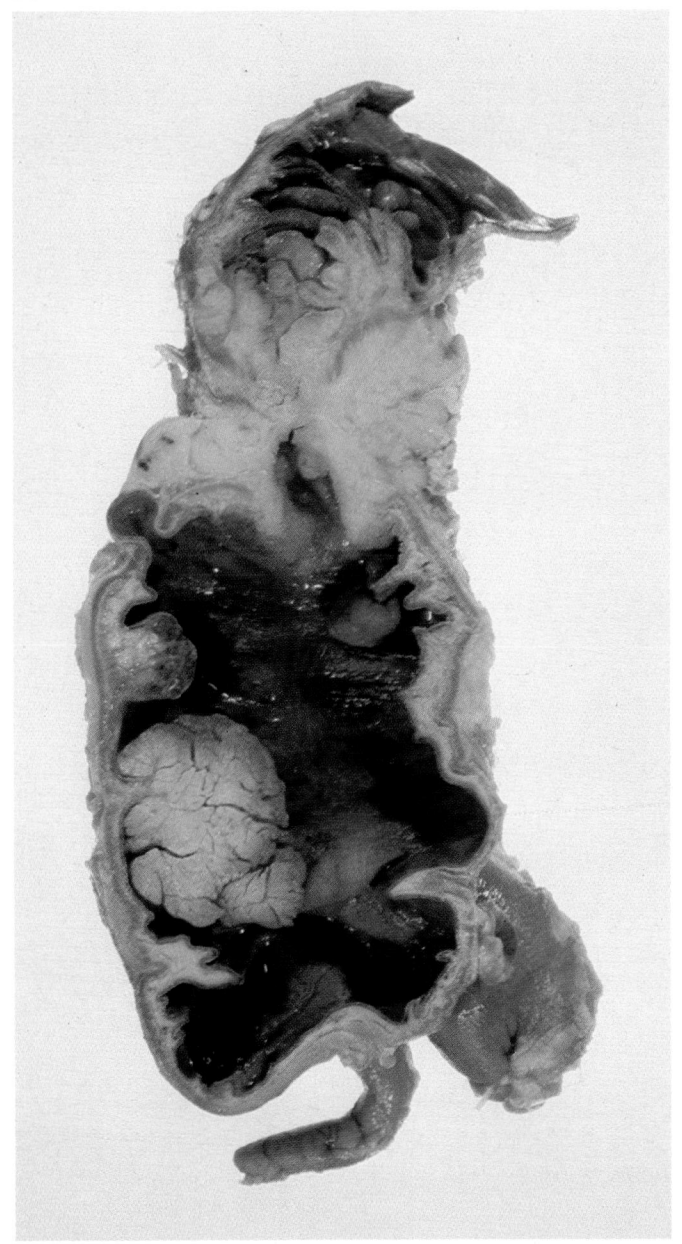

G.C.14672

54 A specimen demonstrating a carcinoma of the hepatic flexure which is causing a degree of obstruction resulting in dilatation of the caecum and ascending colon.

This specimen had the added interest that it demonstrates two separate polypoid tumours proximal to the main mass. The distal tumour is invading and obviously malignant.

The initial evidence of an obstructing carcinoma is colic caused by the increased peristalsis proximal to the lesion. Occasionally, the obstruction is caused by impaction in the narrowed lumen of the gut by a solid foreign body as is illustrated in the case on the preceding page.

Complications *(Continued)*

Intussusception

When the tumour projects into the lumen of the gut and especially if pedunculated, intussusception may occur. This complication is particularly common in tumours of the right colon and is the commonest cause of intussusception in the adult. The condition may run a chronic course and does not present as an acute obstruction.

55

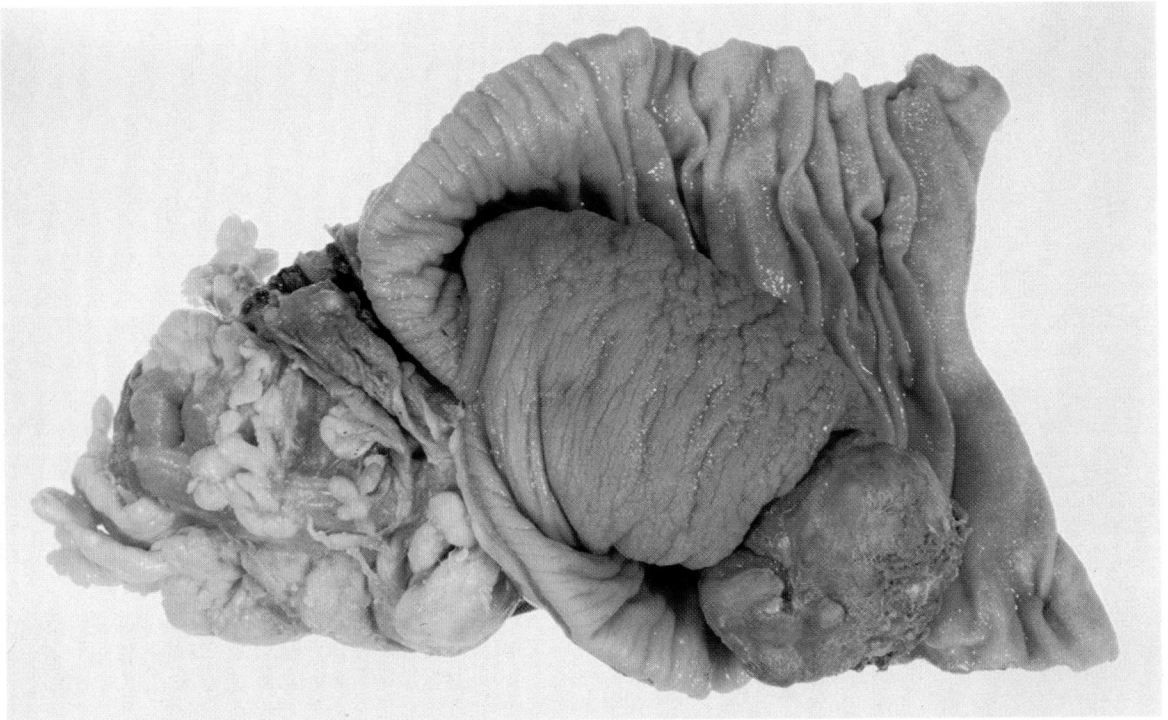

55 From a male aged 68 years with a three month history of chronic intussusception. On examination a palpable mass was found in the left hypochondrium.

The specimen is an intussusception of the transverse colon which has been opened to exhibit the intussusceptum. The intussusceptum is approximately 10 cm long and at the apex is a bulbous projecting and ulcerating carcinoma. There were no palpable lymph nodes indicating secondary disease in the fresh specimen.

Microscopically the tumour is a well differentiated glandular carcinoma.

Ulceration

Ulceration of the tumour with secondary infection leads to increased mucous secretion and may occasion diarrhoea. The ulcerated surface also causes haemorrhage which, although seldom severe, is persistent and may cause profound anaemia.

Perforation

Occasionally in a penetrating carcinoma associated with necrosis a perforation at the base into the free peritoneal cavity occurs. This is relatively rare but occurs with most frequency where the tumour arises in the small intestine.

56a

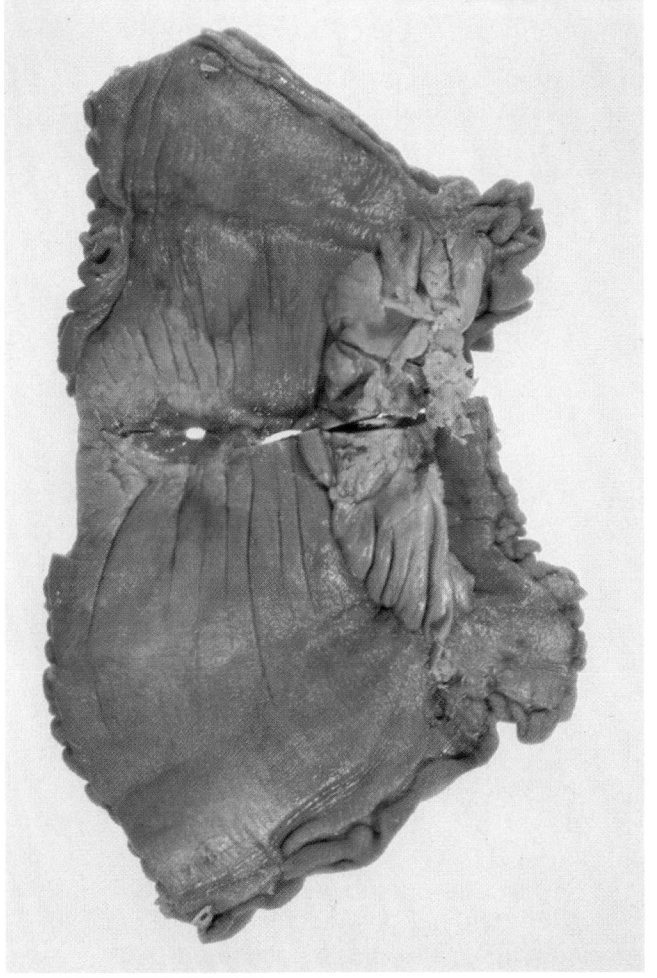

G.C.12234

Perforation

56b

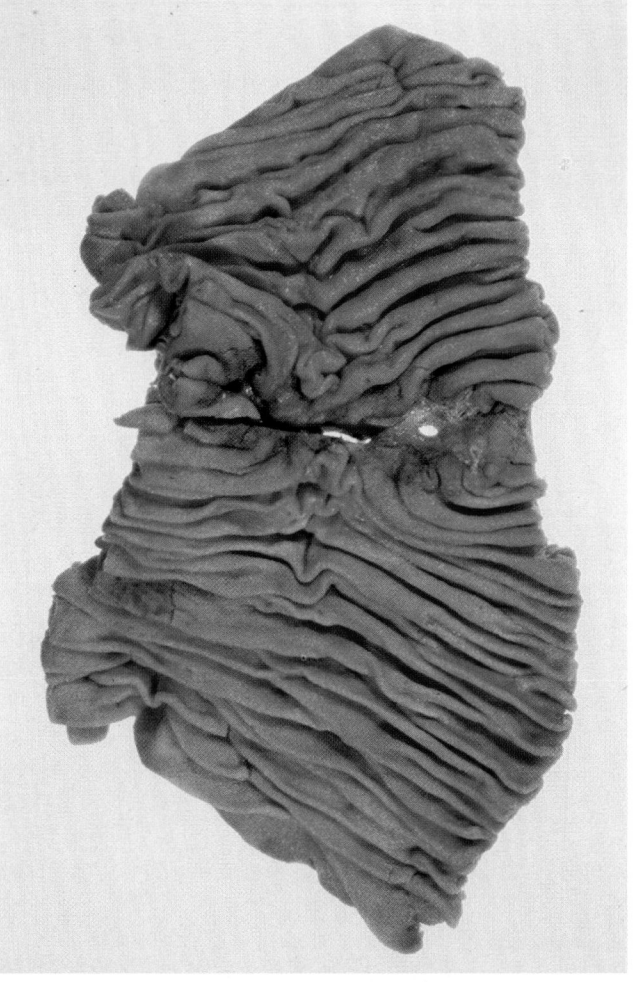

56a and **56b**   From a male aged 58 years who had a long history commencing in 1927 of a duodenal ulcer and which perforated in 1937. Symptoms continued and in 1953 he was admitted for a perforated appendix. In 1959 he was readmitted and the diagnosis of perforated duodenal ulcer was again made. At operation a perforated carcinoma of jejunum was discovered. In 1961 he had a selective vagotomy and gastro-enterostomy. There was no evidence of recurrence of malignancy.

On the serous surface of the specimen (**56a**) the site of the carcinoma is demarcated by a stenosing constriction and the presence of the perforation is clearly seen close to the attachment of the mesentery.

The ulcerated carcinoma (**56b**) has almost completely encircled the circumference of the gut and essentially appears to be extending transversely. The edges are raised and everted. The ulcer base is necrotic.

Microscopical examination showed a differentiated adenocarcinoma with much mucous secretion. It had penetrated the full thickness of the bowel wall. Adjacent to the perforation the peritoneum is acutely inflamed.

Intestinal segmental variations

While the pathological character of intestinal carcinoma is essentially the same, irrespective of which segment of the intestine is affected, variations occur depending on the precise site. These are now noted in the following paragraphs.

Small intestine

Carcinoma is relatively rare but is the most common of all tumours of the small intestine (50%). Polypoid, ulcerating and stenosing are the common types of lesion seen. Jejunum is more frequently affected than the ileum. Obstruction is late but perforation occurs in about one third of the cases. Tumours occur at an earlier age than in the colon (average 46 to 50 years) and examples have been reported in children. In operative series 50% of lesions are found to show involvement of lymph nodes and the prognosis is poor.

57

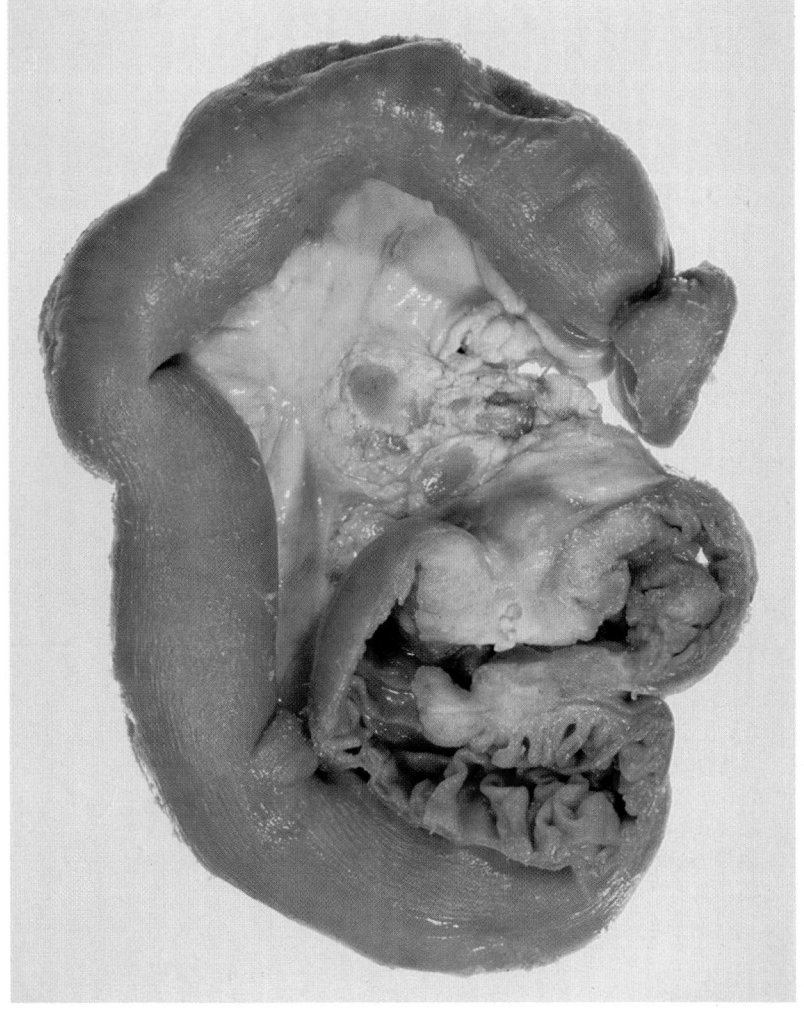

G.C.14414

57 From a female aged 65 years. Subacute intestinal obstruction and the carcinoma of the upper jejunum were diagnosed radiologically. The tumour was located 15 cm distal to the duodeno-jejunal flexure. It projects into the bowel and constricts it. Microscopic examination revealed lymph node involvement.

Ileocaecal valve

Involvement of the ileocaecal valve may result from tumour originating either in the terminal ileum or in the caecum. Obstruction is early and common.

58

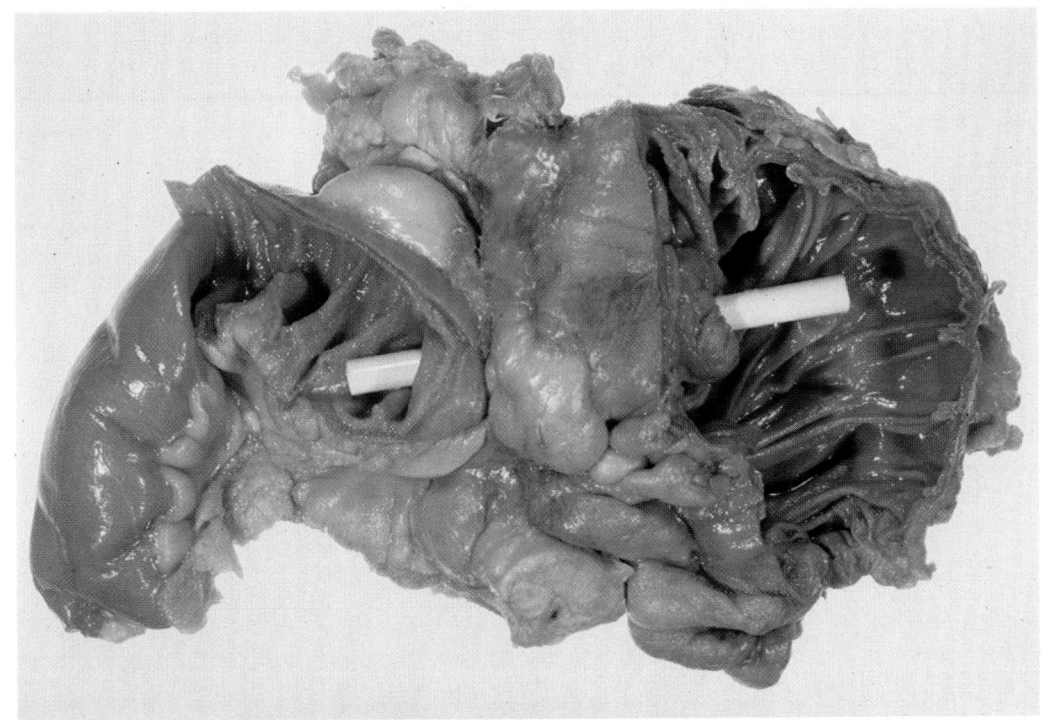

G.C.5129

59

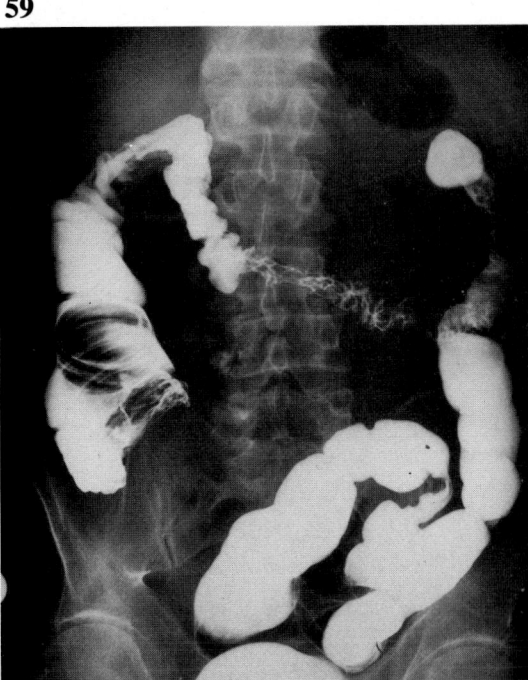

G.C.X.460

58 From an adult. The specimen shows a marked narrowing of the ileocaecal valve and involves both the terminal ileum and aperture. Note how the ileocaecal aperture protrudes into the caecum, a feature which may result in intussusception. The tumour was an adenocarcinoma of the mucoid type and the lymph nodes were invaded.

59 Barium enema shows an intussusception in the ascending colon due to a carcinoma originating at the ileocaecal valve.

Caecum

The most common type of tumour in the caecum is the proliferative, cauliflower, bulky neoplasm which may or may not involve the ileocaecal valve. Many of these tumours are of the mucoid type. Such mucoid carcinomas may give rise to widespread peritoneal involvement and Krukenberg tumours. Since the caecal contents are fluid and the lumen capacious obstruction is late and diarrhoea may be a presenting feature. The surface of the tumour is frequently ulcerated and the bacterial content of the gut high. Bleeding is common and the resulting anaemia may be marked. This is a common mode of presentation. The caecum is also the site occasionally of a malignant ulcer type of neoplasm characterised by the typical raised base and irregular edges.

Intestinal segmental variations *(Continued)*

Appendix

Primary adenocarcinoma of the appendix is rare and presents no special features of pathological interest. It may present as an acute appendicitis following occlusion of the lumen of the appendix. Carcinoma of the appendix is part of the differential diagnosis where appendicitis occurs in elderly patients. Appendicitis may also occur where the carcinoma is located in the caecum leading to retention of appendicular contents.

60

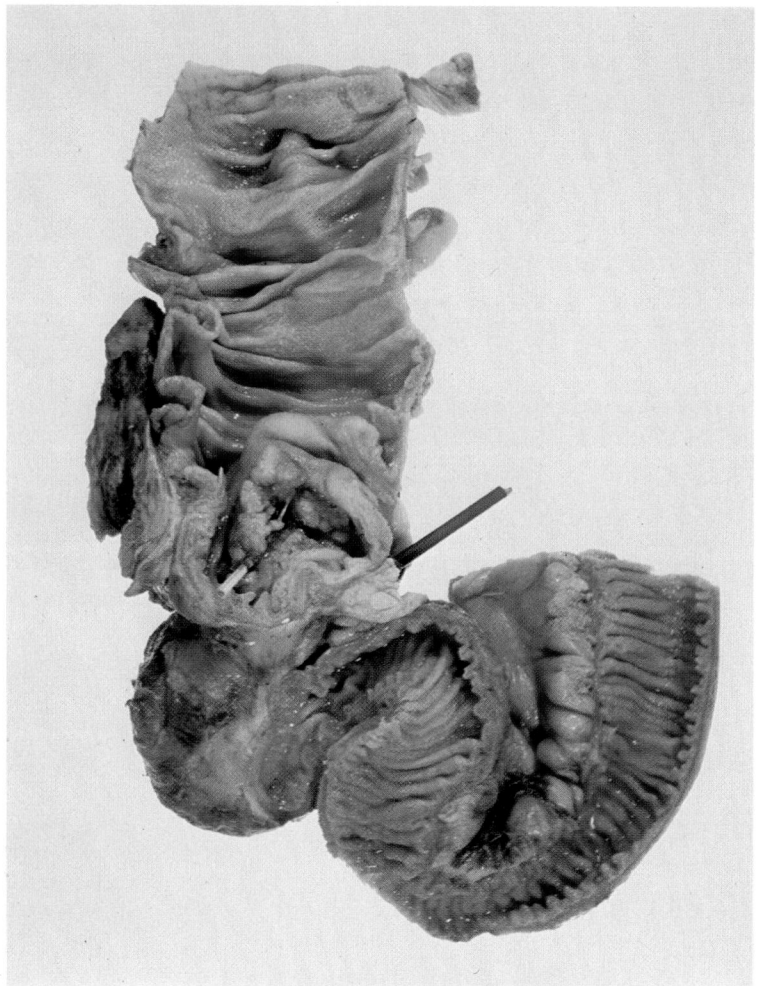

G.C.12088

61

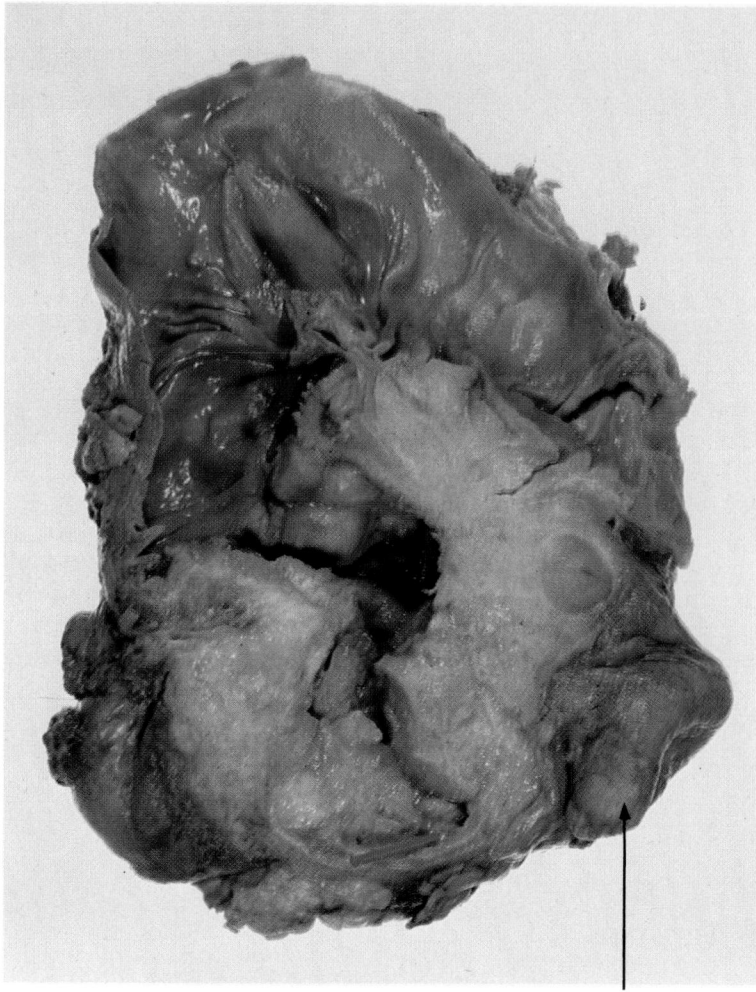

G.C.10708

60 From a male aged 42 years admitted as an acute appendicitis. An immediate appendicectomy was carried out. The base of the appendix was unduly thickened and histology revealed an adenocarcinoma. A right sided colectomy was therefore undertaken. A protruding carcinomatous mass is present in the caput-caeci immediately inferior to the ileocaecal orifice. The lumen of the appendix is indicated by a rod.

61 From a female aged 77 years who was admitted as an emergency on account of a short history of abdominal colic followed by diarrhoea. A palpable mass was present in the right iliac fossa.

The specimen demonstrates a large, bulky tumour of the caecum which has partially occluded the appendicular orifice. The appendix (arrow) is acutely inflamed but is not the site of tumour growth. The specimen exhibits, therefore, an acute obstructive appendicitis secondary to carcinoma of the caecum. This is a diagnostic pitfall when there is apparent acute appendicitis in an elderly patient. The lumen of the appendix communicates with the caecum through the mass of the tumour indicated by a red rod.

Ascending colon

Tumours of the ascending colon and hepatic flexure are commonly of the ring stricture type. When obstruction develops it is often of the closed loop type and the caecum and ascending colon therefore become ballooned with the risk of perforation.

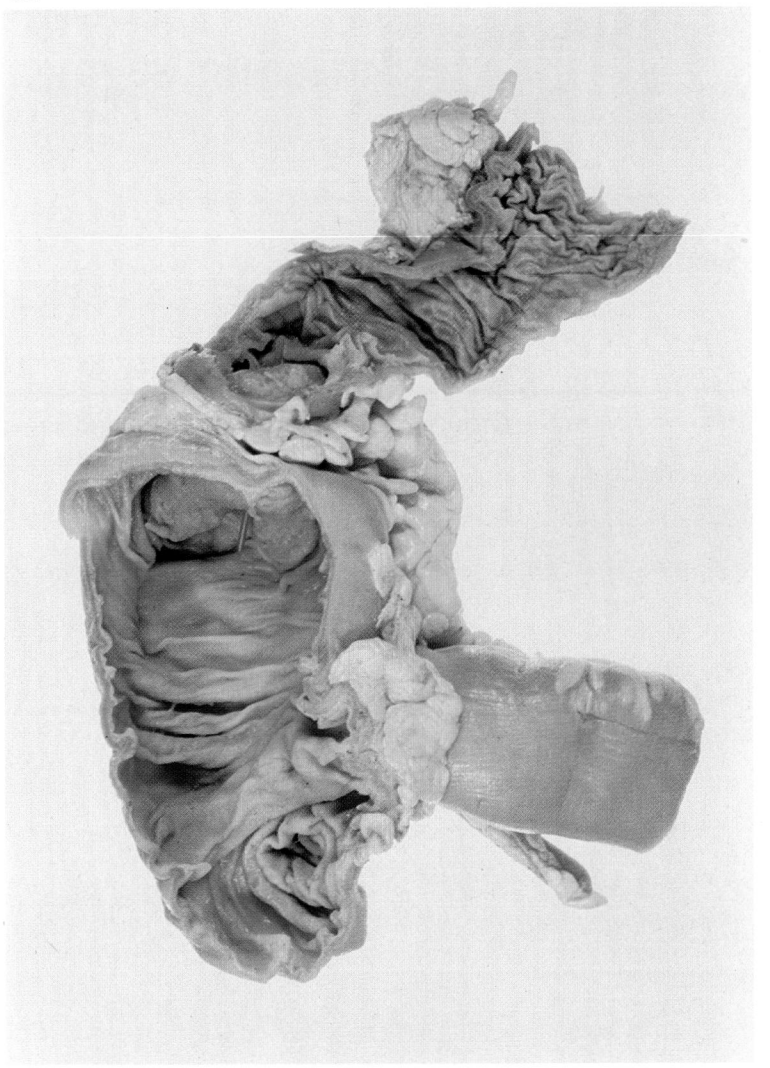

G.C.11374

62 From a female aged 71 years with a 12 day history of acute obstruction.

Two inches distal to the ileocaecal valve an annular carcinoma of the colon is present. The colon proximal to the tumour, the caecum and the terminal ileum are dilated. The tumour, seen either from its proximal or distal aspect forms an irregular ragged ulcer with elevated margins and extending across the lumen of the gut. Only a small central channel (indicated by a red glass rod) remains by which bowel content could pass.

Histologically the tumour was a typical cellular type of adenocarcinoma – local infiltration a prominent feature.

Transverse colon

The transverse colon, splenic flexure and descending colon are less frequently the sites of tumour growth and the neoplasms are usually of the stricture type.

Pelvic colon

The pelvic colon is the second most common site of carcinoma of the colon. The characteristic neoplasm in this segment of the colon is the stricture type and is associated with obstructive features. The presence of inflammatory reaction (fibrosis) around the affected colon is common and adhesions to the bladder, ureter, uterus and vagina as well as small intestine (ileum) which lie in the pelvic cavity are frequent and may lead to the formation of a fistula.

The relationship of diverticulosis/diverticulitis has long been the subject of discussion. The older view that this disease could be a precursor of carcinoma is now discarded but the concomitant occurrence of diverticulitis and carcinoma is not infrequent. Clinically the two lesions, especially in the presence of an inflammatory reaction, are very similar.

Ulcerative colitis occurs in the pelvic colon and rectum with frequency and is related to the subsequent development of carcinoma (vide supra).

Intestinal segmental variations *(Continued)*

Rectum

Carcinoma of the rectum is the most common form of intestinal cancer (65%). In the United Kingdom it is the second most common cause of male deaths from neoplastic disease (12%). It frequently originates in a pre-existing adenoma or papilloma and on occasion multiple independent malignancies may develop. Tumours of the upper part of the rectum close to the pelvirectal junction are generally of the stricture type. Lesions in the ampulla of the rectum may present as bulky tumours or as malignant ulcers.

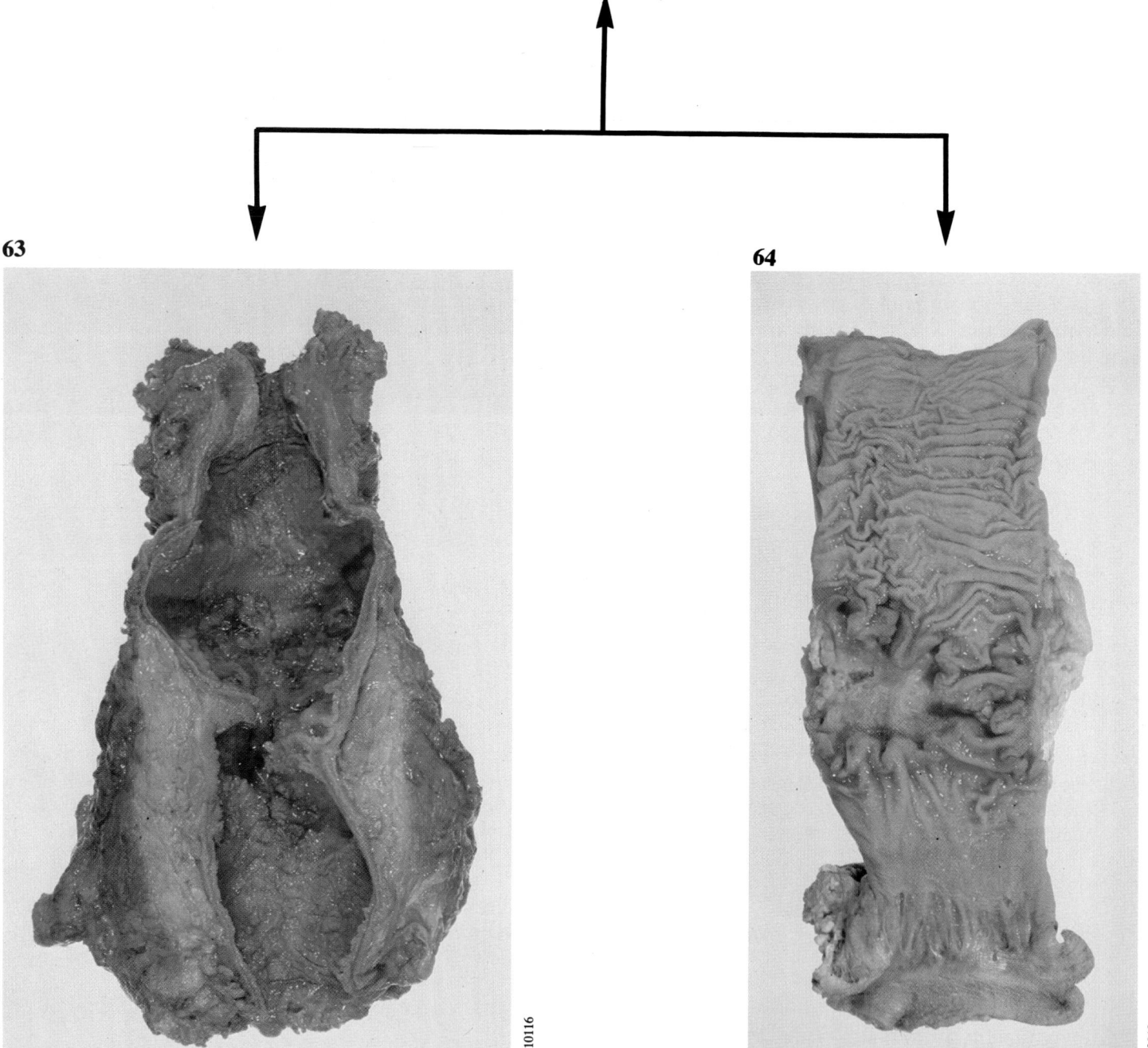

63

High

G.C.10116

64

Low

G.C.12812

Spread

Spread of carcinoma of the rectum has special features of great surgical significance. Spread beyond the rectal wall is early and at operation this will be found in approximately 70 to 80% of cases. It is especially early where the tumour is of colloid type.

Direct spread

Direct spread with involvement of the surrounding fatty tissues and adjacent viscera occurs within 6 to 12 months of the origin of the tumour. Bladder, prostate and uterus are commonly involved. Involvement of the sacral plexus and its branches leads to severe radiating pain.

Lymphatic spread

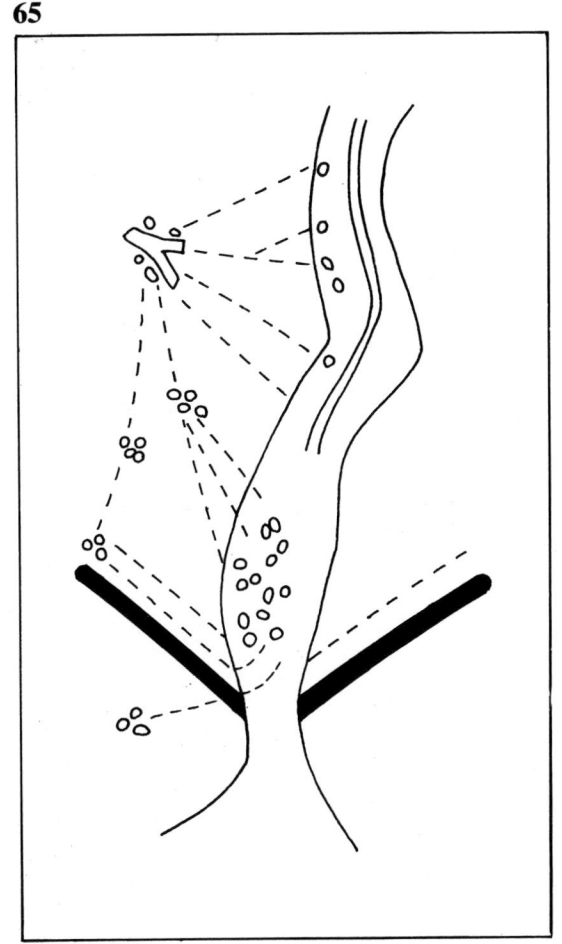

65

65 In the rectum lymphatics run upwards and along the superior haemorrhoidal and inferior mesenteric arteries. Extension to the lateral pelvic nodes also occurs. The major spread in the wall of the intestine from the original tumour is upwards. Downward spread is limited and in operative procedures a margin of 5 cm below the original lesion is regarded as adequate excision. Only when the tumour involves the anal canal and the lowermost segment of the rectum does spread to the inguinal nodes occur.

If both ureters are involved impaired renal function may result.

Intestinal segmental variations *(Continued)*

Rectum – lymphatic spread *(Continued)*

Lymphatic spread is a frequent finding even in cases suitable for excision (50%). The main pathway is by lymphatics which transgress the bowel wall but remain within the perirectal fascia. They extend upwards in the line of the superior haemorrhoidal vessels ultimately spreading to the inferior mesenteric chain. This lymphatic spread was studied in detail by C.E. Dukes and his findings are accepted as authoritative. He carried out meticulous dissection of operative specimens and demonstrated the precise location of involved lymph nodes lying posterior to the rectum and forming an upward chain.

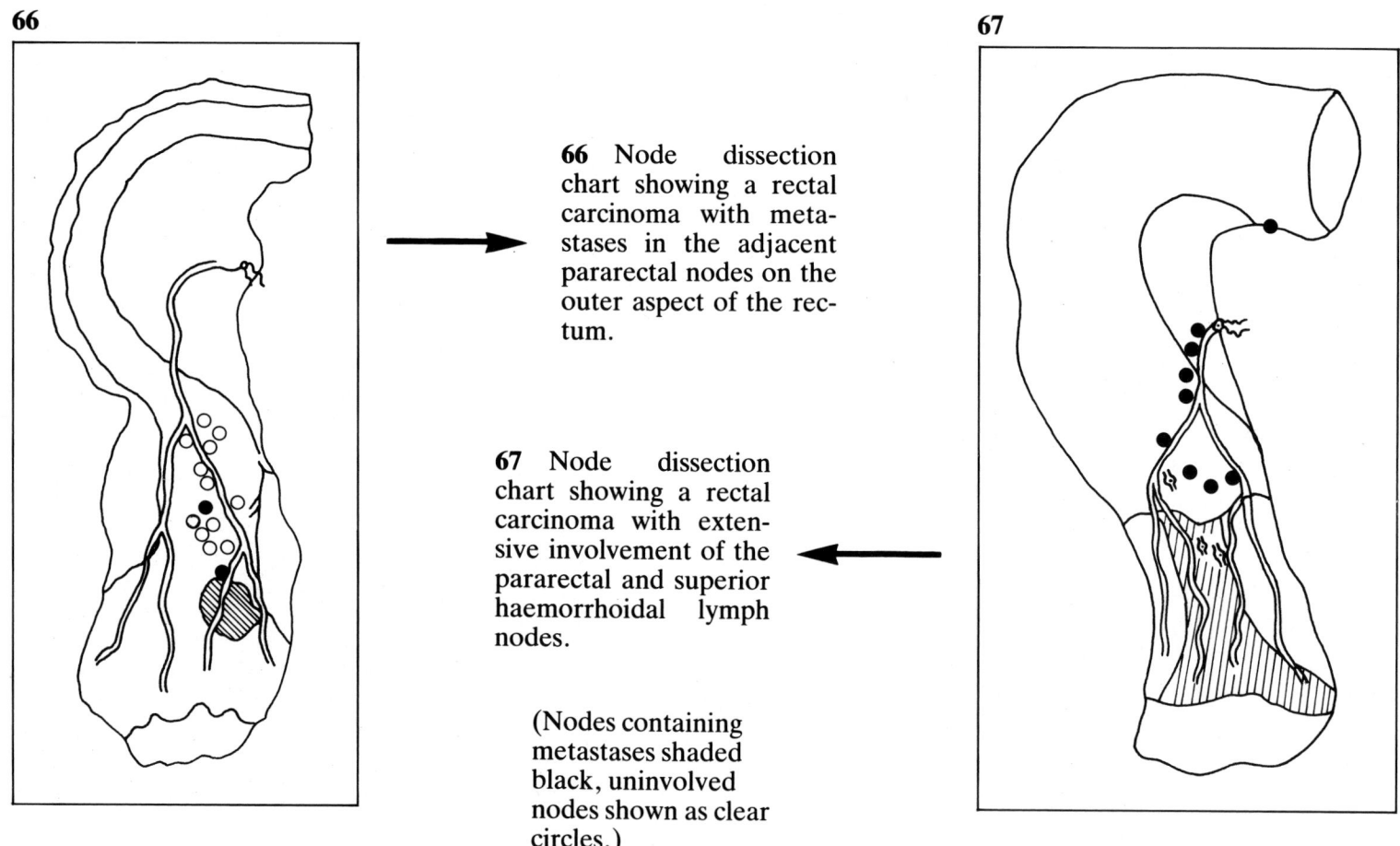

66 Node dissection chart showing a rectal carcinoma with metastases in the adjacent pararectal nodes on the outer aspect of the rectum.

67 Node dissection chart showing a rectal carcinoma with extensive involvement of the pararectal and superior haemorrhoidal lymph nodes.

(Nodes containing metastases shaded black, uninvolved nodes shown as clear circles.)

Lateral spread along lymphatic channels covering the middle haemorrhoidal vessels is rare until the perirectal fascia has been breached. Accordingly the iliac and hypogastric nodes are involved at a later stage.

Downward spread

Downward spread is rare except in tumours low in the ampulla. If the tumour is at a higher level downward spread will only occur if the upward draining lymphatics become blocked.

Haemorrhoids

68

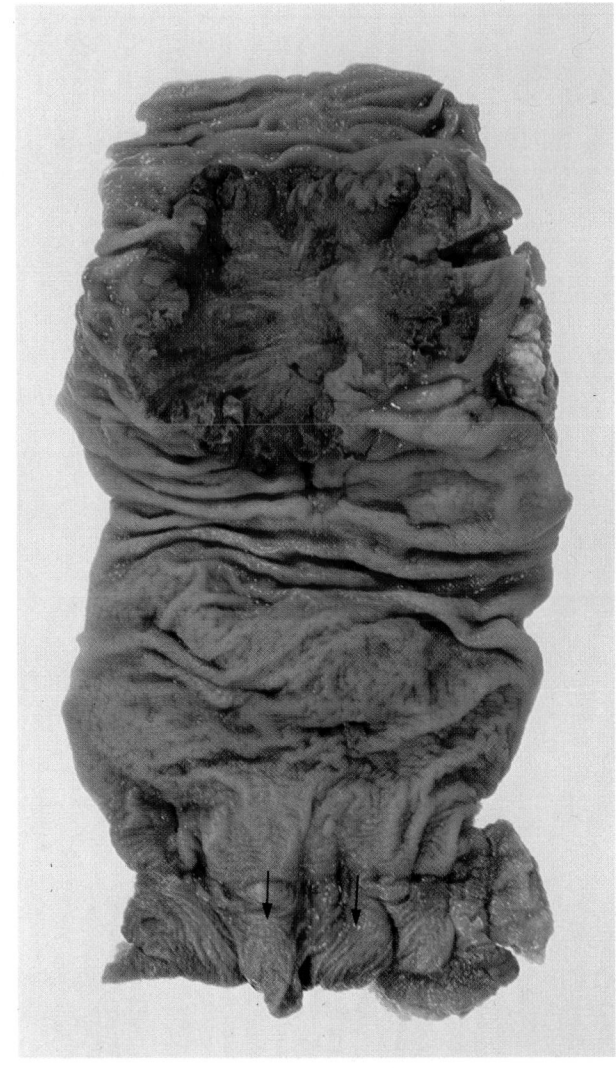

68 Interference by the growth of the tumour with the upward venous drainage into the superior haemorrhoidal veins frequently occurs early. These veins initially run upwards in the submucosa and it is during this part of their course that compression occurs. The blood return from the lower rectum now passes to the inferior haemorrhoidal veins which become dilated. Haemorrhoids may be the initial complaint of the patient and in older persons the sudden development of haemorrhoids should occasion the suspicion of malignancy.

The suspicion illustrates a carcinoma high in the ampulla associated with an internal haemorrhoid (indicated by arrows).

G.C.14796

Blood borne metastases

Blood borne metastases are relatively infrequent and are held to occur most commonly in younger patients. The liver is chiefly affected. Peritoneal metastases may arise as the result of direct spread of a tumour located high in the rectum. Implantation secondary tumours following operation have been recorded.

Radiology

69

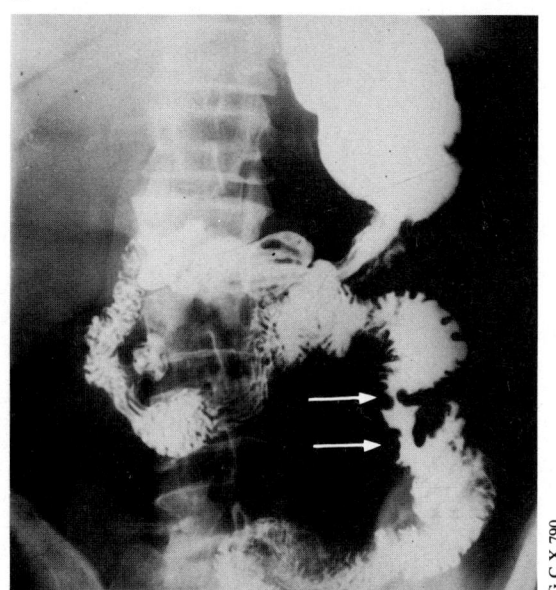

69 Barium follow-through shows an irregular annular malignant stricture in the upper jejunum. There is proximal dilatation.

70

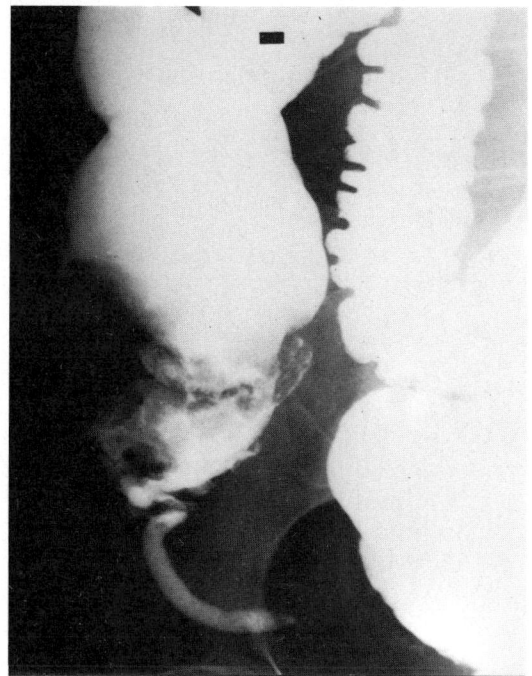

70 Barium enema shows an irregular filling defect occupying and distorting the caecum.

71

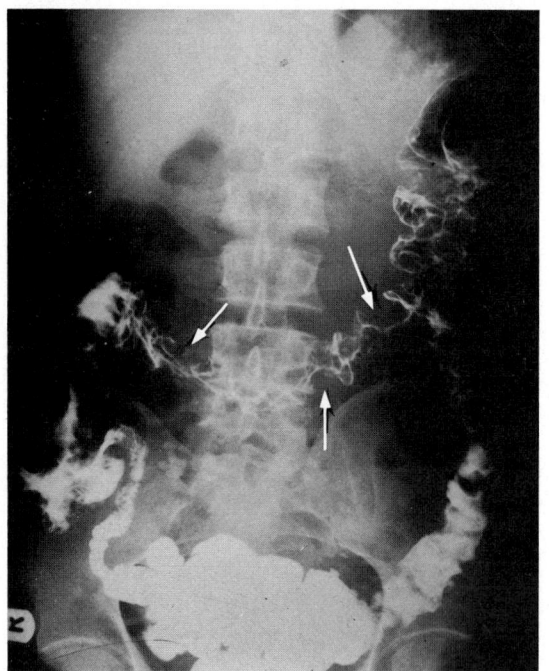

71 Barium enema demonstrating a carcinoma of the caecum. There is a filling defect with marked irregularity. There are polypoid indentations in the transverse colon due to serosal deposits.

72

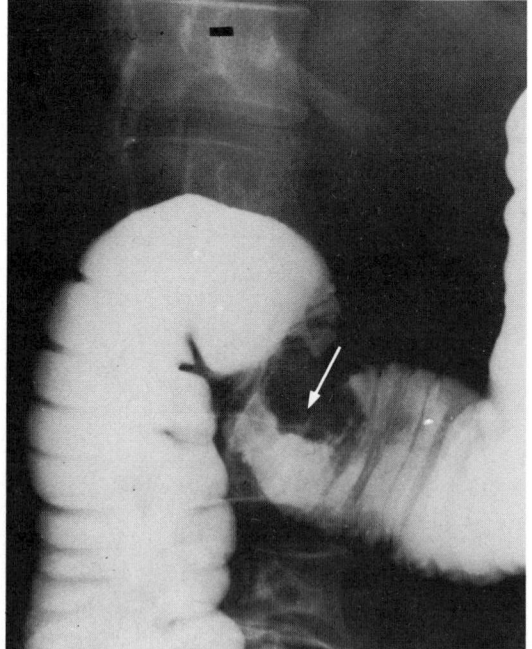

72 Barium enema shows a smooth, lobulated filling defect due to a broad-based polypoid tumour arising from the antero-superior wall of the transverse colon immediately distal to the hepatic flexure.

73

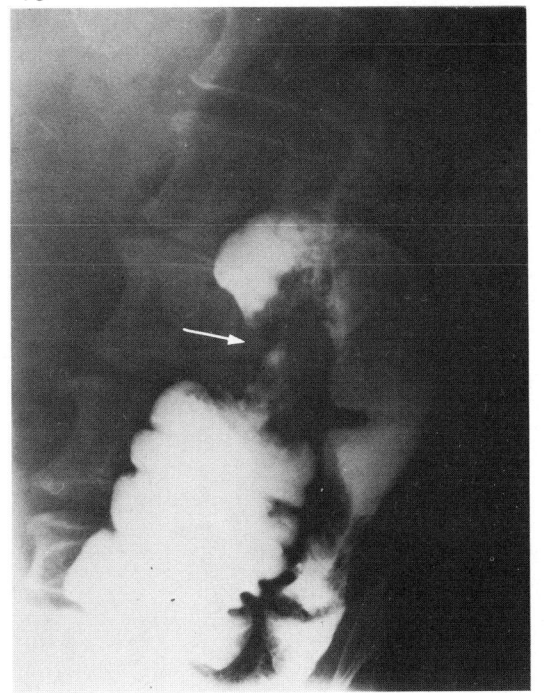

G.C.X.459

73 Barium enema demonstrating an annular carcinoma at the splenic flexure with proximal dilatation of the gut.

74

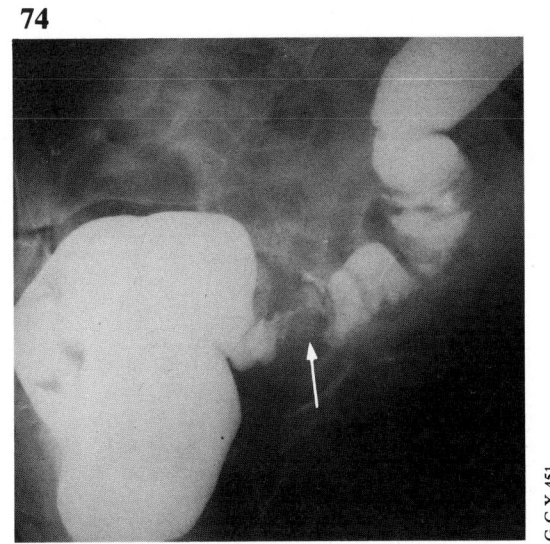

G.C.X.451

74 Barium enema shows an annular localised malignant stricture in the sigmoid colon.

75

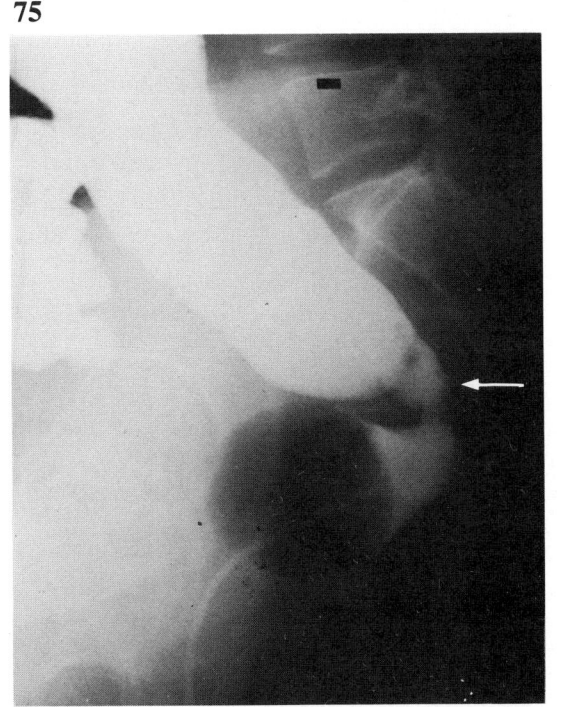

G.C.X.454

75 Barium enema shows an irregular ringlike stricture due to a carcinoma in the upper rectum with proximal distension.

76

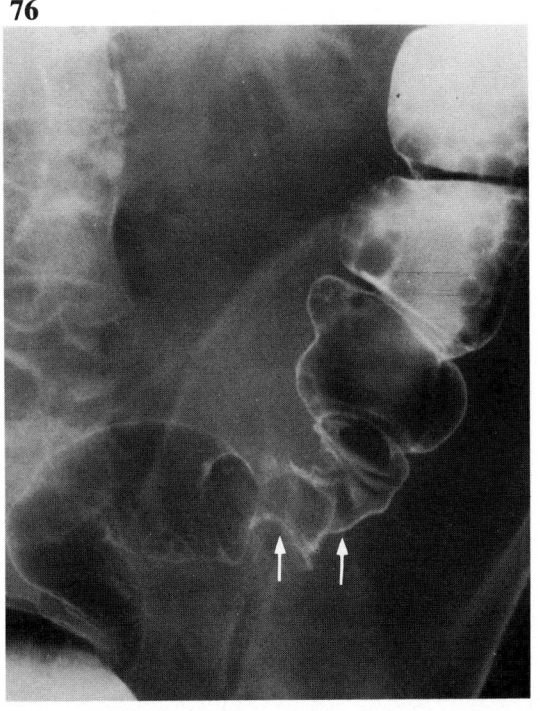

G.C.X.988

76 Double contrast barium enema. There is a 3 cm annular narrowing in the sigmoid colon with shouldering suggesting a carcinoma.

Prognosis

Small intestine

Complications, including obstruction, tend to occur late in the relatively uncommon carcinoma of the small intestine. The tumour has often metastasised before the diagnosis is made and the prognosis is therefore poor. A 5 year survival rate of only 5% has been reported.

Large intestine

The crude 5 year survival rate of carcinoma of the colon and the rectum is under 30%. The disease is often insidious in onset and surgical intervention is therefore late. In 20% of resectable tumours, occult metastases are already present in the liver. Although a fatal outcome is inevitable in such cases it is often compatible with a 2 to 5 year survival if the tumour is of low or average malignancy.

Factors adversely affecting the prognosis

Site   – Carcinoma in the right half of the colon.
Age   – Carcinoma in patients in the younger age group.
Aetiology   – Carcinoma preceded by polyposis coli or chronic ulcerative colitis.

Obstruction

Acute intestinal obstruction occurs in 15 to 20% of all cases of carcinoma of the colon with the greatest risk in those tumours located in the left colon. Even if the acute episode is controlled the occurrence of obstruction is associated with an increased mortality.

Perforation

Perforation of the gut whether as the result of extension of the malignancy or due to stercoral ulceration is less common, occurring in approximately 5 to 8% of all cases. There is a high fatal outcome in the presence of faecal peritonitis.

A.N. Smith

Embryologically the anal canal is formed by two elements, the downward tail projection of the hindgut originating from the cloaca and the upgrowth of the squamous epithelium of the perineum (see Section 15 B4). Tumours derived from the hindgut are essentially rectal tumours and adenocarcinomatous in character as already described.

Those originating in the lower part of the anal canal arise from cells derived from the epiblast of the perineum and are squamous carcinomas comparable to other cutaneous tumours.

1

Tumours at the anal margin and below the dentate line arise from the fully developed squamous epithelium and are differentiated and keratinised neoplasms. They spread downwards and outwards metastasising to the inguinal lymph nodes. Their rate of growth is slow and metastases are late. Tumours of the anal margin have been attributed to trauma and lack of personal hygiene. They have been noted to follow treatment of haemorrhoids and fissure by native practitioners using fire and caustics.

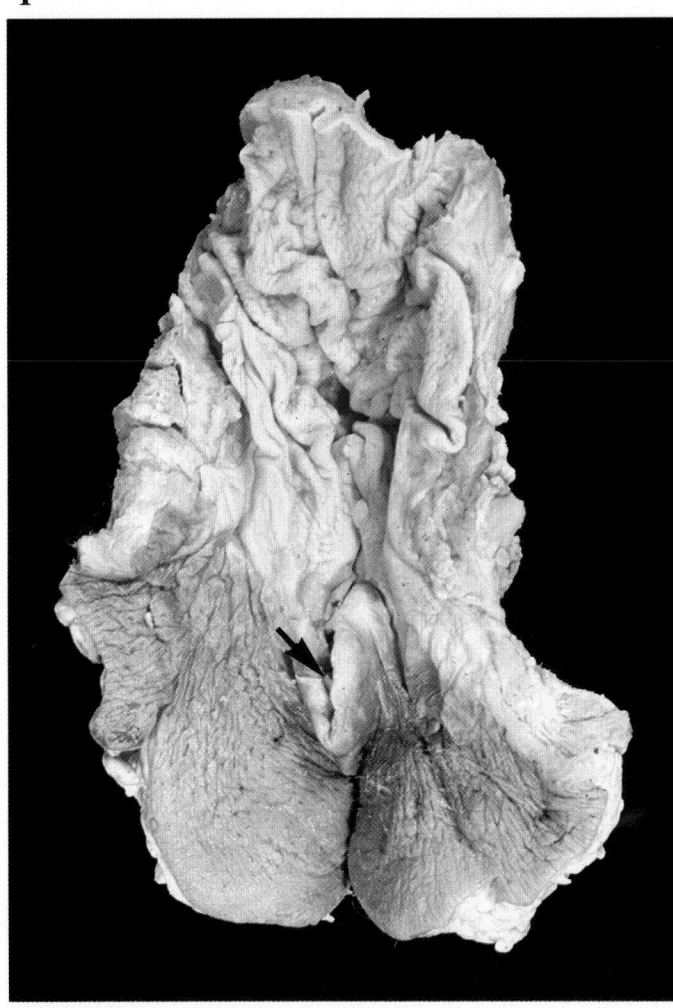

G.C.14340

1 From a female aged 61 years. The patient was admitted to hospital on account of peripheral vascular disease and on routine examination a deep fissure anal carcinoma was discovered. The patient admitted to bleeding after defaecation over a period of 6 months. Histological examination showed a well differentiated squamous carcinoma with some pleomorphism and marked lymphocytic infiltration.

Immediately above the dentate line is an intermediate zone where the epithelial cells, although squamoid, show absence of prickle cell formation. Tumours arising in this area are squamous carcinomas but a majority are of a more transitional cell type (basal carcinoma).

Tumours arising from the anal glands, which are normally lined with stratified columnar epithelium, are also described and these are of adenocarcinomatous character and usually submucous without ulceration. The condition is rare.

Aetiologically tumours of the transitional zone are occasionally preceded by and are attributed to earlier inflammatory lesions notably lymphogranuloma venereum and other non-specific chronic infections.

The histological picture shows a variable mixed pattern. These tumours spread directly in an upward direction in the submucosa and metastasise to the superior haemorrhoidal lymph nodes. Their downward spread is prevented by the obliteration of the submucosa where the dentate line is firmly attached to the underlying muscle.

The majority of these tumours arise in the anal mucosa and the term ano-rectal melanoma is therefore appropriate. They were first described in man in 1857. They had previously been recognised as occurring in animals.

These are rare neoplasms which affect both sexes equally but a number of reports have indicated that the tumour may arise during early pregnancy and in such cases grow rapidly. Most of the tumours occur in the elderly.

The tumour occurs low down in the rectum, arising in the anal canal at the mucocutaneous junction and grows upwards in the submucosa forming an elevated or pedunculated tumour in the ampulla. It may appear as an ulcer or malignant fissure in the anal canal and may simulate a thrombosed haemorrhoid. Melanin is present in only 50% of cases and the tumour may be fleshy in colour or heavily pigmented.

1

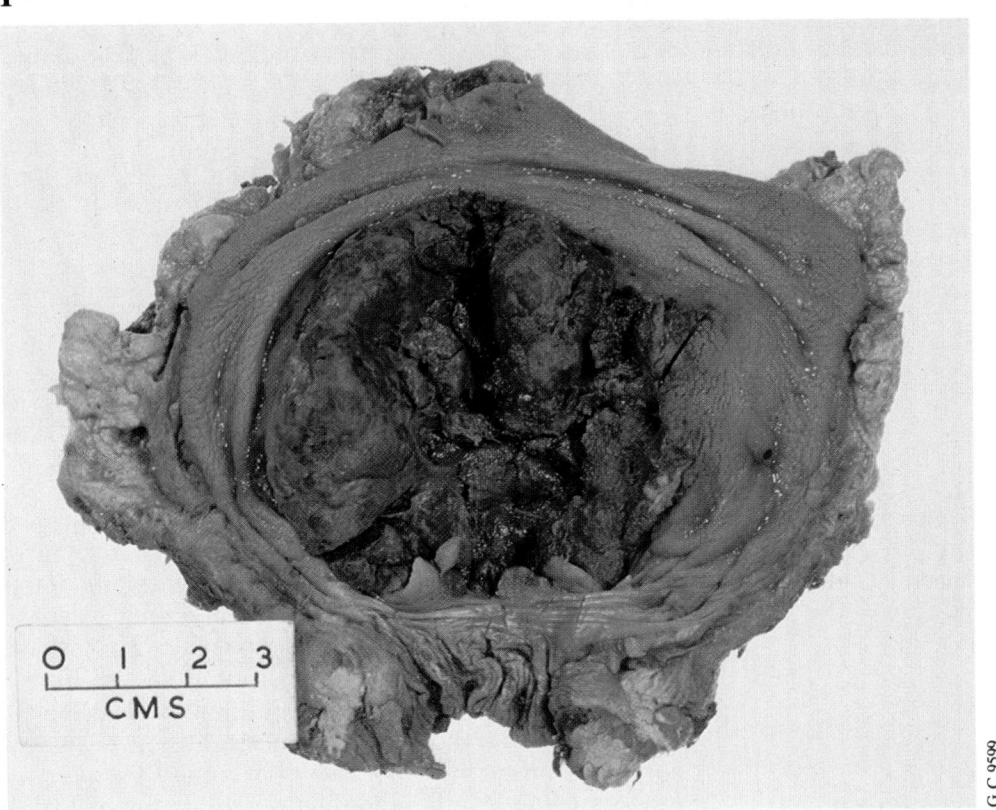

1 From a male aged 67 years in whom frequency of micturition and diarrhoea had existed during nine weeks. Examination showed an irregular ulcer in the posterior wall of the rectal ampulla encircling the rectum and apparently involving the prostate. The neoplasm forms a crateriform circular ulcer 60mm in diameter. Its floor is irregular and nodular. It is wholly black and at the edge black pigmentation is extending into the mucosa.

2

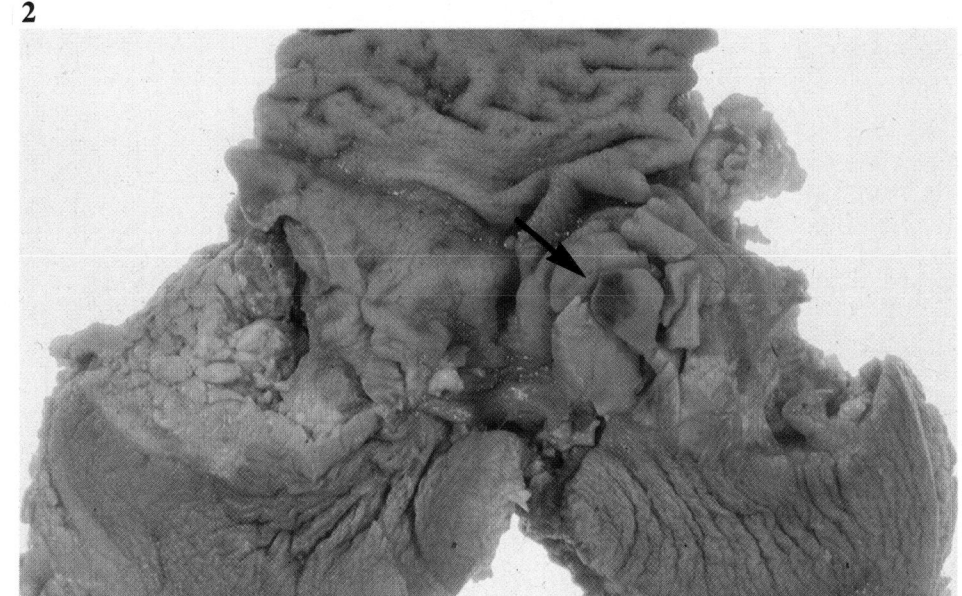

G.C.14326

2 For three months a woman of 48 years had occasionally noticed minor bleeding per rectum after defaecation.

On proctoscopy a slightly pigmented polypoid tumour 2 cm in diameter was found on the right posterior wall of the anal canal adjacent to the muco-cutaneous junction. Microscopic examination of a biopsy specimen revealed that the tumour was a malignant melanoma. An abdominoperineal resection was carried out. The specimen has been opened to illustrate the tumour (arrow).

As in melanomas elsewhere there may be much histological variation and cellular pleomorphism. Many of the pigmented cells, especially in lymph nodes, may be melanophores (phagocytes) which have ingested pigment released by melanotic malignant cells. Some tumours which are non-pigmented may be difficult to distinguish from other poorly differentiated tumours.

3

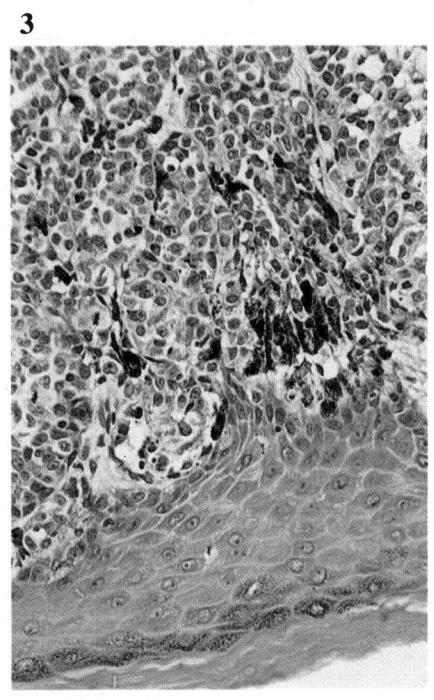

G.C.14398

3 The anal melanoma is covered by squamous epithelium. The cells are poorly pigmented and show numerous mitotic divisions. Most of the pigment in this field is in melanophores. *(H&E ×250)*

Spread

Spread is early, the disease passing both upwards along the rectal lymphatics and laterally to the wall of the pelvis. The inguinal nodes may be involved. Blood spread occurs especially to the liver and lungs and is the ultimate cause of death. The disease is almost invariably fatal.

Secondary melanoma

Metastatic melanoma in the intestine is comparatively rare but is a known occurrence.

4

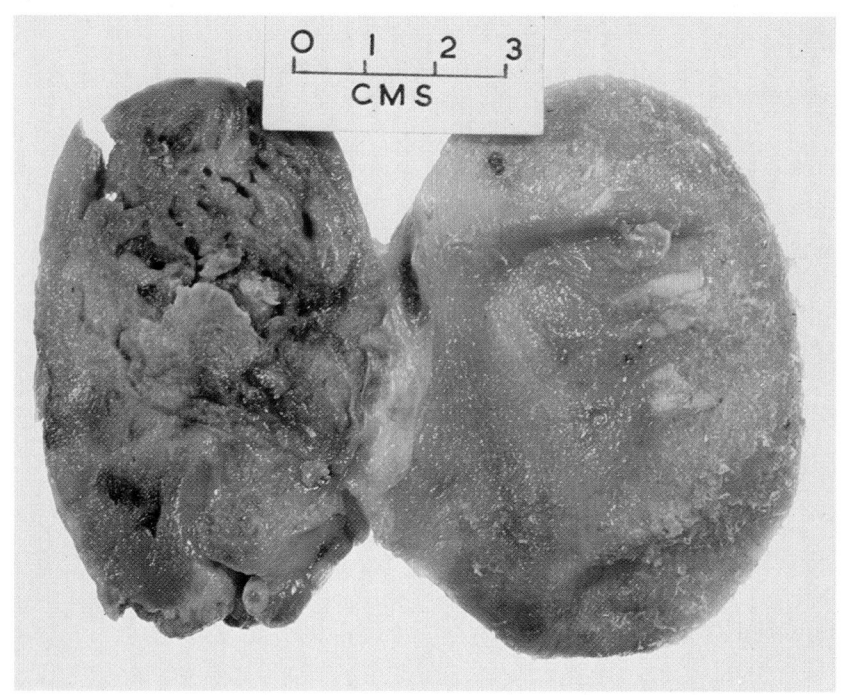

4 From a female aged 37 years who had suffered from a blood-stained discharge per rectum for about two months. A polypoid tumour was found at 14 cm on sigmoidoscopy. At operation the tumour was located in the pelvic colon and a portion of small intestine was adherent to this part of the colon. Part of the descending colon, the pelvic colon and rectum and 15 cm of the affected small bowel were excised. The left half of the illustration shows the cut surface of the tumour.

Previous history: A malignant melanoma of the left forearm had been excised 2½ years previously. Axillary metastases were obvious two months later and a block dissection was performed.

5

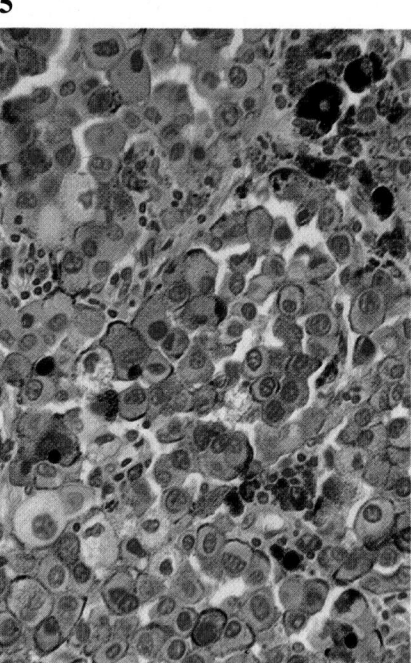

5 The tumour is composed of large round or polygonal cells with eosinophilic cytoplasm. Some of the cells contain dark brown melanin pigment. *(H&E ×312.5)*

Apud system

The term 'Apud system' was introduced to define a widely distributed and diffuse endocrine system signified by the amine-handling qualities of its cells.

The term 'Apud' is ingeniously derived from the common cytochemical properties of these cells:

1 High Amine content
2 Amine Precursor Uptake from their environment
3 Amine acid Decarboxylase (amino acids – amine)

It is known that there is a variety of these cells in the mucosa of the stomach, intestine and pancreas which have specific endocrine actions. The cells, like all polypeptide-secreting cells, have characteristic endocrine granules which show specific immunofluorescence and are probably neuroectodermal in origin. A number of the cells can be recognised by simple histological techniques but many can only be identified by ultramicroscopic or immunofluorescent methods.

Part of this system functions as a producer of gut hormones which are almost exclusively peptides, though serotonin or 5-hydroxytryptamine and prostaglandins may be produced. A list of peptides in the gastrointestinal tract is shown below:

Stomach	Duodenum and jejunum	Ileum and colon	Islet cells
Gastrin Bombesin VIP (Vaso-active Intestinal Peptide) Somatostatin Substance P	Gastrin VIP Secretin Cholecystokinin Somatostatin Motilin Substance P Bombesin	VIP Glucagon-like peptides Neurotensin	Insulin Glucagon Somatostatin Pancreatic polypeptide

The major function of the diffuse endocrine system with the main hormones secreted by its cells is as follows:

(a) Control of secretion, absorption, motility and growth of the stomach and intestine – motilin, gastrin, VIP and glucagon-like peptide.
(b) Control of gallbladder function – cholecystokinin and pancreatic peptide.
(c) Control of exocrine pancreatic function – secretin, cholecystokinin, VIP and pancreatic peptide.
(d) Control of islet-hormone secretion – gastric inhibitory polypeptide (GIP).
(e) Control of metabolism – insulin, glucagon and somatostatin.
(f) Neurotransmitter function – substance P, VIP and enkephalins.

The actions of these hormones and the reaction of this endocrine system in disease may be exemplified by the effects of gut endocrine tumours.

Apudomas

Tumours arising from cells of the Apud system are termed 'Apudomas'.

Classification

I   Ortho-endocrine.
    A.   Tumours secreting normal polypeptides of their cells of origin.
    B.   Tumours secreting normal amines of their cells of origin.

II   Para-endocrine.
    A.   Tumours of endocrine glands secreting hormones of other glands.
    B.   Tumours of tissues not regarded as endocrine in nature secreting hormones.

III   Multiple endocrine adenopathy. More than one gland is the site of neoplasia, which may be either ortho- or para-endocrine.

Most gastrointestinal Apudomas are ortho-endocrine and may be classified as follows:

1A.   Nonenterochromaffin cell tumours

Tumour cell type	Usual site of origin	Product of tumour	Name of tumour	Clinical effect
A cell	Pancreatic islets	Glucagon	Glucagonoma	Hyperglycaemia
B cell	Pancreatic islets	Insulin	Insulinoma	Hypoglycaemia
G cell	Pancreatic islets or stomach	Gastrin	Gastrinoma	ZE syndrome
D cell	Pancreatic islets	Somatostatin	Somatostatinoma	Diabetic type of glucose tolerance
H cell	Pancreatic islets	VIP	Vipoma	Watery diarrhoea
Mixed	Various	Various		Various
Ectopic	Various	Various		ACTH, ADH, MSH, Calcitonin

1B.   Enterochromaffin cell tumours

Enterochromaffin cell	Alimentary tract	Serotonin Motilin Substance P Prostaglandins Kinins Kallikrein Histamine	Carcinoid (Argentaffinoma)	Carcinoid syndrome in metastasising tumours

Carcinoid tumour

Carcinoid tumours were first described in the appendix in 1907 and were regarded as a variant of carcinoma until in 1910 it was realised that they arose from the argentaffin cell. It was also recognised that these tumours could occur in the small intestine and give rise to liver metastases. It was not until 1952 that it was appreciated that these tumours exercised an endocrine effect. This usually occurred only after the tumour had metastasised to the liver. Later it was appreciated that comparable tumours occurred in other parts of the alimentary tract.

The tumour is slightly more common in males. Appendix usual site. Ileum second commonest site closely followed by rectum. In the ileum the tumours are usually small and often multiple.

Appendix – carcinoid

In the appendix the tumours are small and often at the distal end. Elsewhere the tumours may be single or multiple and form projecting nodules or plaques in the lumen of the gut, beneath an intact mucosa. On section the tumours are firm, greyish-yellow or orange in colour. Ulceration of the mucosa occurs in larger and more advanced tumours.

1

G.C.10754

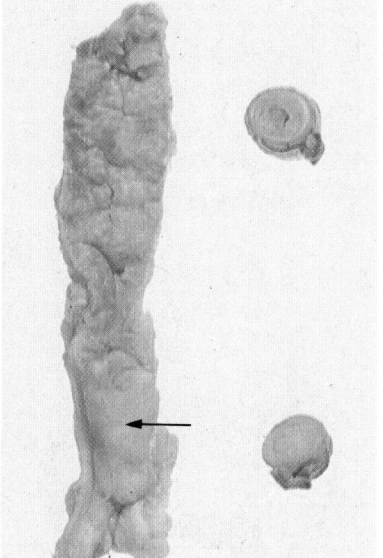

G.C.1441

1 Carcinoid tumour of the appendix. A yellowish rounded carcinoid tumour has encroached upon the lumen and caused acute obstructive appendicitis of the distal end.

2 This preparation exhibits two examples of carcinoid tumour. In the large, long specimen the appendix has been opened and exhibits tumour at the base which shows a degree of submucous infiltration and the distal two-thirds of the appendix shows inflammatory change consequent upon the obstructive element which is present.

The other two small specimens are transverse sections of the appendix of another patient and demonstrate how the lumen of the appendix is completely filled with yellowish homogeneous tumour tissue.

Ileum – carcinoid

3

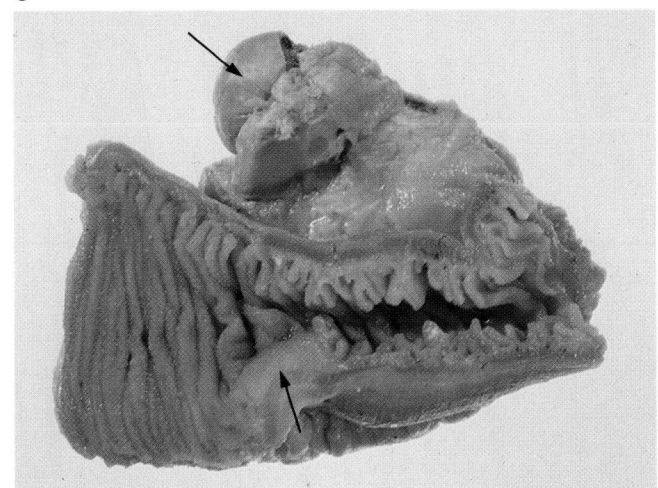

G.C.14646

4

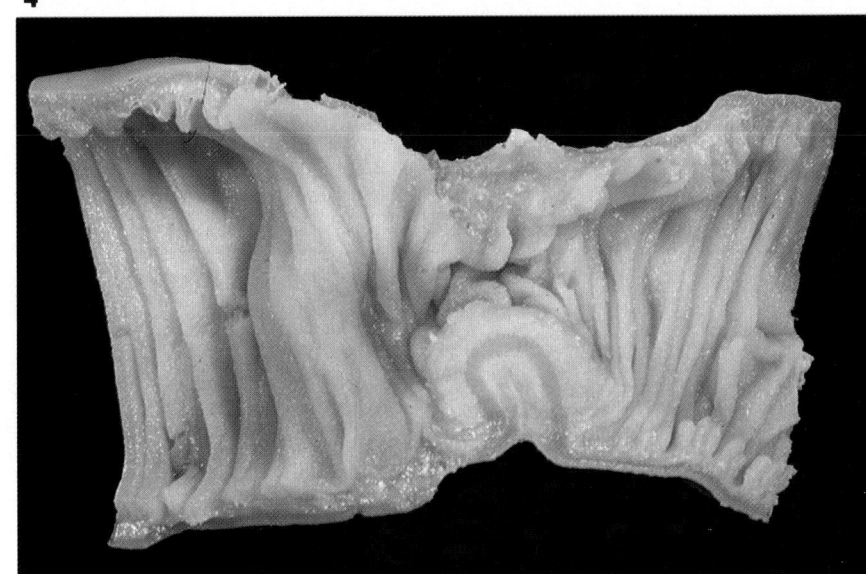

G.C.15180

3 Carcinoid tumour of the ileum resected from a female aged 56 years. The specimen shows a portion of ileum with a distinct constriction approximately 5 cm from one end. The constriction involves one side of the mesenteric aspect of the bowel and is caused by a flat plaque of tumour 1.1 cm in diameter and 5 mm in thickness in the mucosa. Tumour, however, infiltrates through muscularis and appears as a small flat plaque on the serosa. The tumour is yellow and firm. A small lymph node metastasis is present near the mesenteric line of resection and measures 1 cm in diameter. It is enclosed by a fibrous capsule and it lies adjacent to an old calcified lymph node measuring about 2 cm in diameter.

4 A carcinoid tumour of the ileum which caused obstruction in a women aged 62 years.

The yellow tumour infiltrates all coats and has caused obstruction by invaginating the affected part of the wall into the lumen. Proximal to the tumour the bowel is dilated and its mucosa congested. A lymph node on the surface of the ileum contained tumour.

5

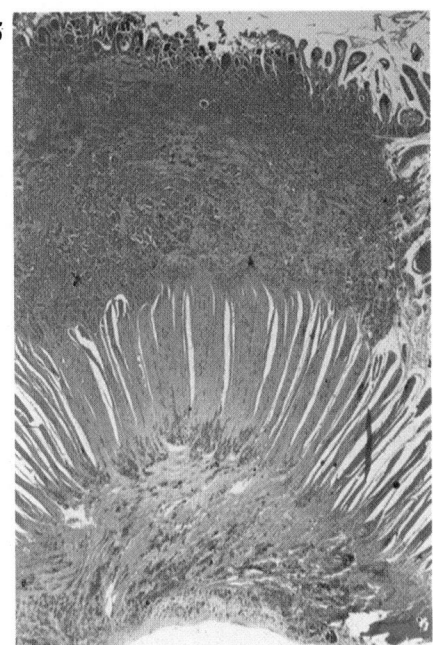

G.C.14646

6

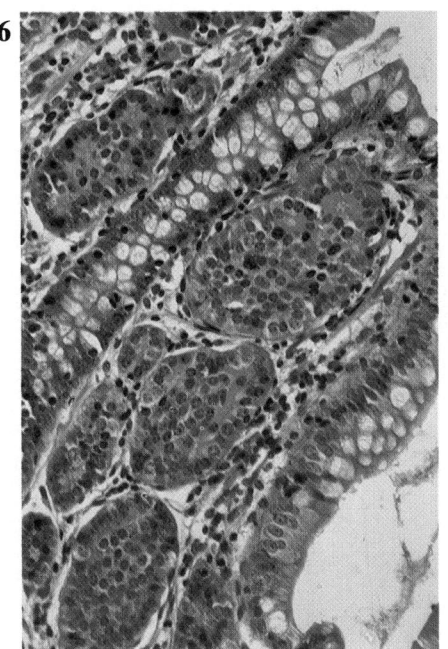

G.C.14646

7

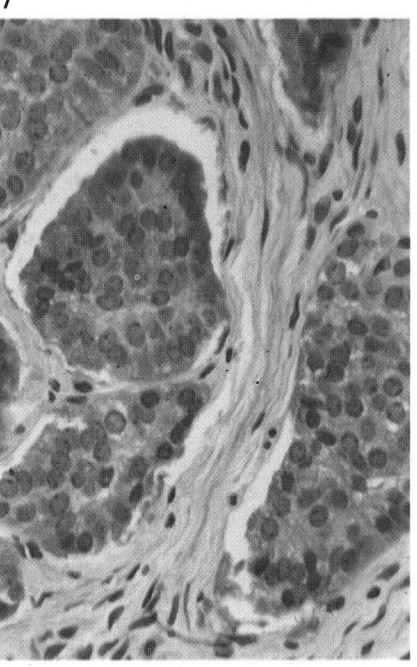

G.C.M.985

5 A portion of the wall showing invasion of all coats by carcinoid tumour. The submucosa is heavily infiltrated and the muscularis hypertrophied and invaginated. Much fibrosis is associated with the tumour in the serosa. *(Red and yellow stain ×12.5)*

6 Same case showing the typical masses of carcinoid tumour cells in the mucosa. *(Red and yellow stain ×250)*

7 Carcinoid tumour. The cytoplasm of many of the cells is crowded with eosinophilic granules. *(H&E ×500)*

387

Carcinoid tumours (Continued)

Microscopic features

Typical sections show solid islands, clusters or cords of compactly arranged, small, rounded tumour cells usually without tubule or mucin formation. Mitotic figures are inconspicuous. The cells show granules which are eosinophilic and give positive argentaffin reaction.

Carcinoid tumours may be recognised in ordinary H&E sections but exhibit distinctive features when special stains are employed.

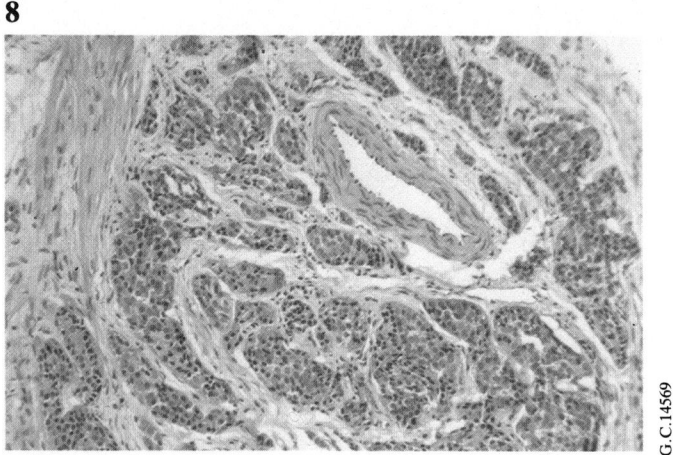

8 Circumscribed groups of tumour cells surround a submucosal vessel and are beginning to infiltrate muscularis. *(H&E ×75)*

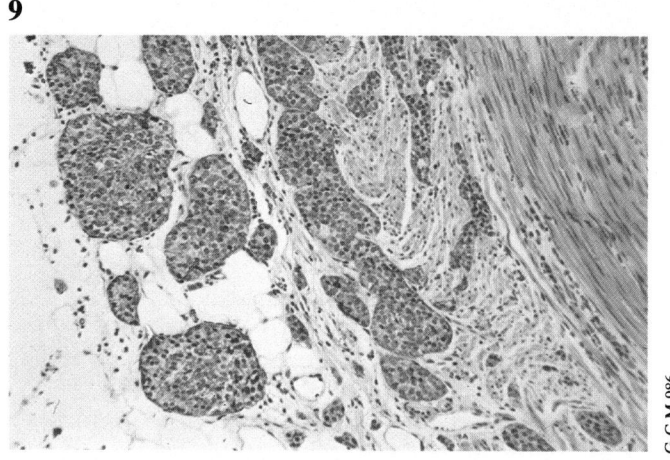

9 The tumour has penetrated muscularis to infiltrate the mesoappendix. *(H&E ×125)*

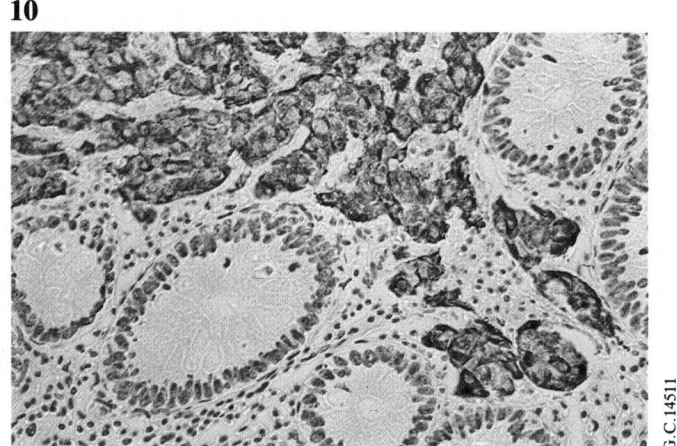

10 The dark silver-impregnated (argyrophil and argentaffin) cells of the carcinoid tumour contrast with the pale cytoplasm of the glandular epithelium. *(Bodian's stain ×250)*

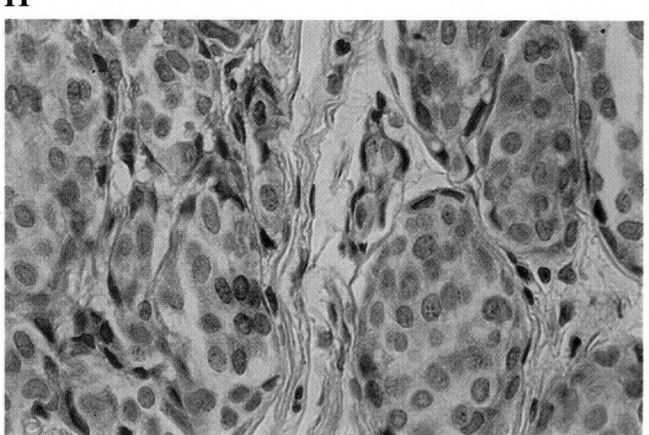

11 The cytoplasmic granules of the tumour cells have stained yellow-brown with a diazonium stain, a positive diazo reaction. *(Fast red salt B ×500)*

Spread

Carcinoid tumours grow slowly. In the narrow appendix they produce symptoms early so that they are met with in the relatively young and are usually removed before spread has occurred. In the small intestine obstruction is late and local infiltration through the muscle coat with involvement of the peritoneum occurs. Lymphatic spread leads to involvement of the mesenteric nodes. Spread to the liver is common and secondary deposits are often considerably larger than the primary.

Other sites

Theoretically carcinoid tumours may develop in any tissue where enterochrom-affin cells are to be found but are uncommon outside the alimentary tract, occurring most often in bronchi and rarely in organs such as ovary, testis and thymus, sites at which teratomas are also sometimes found.

The carcinoid syndrome

In 1952 it was recognised that attacks of diarrhoea, flushing, asthma and signs of cardiac disease could occur in patients with carcinoid tumour. Once metastases reach the liver excessive quantities of 5-hydroxytryptamine (5HT) and kallikrein are secreted into the circulation. In some cases fibrosis of the cusps of the pulmonary and tricuspid valves results and may lead to valvular stenosis. Kallikrein reacts with a serum $\propto$ globulin to produce bradykinin, a vasodilator and powerful smooth muscle stimulant. 5HT is degraded by a hepatic mono-amine oxidase to 5-hydroxyindole acetic acid which can be detected in urine. The syndrome has also been observed in patients with bronchial carcinoma, pancreatic adenomas and teratoma of the ovary and testis.

John Anderson

The appendix commonly points upwards and to the left but it may be retrocaecal or retrocolic passing up behind the caecum and ascending colon being either extra or intraperitoneal, paracaecal or para-ileal, pre-ileal, or it may descend over the brim of the pelvis. Malposition of the appendix to the left iliac fossa is found in a true transposition of the viscera and also in malrotation of the gut.

The appendix is a narrow diverticulum of the caecum and of variable length. It usually arises from the medial posterior aspect of the caecum about 2.5 cm from the ileocaecal valve where the taeniae coli converge to form two complete muscle layers. Rarely there may be a duplication of the appendix while true agenesis is probably unrecorded.

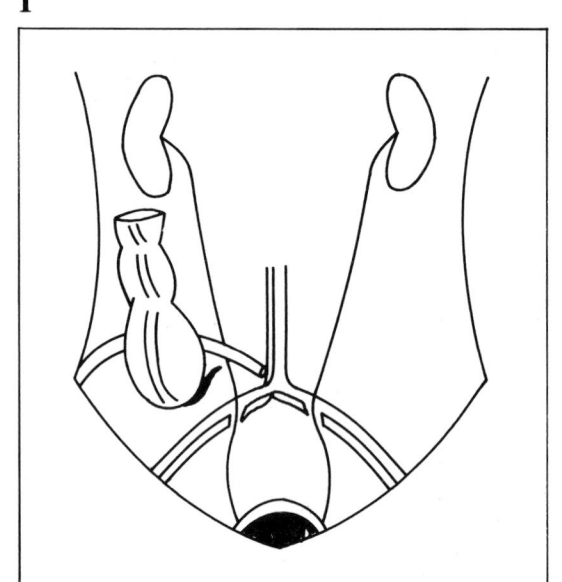

1   Normal.

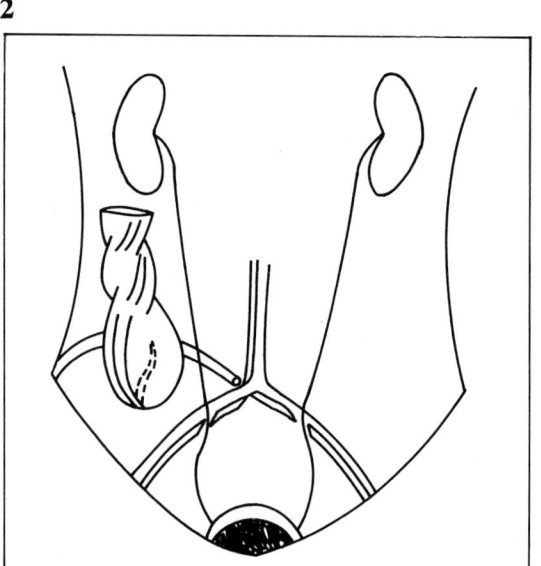

2   Retrocaecal.

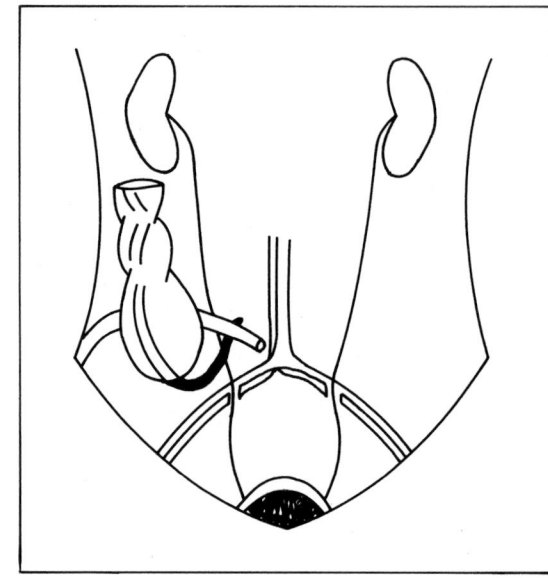

3   Ileal.

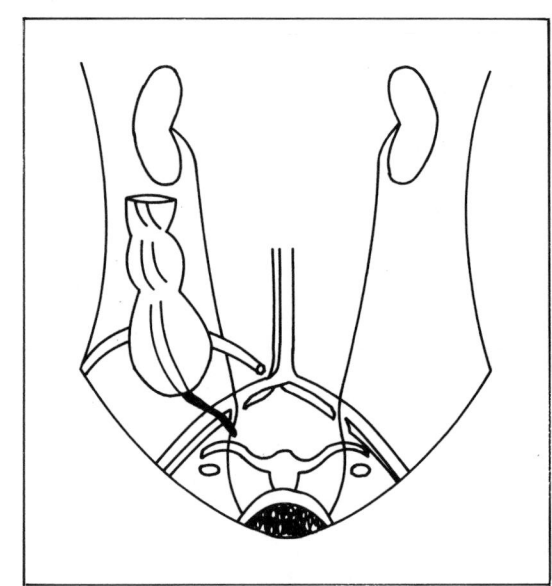

4   Pelvic.

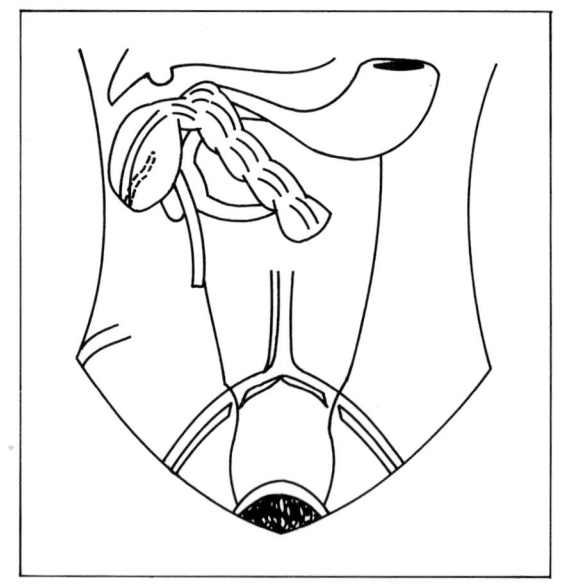

5   Undescended.

Structure

On section the lumen is Y-shaped with a mucous membrane lining consisting of a single layer of columnar epithelium with numerous tubular glands. There are extensive areas of lymphoid tissue below the mucosa arranged partly as a diffuse reticulum and partly as follicles. The mucous membrane acts as the primary barrier against infection but the abundant lymphoid tissue is also a major defence mechanism. The extent and quantity of lymphoid tissue is greatest in childhood but decreases with age probably corresponding to the degree of replacement fibrosis secondary to previous transient inflammatory episodes.

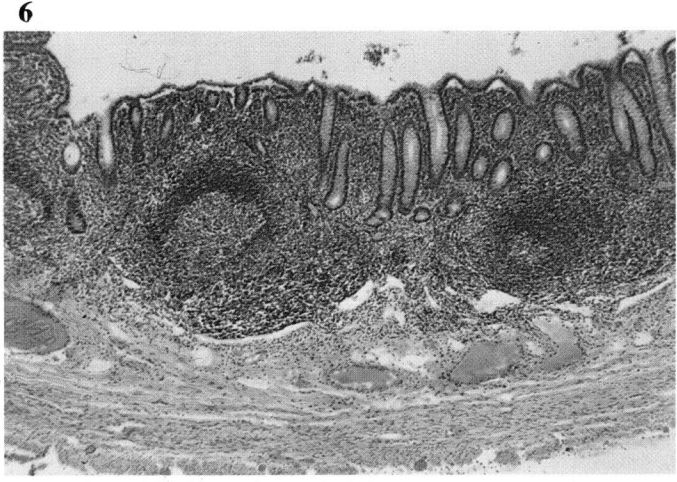

6 Appendix (in childhood). The surface and glandular epithelium is formed by columnar mucin-secreting cells. Lymphoid follicles are prominent in the mucosa. *(H&E ×50)*

Acute appendicitis

Acute appendicitis is a common disease in the United Kingdom, one in 700 of the population being affected in each year. It may occur at any age and there is a steady decline in incidence after the age of 45 years. About 65% of patients are under the age of 30 years and only 5% are aged 60 years or more.

While the aetiology remains obscure it is noted that it appears to be common in industrialised countries and less so in rural communities being exceptionally rare in Asia, Africa and Polynesia unless or until they take to European food. In general it appears to be associated with a low roughage diet and with a high proportion of meat. Overeating, constipation and excessive purgation have been blamed for the high Western incidence. The disease may follow an epidemic pattern but generally in countries with a low incidence it is associated with the fruit season. Thread worms are known to be present in varying frequency in the appendices of children and young adults and may be of aetiological significance.

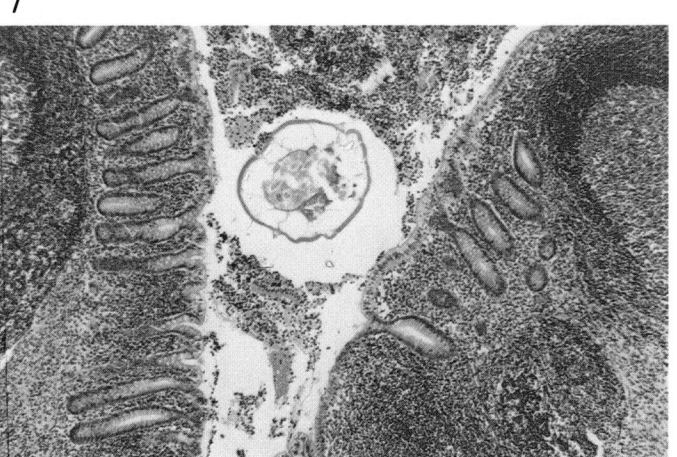

7 Appendix – Enterobius vermicularis. The cross section of a thread worm can be seen in the lumen of the appendix. Occasionally the thread worm penetrates the mucosa and may be found in the substance of the wall. The mucosal lymphoid tissue is hyperplastic. *(H&E ×62.5)*

Acute appendicitis *(Continued)*

Two factors appear to be relevant to the onset of acute appendicitis:
1 Infection
2 Obstruction
It is unlikely, however, that either factor can be responsible on its own.

Infection

Infection usually commences at the bottom of a crypt and extends from the mucosa into the submucosa. There is a progressive inflammatory change which culminates in necrosis of the mucosa, multiple small abscesses within the wall and areas of local haemorrhage and vascular thrombosis. The following organisms are commonly found in the acutely inflamed appendix – *Streptococcus faecalis, viridans* and *pyogenes, Staphylococcus, E. coli* and other coliforms, *Clostridium welchii, Proteus vulgaris* together with bacteriodes. Most of these organisms are derived from the bowel lumen. Infection, especially with streptococci and staphylococci may on occasions be haematogenous as when acute appendicitis occurs during the course of measles or following acute tonsillitis.

Obstruction

Acute obstructive appendicitis has already been described as a form of closed loop intestinal obstruction and reference has been made to the work of D.P.D. Wilkie who first identified this type of appendicitis, described its causation and referred to its high mortality.
The causes of the obstruction are:
(a) a concretion or faecolith lying within the lumen;
(b) a swelling of the intramural lymphoid tissue;
(c) fibrous scarring from previous episodes of inflammation;
(d) acute angulation from peritoneal bands or adhesions;
(e) intraluminal masses of oxyuris vermicularis.

Catarrhal appendicitis

When the obstructive element is minimal or temporary the acute inflammatory phase may resolve with ultimate healing by fibrosis and replacement of the submucosa in varying degree by scar tissue.

8

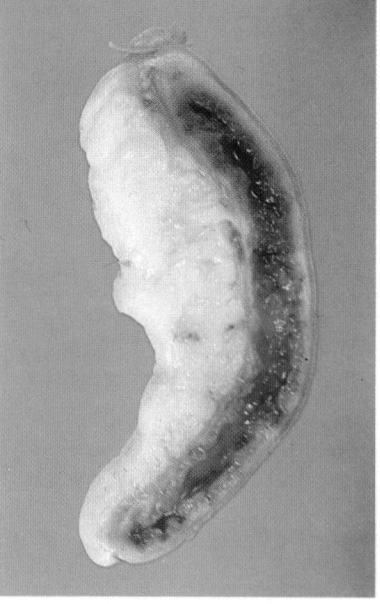

9

8 A typical example of catarrhal appendicitis. Note that the organ is not distended and that the inflammation chiefly affects the mucosa in the whole length of the appendix. The serosa does not show any gross reaction. There is no evidence of concretion or obstruction.

9 Acute appendicitis. Acute inflammatory exudate infiltrates the appendicular wall and covers a mucosal ulcer. *(H&E ×100)*

Obstructive appendicitis

When the obstruction is complete there is progressive local destruction accelerated by local ischaemia from thrombosis and vascular obstruction secondary to an increased intramural tension. The local tissue necrosis will, if localised, result in a perforation of the wall most commonly at the site of the obstructing concretion or if extensive, in gangrenous appendicitis. This process may be hyperacute and perforation occurs within hours of onset.

10

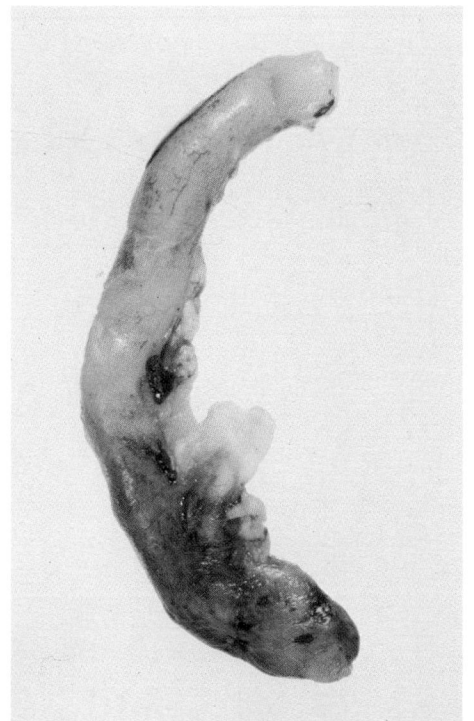

G.C.12118

11

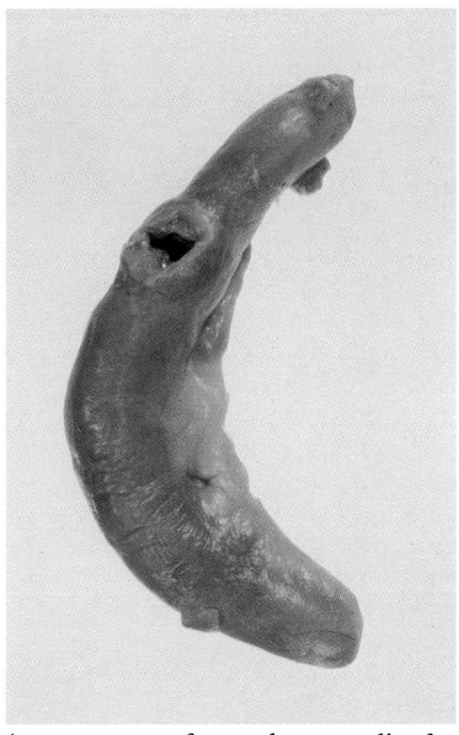

G.C.8196

12

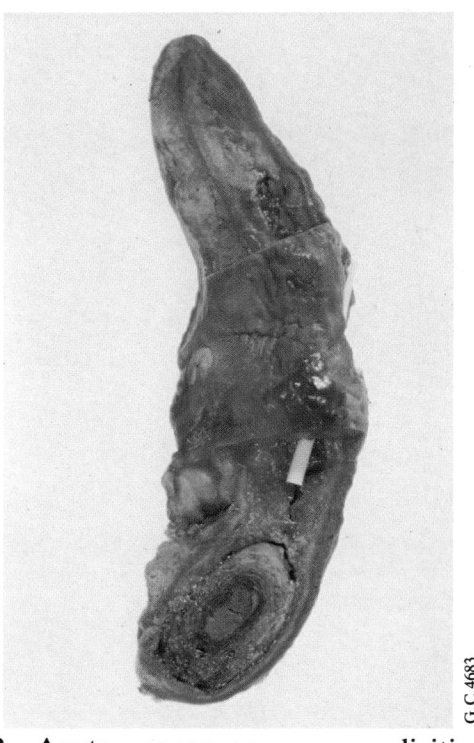

G.C.4683

10 From a male child aged 4 years. This is a typical appendicitis the changes being most marked in the distal half where the peritoneum is acutely congested and covered with a yellowish film of fibrin and the appendix is distended. The swelling at the proximal end of the appendix where there is also slight congestion is the actual site of obstruction of the lumen of the appendix by a small calculus.

11 An acute perforated appendix from a male patient aged 17 years in whom the diagnosis had not been recognised for six days. At operation there was an abscess in the right iliac fossa. The appendix shows a frank perforation close to the base. The appendicular wall is thickened and grossly inflamed but without any adhesion formation. At operation two oval calculi were found in the abscess cavity having escaped via the perforation.

12 Acute gangrenous appendicitis from an adult. The appendix is swollen and inflamed. The serosa is coated with recent exudation and shows several yellow gangrenous patches. The appendicular mesentery is thick. A gangrenous perforation, indicated by a glass rod, has occurred. There is a laminated concretion impacted at the base of the appendix. The mesentery shows inflammation and thrombosis of the vessels.

13

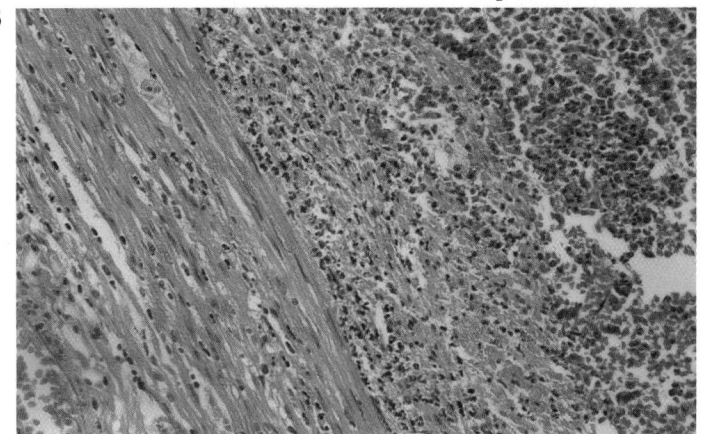

G.C.M.984

13 Gangrenous appendicitis. Part of the muscularis is necrotic and is infiltrated by inflammatory cells. (*H&E ×250*)

Complications

Spread

Following extension of the inflammatory process through the wall leading to gangrene or perforation there is consequent peritonitis, initially localised but later diffuse.

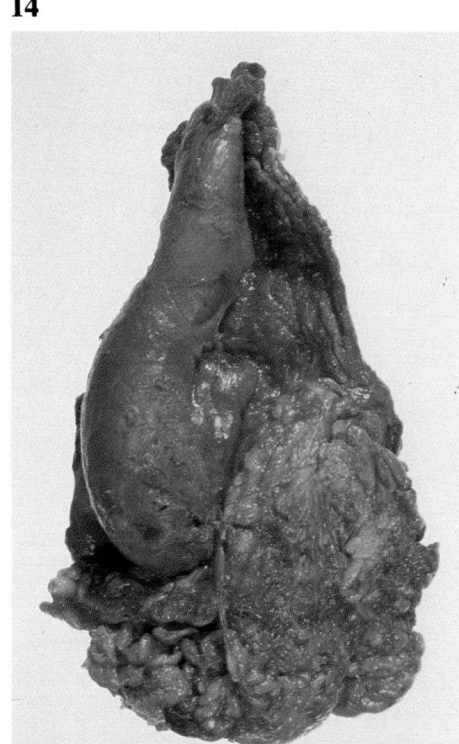

14

14 This specimen demonstrates an acute appendicitis removed from a young adult. The tip of the appendix especially is thick, congested and shaggy and is attached to and practically surrounded by omentum. This is the first stage in the defensive mechanism by which the inflammatory process is limited. This process might well have led to an encapsulated abscess. If the encapsulation were to be delayed the infection could have spread more widely leading even to diffuse peritonitis.

G.C.4675

Appendicular abscesses

Where the appendix lies free in the peritoneal cavity further spread of the infection will be limited by the formation of adhesions between the surrounding loop(s) of intestine and the omentum. The infection may go on to localised abscess formation or resolve.

Where the appendix is retrocaecal in position and the inflammatory process extends through the appendicular wall, the infection may be entirely extraperitoneal or may be intraperitoneal but limited by the fixation of the caecum behind which it lies.

If an abscess forms in this position it becomes therefore strictly localised but expands and if it runs a chronic course may simulate a number of other lesions including carcinoma, tuberculosis, etc.

Where the appendix dips into the pelvis inflammation of the female genitalia or the bladder may result in dysmenorrhoea or cystitis. If the inflammation goes on to abscess formation this will be most readily detected on rectal or vaginal examination.

Variations in the position of the appendix may lead to problems in diagnosis:
1   Where the appendix lies behind the terminal ileum inflammation may lead to a local oedema and paresis. This may simulate an intestinal obstruction. Alternatively the inflammation may cause diarrhoea.
2   If the appendix lies in contact with the ureter it may cause dysuria. Examination of the urine will reveal the presence of both blood and pus cells.
3   Where the appendix is associated with an undescended caecum the manifestations may simulate those of cholecystitis.

Portal pyaemia

Portal pyaemia is a rare and fatal complication. It was, however, known to and described by the surgeons of the 19th century.

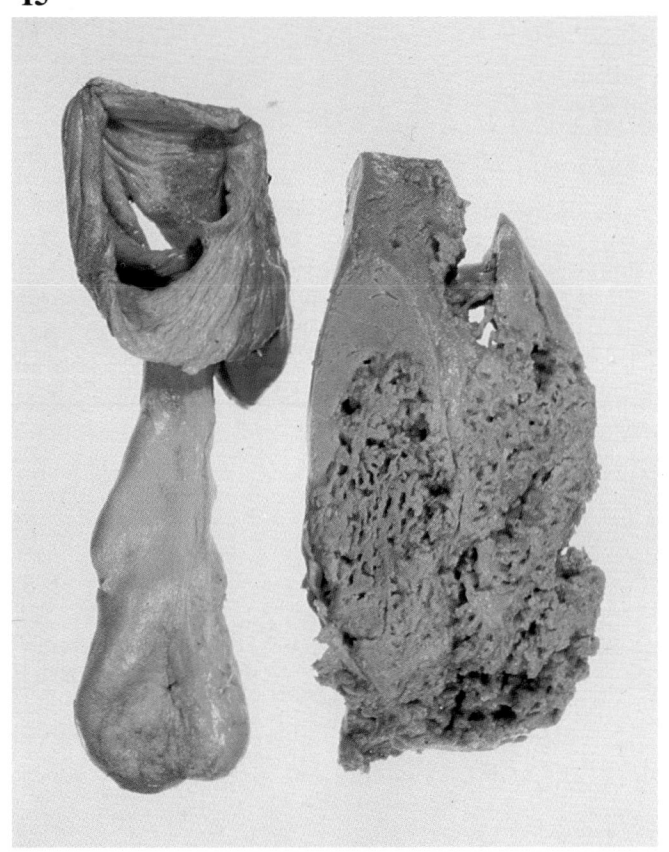

15 This specimen which dates from 1809 illustrates the all too common tragedy observed at that time by disease for which there was no known treatment to the doctors of the day. The patient was a schoolboy aged 11 years who was ill for only 4 days. 'He had symptoms of inflamed bowels with shiverings and costiveness. At post mortem the whole of the appendix caeci vermiformis thickened and ulcerated towards the bottom where it is much enlarged and filled with pus. There was ulceration and suppuration beginning in the interstitial substance of the liver and extending through the greatest part of its substance. The whole of the cavities were filled with purulent matter.'

G.C. 10803

Chronic appendicitis

Chronic appendicitis may result from a chronic inflammation in which there is a persistent low grade infection within the appendix wall and is characterised by a swollen oedematous mucosa with a marked lymphoid hyperplasia. It tends to progress to local or diffuse fibrosis and luminal obliteration. It may also be associated with recurrent episodes of acute obstructive appendicitis usually secondary to a foreign body such as a lead pellet, faecolith, pip or fruit stone, or thread worms.

Although chronic appendicitis has in the past been considered responsible for symptoms of low grade abdominal pain and general ill health, most authorities doubt its relevance in other than recurrent episodes of appendicular colic.

Mortality

The mortality of uncomplicated appendicitis in the United Kingdom has remained stationary for some years at about 0.2%, that of perforated appendicitis with local peritonitis at under 2% while a diffuse appendicular peritonitis is in the order of 5%. In children between 2 and 5 years the mortality in the different types of appendicitis is probably double that of adults but it will reach 30% for those under 2 years of age. Similarly in patients over the age of 70 years the mortality is high being 3 to 4 times that of the younger age group.

Acute obstructive appendicitis carries the gravest risk especially if the rapidity with which perforation occurs is not appreciated on initial examination of the patient.

Mucocoele

16

Obstruction of the lumen of the appendix with little or no associated infection may result in a mucocoele. The appendix becomes distended with a thick tenacious mucous content. The wall becomes thin and the muscle layer may disappear. Usually asymptomatic the mucocoele may rarely rupture into the peritoneal cavity to produce a pseudomyxoma peritonei. As the result of rupture the mucous content is extruded into the peritoneal cavity as whitish gelatinous masses or filament but in such a case there is no evidence of myxoma cell implantation on the exposed peritoneal surface.

16 From a 50 year old female admitted to hospital as a case of probable appendicitis with acute pain in the right iliac fossa where a tender swelling could be palpated. At operation the appendix was found to be enlarged, tense and distended with adhesions to adjacent structures. The appendix contained blood stained mucus. This is a typical mucocoele with minimal inflammatory changes.

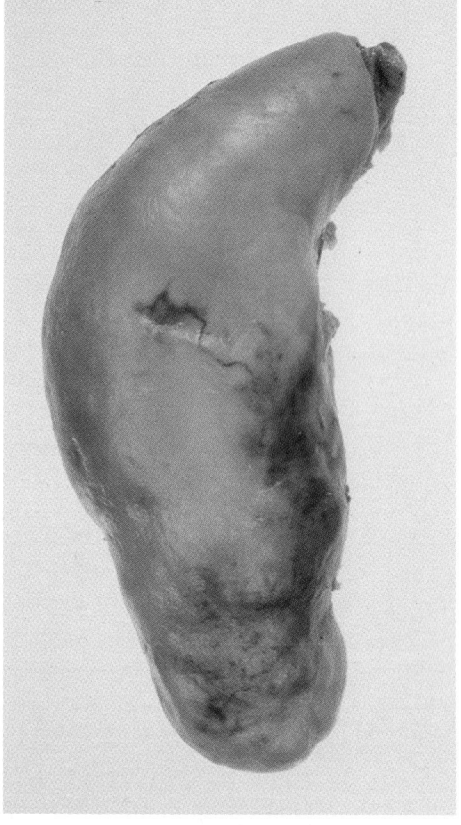

G.C.8503

17

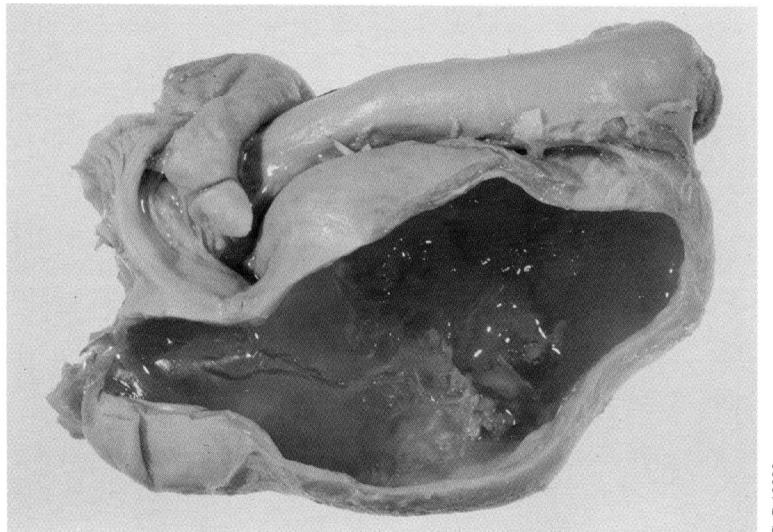

G.C.10099

17 From a female aged 63 years admitted to hospital for recurrent appendicular colic. At operation a mass in the right iliac fossa was mistaken for a tumour and a right colectomy performed. When the mass was opened it was found to contain a large quantity of thick white gelatinous mucus. It was now recognised that the ovoid mass was a grossly enlarged appendix the walls of which were thickened and had become adherent to adjacent parts. There is no evidence of any acute inflammatory reaction or of a neoplasm.

Diverticulosis

18

Multiple acquired diverticula may be found, almost always in association with inflammatory changes.

18 Numerous diverticula are evident. The mucosa has transgressed the muscularis and on reaching the subserosa has dilated into bullous swellings. The wall of these swellings is thin.

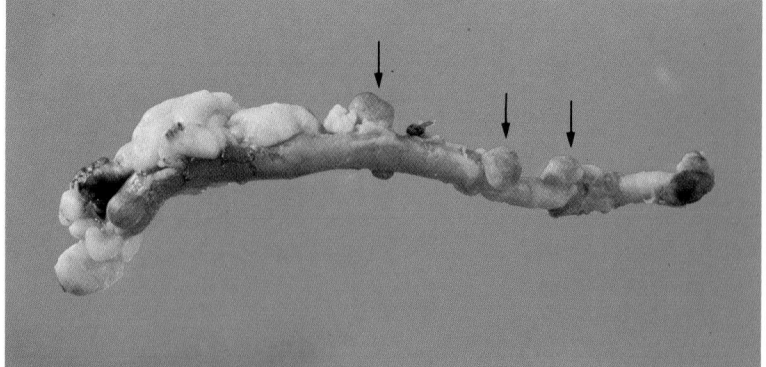

G.C.14331

Foreign bodies

19 and **19a** These are very rare and the accompanying case illustrates an intriguing example in which the appendix was found to be filled with lead shot. The patient, an elderly sportsman, with particular interest in grouse shooting had for many years also enjoyed grouse as an article of diet. It was apparent that the grouse was sometimes eaten together with the shot which had killed the bird and these had come to rest in his appendix. He complained of increasing and recurrent right-sided abdominal pain and the X-ray disclosed the cause of this.

19

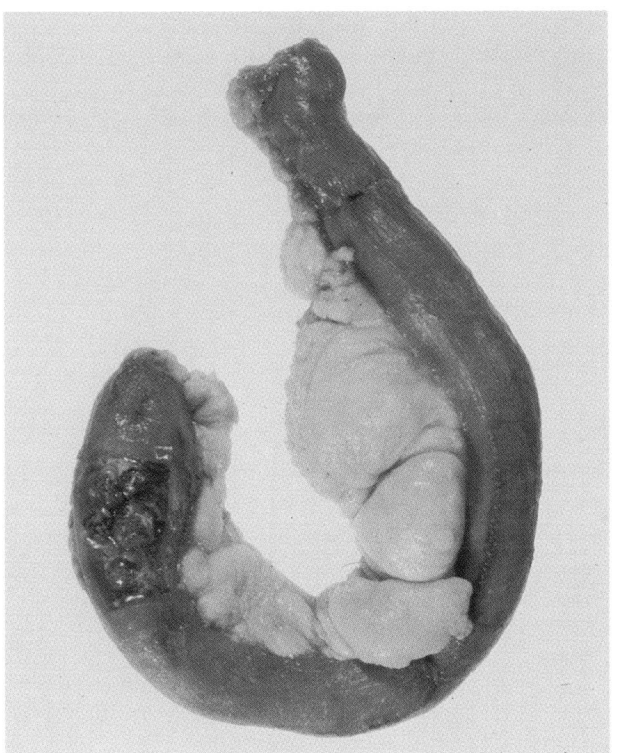

G.C.14421

19a

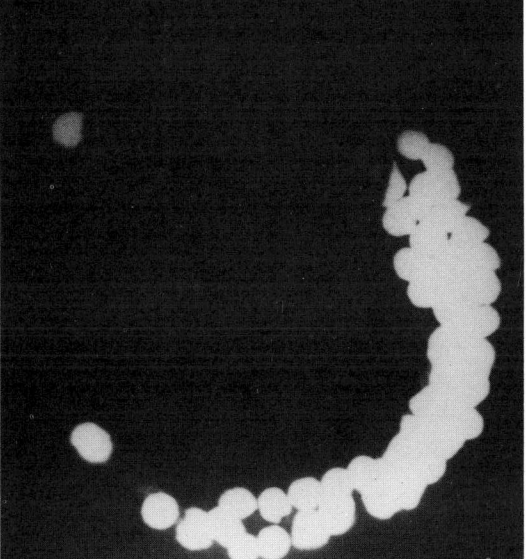

20

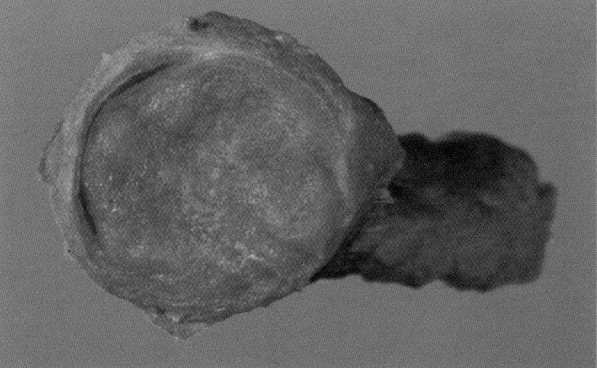

G.C.14646a

Tumours

Tumours of the appendix are rare. The most frequently encountered is the carcinoid tumour which has been described elsewhere (see Section 15 UG). Carcinoid tumours in this situation are usually not associated with evidence of the carcinoid syndrome but occasionally diarrhoea has been noted and may be a minor manifestation of the syndrome.

Adenocarcinoma has also been described elsewhere (see Section 15 U).

Both these tumours are usually associated with some degree of inflammation or obstruction of the appendicular lumen leading to the diagnosis of appendicitis. The true nature of the condition is disclosed at operation or on examination of the appendix after removal.

20 This illustration demonstrates how a carcinoid can almost completely occlude the lumen of the appendix. This therefore predisposes to obstructive appendicitis. The occluding tumour may be so small that the external appearance of the appendix does not suggest a neoplasm but presents the features of the secondary obstruction.

Structure

The liver is a solid organ which lies in the subdiaphragmatic region of the upper abdomen. It is made up of two lobes, a right and a left, the anatomical line of division between the two running from the inferior vena cava on the postero-superior aspect to the fossa for the gallbladder on the inferior surface. The liver has a dual blood supply, from the hepatic artery which is a branch of the coeliac axis and from the portal vein. The total flow through the liver is approximately 1500 ml per minute and the proportional supply is of the order of 20 to 35% arterial to 80 to 65% portal venous depending on the activity of the abdominal viscera, but 60% of the oxygen required by the liver is brought by the hepatic artery. The portal vein carries blood from the whole of the intestine and from the spleen and pancreas to the liver.

Each vessel divides into a right and a left branch for the supply of the corresponding lobe and then subdivides, the subdivisions running together with the bile ductules in the portal triads and in the substance of the liver itself. Finally the mixed blood traverses the sinusoids which are channels lined by the liver cells (hepatocytes) and by cells of the reticulo-endothelial system (Küpffer cells). Drainage from the sinusoids is by the central vein of each lobule through veins of progressively increasing size to the hepatic veins. These are usually three in number, right, middle and left, and drain into the inferior vena cava at or just below the level of the diaphragm.

1

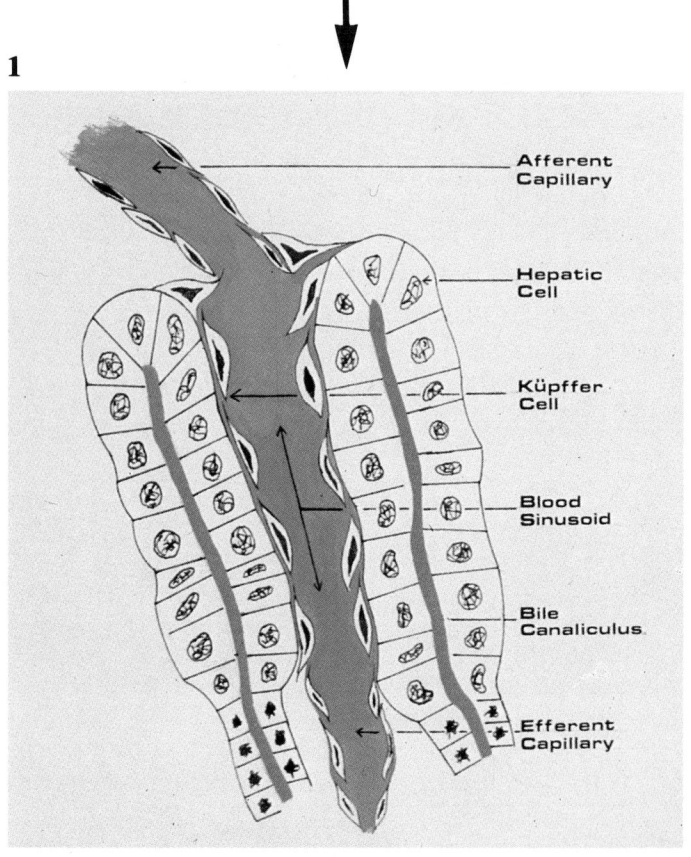

1   Liver – basic structure.

2

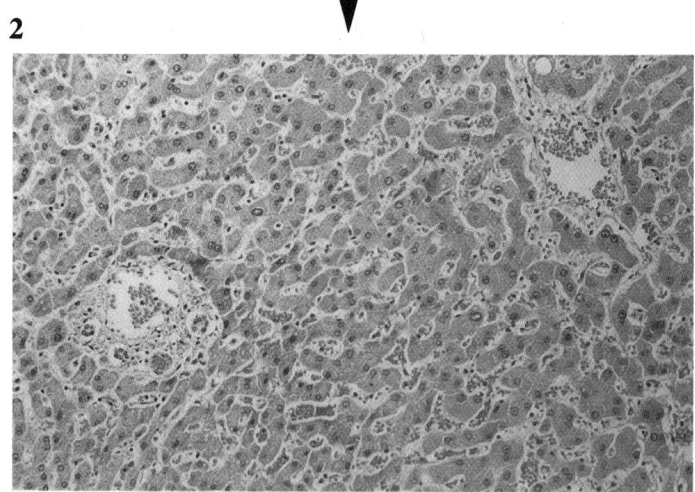

G.C.M.933

2   Part of a liver lobule with a portal tract to the left and a central vein on the right. *(H&E ×125)*

Functions

1 Formation of bile

2 Protein metabolism

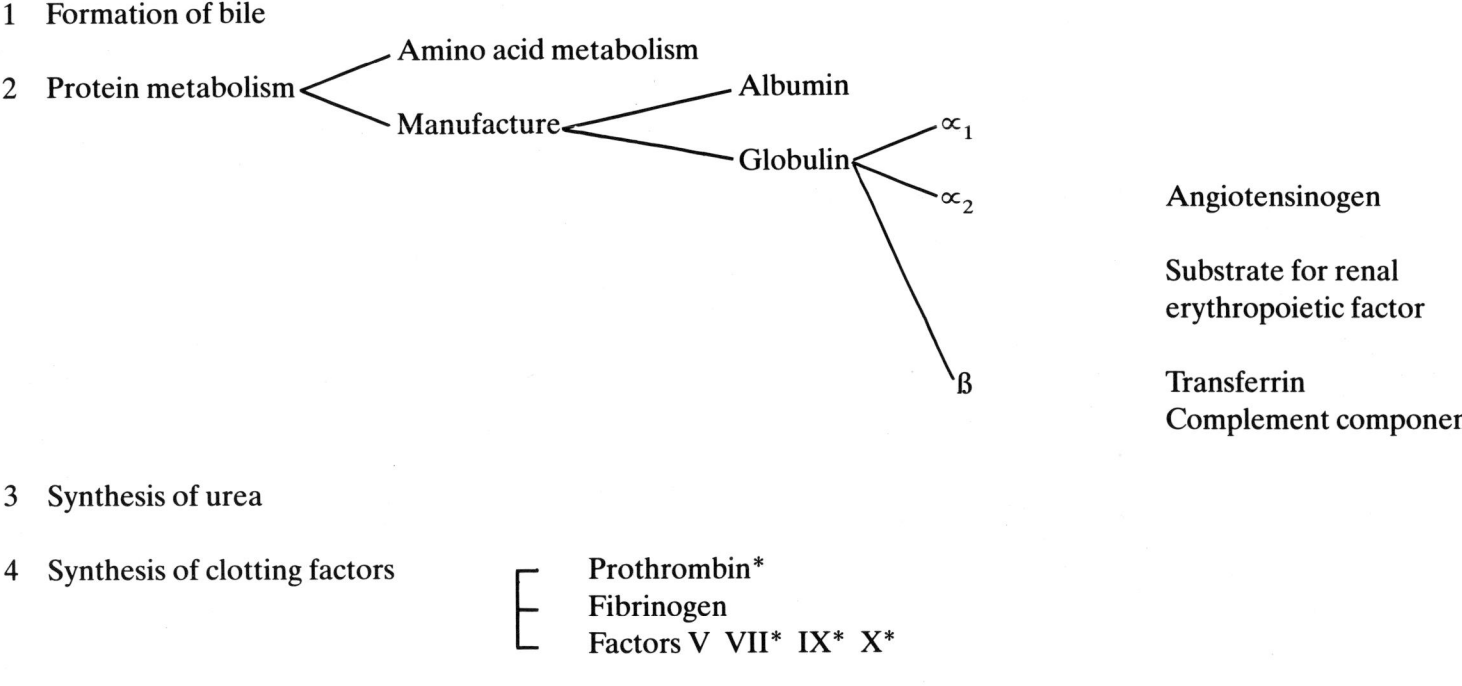

Amino acid metabolism

Manufacture — Albumin

Globulin — α_1

α_2 Angiotensinogen

Substrate for renal erythropoietic factor

β Transferrin
Complement components

3 Synthesis of urea

4 Synthesis of clotting factors

    Prothrombin*
    Fibrinogen
    Factors V VII* IX* X*

    *Requires presence of vitamin K for synthesis

5 Carbohydrate metabolism

    Synthesis and breakdown of glycogen
    Gluconeogenesis

6 Fat metabolism

    Formation of triglycerides
    Formation of pre-β lipoproteins
    Formation and excretion of cholesterol
    Formation of ketone bodies

7 Storage – Vitamins B_{12} ADEK
    Conversion vitamin D $\longrightarrow$ 25 Hydroxycholecalciferol
    Iron and copper

8 Inactivation of hormones

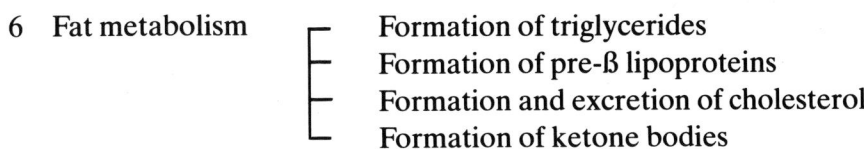

    Adrenal
    Gonadal
    Thyroid
    Peptide hormones: insulin, TSH, ADH

9 Detoxification: drugs and toxins

10 Part of reticulo-endothelial system (Küpffer cells of liver sinusoids)

11 Haematological function in foetus

Bile

Bile is a slightly alkaline fluid secreted continuously by the liver at the rate of 500 to 1000 ml per 24 hours.

Composition of hepatic duct (liver) bile and gallbladder bile

	Liver bile (%)	Gallbladder bile (%)
Water	98	89
Total solids	2.0	11.0
Bile salts	0.7	6.0
Bile pigments	0.2	2.5
Cholesterol	0.06	0.4
Lecithin	0.05 – 0.08	0.2 – 0.5
Inorganic salts	0.7	0.8
pH	8 – 8.6	7 – 7.6

Proteins – albumin, enzymes
— Alkaline phosphatase
— Lactic dehydrogenase

Bile is formed by the secretion of bile acids, inorganic ions and water from the hepatic parenchymal cells into the bile canaliculi, which join to form a continuous three dimensional mesh situated either within the hepatic lobule or near its periphery, closed at one end and draining into larger channels which in turn form bile ducts. In the human liver, the canalicular surface available for movement of water and solute is approximately $10 \, m^2$.

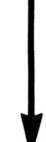

The canaliculus is the primary site of active secretion of conjugated bilirubin, conjugated bile acids, electrolytes and hormonal and drug metabolites.

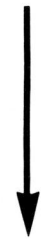

The transport of water, a variety of small solute molecules and the major lipids lecithin and cholesterol are coupled to bile acid transport. Osmotic drive created by the bile acids in the canaliculi may account for the coupled entry of water, while hydrophilic solutes enter by diffusion or bulk flow. The conducting system (bile ductules and ducts) is, however, capable of both secretion and reabsorption of water and inorganic electrolytes.

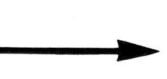

Secretin, gastrin, cholecystokinin and glucagon all have choleretic effects, by acting on the conducting system. Vagal stimulation also increases bile production. Secretion ceases when the pressure in the bile ducts reaches 300 mm H_2O, but this does not normally happen because of the continuous absorption of fluid in the gallbladder.

Bile acids

The two primary bile acids chenodeoxycholic acid and cholic acid are synthesised from cholesterol in the liver. They are then conjugated with glycine or taurine and secreted into the biliary tract where they combine with cholesterol and phospholipid as complexes called micelles. Their action is to aid the emulsification of fat, to take part in the activation of lipases and also to combine with the digested lipid fractions (FFA & monoglycerides) to form the water soluble micelles from which the lipids can be absorbed across the intestinal mucosal cell membrane. The bile salt is split off just prior to absorption. Ninety to 95% of the bile salts are absorbed from the terminal ileum by an active transport process, the remainder being deconjugated by bacteria in the distal ileum and colon. Absorption of part of the deconjugated primary bile acids occurs in both ileum and colon, the remainder being acted on by the intestinal micro-organisms to form secondary bile acids (deoxycholic acid from cholic acid and lithocholic acid from chenodeoxycholic acid). Secondary bile acids are partially reabsorbed in the colon by passive diffusion and the rest are excreted in the faeces (400–600 mg/day).

The synthesis of bile acids is regulated primarily by a negative feedback effect of enterohepatically circulated bile acids on the hepatic enzyme 7 $\propto$ hydroxylase. If bile acids are removed by either cholestyramine or a biliary fistula, activity of the 7 $\propto$ hydroxylase is increased and hence the synthesis of bile acids.

3

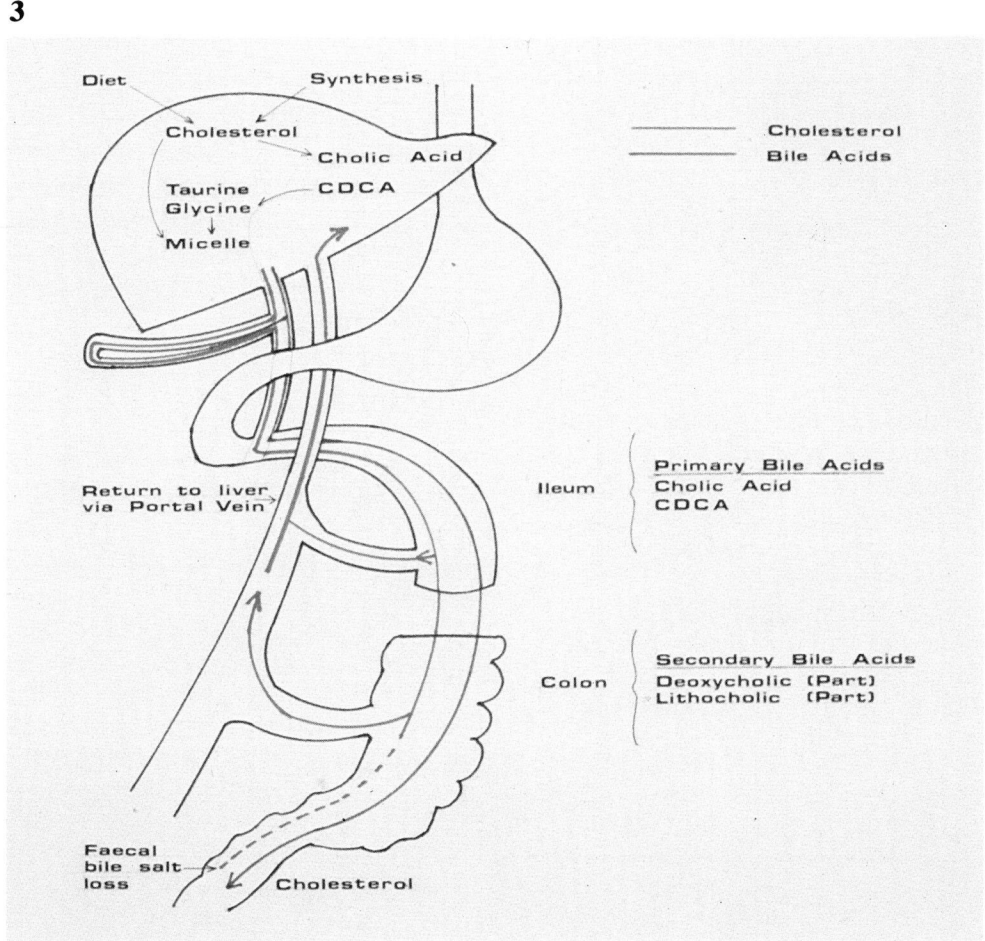

Bile *(Continued)*

Phospholipids

A mixture of substances, the most significant being lecithin (90% of phospholipids). Bile acids in the enterohepatic circulation enhance the synthesis and secretion of lecithin which is predominantly in the liver. Dietary lecithin probably has little effect upon the size of the biliary lecithin pool.

Cholesterol

The cholesterol in bile is derived from the diet and hepatic synthesis from acetate. Bile acids in the entero-hepatic circulation exert a negative feedback action thereby regulating the synthesis of cholesterol. Increased hepatic production is seen in biliary obstruction, when there is loss of bile from the body (biliary fistula), following injury, and during thyroxin medication. Conversely, the secretion of cholesterol and especially of lecithin falls when there is a reduction in the amount of circulating bile acids returning to the liver as a result of increased intestinal bile salt loss.

Admirand and Small produced a triangular co-ordinate graph to demonstrate the interrelationship of the three biliary lipid components. Along the sides of the equilateral triangle are plotted the molar percentages of bile salts, cholesterol and phospholipid (lecithin) as shown.

Biliary micelles

Cholesterol is insoluble in water and to achieve solubility in aqueous bile it is combined with bile salts to form complexes called micelles. The centre of the micelle is rich in hydrocarbon and acts as a solvent which will dissolve fat. Bile salts can render soluble 3 mol of cholesterol per 100 mol bile salt.

The phospholipid lecithin (phosphatidylcholine) also has a hydrophilic residue and when present with bile salts and water an enlarged micelle is formed with an enhanced ability to render soluble cholesterol compared with micelles formed from bile salts alone.

4

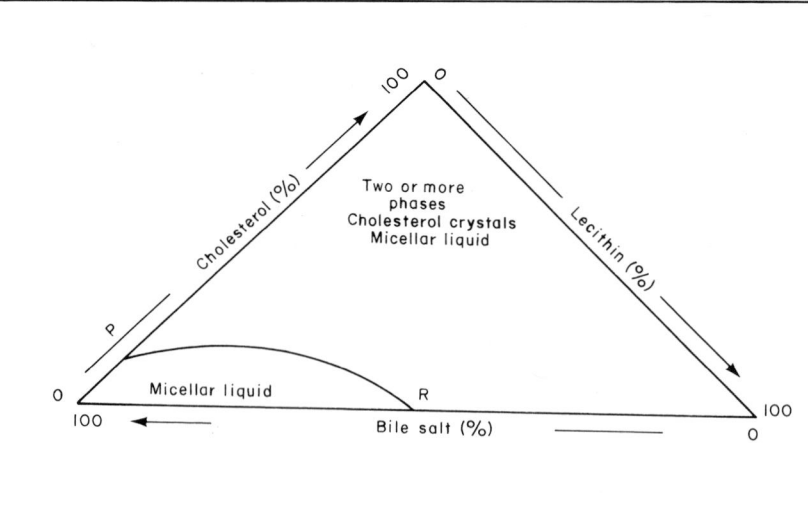

The concentration of cholesterol, lecithin and bile salts can be represented by a point on the triangular co-ordinate graph. Line P R indicates the maximum solubility limit. When bile contains cholesterol in solution in a micellar state, the point on the graph lies below line P R and the bile is unsaturated with cholesterol.

When bile contains a large amount of cholesterol in proportion to the concentration of bile salts and lecithin, the micelles are unable to render soluble all the cholesterol and the bile is saturated or supersaturated and the point for that bile lies above line P R.

Around the line P R is a metastable labile zone of saturation. In this zone cholesterol can exist in one of three phases micellar, liquid crystalline or solid crystalline. The liquid crystalline phase is itself unstable, the cholesterol either returning to micelles or precipitating as cholesterol crystals, the latter occurring more readily with increasing distances above the line P R. Saturated bile is a pre-requisite for gallstone formation (lithogenic bile). The lipid composition of hepatic bile has a diurnal variation, with normal patients secreting a lithogenic hepatic bile at certain times and especially when the bile salt secretion rates are low such as during the overnight fasting state. The maximum secretion levels occur during the day when the bile salt pool is circulating, whereas during the night most of the bile is in the gallbladder with a reduced bile salt and phospholipid secretion. Cholesterol secretion is less dependent upon bile salt return to the liver, hence hepatic bile may be transiently lithogenic, even in normal subjects. The ratio of bile acids and lecithin to cholesterol can be influenced by diet and one high in cholesterol can produce a saturated bile in man, there being little doubt that a diet containing fat, sugar and no dietary vegetable fibres appears to predispose to formation of gallstones. However, most diets contain an excess of refined carbohydrate which suppresses bile salt production, which in turn reduces the bile salt pool and consequently the amount of bile salts in bile.

Obesity has been suspected of contributing to the formation of gallstones, since the saturation of gallbladder bile with cholesterol is significantly higher in obese than in non-obese persons. Women on oral contraceptives also have gallbladder bile which is significantly more saturated with cholesterol than that during the normal menstrual cycle.

Vagotomy has been shown to cause a reduction in secretion of the bile salt fraction of the bile compared with both phospholipid and cholesterol, which in turn leads to a reduction in the ability of the bile to render the cholesterol soluble.

Bile *(Continued)*

Bile pigment

This occurs in the cells of the reticuloendothelial system (liver, spleen, bone marrow)

Blood stream

Liver cell

Biliary tract

Terminal ileum and large intestine

Faeces

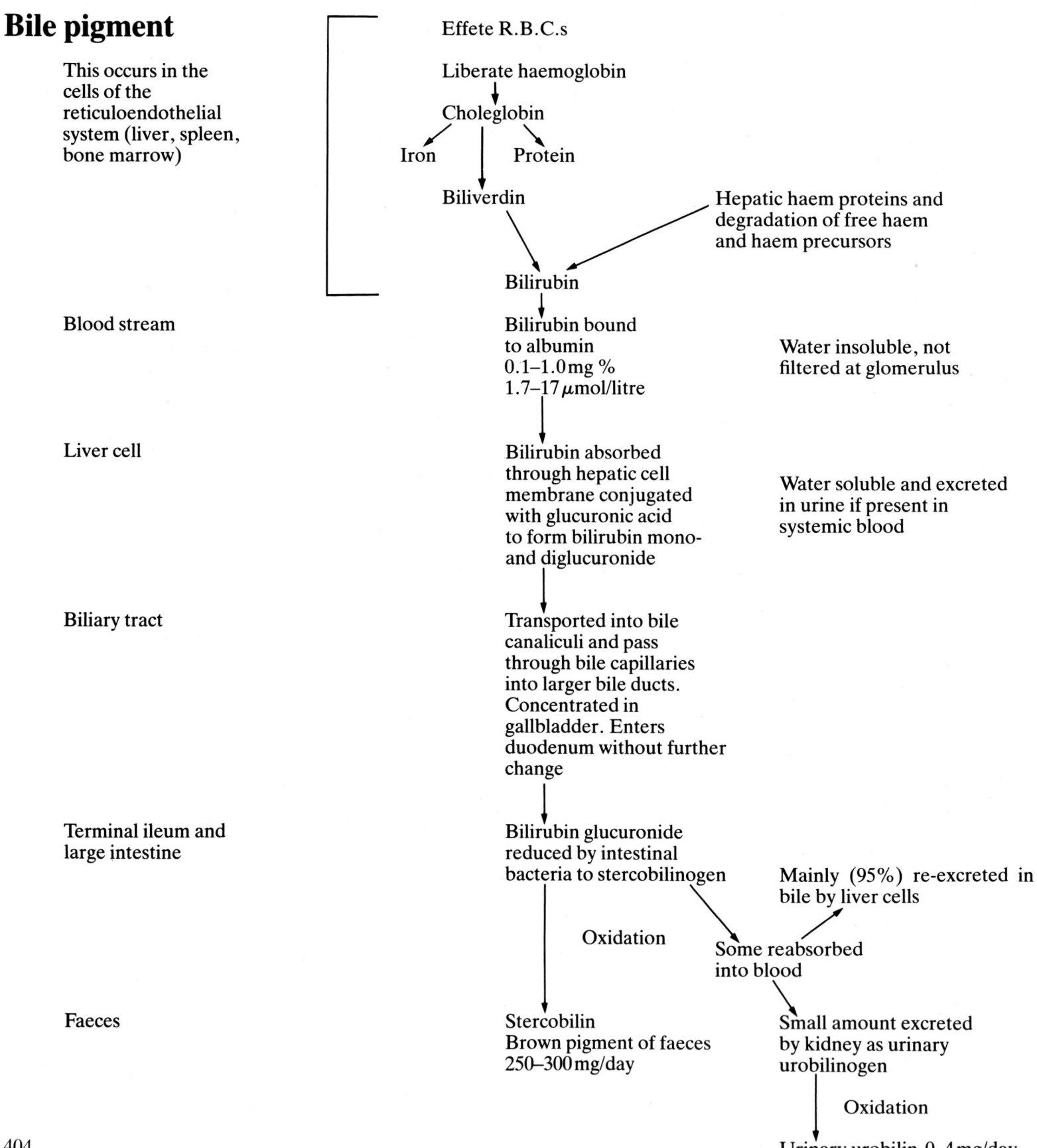

Effete R.B.C.s

Liberate haemoglobin

Choleglobin

Iron   Protein

Biliverdin

Hepatic haem proteins and degradation of free haem and haem precursors

Bilirubin

Bilirubin bound to albumin
0.1–1.0 mg %
1.7–17 μmol/litre

Water insoluble, not filtered at glomerulus

Bilirubin absorbed through hepatic cell membrane conjugated with glucuronic acid to form bilirubin mono- and diglucuronide

Water soluble and excreted in urine if present in systemic blood

Transported into bile canaliculi and pass through bile capillaries into larger bile ducts. Concentrated in gallbladder. Enters duodenum without further change

Bilirubin glucuronide reduced by intestinal bacteria to stercobilinogen

Mainly (95%) re-excreted in bile by liver cells

Oxidation

Some reabsorbed into blood

Stercobilin
Brown pigment of faeces
250–300 mg/day

Small amount excreted by kidney as urinary urobilinogen

Oxidation

Urinary urobilin 0–4 mg/day

Jaundice

Jaundice, which is a yellow staining of the tissues, occurs whenever the plasma bilirubin is significantly higher than $20\,\mu$mol/litre. At $51\,\mu$mol/litre it is clinically obvious in the sclera, skin and palatal mucosa. The seriousness of jaundice depends not on the hue of the skin but on the nature of the underlying pathological process. One serious complication which is rapidly fatal – kernicterus – is due to the staining of the lipids of the basal nuclei by excess lipid soluble unconjugated bilirubin and is a complication of severe jaundice in premature and neonatal infants.

The plasma bilirubin can be elevated because of:
1 An increased rate of production due to haemolysis.
2 Impaired transit through the liver cells due either to specific defects in the mechanism of uptake, transport and conjugation or to liver cell damage.
3 Reduced rate of excretion (a) because of obstruction of the bile canaliculi (intrahepatic cholestasis) or (b) due to obstruction of the large bile ducts (extrahepatic cholestasis).

Haemolytic (pre-hepatic) jaundice

Causes: (1) Abnormal antibodies (a) Rh haemolytic disease of newborn
  (b) Incompatible blood transfusion
  (c) Autoimmune haemolytic anaemia
(2) Defects of R.B.C. (a) Abnormal haemoglobin (sickle cell)
  (b) Abnormal haemoglobin metabolism (Thalassaemia)
  (c) Abnormalities in shape (Spherocytosis, elliptocytosis, megaloblasts in pernicious anaemia)
(3) Extraneous haemolysins (Malaria)

There is increased R.B.C. breakdown with increased production of bilirubin which overloads the liver conjugating mechanism. The patient is anaemic but only slightly jaundiced because the normal liver can rapidly clear large amounts of bile pigment from the blood. Although the plasma bilirubin (unconjugated form) is elevated it seldom exceeds 85 to $170\,\mu$mol/litre (5 to 10 mg%) except in Rh haemolytic disease of the newborn where there is intense jaundice and possible kernicterus. A persistent reticulocytosis is evidence of increased formation of red cells. The dark colour of the stools is due to excess stercobilin resulting from increased haemoglobin breakdown. There is a raised level of urobilinogen in the urine because of increased absorption of stercobilinogen from the intestine. There is no increased reabsorption of conjugated bilirubin and thus no bilirubinuria. There is no retention of bile salts so there is no pruritus. The increased concentration of bilirubin in the bile may lead to the formation of pigment calculi.

Jaundice *(Continued)*

Hepatocellular (hepatic) jaundice

Causes: Neonatal jaudice
Congenital hyperbilirubinaemia
Liver cell destruction
- Infections – Acute infectious hepatitis
  Homologous serum jaundice
  Weil's disease
- Chemical Toxins Carbon tetrachloride, phosphorus, Iproniazid
- Secondary to prolonged biliary obstruction

Intrahepatic cholestasis*
- associated with viral hepatitis
- drugs – phenothiazines, methyl testosterone, oral contraceptives
- late pregnancy – idiopathic cholestasis
  ? hormonal origin
- Cholangitis
- Biliary cirrhosis
- Infiltration of liver   Hodgkin's disease
  Malignancy
- Intrahepatic biliary atresia

*Cholestasis – a syndrome associated with failure of bile to reach the duodenum. Frequently associated with liver cell destruction. Can be due to intra and extra hepatic causes.

Neonatal jaundice

In the first few days of life there is a deficiency of glucuronyl transferase, an enzyme necessary for conjugation of bilirubin. There is an increased bilirubin load because of haemolysis of some foetal R.B.C. and a defective uptake of bilirubin into the hepatocytes by the Y protein. Hepatic excretion is also probably impaired. All of these effects lead to a rise in plasma unconjugated bilirubin level and 'physiological' jaundice of the newborn (Icterus neonatorum). Plasma bilirubin level rarely exceeds 204 μmol/litre (12 mg%). These effects are accentuated in premature infants. When Rh haemolytic disease is also present, kernicterus can easily follow. Breast fed infants may develop jaundice as milk contains the steroid pregnanediol which inhibits glucuronyl transferase.

Congenital hyperbilirubinaemias

In Gilbert's disease, there is a defect in uptake of bilirubin into the cell and a reduction in the conjugating enzyme. This enzyme is also deficient in the Crigler–Najjar syndrome. In both the above conditions the plasma bilirubin is in the unconjugated form and there is mild jaundice. There is no bilirubin in the urine and the faecal pigments are normal or reduced depending upon the severity of enzyme deficiency.

A defect in the failure of transport of conjugated bilirubin into the canaliculi leads to regurgitation of bilirubin glucuronide into the plasma and icterus (the Dubin–Johnson syndrome). The urine contains bilirubin glucuronide and the faeces are pale due to lack of stercobilin. In jaundice due to enzyme deficiency only bilirubin in one form or other is retained in the blood; bile salts are not affected.

Hepatocellular jaundice

Hepatocellular jaundice is complex. It can be due either to a failure of the conjugating mechanism in the liver cells or to obstruction to the transport of bilirubin from cells to canaliculi or from the canaliculi (intra hepatic cholestasis). In a single disease, either or both of these disorders may be present. There is a decreased R.B.C. survival time in liver failure, leading to an increased bilirubin load. Liver cell damage impairs conjugation, disruption of liver structure allows regurgitation. There is jaundice due to a mixture of unconjugated and conjugated bilirubin in the blood (usually more conjugated in the early stages of liver disease such as viral hepatitis since the obstructive element predominates). Bilirubin glucuronide is present in the urine which is dark in colour. There is varying depression of faecal stercobilinogen and the stools are pale. Later there is greatly increased urine urobilinogen, because the diseased liver cells may be unable to excrete the stercobilinogen reabsorbed from the intestine. This leads to an increased excretion of urobilinogen in the urine, even though the hepatic excretion of bilirubin conjugates is itself impaired and the amount of stercobilinogen able to contribute to the entero-hepatic circulation of stercobilinogen is reduced. In hepatic jaundice excess urobilinogen can appear in the urine at the same time that bilirubinuria is present. If the obstruction to bile outflow is complete, no stercobilinogen is formed in the intestine and the enterohepatic circulation of stercobilinogen ceases, leading to the absence of urobilinogen from the urine. In hepatic jaundice with liver cell damage and intra hepatic cholestasis, itching occurs early and then ceases.

Obstructive (post-hepatic) jaundice

Extra hepatic cholestasis

Causes: 1 Obstruction of the common bile duct by calculi
          2 Obstruction by carcinoma of the bile duct or head of pancreas
          3 External pressure on bile duct by tumour or glands
          4 Congenital atresia of the main bile ducts in the newborn

Obstruction by calculus begins suddenly with severe pain following which the patient is jaundiced, the depth of which often fluctuates because the obstruction is intermittent. Associated cholangitis and fever are common. Obstruction by carcinoma is preceded by a period of failing health, and variable amounts of pain, while the jaundice when it appears steadily deepens.

Jaundice *(Continued)*

In complete obstruction of the bile duct the consequences of biliary obstruction result from:
    (a) Retention in the body of the constituents of bile
    (b) Exclusion of bile from the intestine
    (c) Distension of the bile ducts

(a) Obstruction of the biliary system leads to regurgitation of bilirubin glucuronides and bile salts into the blood with consequent jaundice and as the plasma level of water soluble bilirubin glucuronide rises, it is excreted into the urine. The retained conjugated bilirubin is harmless. Absence of the bile pigments from the intestine leads to putty coloured stools and as no stercobilinogen is formed in the intestine none is reabsorbed and there is no urobilinogen in the urine. Retained bile salts lead to itching of the skin which lasts several days and then ceases although the jaundice may deepen. The reason for this may be that when reabsorption of bile salts from the intestine finally ceases, their concentration in the blood falls as the ability of the liver to make new bile salts is limited and may not exceed the excretory capacity of the kidneys. Hypercholesterolaemia may occur due to increased production by the liver and this can lead to cutaneous xanthomata.

(b) The absence of bile salts from the intestine interferes with the digestion and absorption of fat leading to steatorrhoea with bulky offensive stools and loss of weight. Malabsorption of fat leads to malabsorption of the fat soluble vitamins with consequent deficiency of vitamins ADE and K. Deficiency of vitamin K leads after 3 to 5 weeks to a risk of haemorrhage, and deficiency of vitamin D and calcium leads to a combination of osteomalacia and osteoporosis.

(c) When the pressure in the biliary system reaches 30 cm water, secretion of bile ceases. There is distension of the biliary tree and if the obstruction is prolonged, the back pressure of the dammed up bile causes hepatocellular damage.

In long-standing obstruction the bile within the ducts undergoes change. Due to the increased pressure, the liver cells cease bile production, the bile salts are absorbed and there is a replacement of the bile by mucus – white bile.

Post operative jaundice

Many factors are involved:
    (a) Hepatic necrosis following a period of shock
    (b) Hepatitis due to drugs or halothane
    (c) R.B.C. destruction in areas of bleeding
    (d) Haemolysis of transfused R.B.C.

Summary of bile pigment changes in jaundice

Type	Serum bilirubin	Bilirubin glucuronide	Faecal colour	Urine bilirubin glucuronide	Urobilinogen
Haemolytic	++	Normal	Dark	0	+ to ++
Obstructive	+	++	Pale	++	0
Hepatocellular (acute)	+	++	Variable	+	++

M.O. Wright

Vascular abnormalities

The anatomy of the extrahepatic portal system seldom shows variation. However, in 12% of subjects the arterial supply to the right lobe of the liver comes wholly or in part through a separate artery from the superior mesenteric artery which runs to the liver in the free edge of the lesser omentum to the right of and posterior to the common bile duct. A branch of the left gastric artery may go to the left lobe.

The hepatic artery can usually be ligated with impunity proximal to the origin of the gastroduodenal artery. Emboli are very uncommon probably because of the anatomy of origin from the coeliac axis. Occlusion of peripheral intrahepatic branches of the artery is most often due to polyarteritis nodosa which may cause small ischaemic infarcts.

1

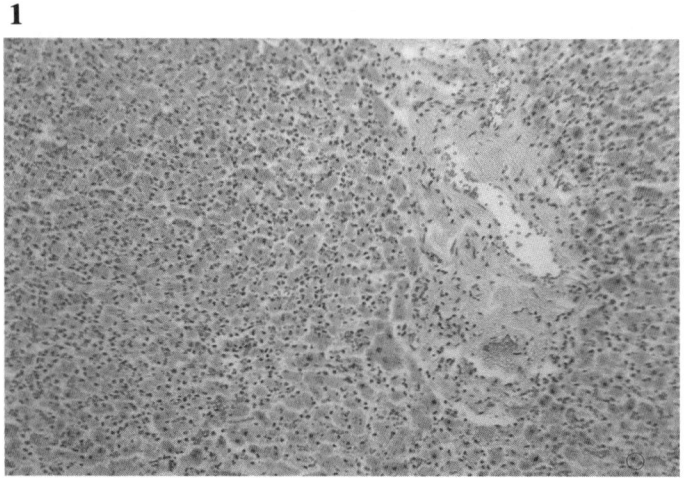

1 Infarction in case of polyarteritis nodosa. Most of the liver cells to the left of the portal tract are necrotic, the cytoplasm is eosinophilic and the nuclei pyknotic. Inflammatory cells infiltrate the area. *(H&E ×125)*

Occlusion of the portal vein may be acute or chronic. In acute occlusion there is stasis, hyperaemia, hypoxia and patchy or more widespread infarction of the gastro-intestinal tract. Slower occlusion allows the development of a porta-systemic collateral circulation which protects the viability of the bowel but is part of the syndrome of portal hypertension.

The liver shows a degree of atrophy with a slight increase in fibrous tissue.

Chronic venous congestion (CVC)

The commonest cause of CVC is congestive cardiac failure. The congestion occurs around central veins. In episodes of peripheral circulatory failure it is often associated with necrosis or atrophy of centrilobular cells eventually resulting in lobular distortion and fibrosis. When CVC is severe and prolonged fibrous portal tracts link up and hepatic cirrhosis results.

2

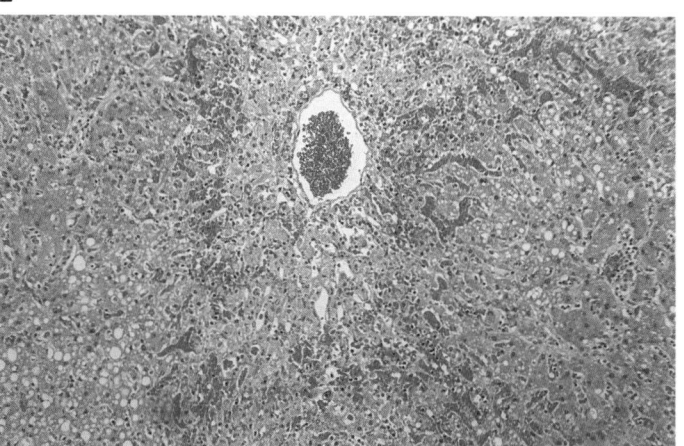

2 Chronic venous congestion. In this case of cardiac failure the central vein is dilated and the necrotic centrilobular cells are surrounded by a zone of dilated sinusoids. Only the periportal cells are relatively normal. *(H&E ×100)*

Other forms of CVC

The main hepatic veins may be occluded by thrombus or tumour (Budd–Chiari syndrome). The tributaries may be involved in veno-occlusive disease following the ingestion of the hepato-toxic alkaloids of herbs such as Senecio and Crotallaria. Endophlebitis of the central veins and congestion of the sinusoids occurs. In severe cases the liver is much enlarged, 'weeps' on its surface, the sinusoids are dilated and centrilobular necrosis and fibrosis may occur.

Rupture of the liver

The liver may be injured by blunt trauma or by penetrating wounds. Blunt trauma may cause contusion, fragmentation of substance especially near the margins, or deep fissuring which may involve some of the larger intra-hepatic vessels and lead to copious bleeding. The effects of penetrating wounds vary with the agent. Knife wounds are generally narrow slits which do not do much damage to the liver provided they do not involve the vessels in the hilum or the hepatic veins. Bullet wounds of low velocity produce ruptures similar to closed injuries whereas high velocity missiles cause extensive and explosive destruction of the substance of the liver and are usually fatal. With any hepatic injury there may be associated trauma to the diaphragm, chest wall or intra-thoracic organs.

4

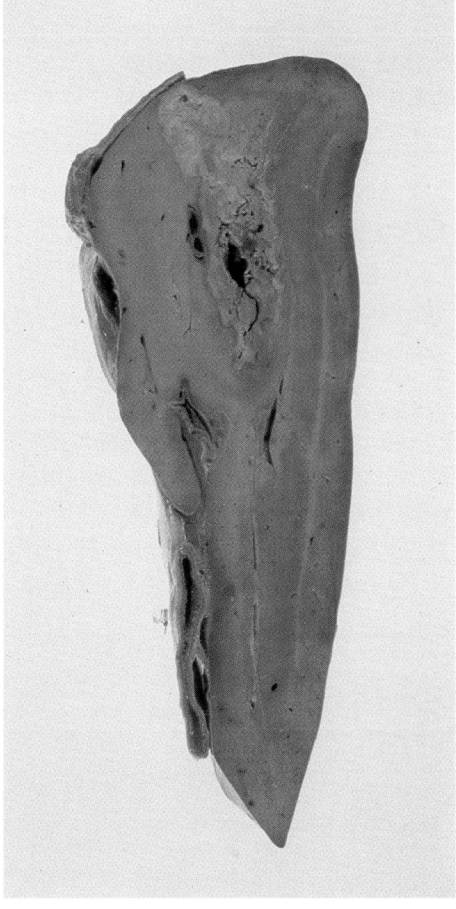

G.C.7755

4 From a soldier wounded in France in 1915. The wound of entry was in the right eighth intercostal space – posterior axillary line. On the 6th day the right chest was aspirated and the fluid on culture demonstrated streptococcal infection. Death occurred on the 16th day.

The section of liver demonstrates the track of the missile which has been cut across transversely. The appearance suggests that this was a low velocity missile. The adjacent parenchyma is contused and necrotic.

3

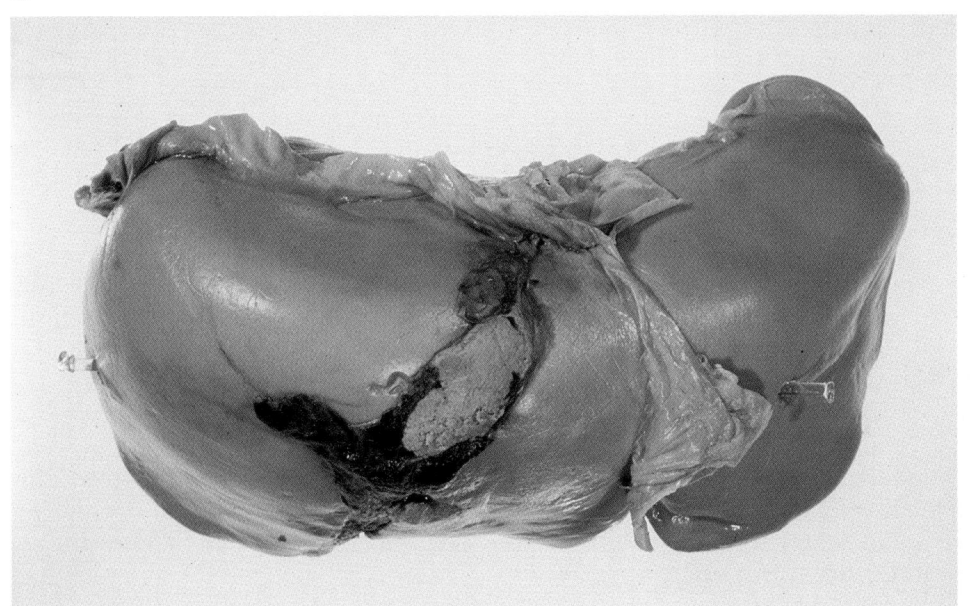

G.C.8524

3 From a 14-year-old boy who was crushed between two hutches in a coalpit. The abdomen was explored and gross bleeding had occurred from a torn branch of the hepatic artery. Death ensued 12 hours later.

There is a gross traumatic triradiate fissure of the right lobe of the liver extending from the anterior border to the superior surface.

Inflammatory and parasitic disease

Pyogenic abscesses are commonly multiple and are due to infection carried into the liver by the portal vein (portal pyaemia) or the hepatic artery, or by ascending cholangitis. Blood-spread infection occurs as a complication of sepsis within the peritoneal cavity, e.g. appendicular or diverticular abscesses or trauma. The causative organisms are those usually associated with such infections, *E. coli,* anaerobic cocci and staphylococci. The liver is enlarged and tender, there are fever and rigors and blood culture is usually positive. If the diagnosis is made early appropriate antibiotics may relieve the condition, but later when the abscesses are larger surgical drainage will also be required.

5 From an adult in whom suppurative pylephlebitis followed appendicitis. A considerable portion of the surface of the liver is covered with recent fibrinopurulent material and throughout the cut surface are numerous irregular cavities of comparatively small size containing pus and tending to become confluent. The abscesses are in relation to the portal canals.

Amoebic abscess

5

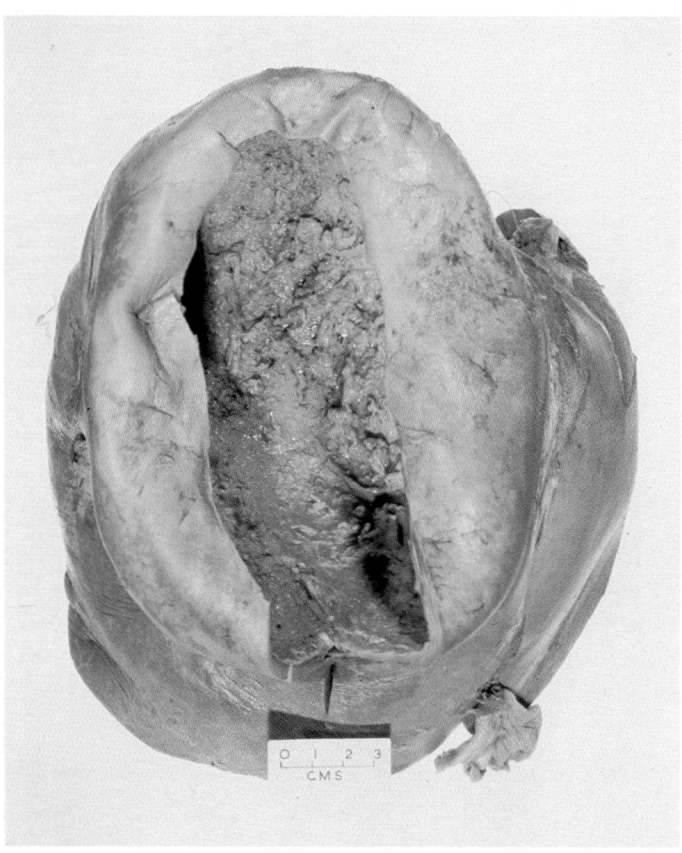

G.C.4623

6

G.C.8210

Hepatic abscesses may be single or multiple. The single abscess is almost always amoebic (due to *Entamoeba histolytica*) and is not initially pyogenic. The abscess grows by the coalescence of multiple areas of infection by the amoeba and is commonly situated in the anterosuperior part of the right lobe. This lobe is enlarged and tender but the rest of the liver is normal. Diagnosis is by X-ray and ultrasound and by the response to specific treatment. Aspirated contents of the abscess cavity do not always show the presence of the entamoeba. The untreated abscess may be secondarily infected by pyogenic organisms and may rupture into the pleural or peritoneal cavities or into one of the larger bile ducts.

6 From a male aged 43 years who contracted dysentery while on army service in South Africa. Apparent recovery was followed some years later by ill health with loss of weight and jaundice. The liver was enlarged. Right pleural effusion. His condition steadily deteriorated until death.

At post mortem the grossly enlarged liver weighed 4.5 kg. The right lobe of the liver is replaced by a large abscess cavity from which 2.5 kg of pus was evacuated. Superficially the cyst is smooth and non-adherent. The lining membrane of the cyst is ragged, irregular and necrotic. Examination of the cyst wall failed to reveal the presence of amoebae but the history is suggestive of an initial amoebic infection.

412

Hydatid disease

The eggs of the tapeworm *Echinococcus granulosus*, if ingested by man, hatch in the duodenum and the embryo passes through the wall of the intestine and is carried by the portal blood to the liver. There the embryo develops into a small cyst which has the characteristic structure of:

1 an inner germinal membrane which lines the cyst and produces the brood capsules where the head or scolex of future tape worms grows, and

2 an outer laminated membrane of fibrous tissue which may become calcified. More than one cyst is found in about 25% of cases. In about 30% the embryos are carried to other sites such as the spleen, muscle, lung or brain.

The right lobe is affected more often than the left and is palpably and firmly enlarged. Otherwise the uncomplicated cyst in the liver is usually symptomless. Complications are:

(1) Pressure on surrounding structures, e.g. the biliary tree, with consequent obstructive jaundice.

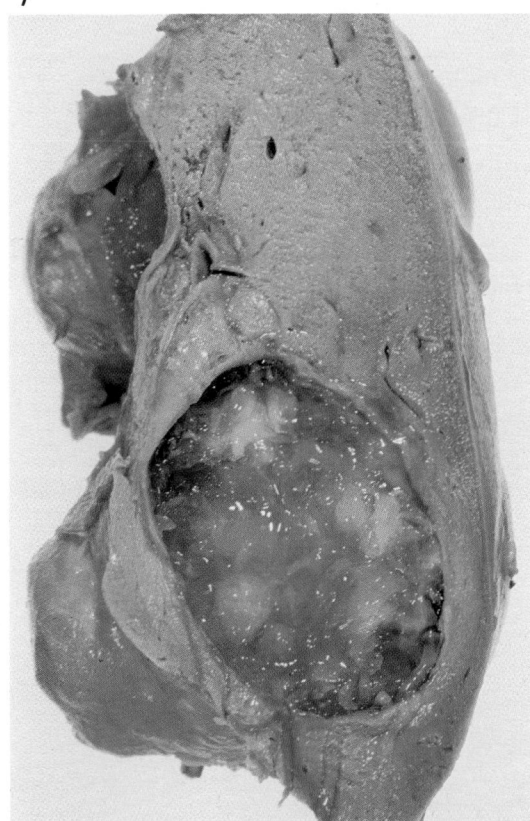

7 Hydatid cyst of liver.

(2) Rupture.
   (a) Into an intra-hepatic bile duct with discharge of cysts into the duodenum and obstructive jaundice in the process.
   (b) Into the peritoneal cavity with widespread dissemination of daughter cysts which will grow slowly and lead to intestinal obstruction and other compression syndromes.
   (c) Through the diaphragm into the pleural cavity with the development of empyema containing pus, bile and daughter cysts.

Therefore, if practicable, excision of the hydatid cyst on diagnosis is advisable. The exception is the symptomless calcified cyst, calcification usually being accepted as evidence of quiescence. Diagnosis may be confirmed by the Casoni test or by a serum complement fixation test.

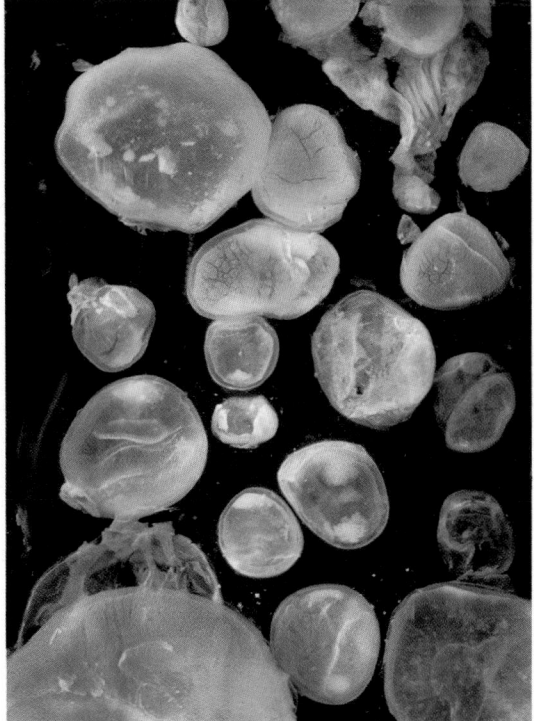

8 Daughter cysts.

Man is usually infected from dogs which are the commonest hosts for the adult worm and pass the ova in the faeces. The intermediate hosts are farm animals such as sheep, pigs and cattle. The geographical incidence of the disease largely corresponds with the sheep farming areas of the globe.

Developmental and anatomical anomalies

Cystic disease

Cystic disease is rare. It is often familial and in two-thirds of cases is associated with cystic disease of the kidneys. The cysts are usually multiple and vary considerably in size. If they communicate with the biliary tree the content is bile-stained. Where there is no communication the content is clear.

9

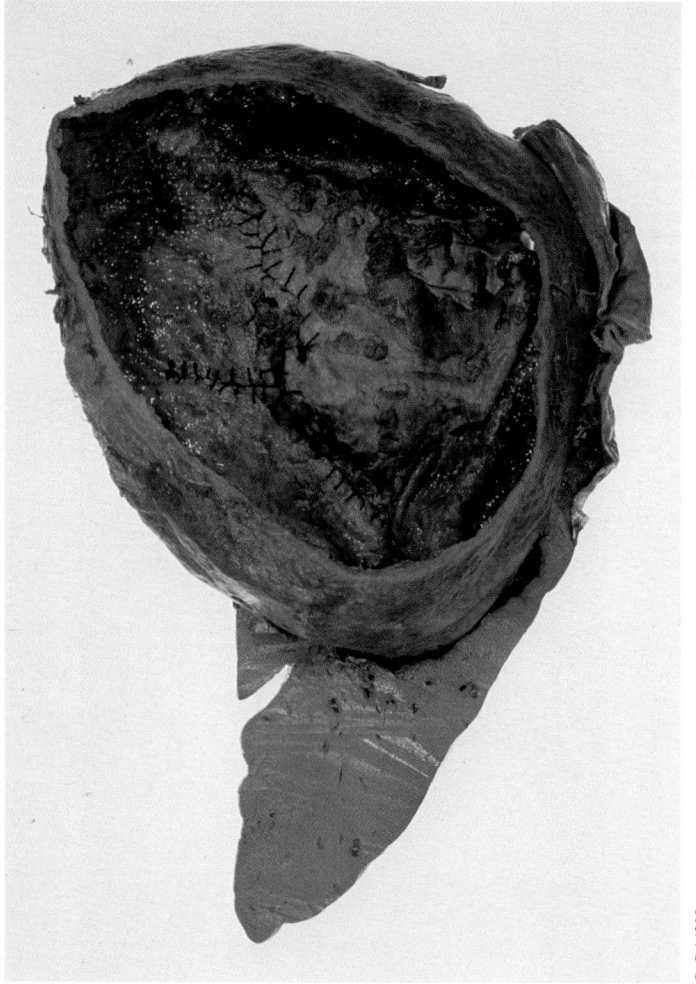

G.C.14288

10

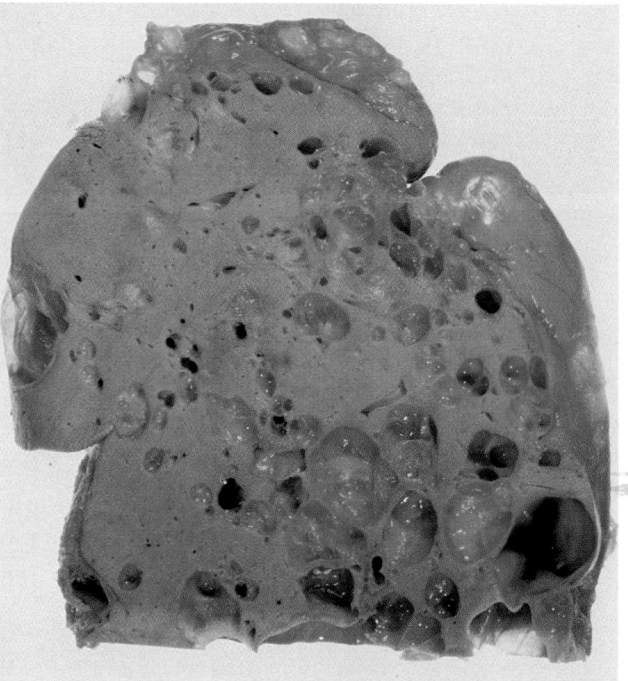

G.C.15170

10   Post mortem specimen demonstrating an enlarged liver due to the presence of numerous cysts scattered throughout the substance of the organ none of which exceed approximately 2.5 cm in diameter. The cysts are lined with a smooth membrane and the appearances are those of multiple cystic disease of congenital origin.

The cysts are lined with simple cuboidal epithelium. The liver tissue between the cysts may be normal, but often the portal triads are enlarged and contain an excess of fibrous tissue in which there are tortuous dilated biliary ductules some of which contain biliary thrombi.

11

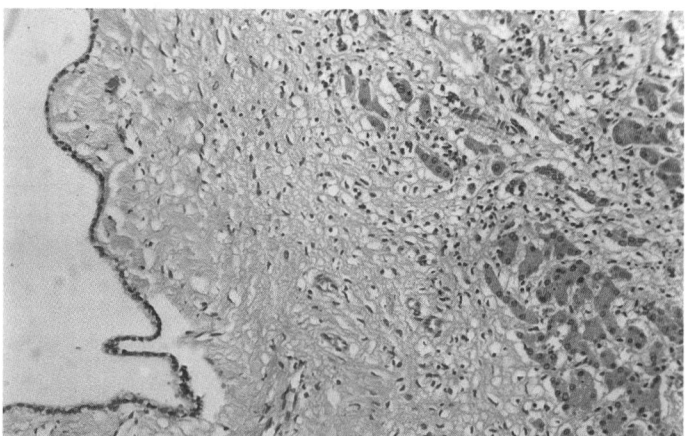

G.C.M.936

11   Part of the wall of a large cyst lined by a single layer of cuboidal epithelium. Fibrous tissue separates it from the hepatic parenchyma. (*H&E ×150*)

9   No clinical details are available.
The illustration shows the liver and a large thick walled cyst involving the subdiaphragmatic portion of the liver and extending under the diaphragm. The brown staining on the inner wall of the cyst indicates that there has been bleeding into it; otherwise the wall is smooth and shows no specific features. The condition appears to be a large long-standing cyst of the liver of unknown origin.

Congenital hepatic fibrosis

Congenital hepatic fibrosis. When this is well developed the liver is enlarged, firm, regularly lobular. The presenting features are usually those of portal hypertension. The portal triads are enlarged and obvious and are joined by coarse fibrous tissue tracts which surround but usually do not distort the hepatic lobules. The triads contain many bile ductules some of which appear to be small blind tubes and others are greatly dilated and tortuous. Hepatic function is little disturbed.

It is arguable that polycystic disease of the liver and congenital fibrosis are different degrees of the same congenital abnormality and may also be related embryologically to intra-hepatic and extra-hepatic biliary atresia and choledochus cyst.

Von Meyenburg complexes

Von Meyenburg complexes have affinities both with congenital hepatic fibrosis and polycystic disease. They are congenital abnormalities presenting as small fibrous nodules which may be single or multiple.

Histologically they consist of numerous abnormal bile ductules set in fibrous tissue. The ductules may form microcysts and may contain darkly pigmented biliary thrombi.

12

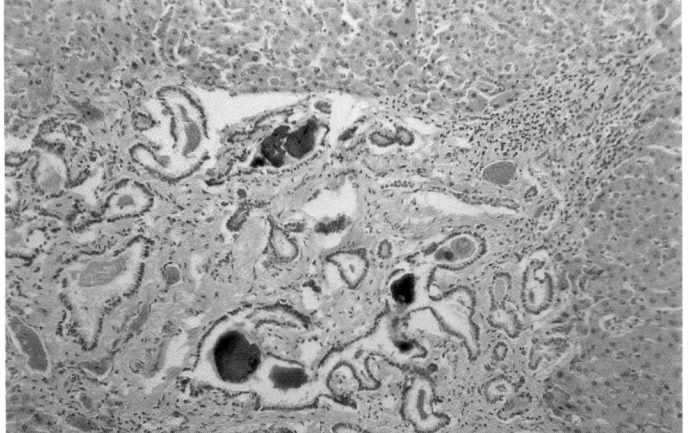

G.C.M.934

12   Von Meyenburg complex. *(H&E ×100)*

Ultrasound examination

13

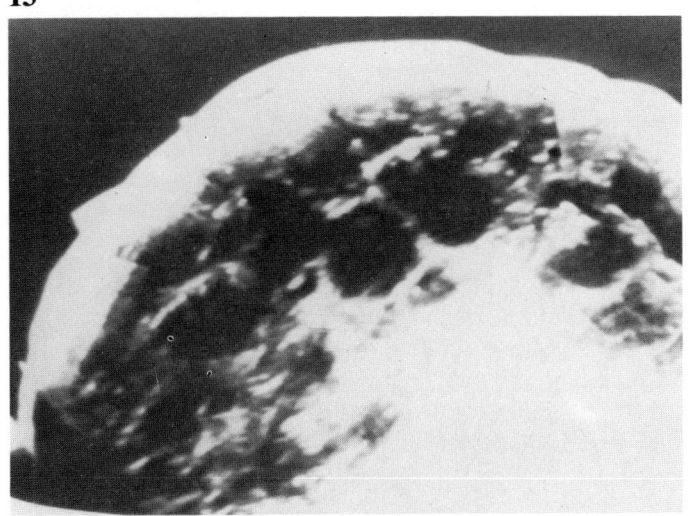

G.C.X.787

13 Ultrasound examination is a modern technique whereby internal lesions can be defined. Cysts and other tumours of the liver can thus be demonstrated. The illustration shown is polycystic disease of the liver.

Metabolic disorders

The liver is involved in glycogen storage disease and in defects in the metabolism of such heavy metals as iron and copper. All are rare. Glycogen storage disease is diagnosed by enzyme analysis of hepatic biopsies. Its surgical importance is that a few cases can be improved by porta-caval transposition whereby glucose absorbed from the alimentary tract is diverted past the liver and becomes immediately available to other body tissues.

Excessive deposition of iron occurs as a result of a metabolic defect within the hepatic cells and the Küpffer cells in Idiopathic Haemochromatosis. The deposit, mainly of haemosiderin, damages the parenchymal cells and induces changes which progress to cirrhosis.

Similar changes occur in the pancreas. Diabetes is present in 50% of cases and bronze pigmentation of the skin is almost invariable.

14

14 Haemochromatosis. Excessive amounts of the brown pigment haemosiderin accumulate in the liver cell cytoplasm. As liver cells break down haemosiderin is carried to the fibrotic portal tracts by phagocytes. *(H&E ×125)*

Hepato-lenticular degeneration (Kinnier Wilson's disease) is an inherited disturbance of copper metabolism in which the total body copper is increased, urinary excretion of copper is high, the copper binding globulin (Caeruloplasmin) is abnormally low and copper is deposited in the liver, the renal tubules and the basal ganglia of the brain. A persistent chronic hepatitis ensues and usually progresses to a coarse nodular cirrhosis. Portal hypertension may complicate the cirrhosis. Neurological signs are prominent.

15

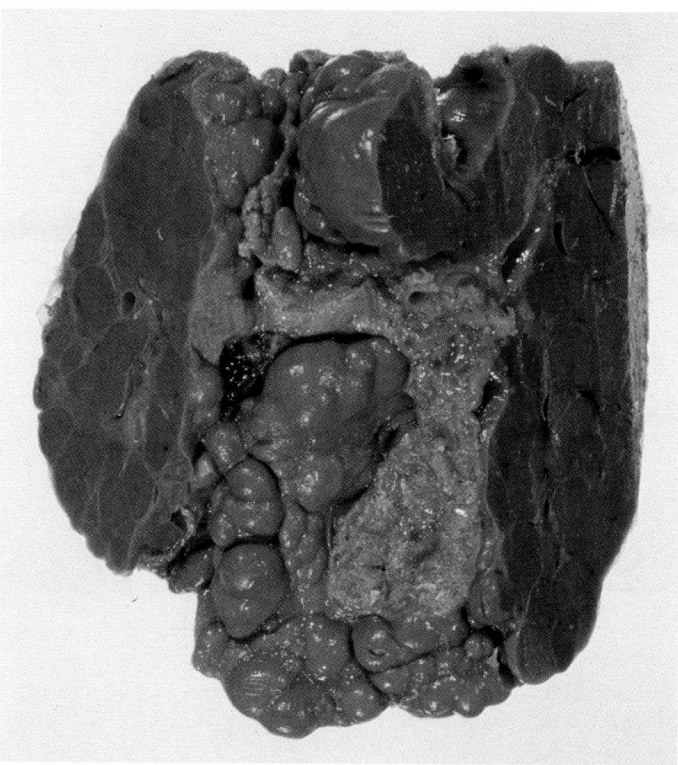

15 From a female patient in whom the diagnosis of hepato-lenticular degeneration was established. The peritoneal surfaces are irregular with nodules of different sizes, varying from 0.5 to 2cm in diameter and separated by deep clefts which on the cut surface can be seen to be continuous with fibrous septa which traverse the whole thickness of the liver. No areas of necrosis or infarction are evident and there is no bile staining.

Viral hepatitis (infectious jaundice)

Three different forms of this disease can be distinguished:

Viral A Hepatitis has a relatively short incubation period (2 to 6 weeks), generally a mild and fairly short course and seldom has any complications or sequellae (2 to 5%). It is transmitted by contact and ingestion of contaminated food, etc.

Viral B Hepatitis (serum hepatitis) has a longer incubation period (7 to 23 weeks) and varies in severity from an almost symptomless hepatitis to acute hepatic necrosis and failure. Transmission is parenteral by direct contact or inoculation with infected material. Hepatitis B antigen (HBAg) can be demonstrated in the serum of patients both immunologically and by the electron microscope within ten days of the onset of the disease and usually until about four weeks later.

Hepatitis B may resolve completely, may persist, the patient becoming a symptomless carrier, may progress to chronic hepatitis with persistent virus B infection or to acute hepatic failure and death.

The importance of hepatitis B to the surgeon lies first in the differential diagnosis of upper abdominal pain with fever, nausea and vomiting before jaundice has appeared; and second in the danger of cross-infection by the blood or secretions of a patient or a symptomless carrier. All precautions must be taken to prevent contamination of skin, mucous surfaces or conjunctiva at venepuncture, wound dressing, transfusion or operation on known infected patients and carriers.

Non-A non-B Hepatitis. This diagnosis is made by exclusion of Virus A and Virus B infection. The causative agent is not yet known. The usual route of infection is parenteral and it is the most frequent cause of post-transfusional hepatitis.

16

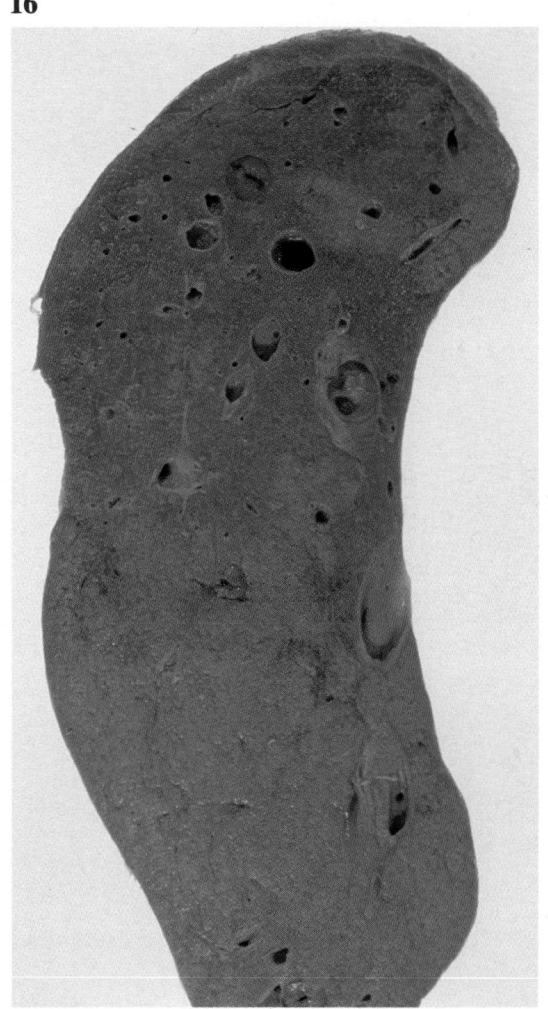

The naked eye appearance of the liver in the presence of hepatitis varies greatly. The liver may be enlarged and smooth when the hepatitis is diffuse and in its early stages. In fatal cases, where the destruction of the liver cells is massive and rapid, the liver is small, shrunken and yellowish (acute yellow atrophy).

16 The illustration shows the liver of an elderly female who died following massive hepatic necrosis. Microscopic examination revealed that most of the hepatic parenchyma of the darker upper portion of the liver had undergone necrosis and resorption leaving highly vascular portal and stromal tissues. The pale swollen lower portion was already showing signs of regeneration.

Viral hepatitis *(Continued)*

The principal histological lesion is necrosis of the hepatocytes which may be focal and widespread but retaining the architecture of the lobules, or massive with patchy haemorrhages and lobular disintegration. Regeneration after focal necrosis restores the liver apparently to normal, but the collapse of the lobule and the subsequent fibrous tissue scarring after massive necrosis lead to irregular areas of regeneration and the formation of nodules of hyperplastic liver tissue which does not have the normal portal/central vein relationship.

17

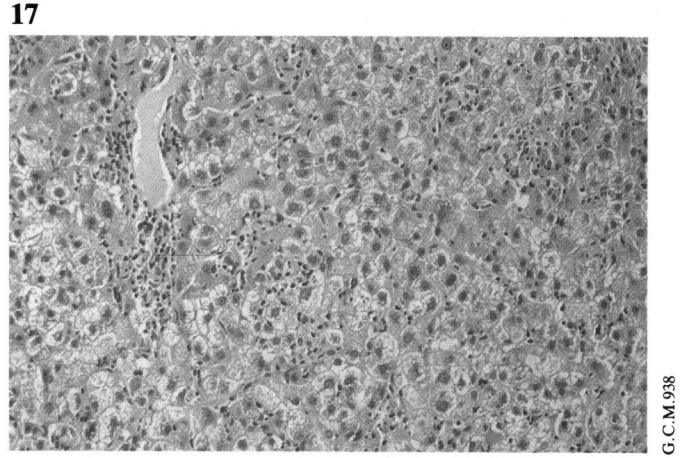

18

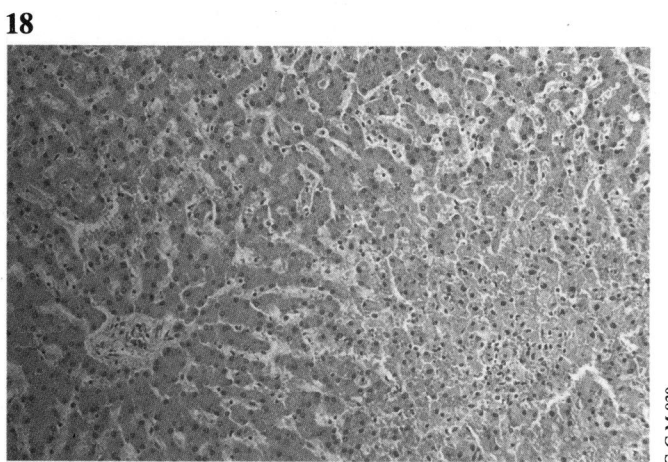

17 Viral hepatitis. Active chronic phase of the disease. Many of the hepatocytes show degenerative change. Groups of inflammatory cells indicate foci of former necrosis and also infiltrate portal tract and centrilobular zones. *(H&E ×150)*

18 Focal necrosis in a case of circulatory failure. The centrilobular cells are necrotic and eosinophilic. Periportal cells are relatively normal. *(H&E ×125)*

Massive necrosis. Whole lobules are destroyed and the normal architecture is not restored. The groups of liver cells which survive may later form centres of regenerative nodules.

19

20

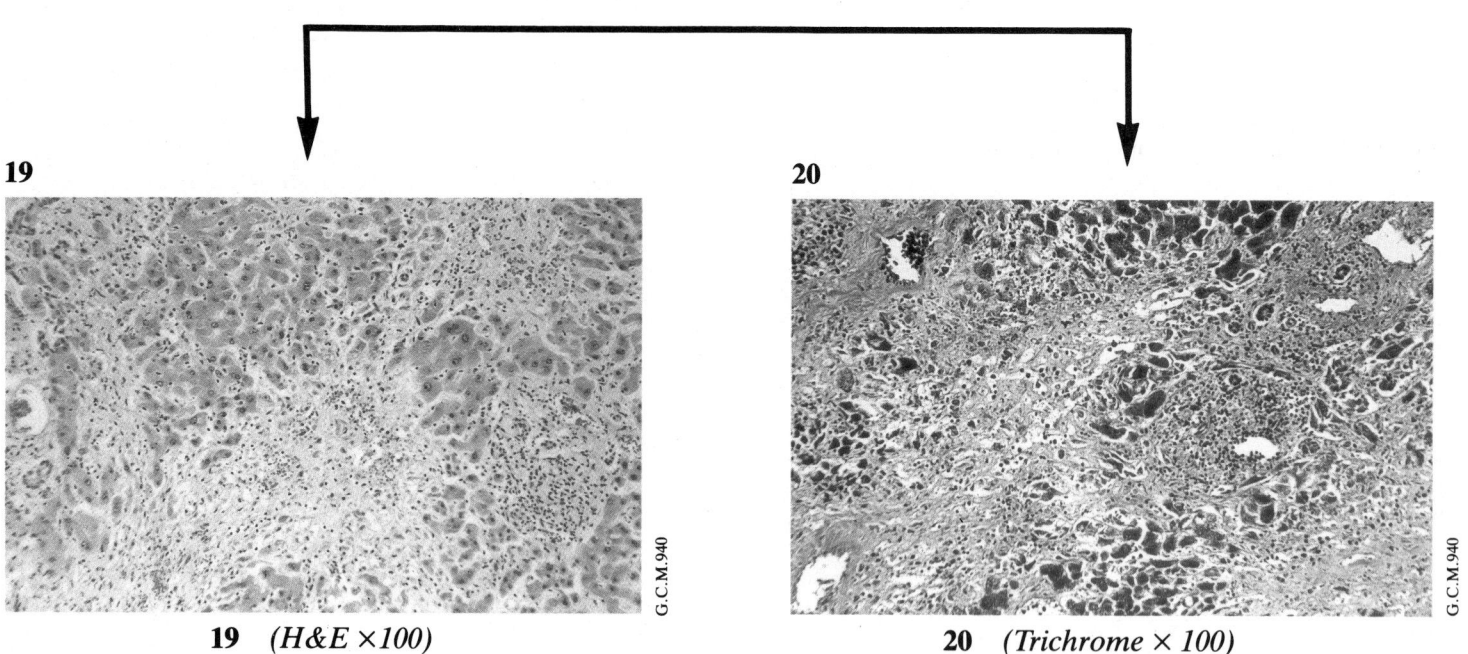

19 *(H&E ×100)*

20 *(Trichrome × 100)*

418

Cirrhosis

The end result of either a single episode of massive acute hepatic necrosis which the patient survives, or more often of repeated episodes of less severe liver damage, is cirrhosis of the liver. The essential pathological features of cirrhosis are:

1   irregular degeneration and regeneration of hepatocytes, giving rise to nodules of hyperplastic liver tissue in which the normal portal/central vein relationship is lost and

2   increase in fibrous tissue which surrounds these lobules and interferes with the flow of portal blood through the liver.

21

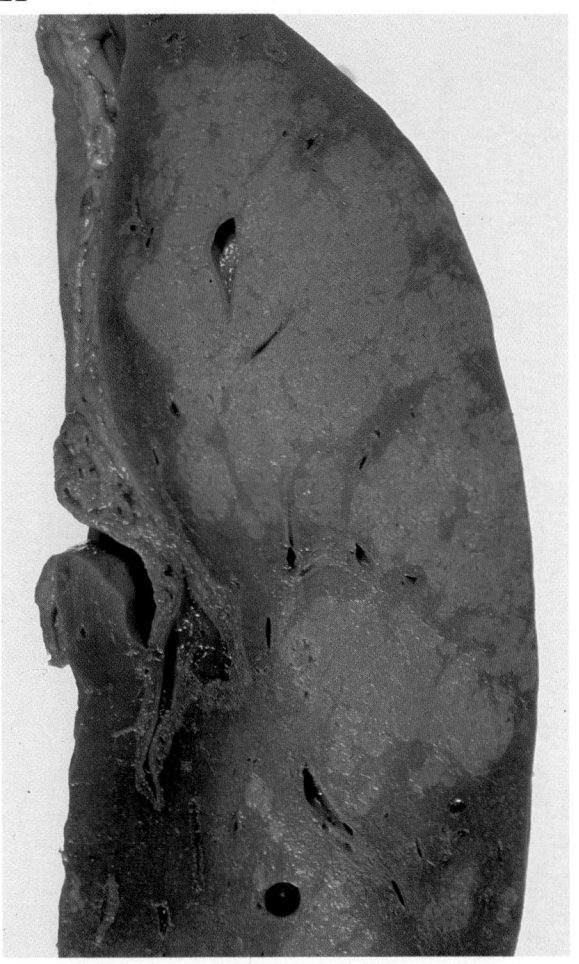

22

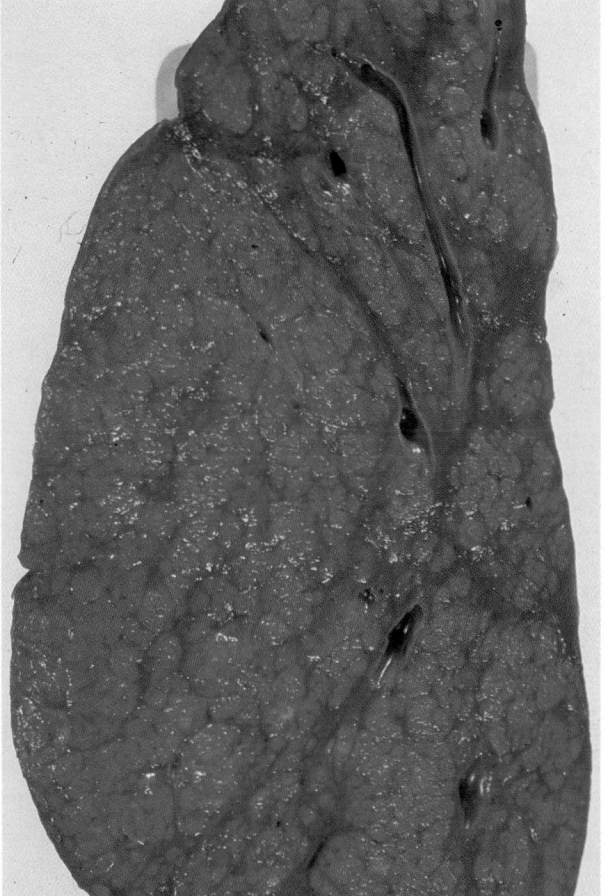

21 Subtotal hepatic necrosis. From an adult male the subject of acquired syphilis who in the course of 3 weeks had eight intravenous injections of novarsenobillon alternating with seven intramuscular injections of mercury.

The cut surface of the liver shows large pale irregular areas of surviving and regenerating liver contrasting with darker tissue where most of the liver cells have been lost. Had the patient recovered large regenerative nodules would have developed in a grossly irregular liver.

22 From a female aged 47 years who died in hepatic coma 4 days after drainage of ascitic fluid.

Here regenerative nodules predominate in the 'cirrhosis' following less severe massive necrosis. Dark shrunken hepatic stroma can still be seen between aggregates of regenerative nodules.

Types of cirrhosis

The two main types of cirrhosis are portal (syn. Laennec's) and biliary.

23

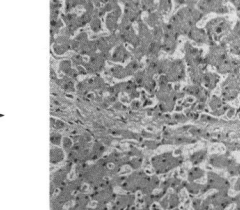

Portal cirrhosis is currently classified as:

1 Micro-nodular in which the nodules are small (about 1 to 2 mm in diameter) and seldom show a central vein. This type is the commonest end-stage of alcoholic cirrhosis and haemochromatosis.

23 Micro-nodular cirrhosis. Condensed portal tracts and fibrous tissue surround small nodules of liver without normal central veins. *(H&E ×100)*

24

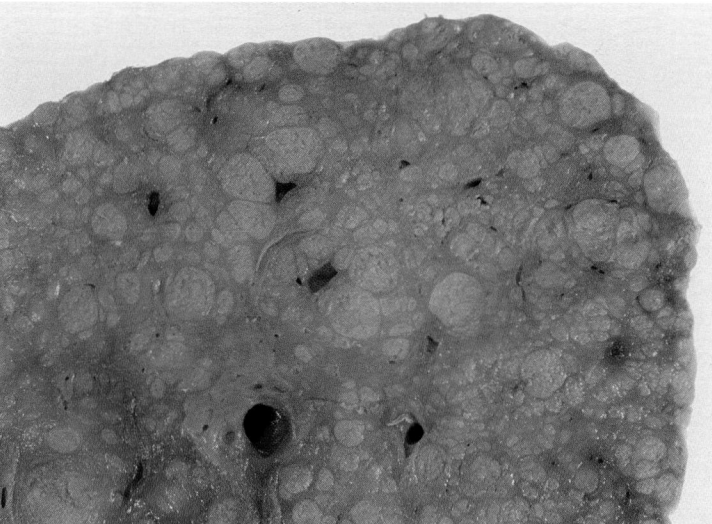

2 Macro-nodular. Here the nodules vary in size and structure, sometimes the anatomical pattern in the nodules being lost and sometimes nearly normal. Fibrosis may be coarse and dense and in the fibrous bands there may be bile duct proliferation and islets of liver cells. This is the common pattern in post-hepatic cirrhosis.

3 Mixed micro- and macro-nodular is characteristic of cryptogenic cirrhosis and is found in varying degree in most cirrhotic livers even though they may be predominantly either micro- or macro-nodular.

Complications

Three complications are recognised sequellae to portal cirrhosis.

    1 Portal hypertension
    2 Encephalopathy
    3 Hepatocellular carcinoma

These are discussed separately (see pages 424, 428 and 430).

24 The patient suffered from portal hypertension and the spleen was enlarged.

The pale nodules of hyperplastic liver parenchyma vary greatly in size, and the large nodules are formed by the components of several regenerated hepatic lobules. Septa of vascular stromal tissue containing fibrosed portal tract elements intervene between the nodules.

Aetiology

The aetiology of hepatic cirrhosis differs in different parts of the world. In the U.S.A. and France about 90% of cases have an alcoholic background whereas in Scotland this is found in about 50%. In North African countries it very seldom occurs.

25

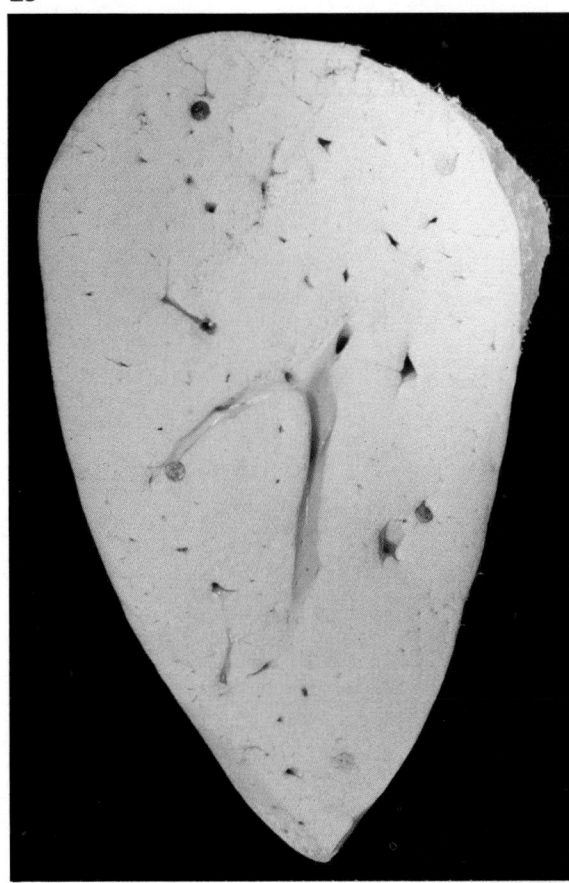

G.C.14582

Fatty degeneration of the liver is seen as the result of a variety of factors but is commonly and correctly associated with beer drinkers. It represents a disturbance of the liver cells and their ability to deal with absorbed fat. The condition may go on if unchecked, to the death of the liver cells and the development of cirrhosis.

26

G.C.15062

25 The illustration shows a section of a grossly enlarged liver. The capsule is thin and smooth and no adhesions are present. The cut surface is pale yellow in colour and uniform throughout in structure. The condition is one of gross fatty degeneration of the liver.

26 Hepatitis Cirrhosis (Alcoholic). Two sections of liver demonstrating advanced cirrhosis. The cut surface of the liver shows diffuse cirrhosis with multiple small lobules set in fibrosed portal tracts. The outer surface is nodular (the hobnail liver) and the liver is pale.

27

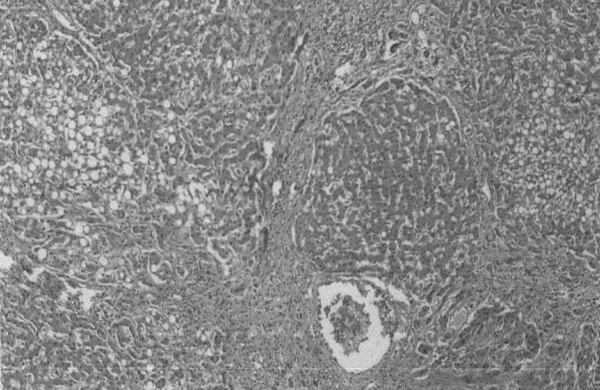

G.C.M.942

27 Alcoholic Cirrhosis. The liver is divided into nodules of varying size and the normal architecture is lost. Some of the liver cells are vacuolated due to accumulation of fat in the cytoplasm. The portal tracts are infiltrated by lymphocytes. *(H&E ×50)*

Cirrhosis *(Continued)*

Schistosomiasis

In Egypt the almost universal cause of cirrhosis is schistosomiasis, the eggs of the larvae being trapped in the portal venules, stimulating a great overgrowth of fibrous tissue in the portal triads.

28

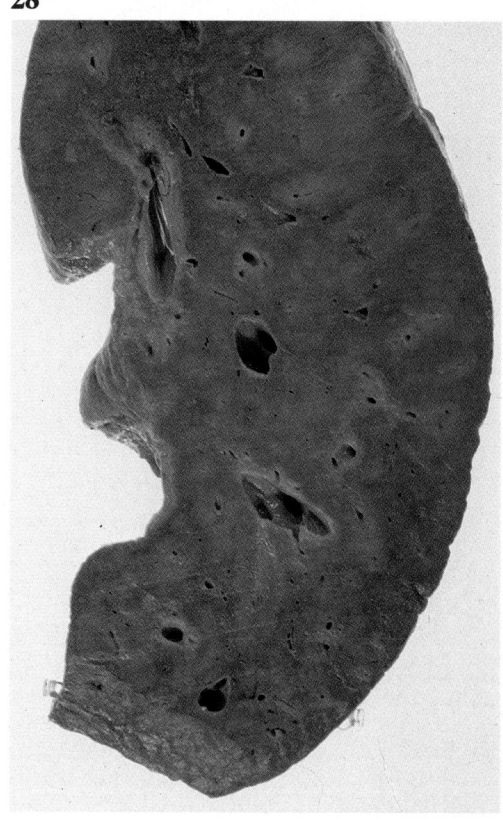

G.C.5170

28 From an adult the subject of schistosomiasis. The liver does not appear to have been increased in size. The capsule and serosa are normal. On section the liver parenchyma is mottled with lighter areas of fibrosis particularly around larger portal tracts.

Two ova have caused chronic inflammation and fibrosis in portal tracts. Later extensive fibrosis and cirrhosis develop.

29

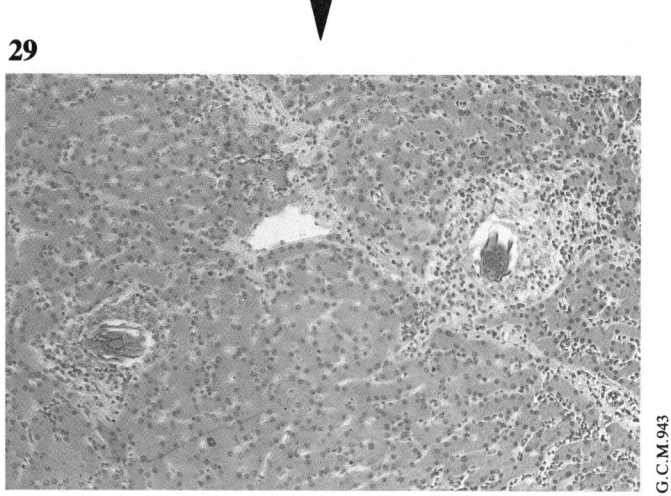

G.C.M.943

30

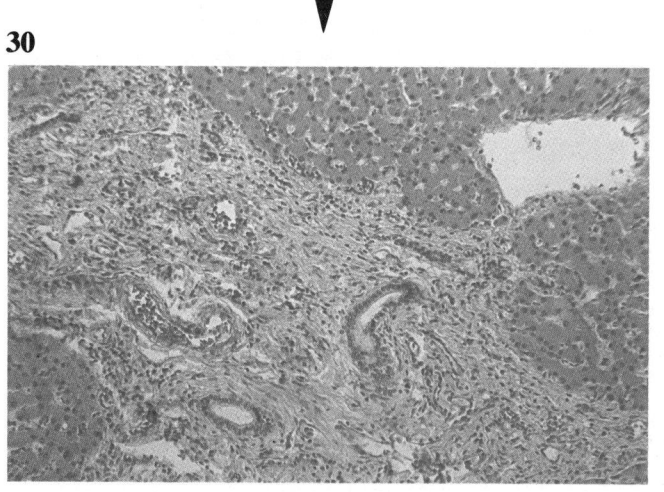

G.C.M.943

29 *(H&E ×125)*   **30** *(H&E ×125)*

In the United Kingdom 10 to 15% of cases of cirrhosis follow viral hepatitis or the ingestion or absorption of hepatotoxins and the remainder are classed as cryptogenic because no obvious factor can be incriminated.

Biliary cirrhosis

Primary

Primary biliary cirrhosis affects predominantly middle-aged women (sex ratio F:M – 8:1). It appears to be an autoimmune disease, the basic lesion being destruction of the intra-hepatic bile ducts. The disease runs a chronic and slowly progressive course. At first the liver is enlarged and smooth and histologically shows:

1 aggregations of lymphocytes and plasma cells in the portal triads and

2 in about 40% of cases granulomas either in the triads or in the parenchyma.

Later there is infiltration into the parenchyma by the lymphocytes and plasma cells, destruction of the hepatocytes and replacement by fibrous tissue.

The clinical features are jaundice and itching and laboratory tests indicate an obstructive jaundice, hypergammaglobulinaemia and a high titre of anti-mitochondrial antibodies in the serum. This finding virtually excludes a diagnosis of jaundice due to obstruction of the common hepatic or common bile ducts.

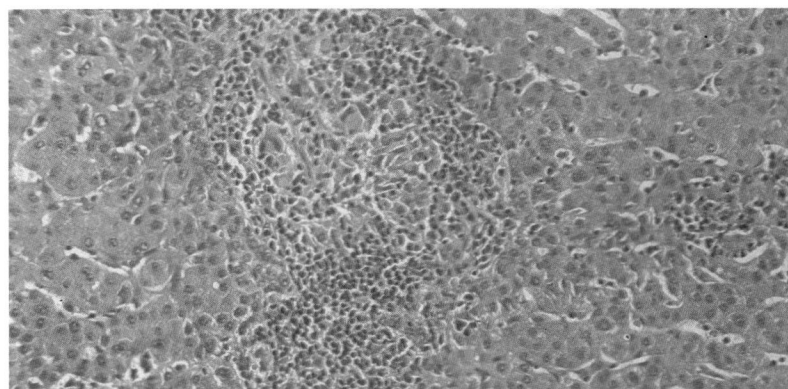

31 Primary biliary cirrhosis. A portal tract is heavily infiltrated by lymphocytes and plasma cells and a giant cell granuloma has developed. Bile ductules are inconspicuous. *(H&E ×180)*

Secondary

Secondary biliary cirrhosis is a complication of long-standing obstruction of the bile ducts and cholangitis.

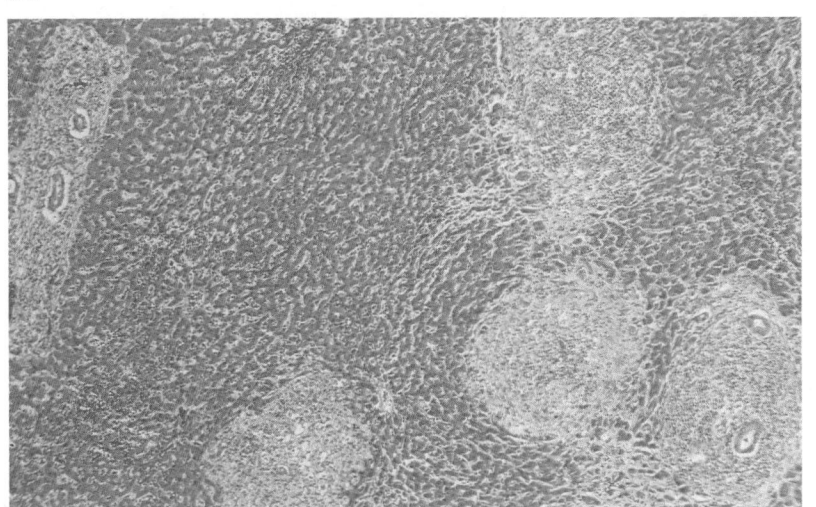

32 Biliary cirrhosis due to obstruction of common bile duct. The portal tracts show 'nodular' thickening due to chronic inflammation and fibrosis. Later the tracts join up to cause a fine grain cirrhosis. *(H&E ×48)*

A.I.S. Macpherson

The portal vein is formed behind the neck of the pancreas by the union of the splenic and superior mesenteric veins. At or near this junction it is joined by the left gastric vein and pancreatico-duodenal veins. The inferior mesenteric vein is usually a tributary of the splenic vein.

The portal vein is thus the common pathway for all the blood from the small and large intestines, the stomach, pancreas and spleen. It runs a short course in the free edge of the lesser omentum behind the common bile duct and the hepatic artery and ends in the porta hepatis by dividing into right and left branches which go respectively to the right and left lobes of the liver.

The left branch of the portal vein receives the umbilical vein which normally becomes occluded shortly after birth. Often a potential lumen remains which, together with veins on its surface (para-umbilical veins), may reopen later in life if the flow of portal blood through the liver is obstructed.

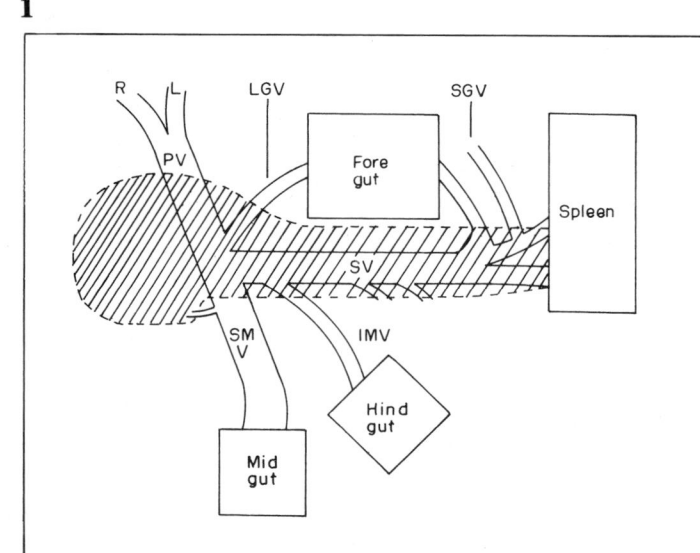

1 Diagram of anatomy of portal venous system.

A rise in blood pressure in the portal venous system (portal hypertension) occurs when there is an obstruction to the flow of portal blood into or through the liver. The obstruction may be outside the liver (extra-hepatic) or within it (intra-hepatic).

Extra-hepatic obstruction

Extra-hepatic obstruction accounts for about 50% of cases in childhood but not more than 10% in the adult. The commonest cause is occlusion of the portal vein by thrombosis which may follow umbilical sepsis or catheterisation in the infant or intra-peritoneal sepsis in the adult. A network of small collateral veins may develop in the lesser omentum to carry some portal blood to the liver. This is called cavernous transformation. Occasionally the right and left branches of the portal vein may be congenitally narrowed or occluded. In about 2% of cases the block is in the splenic vein.

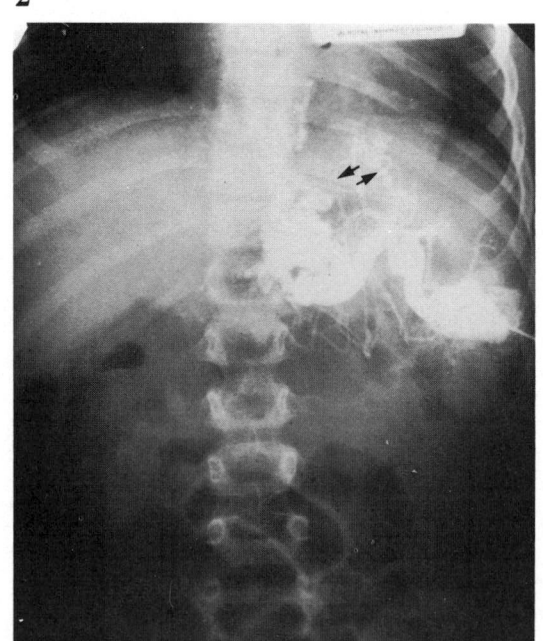

2 Trans-splenic portography in a girl aged 9 years showing occlusion of the portal vein and extensive collateral development in the cardio-oesophageal area. The splenic vein is dilated and tortuous.

Intra-hepatic obstruction

Intra-hepatic obstruction is almost always due to some form of cirrhosis, the cause of which in Western countries may be alcoholic, post-hepatitic or cryptogenic.

Schistosomiasis in endemic areas may lead to chronic inflammatory changes and fibrosis in the portal tracts obstructing the portal flow before it reaches the sinusoids (pre-sinusoidal obstruction). A rare cause is veno-occlusive disease affecting the tributaries of the hepatic veins leading to an enlarged congested liver, ascites and portal hypertension (post-sinusoidal obstruction). This has been described in the West Indies where it was associated with the drinking of herbal teas especially of the Senecio family.

A similar picture may result from obstruction of the hepatic veins (Budd–Chiari syndrome) by thrombosis, tumour or retroperitoneal fibrosis.

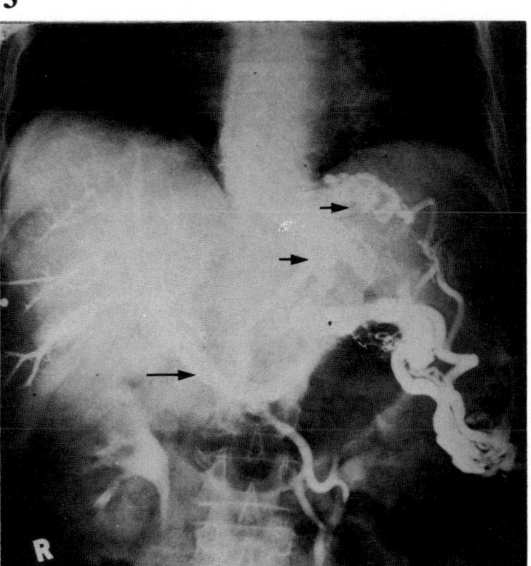

3 Trans-hepatic portography. The portal vein is patent and there is collateral development through the left and short gastric veins. The intra-hepatic portal branches are irregular and tortuous indicating intra-hepatic portal obstruction due to cirrhosis.

Pathology

The pathological consequencs of portal venous obstruction are similar, no matter what the cause of the obstruction. The pathological changes are:

1 A sustained rise in the portal venous pressure distal to the obstruction
2 Dilatation and congestion of portal tributaries
3 Splenomegaly
4 Development of porta-systemic venous anastomoses.

1 Elevated portal pressure

A sustained rise in the portal venous pressure distal to the obstruction. Normal portal pressure is in the region of 100 mm of saline. A persistent pressure over 250 mm is diagnostic of portal hypertension.

2 Portal congestion

Congestion, dilatation and elongation of all the portal tributaries. Veins in the omenta and on the serous surfaces of organs and parietes are enlarged, tense and tortuous.

425

3 Splenomegaly

Splenomegaly is due to a combination of sinusoidal congestion and reticulo-endothelial hyperplasia. There is a great increase
in fibrous tissue making the spleen firm and incompressible and on
the cut surface can be seen numerous grey or brown spots (siderotic
or Gamna–Gandy nodules). These are fibrotic areas in the pulp
where small haemorrhages have occurred in the past with subsequent deposition of iron. Many vascular adhesions bind the spleen
to the abdominal wall and the diaphragm. In about 50% of cases the
enlarged spleen is associated with greatly decreased numbers of
circulating platelets and/or granulocytes (Hypersplenism).

The naked eye appearance of the spleen is described and illustrated
in Section 18.

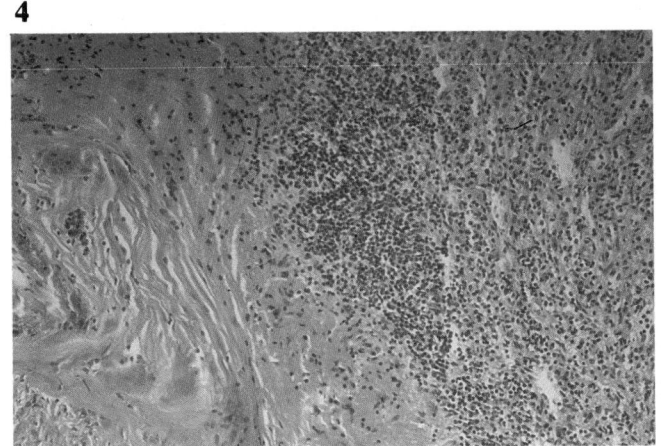

4 Gamna–Gandy Body. A focus of grey-brown
haemosiderin (left margin) is separated by dense
fibrous tissue from the peripheral lymphocytes of the
Malpighian body. The splenic pulp (right) is congested.
(H&E ×125)

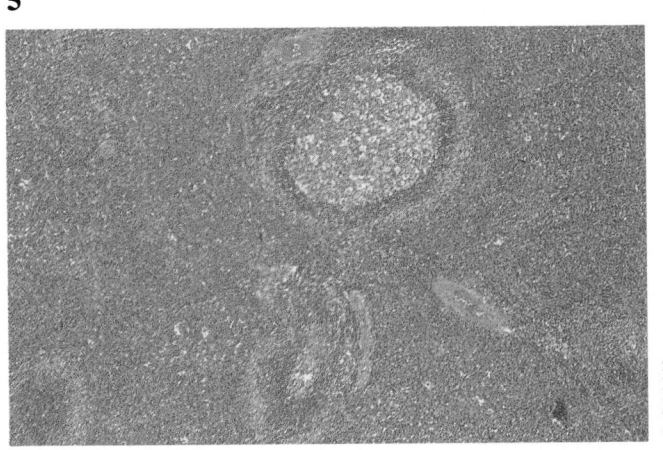

5 Splenomegaly – Hepatic cirrhosis.
The red pulp is engorged with blood as a
result of portal hypertension. A germinal centre is prominent in one of the
three Malpighian bodies. *(H&E ×37.5)*

4 Porta-systemic venous anastomoses

Development of porta-systemic venous anastomoses.
Two main areas in which these occur have been defined:

(a) Protected and beneficial anastomoses such as those
on the posterior abdominal wall where viscera are in
direct contact with the parietes, and along or through
the obliterated umbilical vein. These are beneficial
because they serve to return the portal blood to the
general circulation and are not at risk of bleeding.

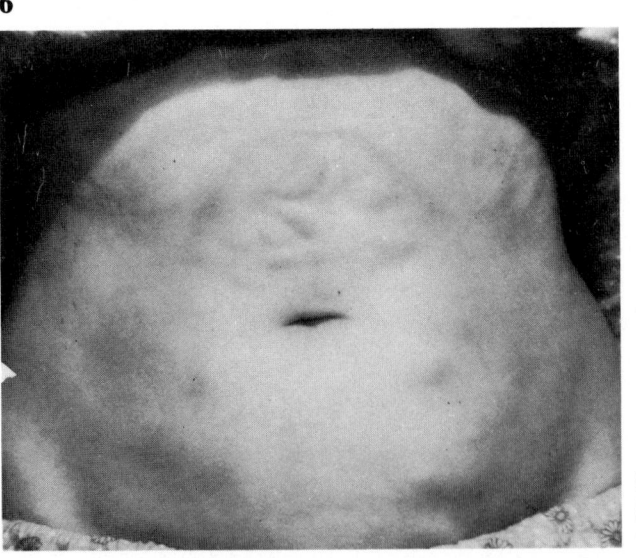

6 Beneficial anastomoses on the anterior abdominal
wall between recanalised para-umbilical veins and epigastric veins (Caput Medusae).

(b) Superficial and dangerous anastomoses, so called because they lie immediately under the epithelium or the mucosa of the stomach and oesophagus and consequently are exposed and unprotected on one aspect. These cardio-oesophageal 'varices', which are anastomoses between the gastric veins which drain into the portal vein and the oesophageal veins which are systemic venous channels, may rupture and give rise to the bleeding that is the most serious and lethal feature of portal hypertension.

7

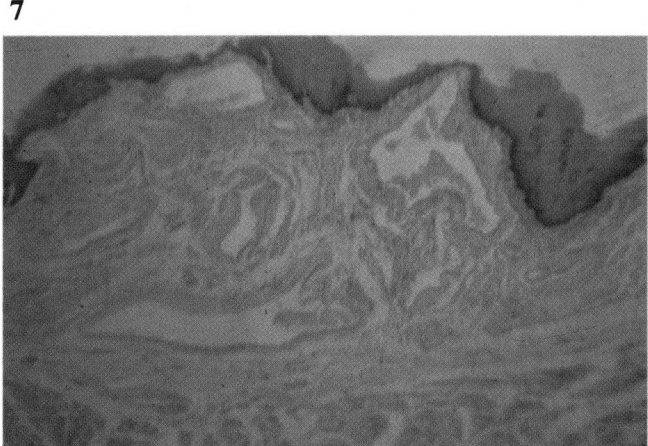

7 Transverse section of oesophagus showing sub-epithelial and submucous venous channels.

8

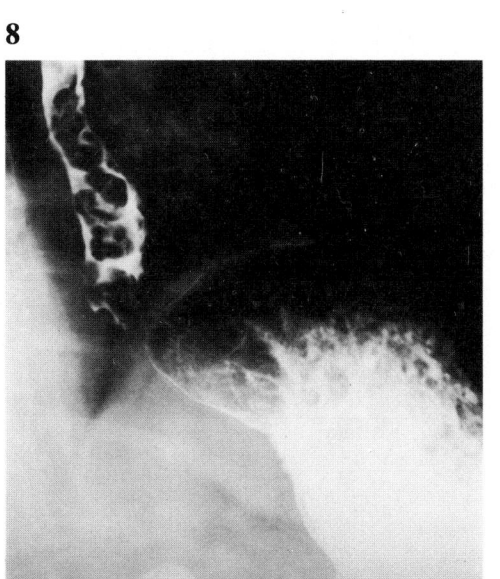

8 Oesophageal varices. From a female aged 63 years. No special treatment in view of her age and poor condition. Patient died of haematemesis 9 months later.

The X-ray reveals large varices due to portal hypertension as a result of portal cirrhosis.

9

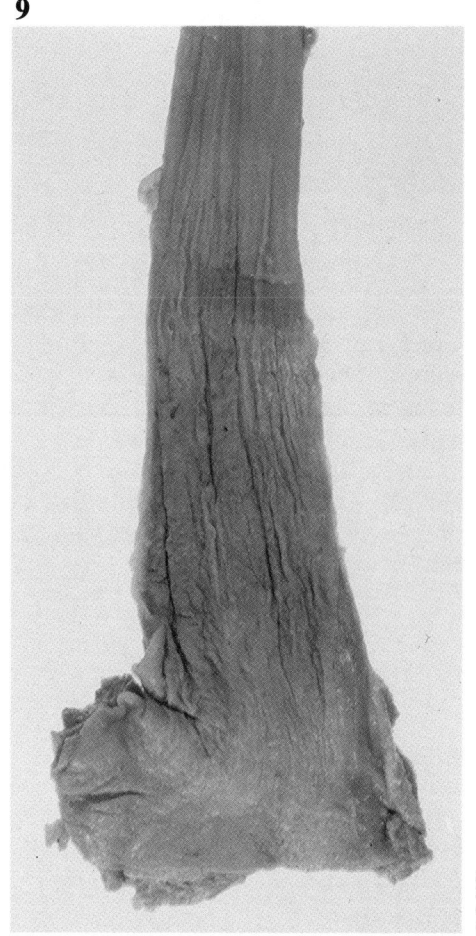

9 From a female aged 58 years who suffered from recurrent ascites and who died of haemorrhage from varicosity of the oesophageal veins.

At post mortem examination cirrhosis of the liver was found to be present. The spleen showed enlargement.

The oesophagus has been opened longitudinally to show raised ridges of the enlarged oesophageal veins.

There is also an anastomosis between the rectal veins which run in the submucosa of the rectum and the systemic veins which drain the anal region. The submucous veins in the rectum become dilated and can be observed by proctoscopy.

True haemorrhoid formation, however, is rare.

Complications of portal cirrhosis

Encephalopathy

Four factors appear to influence the development of encephalopathy in cirrhosis:
(a) the degree of hepatic dysfunction.
(b) the protein content in the lower ileum and proximal colon.
(c) the bacterial flora in the ileum and colon, particularly the presence of urea-splitting organisms.
(d) the presence of extensive porta-systemic venous shunts.

By flowing through these anastomoses the portal blood bypasses the liver and the total hepatic blood flow is significantly reduced. Amino acids and other substances which are absorbed from the small intestine and normally go to the liver to be metabolised are carried directly into the circulation and may have injurious effects.

Clinically the most obvious and important of these is encephalopathy which can vary from clumsiness and disorientation to coma. The pathological features in the brain are spongy demyelination, particularly at the junction of the grey and white matter, and the presence of Alzheimer II astrocytes in the basal ganglia and cerebellum. The electro-encephalogram shows a marked increase in slow waves and therefore a fall in the Mean Dominant Frequency (average number of cycles per second).

Ascites

Ascites in portal hypertension is due to the combination of impaired venous return and the presence of hepatic parenchymal disease. The effect of the former is mechanical, an increased transudation into the peritoneal cavity, and it determines the location of the generalised fluid retention which is a feature of the impaired metabolism of advanced hepatic disease. Ascites is a common feature of portal hypertension due to cirrhosis of the liver but is rare when the obstruction is extra-hepatic.

Prognosis

The prognosis in portal hypertension is different in extra-hepatic and intra-hepatic obstruction. In the former the liver is usually functionally normal and the patient young, and if bleeding from cardio-oesophageal varices can be prevented the outlook is good. In a personal series of children with extra-hepatic portal obstruction 50% were alive and well 20 years after operation. The prognosis in intra-hepatic obstruction depends on the type of liver disease, its functional and histological severity and the incidence of gastro-oesophageal haemorrhage. Features with a poor prognosis are active hepatitis, continued excessive consumption of alcohol, severe hepatic dysfunction, persistent ascites and recurrent haemorrhage. Most patients progress to and die from hepatic failure with jaundice, ascites and coma, often precipitated by a bleeding episode.

A.I.S. Macpherson

428

Benign tumours are rare. Adenoma, either biliary or hepatocellular, is usually symptomless. An association of adenoma with the prolonged use of oral contraceptive pills has been reported.

Hepato-cellular carcinoma

Hepato-cellular carcinoma in 80% of cases is secondary to hepatic cirrhosis or haemochromatosis. The tumour may form a single mass, be multicentric in origin, or infiltrate diffusely. It grows slowly and shows a marked tendency to blood spread within the portal and hepatic veins. The geographical incidence is striking, being far higher in certain areas in Central and South Africa and in the Far East than in the Western world. The tumour cells elaborate alphafoetoprotein and a very high level of this substance in the serum is characteristic of hepatoma but not diagnostic. It may be elaborated by other tumours, e.g. teratoma.

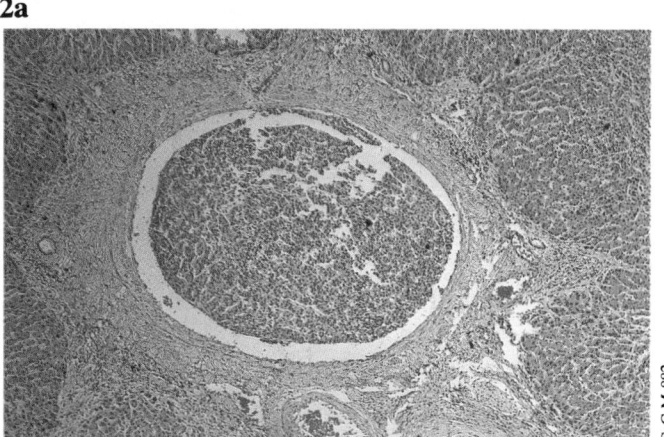

2 Hepato-cellular carcinoma. In a well differentiated tumour the cells are regular, show little mitotic activity and may be arranged in pseudo-lobules. *(H&E ×250)*

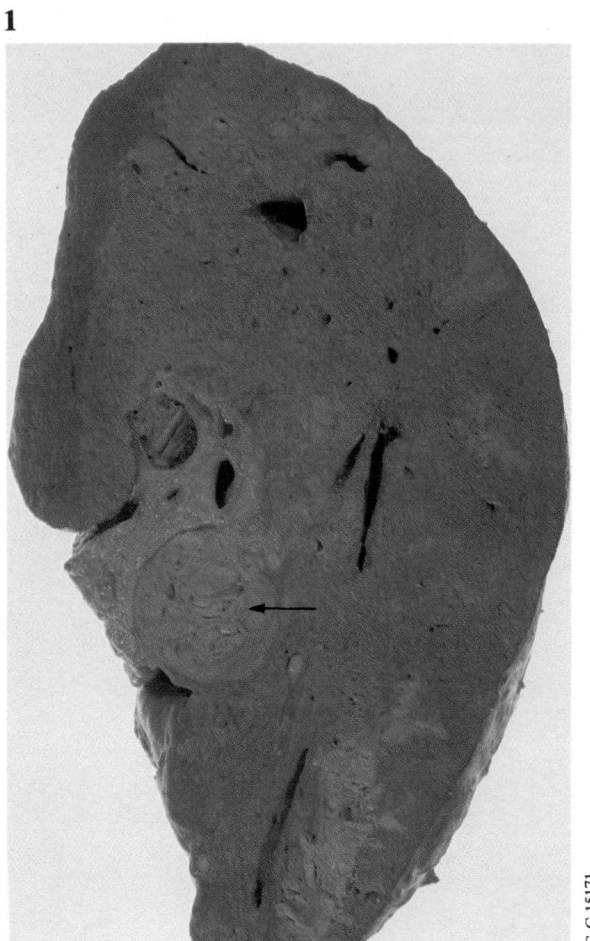

2a Hepato-cellular carcinoma permeating a portal vein radicle in the liver. *(H&E ×40)*

1 Haemochromatosis with cirrhosis and hepato-cellular carcinoma.

On the dark surface of the affected liver several pale areas can be seen. In the smaller pale areas it is difficult to distinguish between regenerative and neoplastic nodules. The larger nodules are undoubtedly malignant – multicentric hepato-cellular carcinoma. The portal veins have been invaded and a large radicle at the hilum contains tumour-thrombus.

Cholangiocarcinoma

This adenocarcinomatous tumour of the bile ducts has a marked scirrhous tendency which leads to obstruction of the duct in which it originates. It is often multicentric.

3 Liver – cholangiocarcinoma. On the left the parenchyma is invaded by poorly differentiated tumour. In the portal tract the carcinoma shows ductal differentiation. *(H&E ×100)*

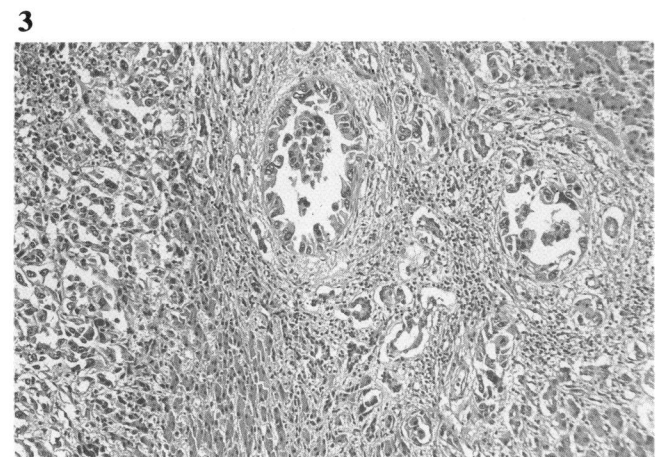

Hepatoblastoma

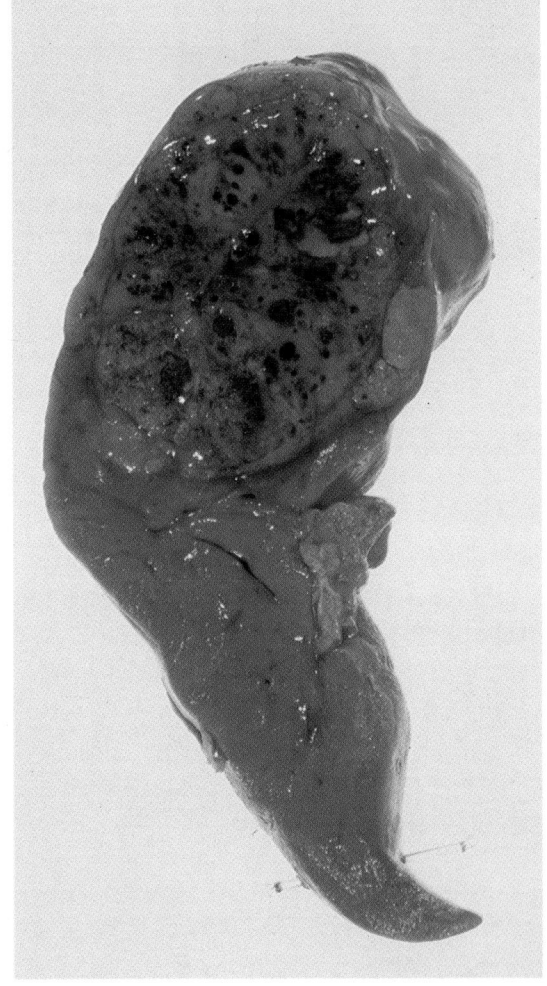

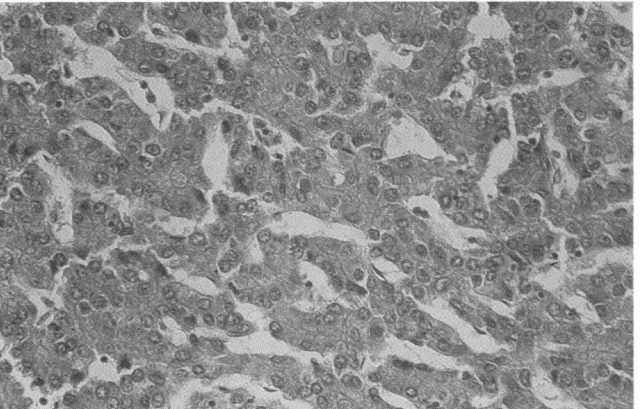

4a Liver – hepatoblastoma. A tumour composed of well differentiated cells forming columns and sinusoids. The structure resembles that of embryonic liver. *(H&E ×250)*

Hepatoblastoma is a rare and highly malignant tumour found only in infants and young children. It is derived from embryonal hepatic cells and occurs in an otherwise normal liver. Mitoses are frequent. The tumour metastasises early to regional lymph nodes, lung and brain. Sometimes the tumour may produce ectopic hormones leading to a degree of virilism.

4 From a male child aged 3 years 6 months who suffered from loss of energy associated with loss of weight and occasional upper abdominal pain. On clinical examination a firm tumour extended below the right costal margin. Exploratory examination revealed an inoperable hepatic tumour with adherent omentum which bled readily. Death ensued some hours after. The cut surface of the liver exhibits a large lobulated tumour in the upper part of the specimen. The tumour is hemispherical with a wrinkled lobulated surface. There has been much necrosis of the centre of the tumour with haemorrhage. Some of the lobules which have been cut across are fleshy in appearance.

Haemangioma

Haemangioma is a congenital vascular anomaly which may occur as a single lesion in the liver in cavernous or capillary form. It presents as a purplish mass which on section shows large endothelial-lined spaces filled with blood. When near the surface a haemangioma may bleed either spontaneously or following minor trauma. Haemangiomas may be found simultaneously in the liver and the spleen. Whether these are multifocal hamartomas or a sarcomatous change in the spleen with secondary deposit in the liver is difficult to determine pathologically and may be resolved only by the course of the disease.

Haemangiosarcoma

Haemangiosarcoma has been observed many years after the injection of thorotrast, a radioactive compound of thorium which was formerly used as the opaque medium in angiography.

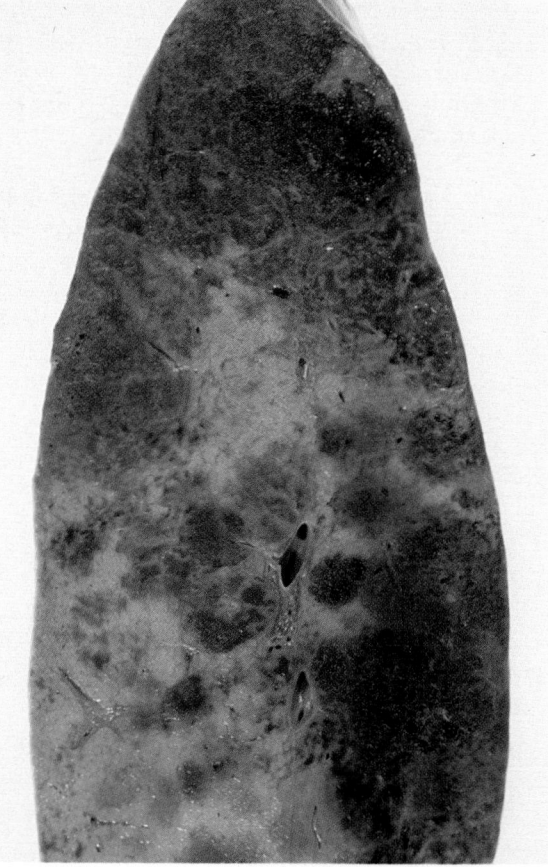

7 From a male aged 39 years who died 2 days after admission to hospital. The liver was grossly enlarged weighing 5 kg. The surface of the liver is smooth and mottled with large blue coloured areas interspersed with yellowish patches. On section the greater part of the liver appears replaced by dark coloured areas which are very haemorrhagic. Between the nodules the liver substance is paler than normal. Subepicardial and subpleural haemangiomas were also present.

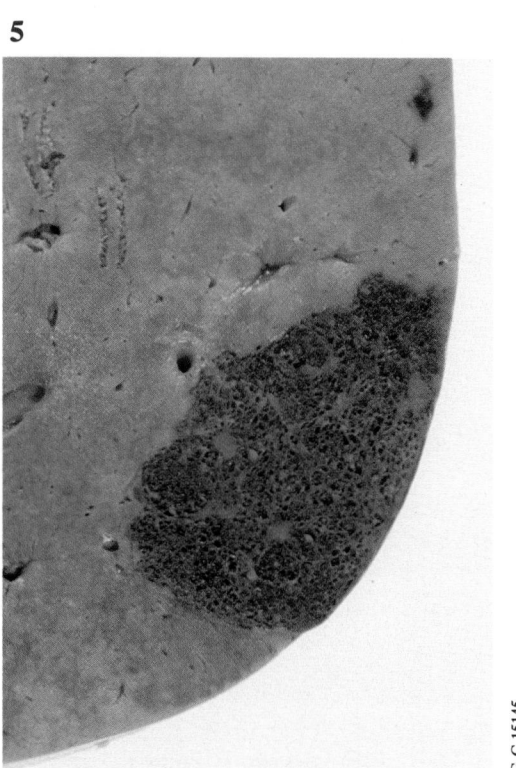

5 Subcapsular haemangioma.

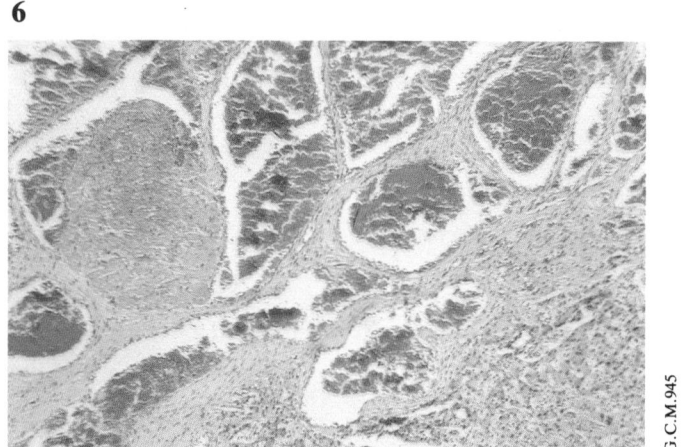

6 Cavernous haemangioma. Large vascular spaces replace the liver substance. They are lined by endothelial cells and some of the spaces may contain thrombus. *(H&E ×50)*

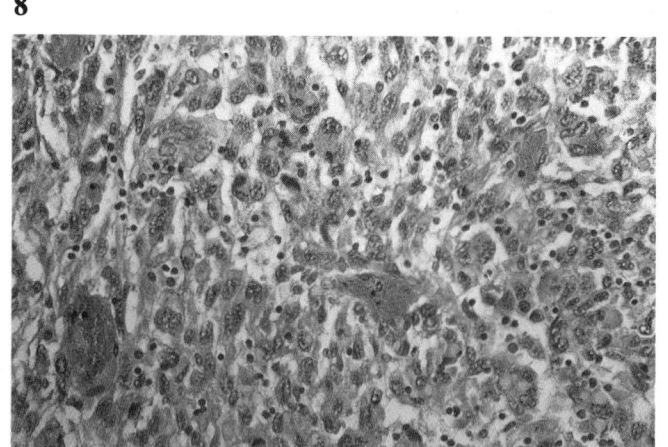

8 Haemangiosarcoma following thorotrast injection. Poorly differentiated vaso-formative tumour infiltrates the liver. *(H&E ×250)*

Secondary tumours

Secondary malignant tumours are common in the liver and are generally multiple. They may be demonstrated by radio-nucleide scanning. The commonest are metastatic carcinomas from the alimentary tract and when subcapsular these are characteristically umbilicated due to central necrosis. In the lymphomas and in leukaemia diffuse infiltration may occur.

Aneurysm of the hepatic artery

9

This rare lesion may be intra- or extra-hepatic, single or multiple, and when extra-hepatic may involve the main trunk or one of its branches. Aneurysm of the hepatic artery seldom causes symptoms until it leaks or ruptures. Intra-hepatic rupture gives rise to pain, fever, fluctuating jaundice and haemobilia. Extra-hepatic rupture is into the peritoneal cavity or the retroperitoneal spaces and carries the features of an upper abdominal emergency and of internal haemorrhage.

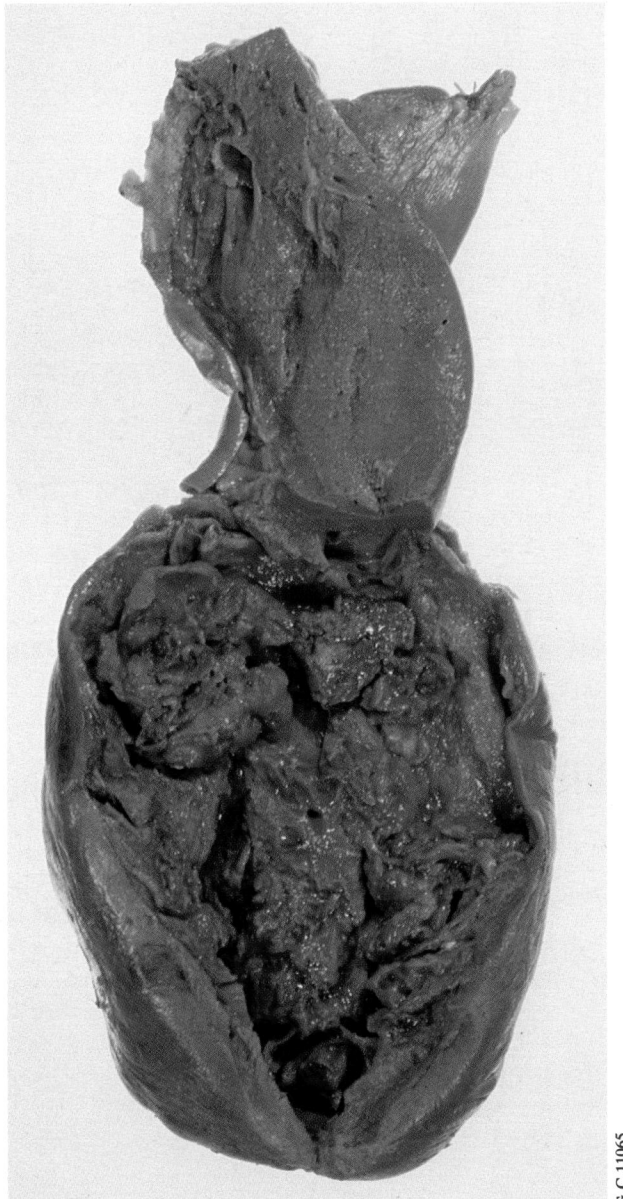

9 Aneurysm of the hepatic surgery. This historic specimen was originally prepared and described by Sir Charles Bell (cat. 1823). The patient was a male aged 50 years who was ill in health for 7 years.

The specimen demonstrates an aneurysm of the hepatic artery (possibly intrahepatic) which has ruptured and burst into the liver substance there forming a large thin walled sac in which there is much coagulum.

A.I.S. Macpherson

1

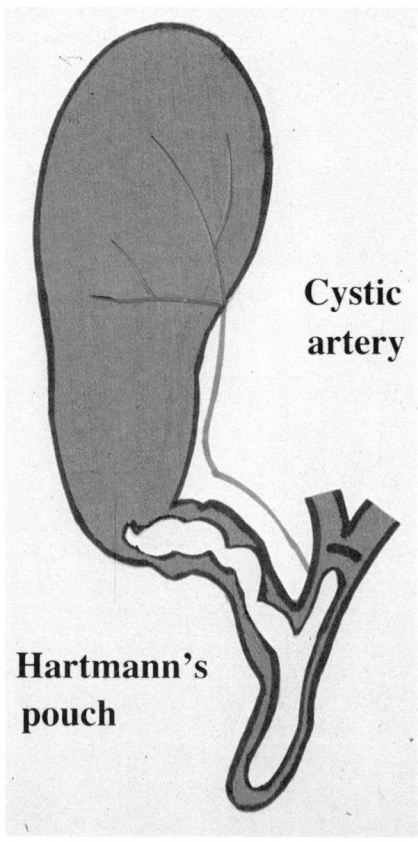

Cystic artery

Hartmann's pouch

The gallbladder is a pear shaped sac with a potential capacity of 50 ml.

The mucosa at the neck of the gallbladder is arranged in a series of folds sometimes known as the valves of Heister. An eccentric dilatation of the neck of the gallbladder is found so that the duct appears to leave the gallbladder laterally rather than from the apex. The dilatation is called Hartmann's pouch in which a calculus, if present, may become impacted. The cystic duct runs an S-shaped course 4 cm in length. It runs obliquely downwards close to the right hepatic artery and joins the common hepatic duct at an acute angle to take part in the formation of the common bile duct.

The gallbladder lies in a fossa on the inferior surface of the right lobe of the liver. The free surface of the gallbladder is covered by peritoneum by which it is firmly attached to the liver. The degree to which the gallbladder is embedded in the liver varies. In some instances the fossa is relatively deep. In others it is shallow and the gallbladder therefore acquires a mesentery of varying size. If the mesentery is long there is a predispositon to torsion of the gallbladder.

Histology

The gallbladder wall has four layers.

1 The mucosa formed by the inner covering epithelium set upon stroma and normally consisting of a single layer of tall columnar epithelium. The mucosa is thrown into folds so that on section it shows a gross villous-like pattern. Its stroma is an upward extension of

2 The lamina propria, a layer of vascular connective tissue

3 Bundles of longitudinal and transverse muscle fibres – the muscularis – separate the lamina propria from

4 The serosa where the peritoneal covering is set upon a layer of loose connective tissue containing blood vessels and nerves.

Common bile duct

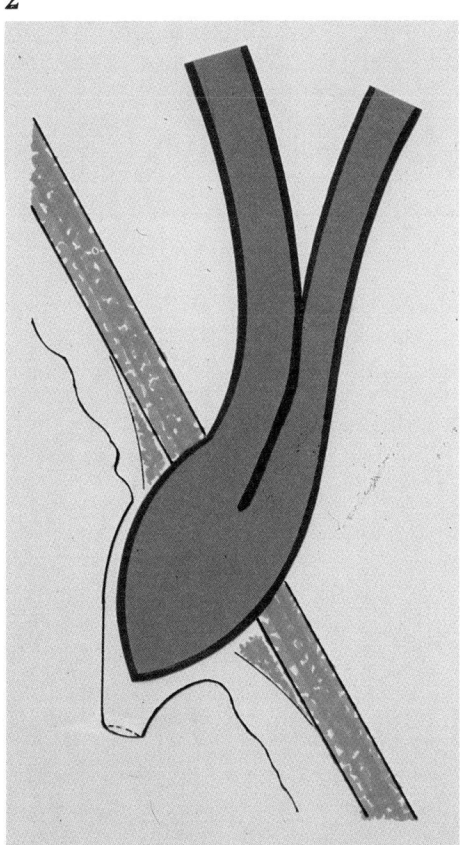

2 The common bile duct is formed by the junction of the common hepatic and cystic ducts. It runs downwards in the free border of the lesser omentum and after passing on the deep surface of the first part of the duodenum and the head of the pancreas, opens into the second part of the duodenum on its postero-medial wall. Normally the common duct and pancreatic duct join in a dilated ampulla (Ampulla of Vater). The ampulla opens on a raised papilla lying between adjacent folds of mucosa.

At the ampulla the muscle coat of the common bile duct, which now surrounds the ampulla, is increased in thickness, constituting the Sphincter of Oddi.

The common bile duct has relatively little muscle in its wall compared with the gallbladder. This explains the greater severity of biliary pain when a calculus is located in the gallbladder and the lesser pain, or its absence, when the calculus lies in the common duct.

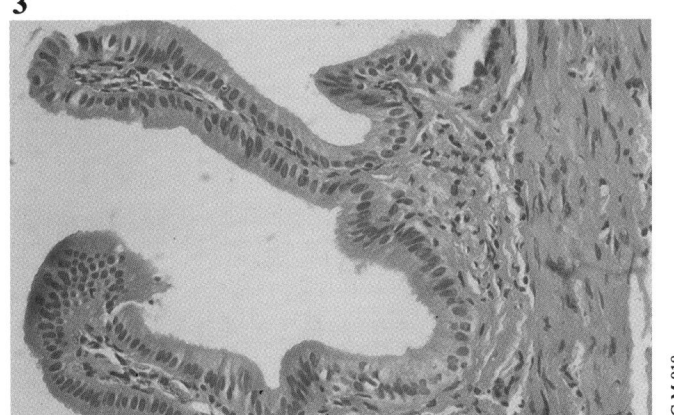

3 A section of gallbladder showing villous processes of mucosa separated by the lamina propria from the muscularis. *(H&E ×100)*

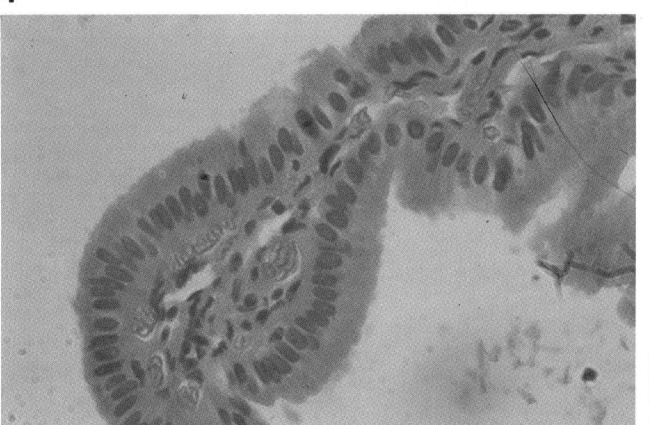

4 Gallbladder mucosa showing tall columnar epithelium set upon its vascular stroma. *(H&E ×500)*

Anatomical anomalies

There are many anatomical anomalies both of the arterial supply to the gallbladder and of the cystic and common ducts. These are of special interest to the operating surgeon since full exposure of the arteries of supply to the gallbladder and the relationship of the cystic to the common duct as an initial step in the operation of cholecystectomy is essential. Failure to do so may result in damage especially to the right hepatic artery or the common duct.

Blood supply

Arterial

The classical description of the blood supply to the gallbladder is that of a single artery arising from the common hepatic or the right hepatic artery, close to the bifurcation. It lies superior and posterior to the cystic duct. Certain variations of this arrangement are illustrated.

5

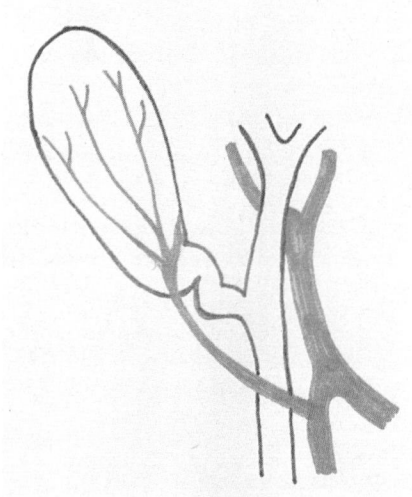

6

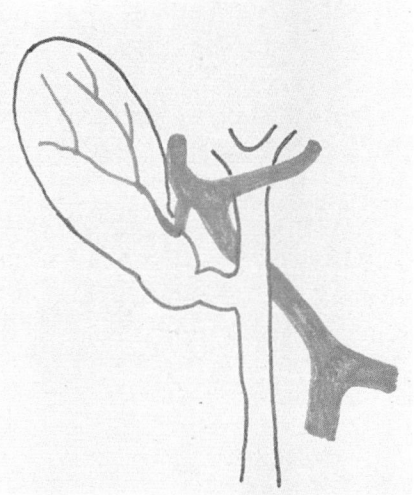

7

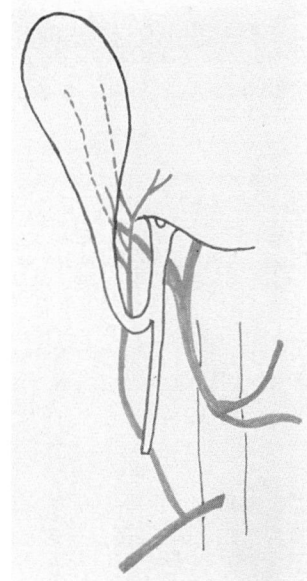

5 Origin from gastro-duodenal artery.

6 Left hepatic artery lying anterior to duct.

7 Origin from superior mesenteric or superior pancreatico-duodenal artery.

8

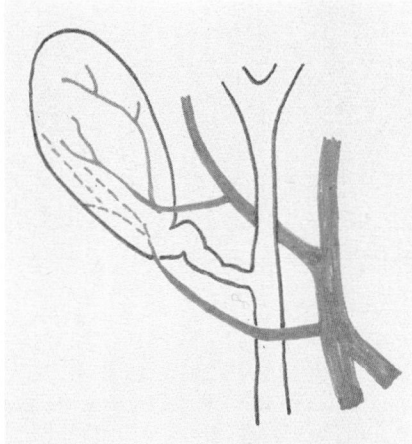

9

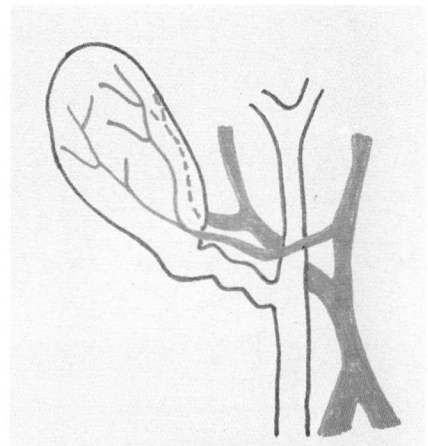

8 Duplication of cystic artery. Origin from right hepatic and common hepatic arteries.

9 Duplication of cystic artery. Origin from right and left hepatic arteries.

Bile duct

Anomalies of the cystic and common duct are numerous and certain typical examples are illustrated.

10

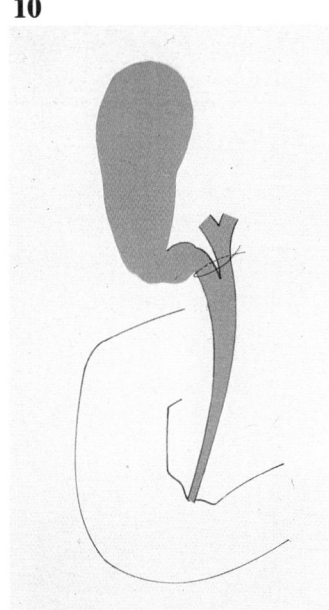

11

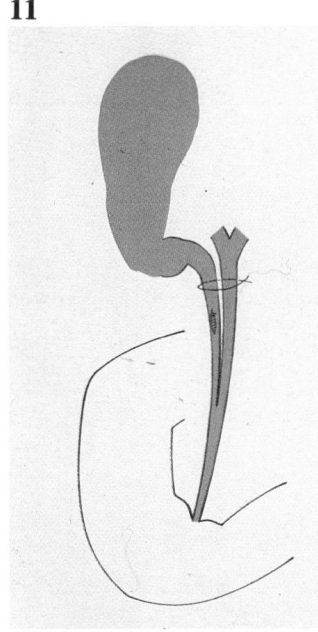

12

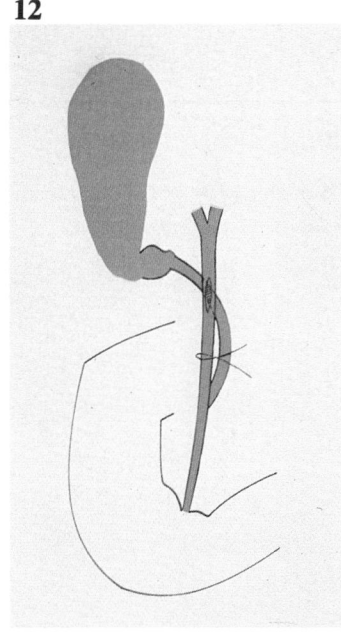

10 Short cystic duct.
   Danger – Ligature or section of the cystic duct is liable to include the common duct.

11 Low entry of cystic duct. Danger – Simultaneous ligature of cystic and common duct. Attempted choledochotomy may open cystic duct only.

12 Left sided entry cystic duct. Danger – Cystic duct runs behind the common duct and enters on left side. Ligature of common hepatic duct instead of cystic duct.

13

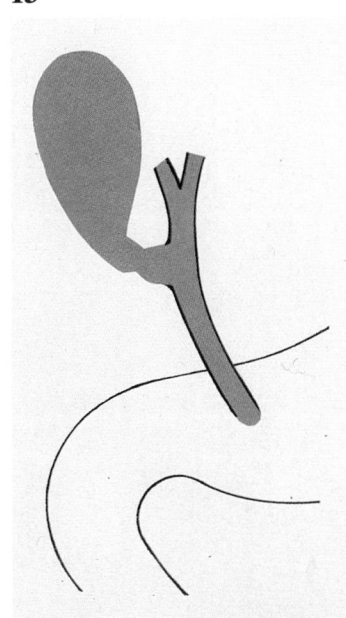

14

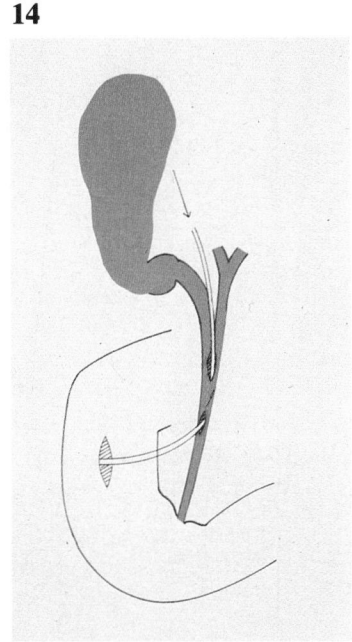

15

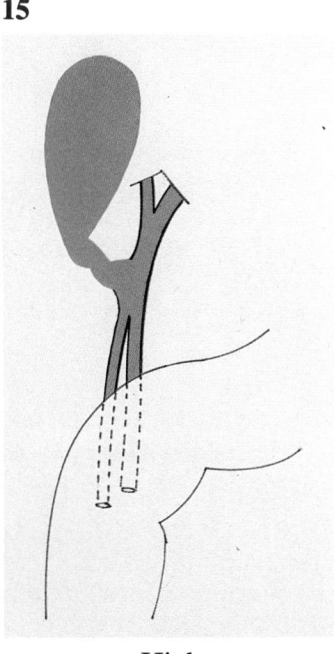

16

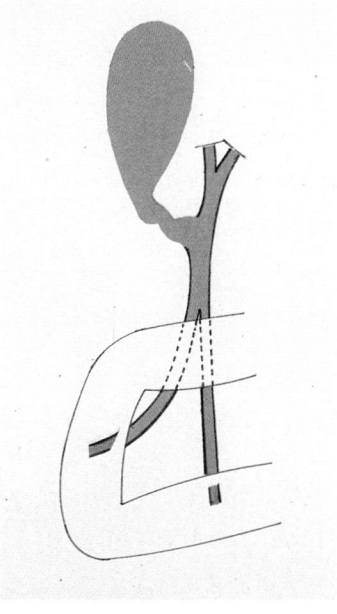

13 The common bile duct opens into the pyloric canal.

14 Low entry common duct into duodenum.
   Danger – False passage by bougie leading to fistula.

High

Low

15 and **16** Bifurcation of the common bile duct with anomalous openings into the duodenum.

Functions of gallbladder

1 The storage and concentration of bile – Bile is produced continuously by the liver, but is required in the intestine only intermittently. Between meals, the sphincter of Oddi is contracted. This prevents the outflow of bile from the common duct and when the pressure of bile in the common bile duct exceeds 7 cm bile, bile passes along the cystic duct to the gallbladder where it is stored and concentrated by selective reabsorption to a small fraction (1/10) of its original volume. The reduction in volume is caused by the isosmotic reabsorption of sodium chloride and water. Potassium, bicarbonate and some calcium ions are also absorbed and the pH falls from 8–8.6 to 7–7.6. There is little if any absorption of bile salts, cholesterol, phospholipid or bilirubin and these are concentrated from 5 to 10 times. Both hepatic and gallbladder bile are isotonic with plasma, even though bile is concentrated × 10 in the gallbladder.

2 The secretion of a thick mucous material.

3 The equalisation of pressure in the biliary duct system. The loss of gallbladder equalising action within the duct system may be a factor leading to the dilatation of the bile ducts following cholecystectomy.

17

17 During the process of concentration of bile in the gallbladder, micelle formation occurs. This process has already been described (see Section 16/1).

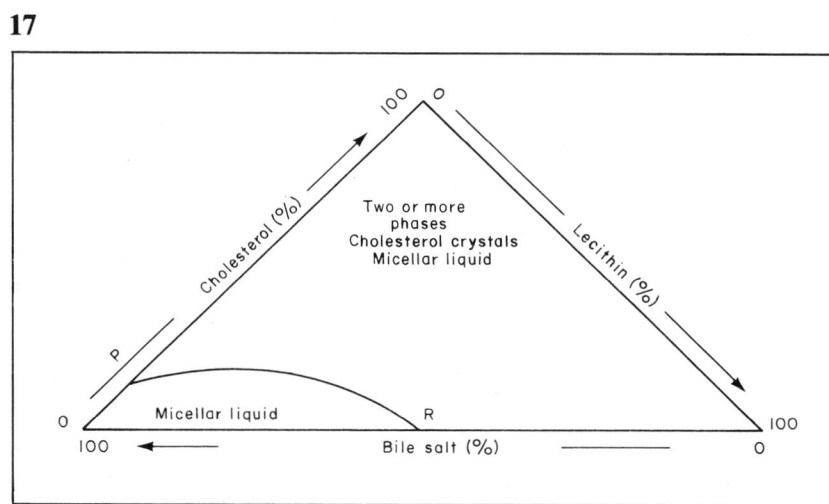

Fatty acids and to a lesser extent the products of protein digestion and calcium stimulate the release of Cholecystokinin/Pancreozymin (CCK/PZ) from the upper intestinal mucosa, which causes simultaneous contraction of the gallbladder and relaxation of sphincter of Oddi. Vagal stimulation as part of the cephalic phase of gastric secretion or of several intestinal reflexes produces a weak contraction of the gallbladder and relaxation of the sphincter. Many other substances such as adrenaline, histamine and bombesin produce contraction of the gallbladder and relaxation of the sphincter while morphine, atropine, somatostatin and vaso-active intestinal peptides relax the gallbladder.

Gallbladder motility

The gallbladder contracts to provide the force required to move the bile along the common bile duct, and the sphincter of Oddi relaxes to allow bile to flow from the common bile duct into the duodenum. The control of the gallbladder and sphincter is nervous and hormonal, the latter being the more important.

By the administration of Telepaque the gallbladder can be visualised. The concentration of the dye within the gallbladder varies and is a measure of the absorptive function of the gallbladder. A defective shadow therefore is indicative of gallbladder wall disease.

The emptying of the gallbladder can be visualised and if defective is also indicative of gallbladder wall pathology.

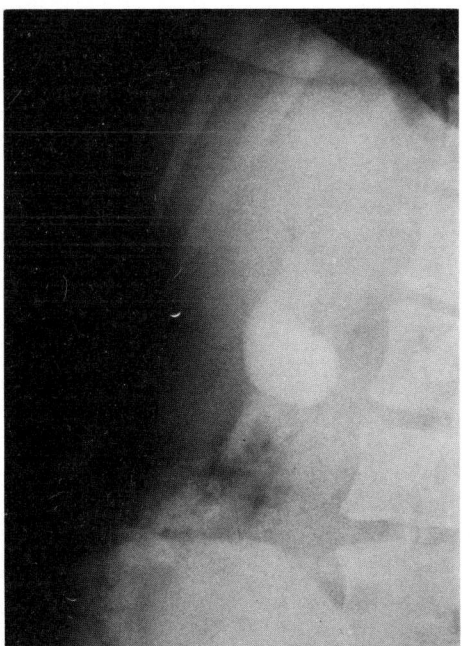

18 Oral cholecystogram. Normal gallbladder 12 hours after ingestion of Telepaque.

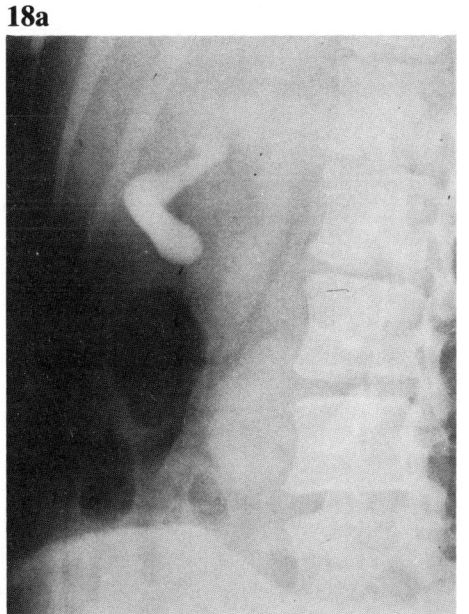

18a Oral cholecystogram (same patient) 30 minutes after fatty meal showing contraction of the gallbladder.

The presence of calculi within the gallbladder and lesions of the gallbladder wall can be demonstrated by cholecystography.

The terms cholecystitis and cholelithiasis refer to pathological conditions of the gallbladder which may be identified as separate lesions but more frequently occur together as a mixed lesion. In common parlance the term 'cholecystitis' covers both conditions.

Gallbladder disease presents in a variety of forms:
1   The presence of calculi in the gallbladder without inflammatory change in the wall of the viscus.
2   Inflammatory change in the mucosa and the wall of the gallbladder unassociated with the presence of calculi.
3   The occurrence of a mixed lesion in which both calculi and inflammatory change are present.

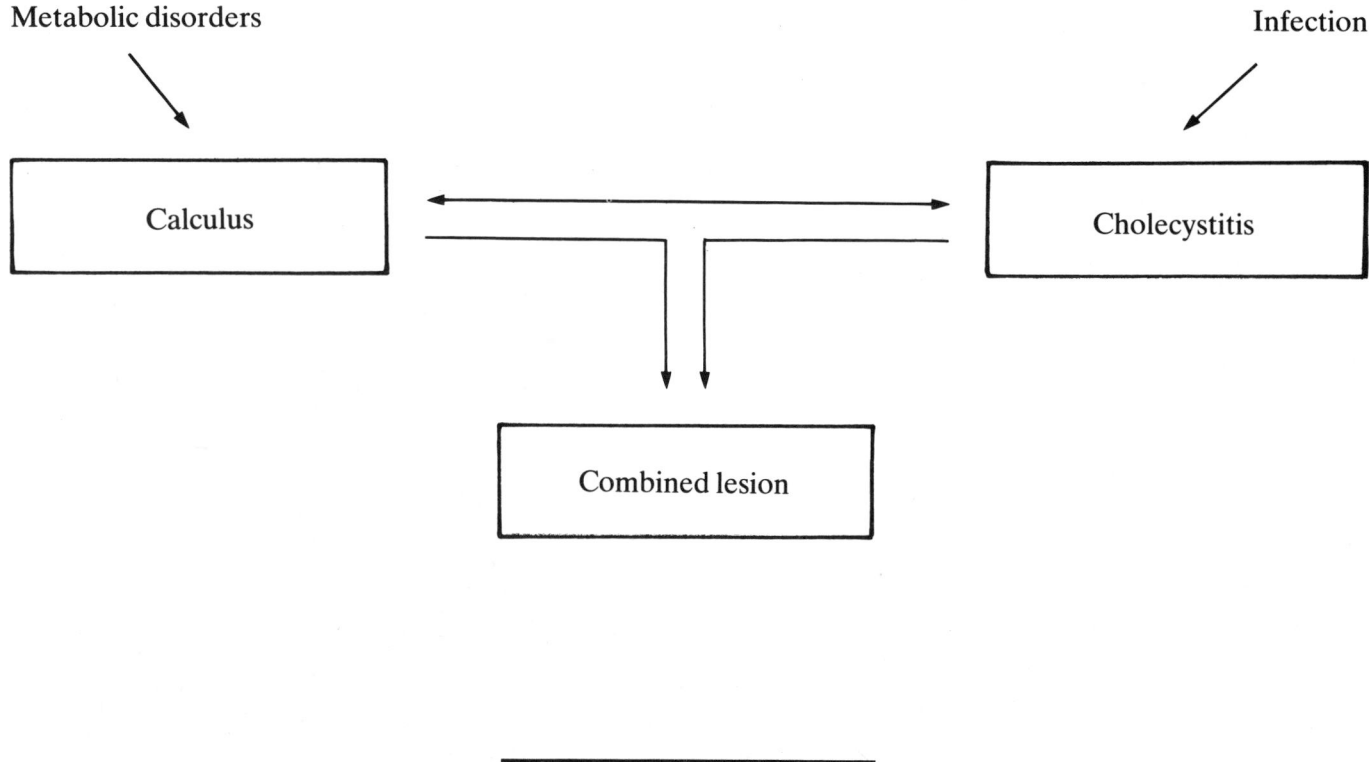

The aetiology is complex since several factors have been identified. Earlier workers considered that bacterial infection was the principal cause but there is a growing appreciation that pathological changes at least initially may be attributable to metabolic disorder. The presence of a gallstone within the lumen of the gallbladder causes further change by reason of the physical trauma it exercises on the wall of the viscus or by causing obstruction to the outflow of bile. In many instances all factors play a part.

For clarity of presentation both the pathological variants with their complications and the several aetiological factors are described in separate paragraphs.

Incidence

The incidence of gallbladder disease is unknown. There has been a marked increase in cholecystectomy in many countries over the last 15 years although there is considerable variation. The figures for the Scottish Regional Hospital Boards demonstrate the change. The variation could reflect differences in the prevalence of the disease or in the threshold level for treatment. The former is difficult to measure because many gallstones may not cause sufficient symptoms to make the patient report to the doctor. Autopsy studies do not necessarily furnish a true estimate as these patients form a selected group. However, the incidence is similar in countries with very different cholecystectomy rates, indicating that other factors must play a part.

The threshold for surgery is determined by the balance of demand for and the supply of health resources. These vary with factors such as awareness and tolerance of symptoms, the accessibility and availability of primary care and surgical services, and the indications for surgical treatment. There is an increased belief in surgical treatment for patients with acute cholecystitis and there has been a marked increase in surgical treatment for women under the age of 40 years with the suggestion that the increased use of the contraceptive pill may be important.

Post mortem studies show that in subjects over 70 years of age gallstones are found in 20% of cases.

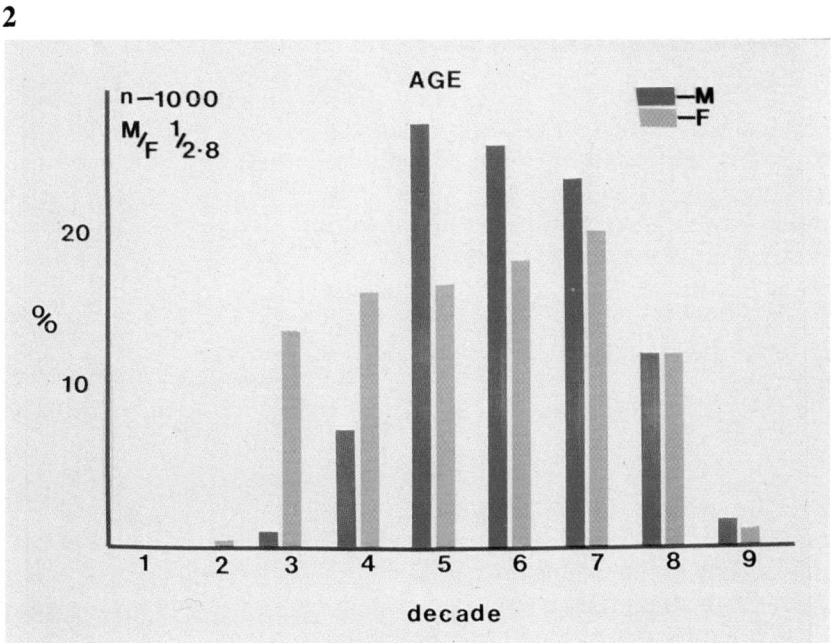

1

2

The sex ratio is 1 male to 3 females and the disease presents later in men. It is commonest in the seventh decade but many patients have a long history of preceding dyspepsia. There is evidence of a familial tendency.

In childhood cholecystitis and cholelithiasis are uncommon but appear to be increasing. Clinically the main presenting feature is abdominal pain, often recurrent, and a gallbladder lesion has to be differentiated from intestinal obstruction and appendicitis. The bile pigment stone is the variety most commonly found and may be associated with a haemolytic anaemia. It has also been held that calculus formation may result from a congenital narrowing of the outlet of the gallbladder with resulting biliary stasis.

441

Metabolic disturbances

Two of the obvious initiating factors in cholelithiasis are the process of bile concentration within the gallbladder (see Section 16/1) and impairment of micellar formation by reduction in the bile salt/cholesterol ratio. All the main constituents of bile including cholesterol are concentrated in the gallbladder. Bile pigments are concentrated most of all. In the presence of stasis or excessive production of bilirubin resulting from haemolysis bile pigments may be precipitated.

Cholesterol

The significant errors of cholesterol metabolism are supersaturation in the bile and disturbance of resorption of cholesterol by the biliary mucosa.

The cholesterol content of human bile is near saturation point. The stability of the solution is dependent upon bile salt and protein content. The bile cholesterol content may be raised by:
1 A high fatty intake in diet with resulting hypercholesterolaemia.
2 Pregnancy, especially in multiparae.
3 By hormonal imbalance which may be occasioned by the contraceptive pill.

Cholesterol stone formation is enhanced if the bile salt content in the gallbladder is diminished. It has been found that when bile salt absorption is impaired by the administration of drugs such as cholestyramine and clofibrate or by disease or resection of the terminal ileum, the incidence of gallstones is increased.

3 Cholesterol calculi and cholesterosis have been produced experimentally in animals by dietary methods.
In man the effects of diet can be illustrated by reference to Japanese statistics.

3

Effect of race, social status and diet on gallstone formation (cholesterol and pigment) Japan

(60 to 80% of all gallstones are pigment stones. Half or more form in bile ducts)

	Cholesterol	Pigment	Diet
Professional	32	29	Similar to occident
Labouring	8	62	Low in fat and protein

Japanese resident in U.S.A. show the same incidence and character of gallstones as the indigenous general population.

Cholesterol metabolic disturbances may result in the deposition of
1 Cholesterol in the wall of the gallbladder – Cholesterosis.
2 The formation of intraluminar calculi – Cholesterol stone.

Cholesterosis

The essential error is a precipitation of cholesterol during resorption through the gallbladder wall. The cholesterol accumulates in subepithelial macrophages in the mucosal ridges. The yellow streaks which result contrast with the darker surrounding mucosa giving an appearance which has been likened to an unripe strawberry (Strawberry gallbladder). The gallbladder wall is thin and is not inflamed. The contractile and absorptive function of the gallbladder may be impaired.

4

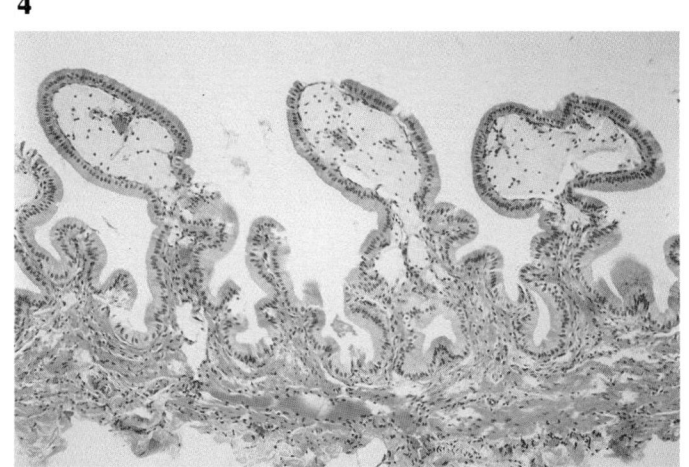

G.C.M.918

4 A section of gallbladder showing three mucosal ridges distended by accumulation of foamy macrophages in their stroma. *(H&E ×100)*

5

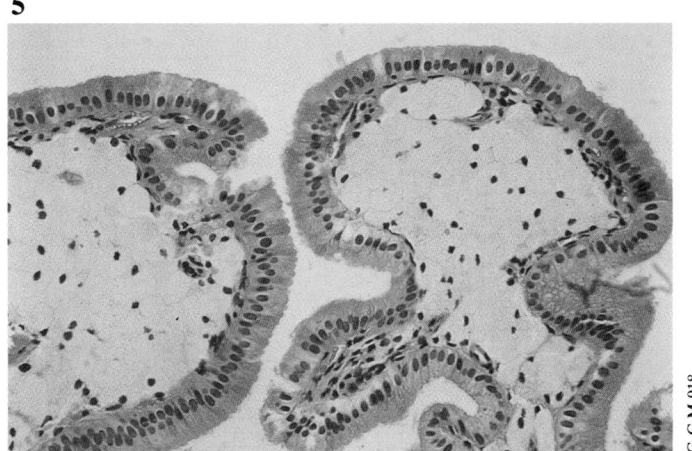

G.C.M.918

5 Macrophages distended by cholesterol lie tightly packed in the subepithelial stroma of the mucosal 'villi'. *(H&E ×250)*

6

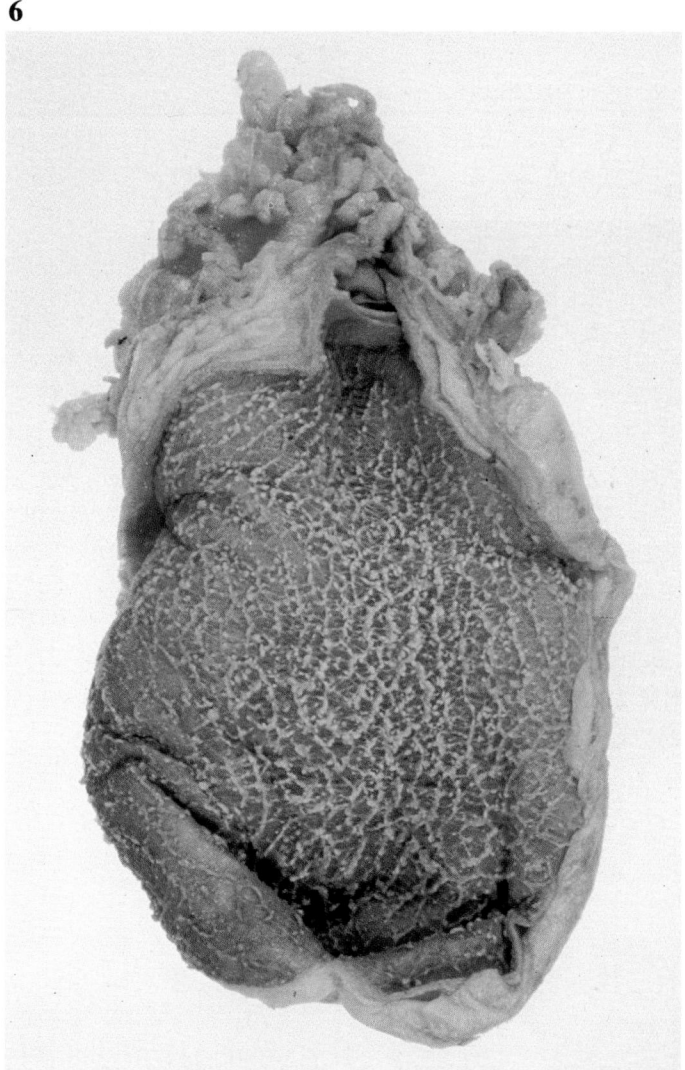

G.C.10479

6 From a multipara aged 63 years. Nine month history of flatulent dyspepsia. Cholecystography demonstrated a non-functioning gallbladder. When the specimen was examined after operation no stone was present. The mucosa shows numerous deposits of cholesterosis either in small isolated masses or in ridges. The gallbladder wall is not grossly abnormal.

By the use of the stain Sharlach R the presence of cholesterol can be more readily observed.

Cholesterol calculi

Precipitation of cholesterol within the gallbladder is facilitated by the presence of a nidus. It has been suggested that a cholesterol polyp from a preceding cholesterosis becomes detached and forms a nidus. In many instances what appears to be a pure cholesterol stone nevertheless has a small pigmented spot at its centre. This suggests that there is a nidus of bile pigment.

7

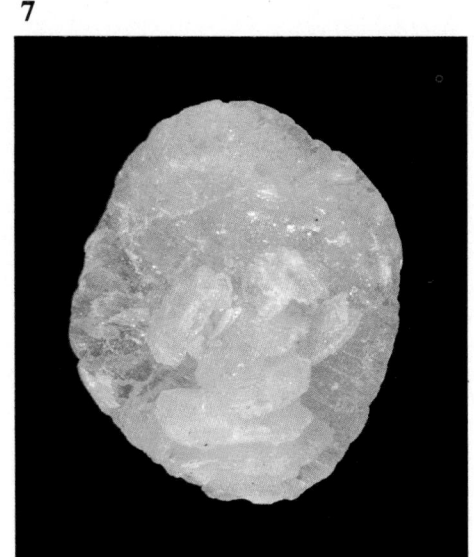

G.C.11442

7 The characteristic cholesterol calculus is the 'solitaire', an ovoid, white calculus with a slightly roughened and obviously crystalline surface.

8

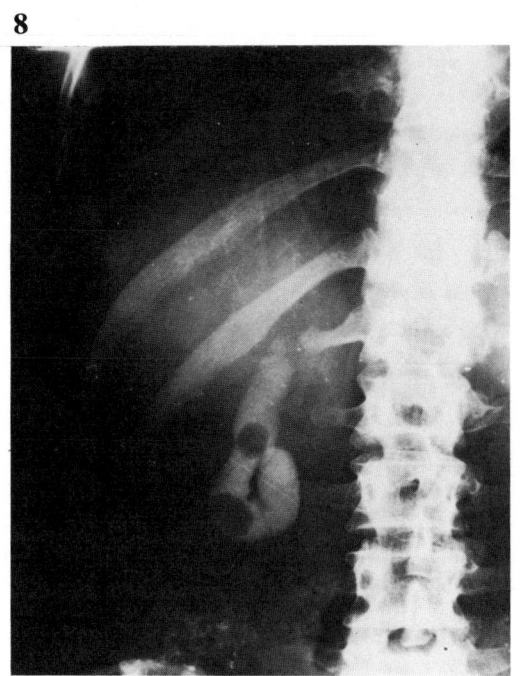

G.C.X.50

8 The calculus is radiotranslucent.

9

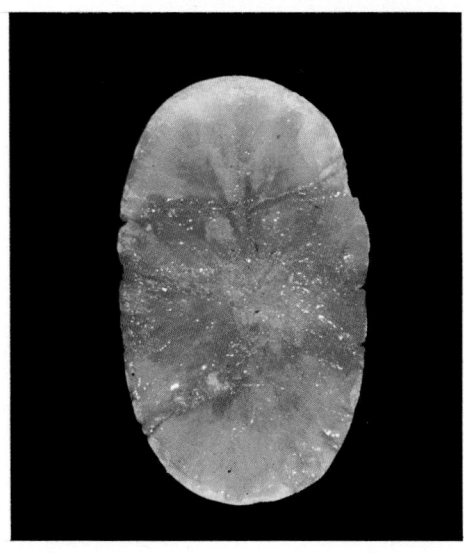

G.C.10809

9 On section the calculus is yellow/white in colour, crystalline in nature and the crystals appear to be radiating from its central point.

10

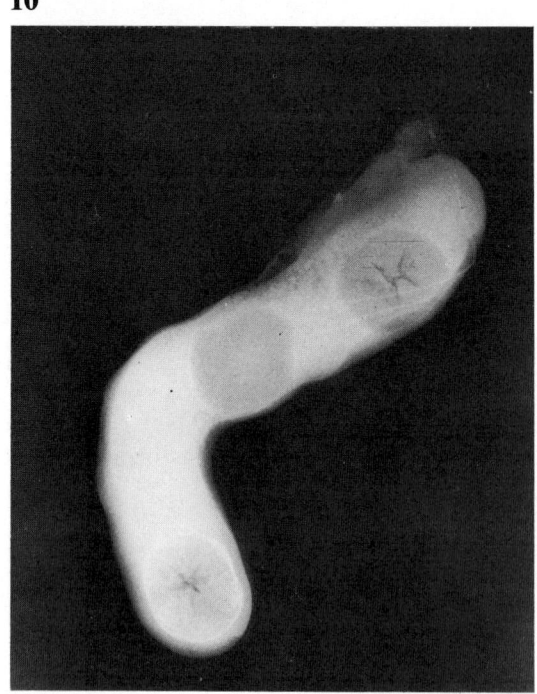

G.C.X.1000

10 Rarely there is fissuring of the calculus which can be demonstrated radiologically.

444

11

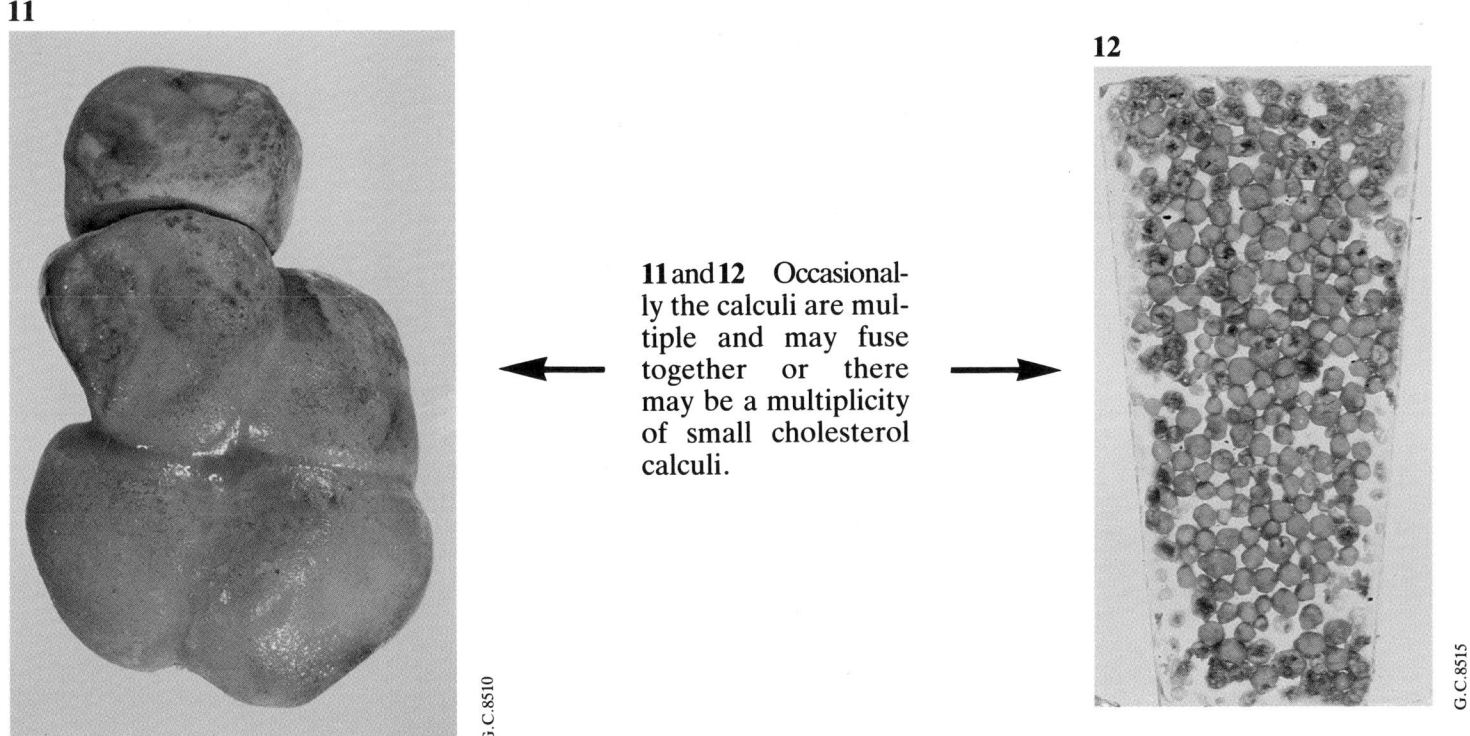

11 and **12** Occasionally the calculi are multiple and may fuse together or there may be a multiplicity of small cholesterol calculi.

12

G.C.8510

G.C.8515

13

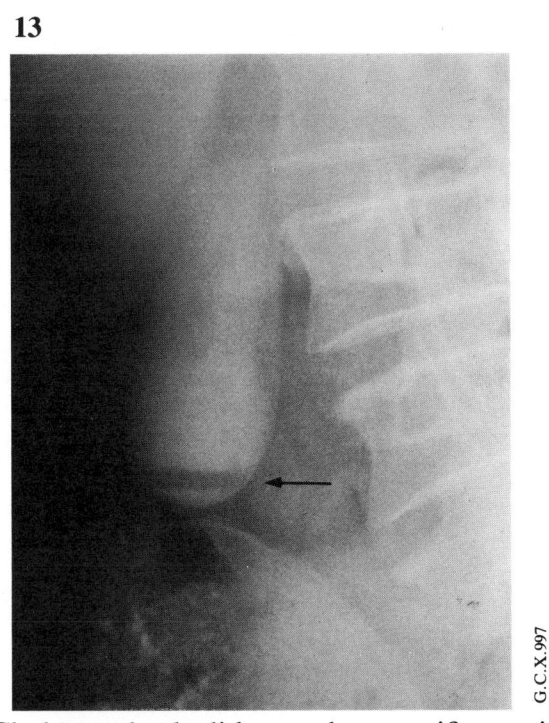

G.C.X.997

14

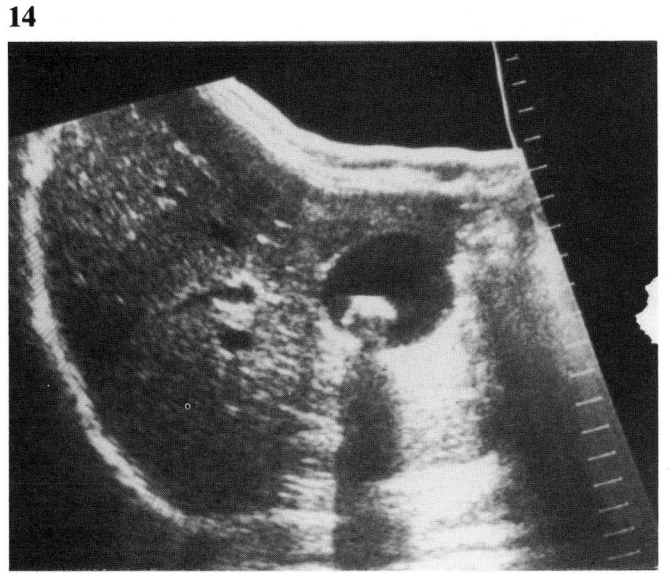

G.C.X.998

13 Cholesterol calculi have a low specific gravity and when the patient stands erect, float upwards. This can be demonstrated during radiological screening. Where there are multiple small cholesterol calculi these may form a horizontal line of translucency across the shadow of the gallbladder. This depends upon layering according to specific gravity.

14 Gallstones can be demonstrated using the modern technique of screening by ultrasound.

Cholesterol calculi *(Continued)*

Mulberry calculi

15 This is an alternative type of cholesterol calculus. The calculi are frequently multiple and have a bossed contour justifying the name mulberry stones. They are believed to arise as the result of the detachment of small polyps since they are most often associated with cholesterosis of the gallbladder wall.

15

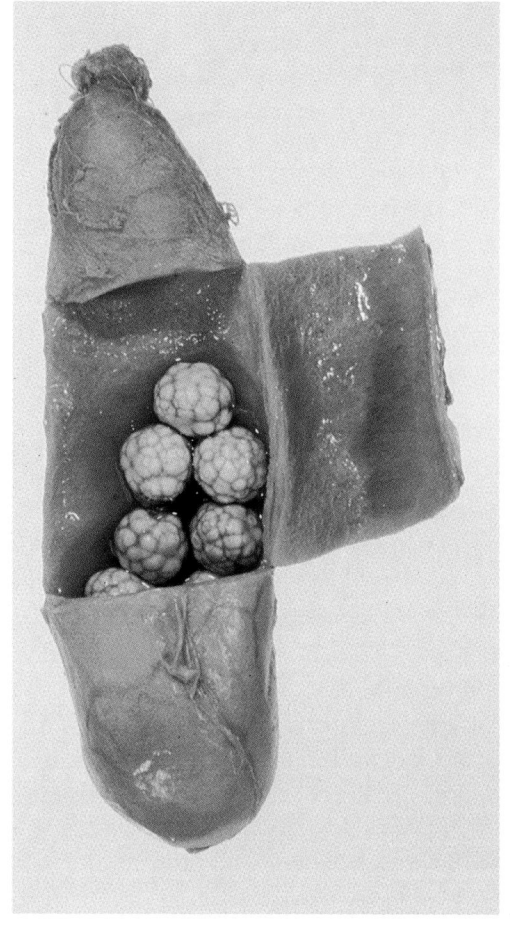

G.C.6109

Mucocoele

16

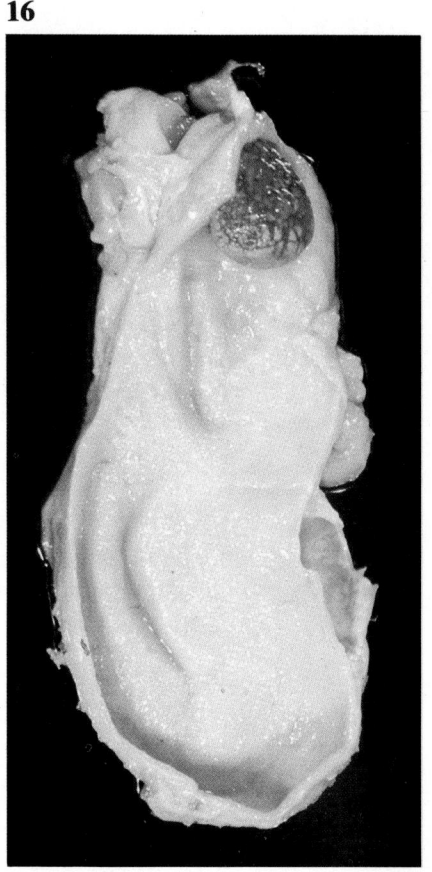

G.C.14562

A mucocoele occurs when a cholesterol calculus has become impacted at the neck of the gallbladder without associated infection. This is followed by a rapid outpouring of mucus and absorption of biliary salts. The gallbladder wall is thin, the mucosa shows no signs of inflammatory reaction and may be flattened, and the serous coat shows no reaction. The gallbladder becomes distended. If the mucocoele subsequently becomes infected it constitutes a dangerous type of empyema of the gallbladder.

16 The clinical features of mucocoele are frequently dramatic. A large ovoid swelling extending down below the left costal margin which may even reach the level of, or below, the umbilicus. This swelling is smooth and tense. Mucus may empty with great rapidity and the abdominal swelling disappears following the administration of a relaxant. The calculus may move forward into the common duct or slip back into the lumen of the gallbladder. The condition may recur.

Bile pigment calculi

Pure bilirubin calculi are multiple, irregular in outline, greenish, reddish or black in colour and always small in size. Such calculi are probably formed originally in the canaliculi of the liver. Chemically the calculi also contain calcium present as calcium bilirubinate.

Small aggregations of bilirubin are frequently found as the nidus about which a cholesterol calculus has formed as noted previously.

Pigmented calculi are frequently an incidental finding in the gallbladders of aged persons.

More significantly they are associated with a high secretion of bile pigment as occurs in haemolytic disease:

(a) Haemolytic jaundice of the congenital type in which there is a long continued increase of circulating bilirubin present in 50% of patients.

(b) Sickle cell anaemia.

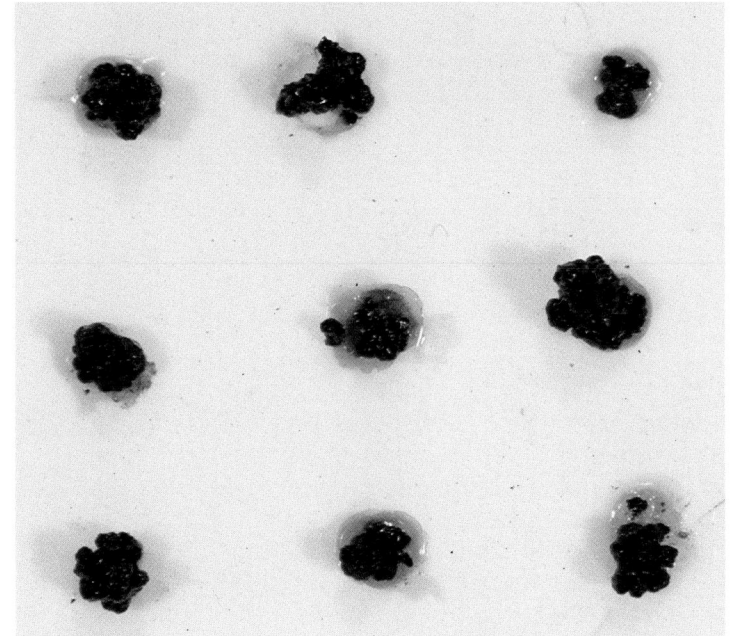

17

G.C. 10810

17 An incidental post mortem finding. There were a total of 102 pigmented calculi found in the gallbladder of which nine typical examples are illustrated.

Calcium carbonate calculi

Pure calcium carbonate calculi are very rare. They occur in the absence of overt inflammatory change in the gallbladder wall but apparently their formation is favoured by cystic duct obstruction causing retention of gallbladder content.

A calculus may form in the lumen of a gallbladder without evident inflammatory change in the wall (cholelithiasis). Later it may cause damage of the gallbladder wall and the development of an inflammatory reaction in it (cholecystitis).

The combined lesion

The commonest lesion of the gallbladder is one in which both calculus formation and infection of the gallbladder wall are present.

The initial lesion may be either of these two conditions and each may be the cause of the other. The calculi found in a combined lesion are always of a mixed type.

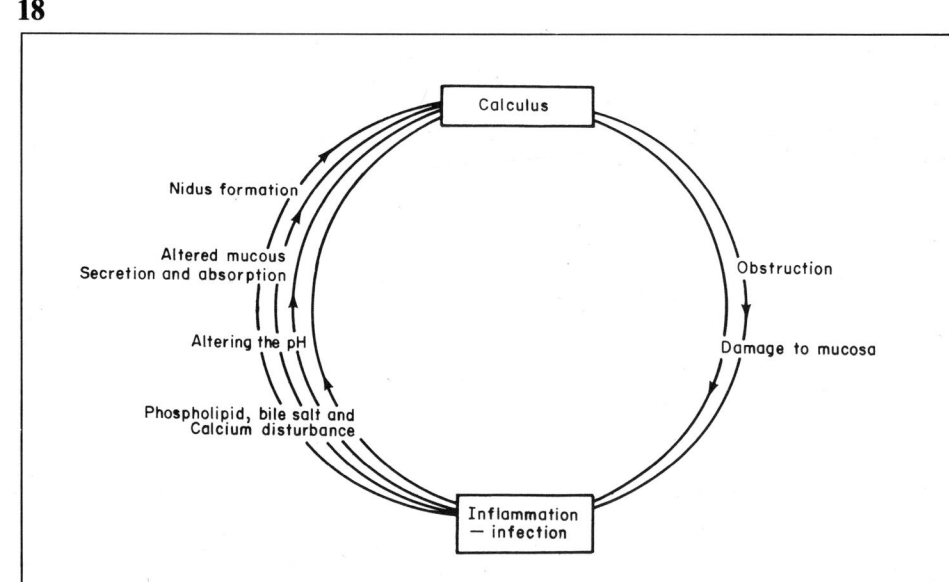

18

Physical factors

The older view that an inflammation of the gallbladder and the presence of gallstones was always attributable to infection is no longer tenable. It is now clear that calculi may result in mural changes as the result of physical factors which also render the gallbladder more liable to invasion by organisms (infection).

It is evident from more recent bacteriological studies of gallbladders showing inflammatory change that in many instances the presence of organisms cannot be demonstrated. Inflammatory reaction therefore must be attributed to other non-organismal factors.

Changes directly attributable to the presence of a calculus result from:

1   Direct pressure

Direct pressure causes ulceration and necrosis of the mucosa, exposing the underlying tissues to the irritant effect of the bile salts.

2   Obstruction

Caused by impaction of a calculus at the neck of the gallbladder or in the common bile duct.

3   Tension

The intraluminal pressure rises causing ischaemia of the mucosa which may proceed to gangrene.

Other causes of obstruction and/or stasis

In addition to calculi, obstruction to the cystic duct leading to bile stasis and therefore favouring infection may also be due to:
- (a) Torsion
- (b) Anomalous vessel
- (c) Inflammatory adhesions – Fibrosis
                          Periduodenitis
- (d) Enlarged lymph nodes
- (e) Neoplasm
- (f) Congenital stenosis
- (g) Regurgitation of pancreatic juices due to blockage at the lower end of the common duct
- (h) Disturbed neural control of gallbladder function. This occurs after vagotomy and other operations on the stomach.

This may also be the cause of dysfunction in association with duodenal ulcer.

Other effects of stasis

Where a pure cholesterol calculus has been retained in the gallbladder a further deposition of other salts on its surface may occur. Usually the original cholesterol calculus is covered by a thin shell of calcium. The cholesterol calculus has acted as a nidus and if there has been obstruction to the outflow of bile the concentration of bile is disturbed.

These two factors lead to the precipitation of other salts. These changes can occur without any evidence of inflammation of the wall and represent purely metabolic disturbance.

This is thus a non-infective type of mixed calculus.

20

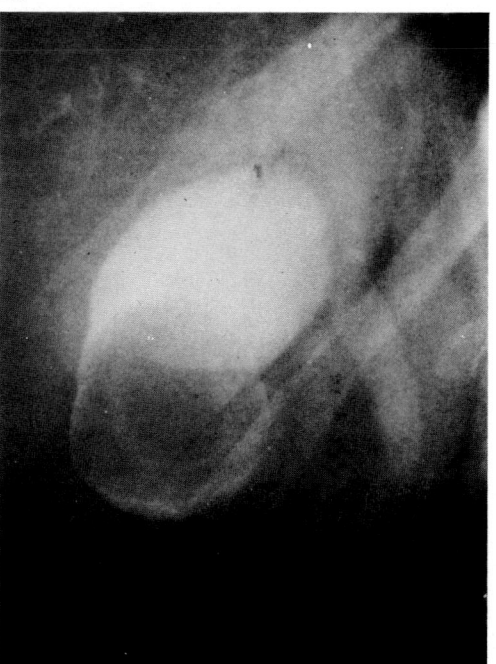

G.C.X.100

20 Cholecystogram showing a large cholesterol calculus with thin layers of superimposed calcium salts.

19

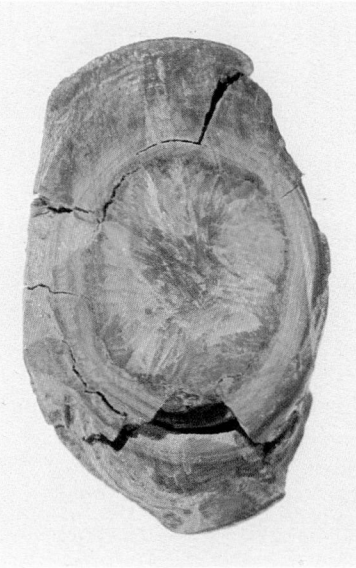

G.C.10055

19 The specimen is that of a large cholesterol calculus with the typical radiate deposition and the thick surrounding lamina of calcium salts which is laid down concentrically about the cholesterol nucleus.

The combined lesion *(Continued)*

Infection

Older observations were concerned with the identification of organisms recovered from the bile, the interior of gallstones or the wall of the gallbladder in cases of cholelithiasis.

It was held by such investigators as Rosenow (1921) and others that cholecystitis was due to a specific haematogenous streptococcal infection. Illustrative of the thinking at this time was the often quoted aphorism of Moynihan, 'Every gallstone is a tombstone erected to the memory of organisms dead within it but the organisms are sometimes buried alive'.

Secondary infection

A gallbladder wall damaged by calculi is prone to secondary bacterial infection.

In the presence of overt infection any calculi present will be of a mixed variety.

Route of infection

The possible routes of infection are shown diagrammatically.

Vascular	Hepatic artery
	Portal vein
Lymphatic	Ascending
	Descending
Bile duct	Ascending
	Descending

In a series personally studied the following findings were recorded:

Bacteriological findings   112 patients – 146 organisms

E. coli	76	Ps. pyocyaneus	2
Strep. faecalis	36	B. proteus	2
Staph. aureus	10	Enterococci	1
Cl. welchii	9	Non-haem strept.	1
H. strept.	8	Candida	1

Positive culture (%)	
Emergency cholecystectomy	35%
– Acute	30%
– Acute and chronic	38%
– Chronic	20%
Elective cholecystectomy	19%

In areas where typhoid fever is endemic the recovery of typhoid bacilli from the gallbladder is common. The organisms are found in the wall, in the bile and also in the interior of gallstones, if present, and in the intestine.

The infection may persist lasting for years and in many cases is symptomless; such persons are dangerous carriers of the disease.

Infection may predispose to calculus formation in several ways:
(a)   Bacteria may act as a nidus for calculus formation.
(b)   Mucus secretion may be disturbed.
(c)   The chemical structure of the phospholipids and the bile salts may be upset.
(d)   The pH may be altered.
(e)   Insoluble calcium salts may be formed.
(f)   Mucosal damage may lead to loss of resorption.

Mixed calculi

In cholelithiasis associated with infective cholecystitis the calculi are generally multiple, small, faceted and of similar size. Large calculi are occasionally found and sometimes 'families' of smaller stones of different size may be present.

The bile content may be thick containing much mucus or be purulent.

The gallbladder wall will show evidence of inflammatory change (cholecystitis – which is described in subsequent paragraphs).

On section the surface of the calculus is seen to be laminated. Alternating layers of white or light brownish colour represent the deposition of cholesterol or calcium carbonate. Layers of deep pigmentation represent the deposition of biliverdin and bilirubin. The thickness of the layers varies. There may be evidence of a central nucleus or the layers may be deposited around a pre-existing cholesterol calculus. The calculi have a protein matrix or network which demonstrates the same laminar formation as can be seen on the cut surface of the calculus. Organisms may be recovered occasionally from the interior of such calculi.

21

G.C.11430

21 Specimen showing multiple mixed calculi. The gallbladder is shrunken and the wall shows evidence of inflammatory change. The serosa is thickened, opaque and with shaggy fibrinous adhesions. The mucosa is thickened, velvety and congested.

22

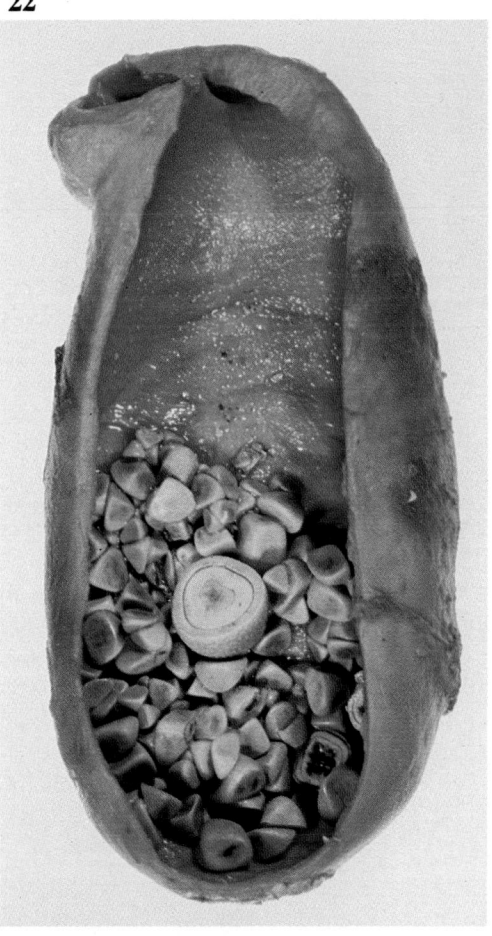

G.C.10086

22 The gallbladder contains a large rounded calculus and many smaller calculi. Much of the large calculus is formed by cholesterol crystals radiating around a slightly pigmented centre. The cholesterol nucleus is covered by partly calcified laminae. The smaller calculi vary in size, are faceted and have a pigmented nucleus covered by outer calcified laminae.

451

Chronic cholecystitis

Clinico-pathological features

Patients suffering from gallbladder disease, whether the dominant feature is the presence of a calculus or the associated histological features of chronic cholecystitis in the gallbladder wall, report to their doctor complaining of recurrent attacks of biliary pain. This is experienced in the right upper quadrant (anterior branch of the intercostal nerve) or in the epigastrium due to the developmental origin of the gallbladder. The pain is commonly referred to the tip of the right scapula (posterior branch of the intercostal nerve). These attacks are intermittent and may be provoked by fatty meals (cholecystokinin response). Such symptoms are due to obstruction to the outflow of bile from the gallbladder. The symptoms are relieved if the obstruction is cleared by the stone falling back into the gallbladder or entering the common duct.

Cholecystitis usually presents as a chronic illness characterised by progressive changes in the wall of the organ caused by a combination of the effect of calculi and recurrent attacks of inflammation.

Inflammatory lesions of the gallbladder without stone formation are relatively uncommon. Most usually the picture is seen in an early acute lesion, often in a young person, but later secondary stone formation will occur and the result is a lesion in which both inflammatory and calculus formation are found.

The differentiation between cholelithiasis and cholecystitis is really artificial in such lesions but is convenient only as a matter of presentation to the students.

In the following paragraphs emphasis is placed on the inflammatory changes in the gallbladder wall.

23 The appearance of the gallbladder varies greatly. It may be distended or enlarged but later may become shrivelled and small. Characteristically in the early stages the peritoneal coat of the enlarged gallbladder loses its normal sheen, and its normal bluish colour disappears as the wall thickens and becomes less translucent. Adhesions may develop between the gallbladder and adjacent organs such as the hepatic flexure, duodenum and omentum. At the same time fibrosis attaches it more firmly to its hepatic bed. The gallbladder may be especially tense if a calculus, by impacting in Hartmann's pouch, causes obstruction to the outflow of bile.

23

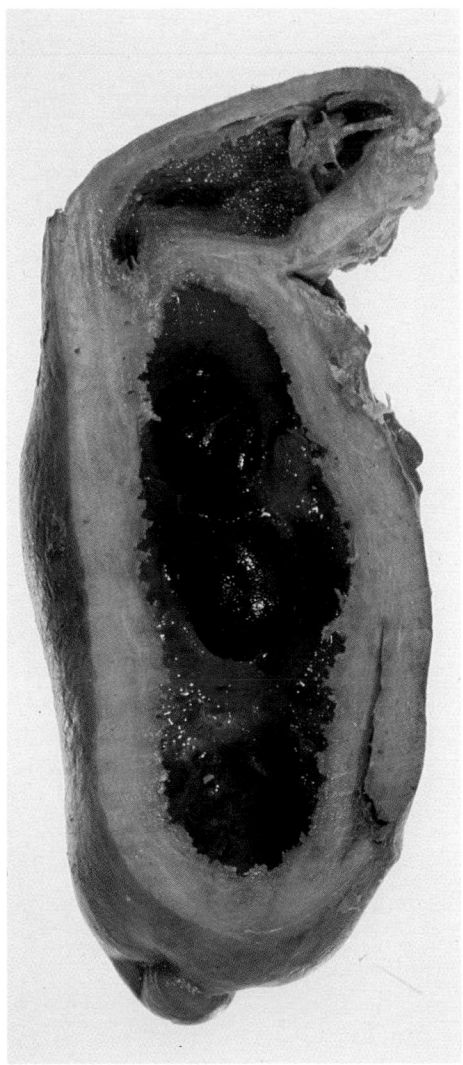

24 Between these appearances of comparatively early chronic cholecytitis and those of the late stages of fibrosis and contracture, there are innumerable variations depending upon the stage of the disease, the number and character of the calculi, the degree of obstruction and the intensity of inflammation and fibrosis. These variations are reflected in the appearances of the opened viscus. The wall may measure up to 1cm in thickness as a result of fibrosis and muscular hypertrophy and may show evidence of mucosal diverticulation and cystic change and occasionally calcification. The mucosal surface may be smooth or trabeculated and indented or eroded by pressure of the calculi. The mucosa may show atrophy or hyperplasia and will vary in colour according to the activity of the inflammation.

24

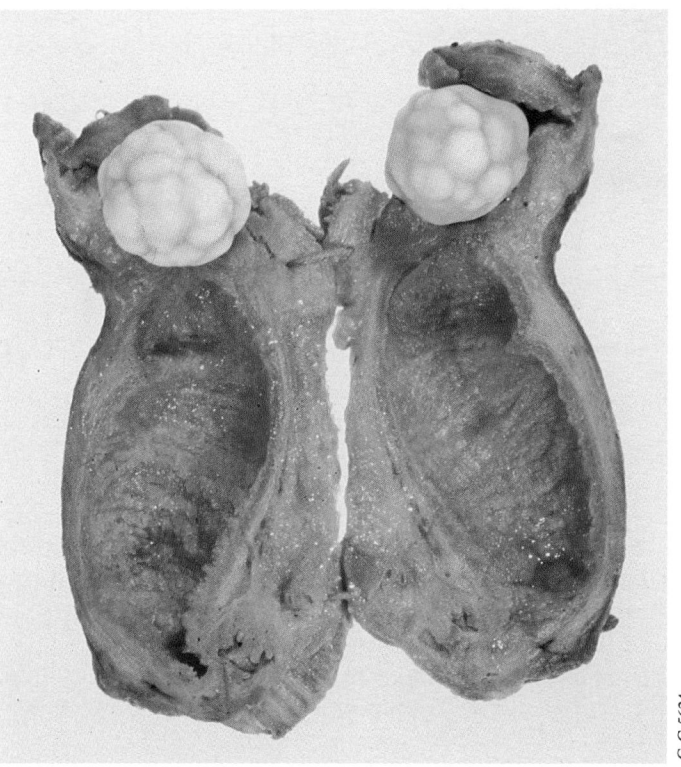

Chronic cholecystitis *(Continued)*

Microscopic features

Calculi in the gallbladder which are responsible for most cases of chronic cholecystitis bring about the changes in a variety of ways:

1   They may, if they are sufficiently large, cause pressure atrophy of the mucosa.
2   They predispose to inflammation, with or without superadded infection, by causing obstruction to the outflow of bile from the gallbladder.
3   They cause obstruction which leads to hypertrophy of muscularis and diverticulation of mucosa.

25

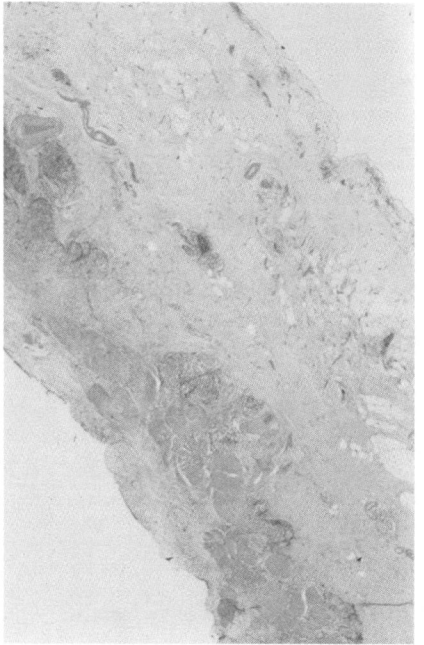

26

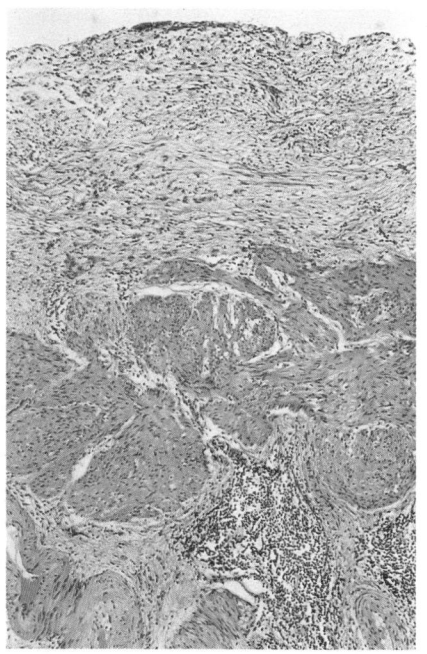

27

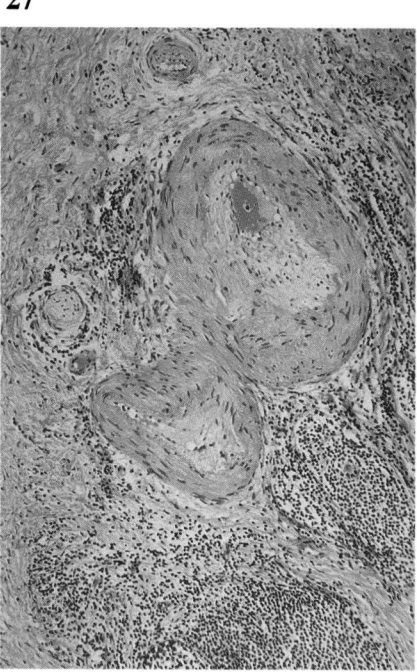

25 A full thickness section of gallbladder wall showing epithelial atrophy, hypertrophy of muscularis, foci of chronic inflammatory cells mainly external to the muscularis, and marked fibrous thickening of the extramuscular connective tissue. *(H&E ×15)*

26 A higher-power view: mucosal fibrosis, muscular hypertrophy, and chronic inflammatory infiltrate. *(H&E ×62.5)*

27 An artery in the outer part of the muscularis is almost occluded by intimal fibrosis resulting from involvement by chronic inflammation (endarteritis). *(H&E ×100)*

The combination of diverticulation with mucosal and muscular hyperplasia gives rise to a variety of appearances. Many names such as adenomyosis, cholecystitis glandularis proliferans, etc., have been attached to the varying manifestations of this process. Bile may be trapped in diverticula deep in the gallbladder wall. If inflammation and ulceration of a diverticulum ensue the bile constituents liberated into the connective tissue give rise to a granulomatous reaction particularly in the case of cholesterol. Occasionally in chronic cholecystitis the epithelium lining the gallbladder shows metaplasia. Transition to intestinal, duodenal and squamous type epithelium have all been described. Dysplastic changes also occur and may be premalignant.

The changes resulting from recurrent attacks of cholecystitis with attendant fibrosis and epithelial atrophy or hyperplasia are therefore complex and only certain aspects of their microscopic appearances can be illustrated.

28

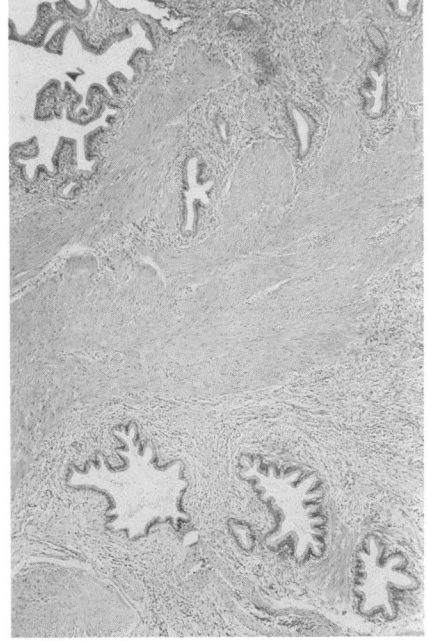

G.C.M.875

29

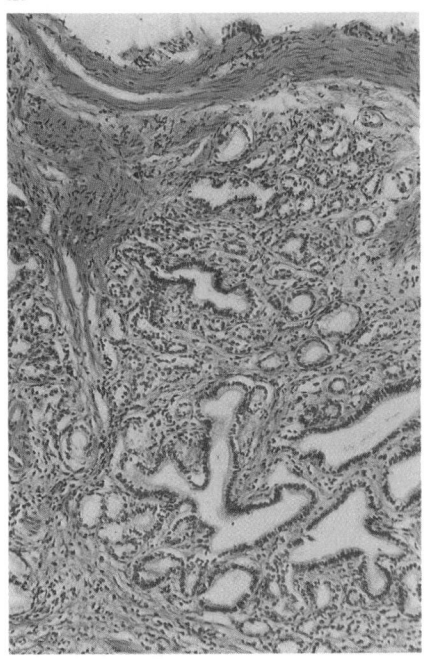

G.C.M.874

30

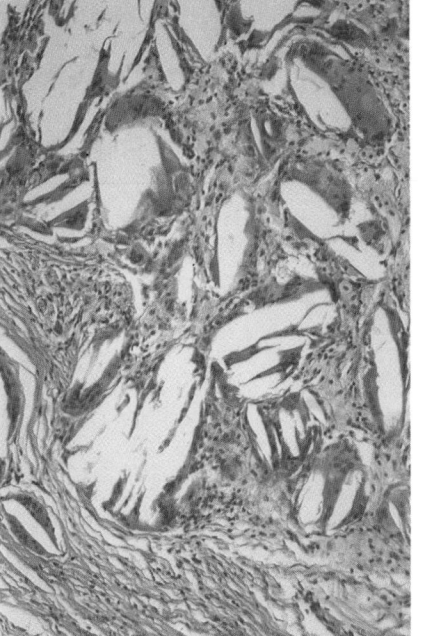

G.C.M.919

28 Mucosal diverticula (Rokitansky–Aschoff sinuses) are present both in muscularis and extramuscular connective tissue. *(H&E ×40)*

29 'Cholecystitis glandularis proliferans'. Numerous epithelial channels have formed in the muscularis. *(H&E ×100)*

30 Cholesterol crystals are surrounded by multinucleated giant cells. The cholesterol granuloma has resulted from escape of bile into the connective tissue of the gallbladder. *(H&E ×125)*

Acute cholecystitis

Patients with an acute attack of pain have obstruction which has persisted. Some surgeons believe in operating on these patients and have found that not all patients with acute biliary pain have the histological changes of acute inflammation.

Chronic cholecystitis with acute inflammation	65%
Chronic cholecystitis without inflammation	25%
Acute inflammation without chronic change	10%

90% have chronic cholecystitis with irreversible change.

When the disease commences as an initial acute lesion the changes observed are those of acute inflammation, the gallbladder wall is thin, stretched and may still retain its translucency. The congestion may be marked and early adhesion formation may be observed.

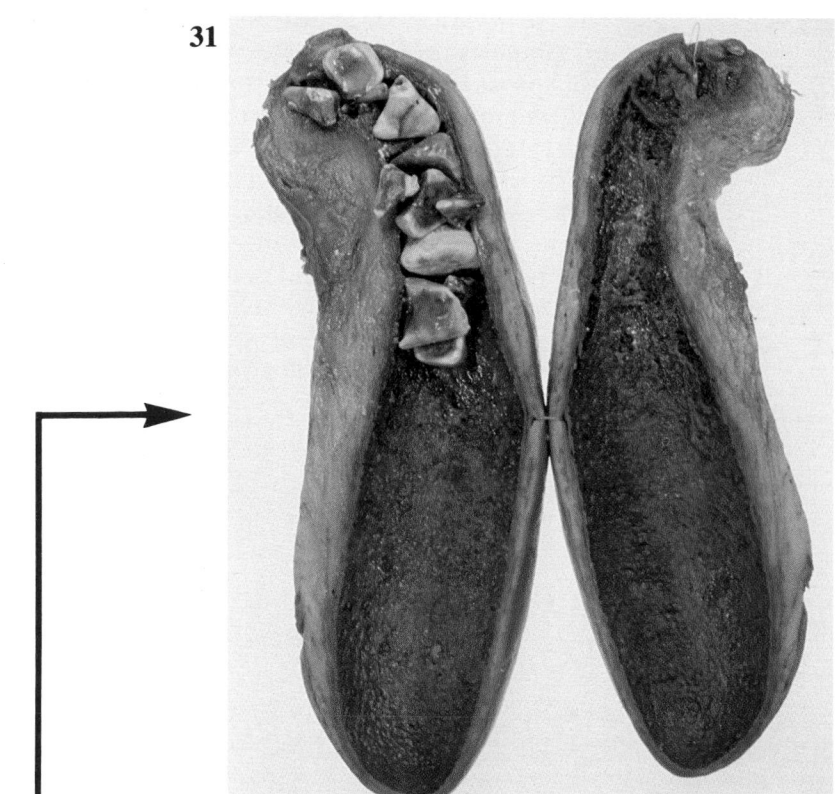

31 From a female aged 42 years. Her clinical history was limited to a single acute attack diagnosed as cholecystitis. The gallbladder is enlarged, smooth on its serous surface but of a dusky-red colour. The wall is slightly thickened and the mucosa congested, haemorrhagic and necrotic. A number of angular medium sized gallstones of mixed composition occupy the cavity of the gallbladder.

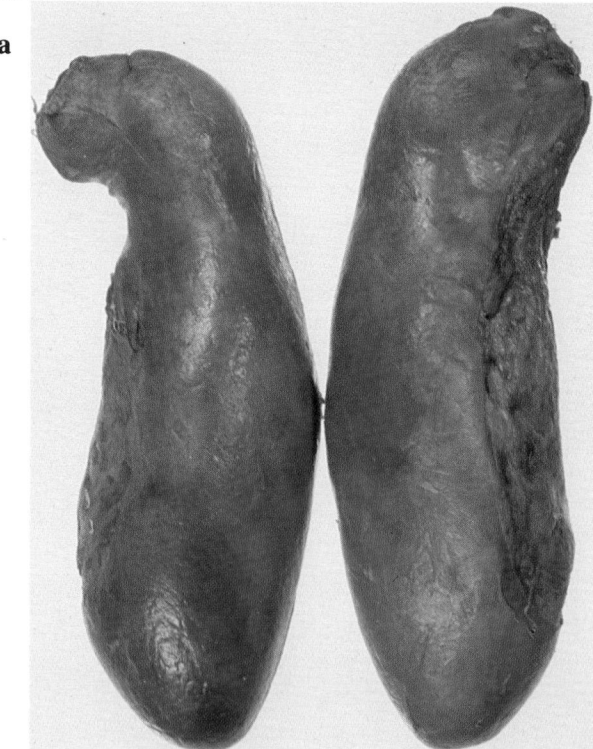

31a Macroscopically oedema is obvious in the surrounding tissues including the gallbladder bed (a fact that makes mobilisation of the gallbladder easy in the early stages of the attack). Oedema in the free border of the lesser omentum can sometimes be responsible for jaundice. The wall of the gallbladder may be surrounded by omentum or neighbouring intestine – particularly the hepatic flexure of the colon. Other organs can be easily separated in the first week of the attack but get progressively fixed by granulation tissue and fibrosis thereafter.

When there is an acute exacerbation of a pre-existing lesion the signs of acute inflammation, congestion and oedema, are superimposed upon the evidence of the preceding chronic cholecystitis. When the gallbladder is opened the mucosa will show acute inflammation and probably ulceration while the contents will be thick and may be purulent. The most common cause of the acute episode is obstruction at the outlet of the gallbladder. The acute manifestations will subside if the obstruction is relieved.

The natural progression of untreated cholecystitis is empyema – chronic cholecystitis with acute changes including the formation of pus.

▼

Ischaemia and gangrene – venous followed by arterial obstruction.

▼

Perforation – this may remain localised as an abscess adherent to surrounding tissues or give rise to biliary peritonitis.

32

33

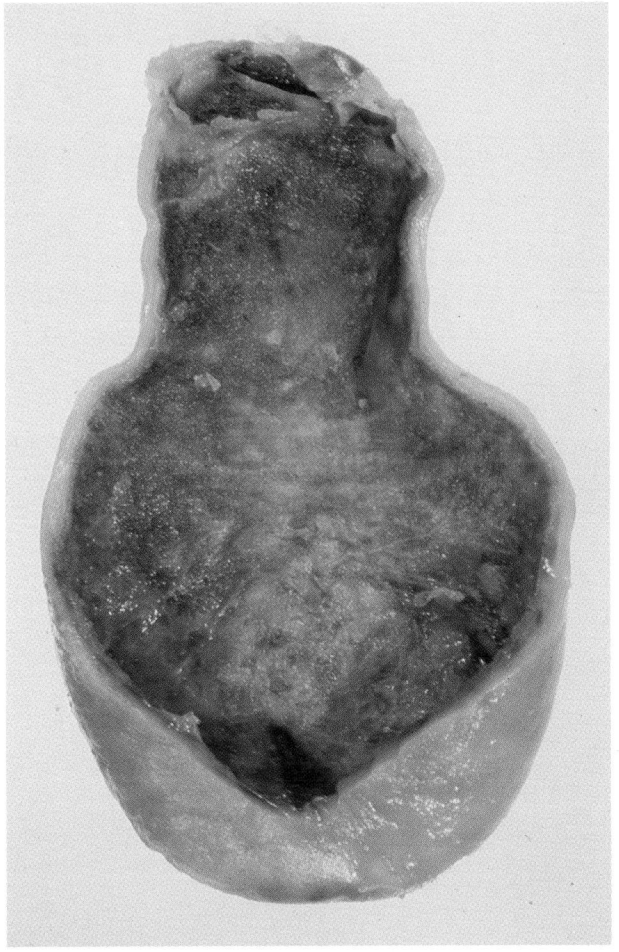

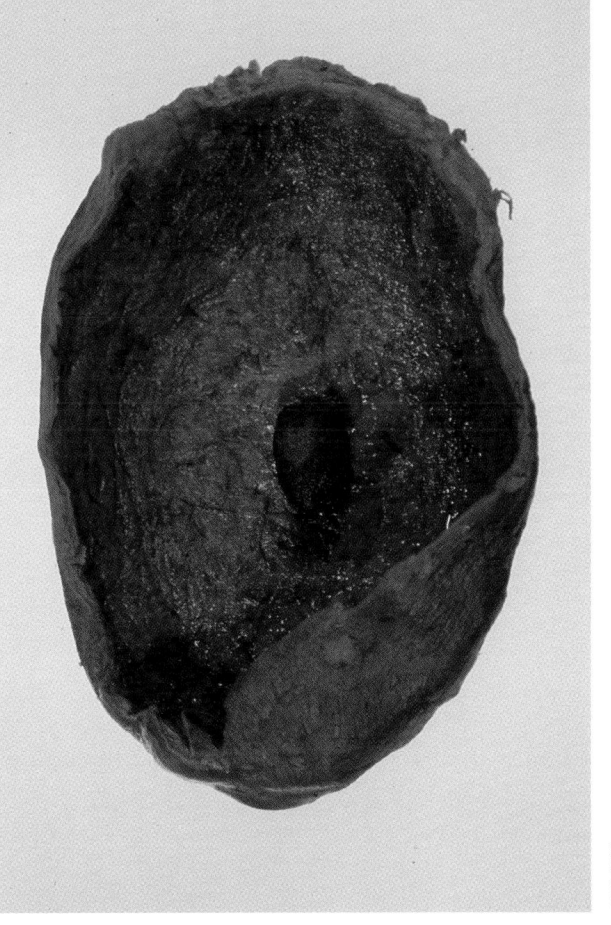

G.C.15133

G.C.8504

32 From a male aged 76 years with a history of two attacks of acute abdominal pain separated by a period of 5 months.

In the illustration the calculi which filled the gallbladder have been removed to show the severe inflammation of the mucosa. Most of the mucosa has been destroyed and replaced by granulation tissue covered here and there by inflammatory exudate. The gallbladder is greatly enlarged and its wall is thickened by muscular hypertrophy and by fibrosis.

33 From a male aged 35 years who had a history of three separate attacks of acute pain associated with vomiting and fever.

The illustration shows the gallbladder which has been opened and demonstrates a small, dark, oval calculus. The surface of the gallbladder is intensely congested and irregularly coated with recent lymph. The wall is slightly thickened. The inner surface is intensely congested and its mucosa has a finely granular appearance in places while elsewhere it is grey, more smooth and necrotic.

Acute cholecystitis *(Continued)*

Microscopical features

34

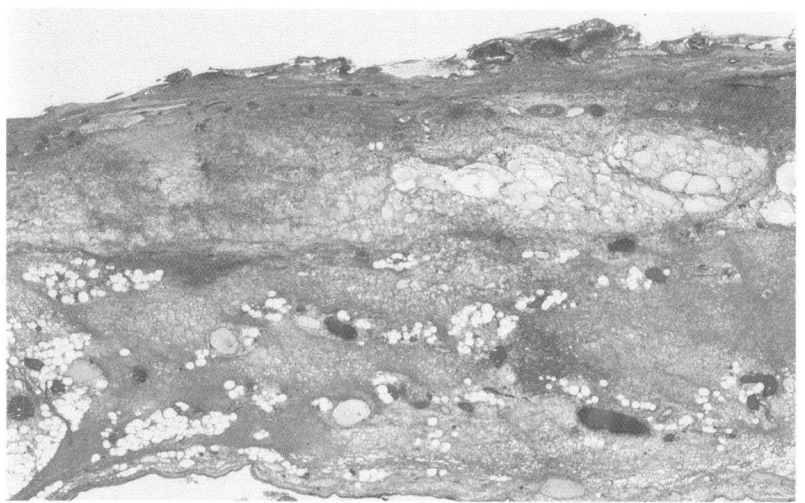

G.C.M.876

34 A full thickness section of an acutely inflamed gallbladder. The wall is swollen by inflammatory congestion and oedema. There is no gross fibrosis. *(H&E ×15)*

35

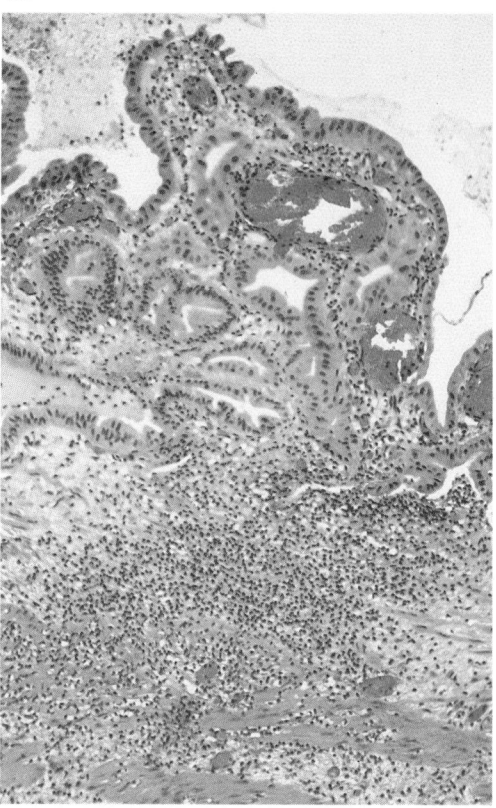

G.C.M.876

35 Same case. At least part of the inflamed mucosa is preserved. The lamina propria and the muscularis are infiltrated by inflammatory cells. *(H&E ×120)*

36

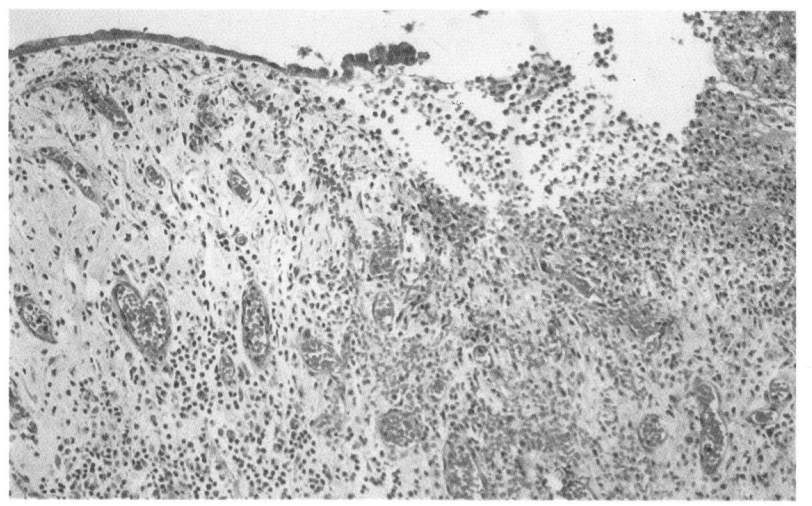

G.C.M.920

36 Acute exacerbation of chronic cholecystitis. A thin layer of regenerating epithelium covers granulation tissue at the margin of a small ulcer. *(H&E ×150)*

Distinctive varieties

A number of lesions presenting distinctive appearances have been reported and have been given individual names. They are, however, essentially variations of cholecystitis/cholelithiasis.

Calcified gallbladder

The deposition of calcium in the wall of the gallbladder is sometimes relatively diffuse and occurs in a viscus not showing gross mural changes. The appearances justify the name of 'eggshell' gallbladder. The calcium is laid down as a thin plaque in the submucosa and the overlying mucosa, becoming ischaemic, is ultimately lost. A calculus may or may not be present within the gallbladder. The condition is regarded as the sequel to an inflammatory change in the wall of the gallbladder but the precise mechanism leading to this pattern of lesion is unknown.

38

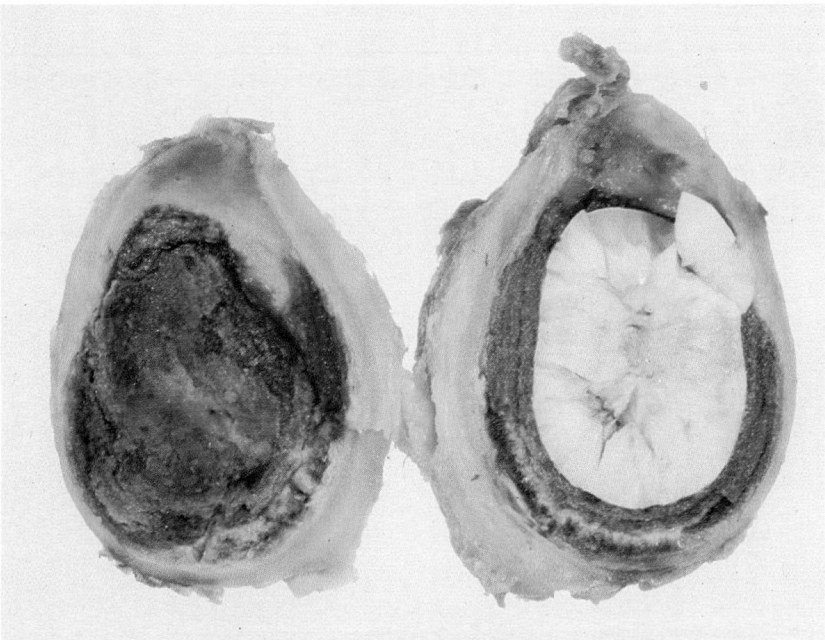

G.C.11838

38 From a female aged 46 years. Following an accident radiological examination of the lower chest demonstrated a calcified gallbladder as an incidental finding. Cholecystography demonstrated a non-functioning gallbladder. The only feature on clinical examination was a point of tenderness over the fundus of the gallbladder.

The illustration is that of the gallbladder which has been opened to demonstrate its contents. It is largely filled by a single cholesterol calculus the size of a walnut. The wall of the gallbladder is thickened and fibrous and contains calcium except in the region of the neck. Between the calculus and the wall there is a layer of brownish pigment material.

Histological sections show loss of mucosa and replacement of the constituents of the gallbladder wall by dense fibrous tissue in which there were areas of calcification. The gallbladder was adherent to the adjacent liver.

37

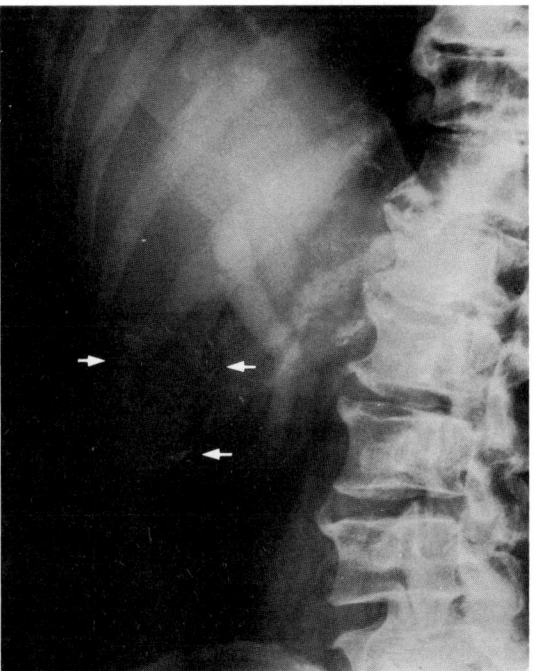

G.C.X.992

37 Cholecystogram. The gallbladder has not filled with contrast and is occupied by a very large calculus. The surface layers of the calculus are calcified.

Distinctive varieties *(Continued)*

Diverticulosis (cholecystitis cystica)

Note has already been made of the occurrence of dilated Rokitansky–Aschoff sinuses and the appearance of small cysts in the wall of the gallbladder. Rarely clearly evident macroscopic cysts and diverticula are found and controversy has existed as to their aetiology.

This is a very typical example of diverticulosis in a gallbladder which has presented as a thin walled viscus containing a calculus. The calculus has impacted previously in the neck of the gallbladder but note that while there is some trabeculation there is no evidence of acute inflammatory reaction. It is probable therefore that during the period of obstruction by the gallstone the tension within the gallbladder was elevated and was the cause of the dilatation of the sinuses. This was associated with muscular hypertrophy. Note how the diverticula are limited to the fundal part of the gallbladder.

39

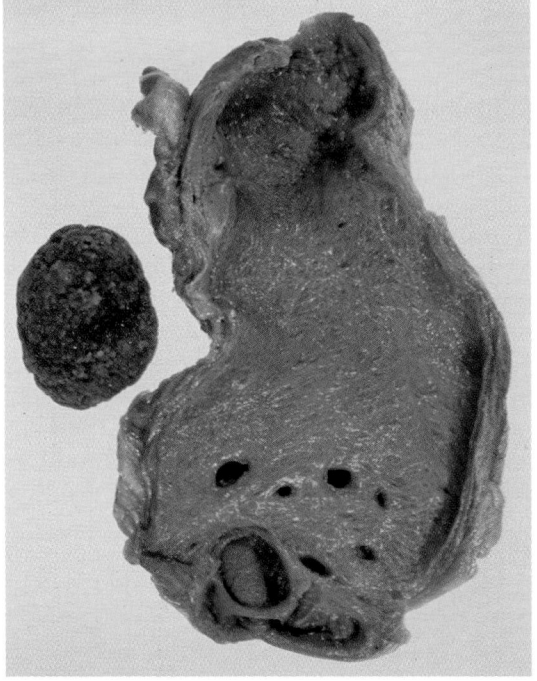

40

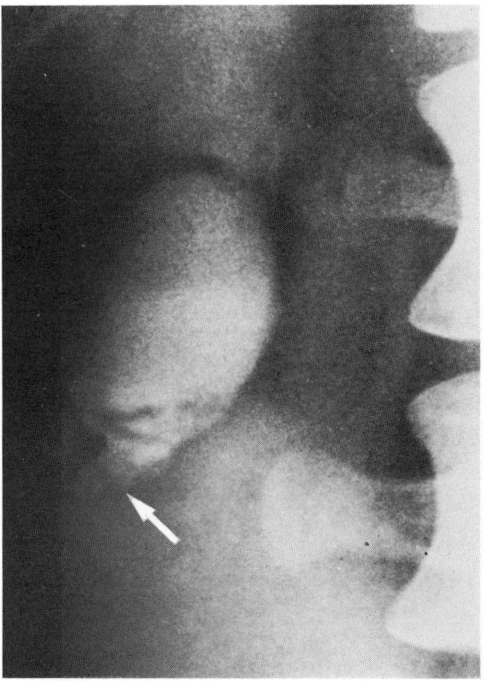

39 From a male aged 52 years who over the preceding 24 years had had three brief attacks of subcostal pain associated on the last two occasions with nausea and vomiting. In the interval between the attacks he had no dyspepsia or other features of gallbladder disease. Radiological examination showed the presence of a calculus and impaired gallbladder function.

40 Cholecystogram from another patient in whom the diagnosis was made of fundal diverticula of the gallbladder.

41

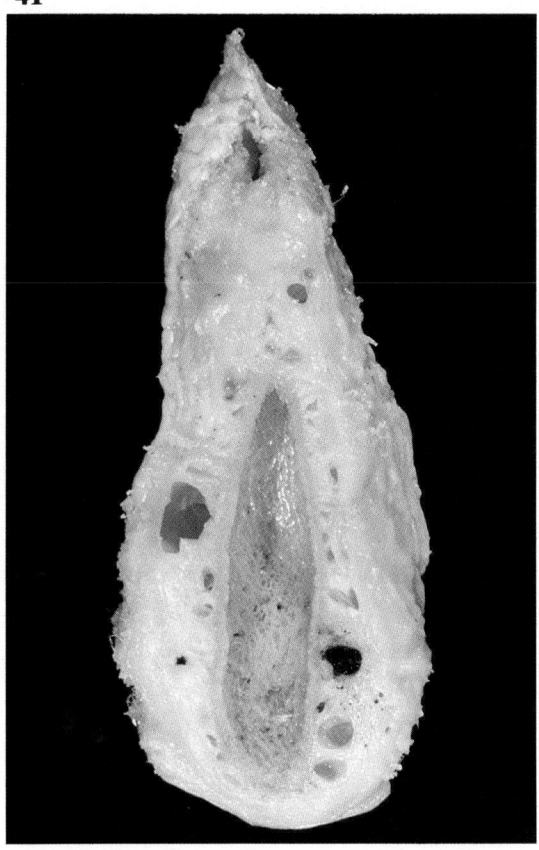

G.C.14883

41 From a female. Clinical notes are not available. The gallbladder has been sectioned and demonstrates the gross thickening of the wall of the viscus with numerous cysts. The majority are located towards the fundus of the gallbladder but one is seen close to the neck of the organ. Most of these cysts contained bile. Note the shaggy thickened serosa. Microscopic studies showed gallbladder mucosa atrophy. The cysts were generally lined with similar epithelium but occasionally are devoid of a mucosal lining and contain bile pigment or cholesterol debris. The thickness of the wall results from fibrosis and is clear evidence of a pre-existing chronic cholecystitis. These cysts are usually associated with inflammatory changes. For this reason the term cholecystitis cystica has been used.

Septate gallbladder

42

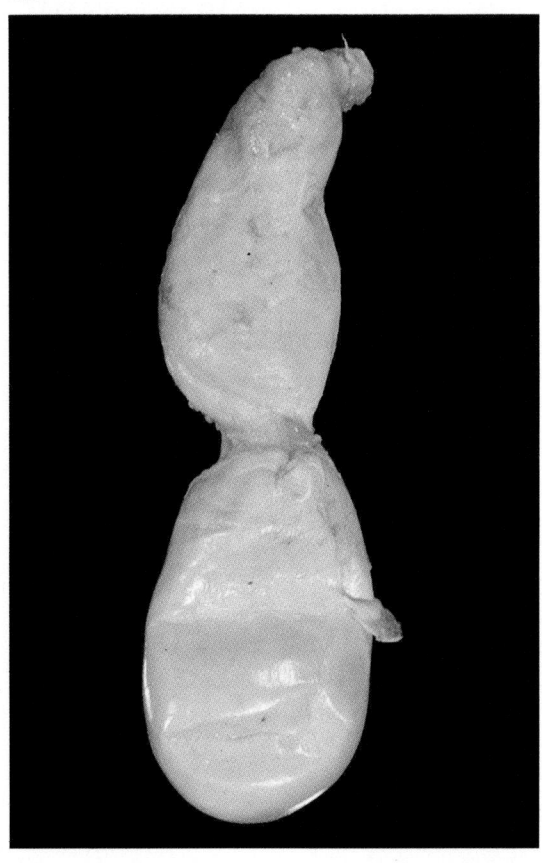

G.C.9669

42 From a female aged 50 years. At operation for a chronic cholecystitis the cystic duct was blocked by a single calculus. The gallbladder was enlarged and contained clear mucoid fluid. The wall of the gallbladder was thickened and constricted at its mid-point. The appearances are those of an hour-glass constricture of the gallbladder.

43

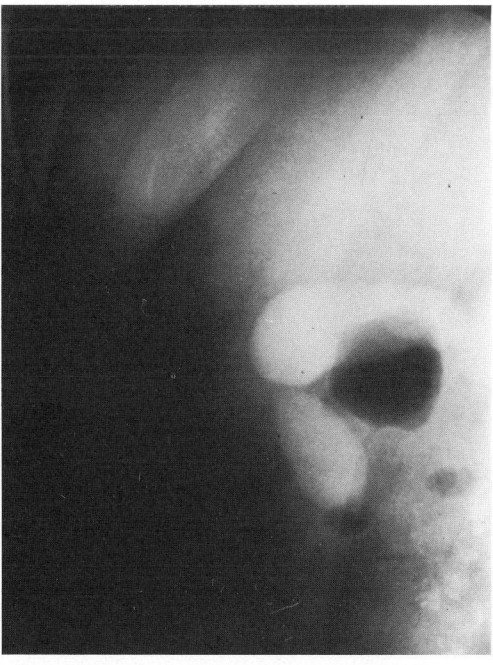

G.C.X.73

43 From a female aged 46 years. This X-ray shows a 'septate' gall bladder. It would appear that the deformity follows a chronic cholecystitis in which epithelial proliferative changes have been marked – the so-called cholecystitis glandularis proliferans. Radiologically associated with the localised area of narrowing, evidence of 'diverticulosis' of the gallbladder is found.

Calculus migration and obstruction

A calculus obstructing the outlet of the gallbladder may:
1 Fall back into the gallbladder with relief of symptoms.
2 Proceed into the common bile duct (choledocholithiasis). This occurs in 1/5 of patients coming to surgery.
3 Remain fixed and erode into neighbouring organs creating a fistula (approx. 1% of patients).

Common duct calculi or a fistula increase the mortality of surgery by a factor of 4.

Choledocholithiasis

Normally calculi in the common duct originate in the gallbladder but calculi can form in the duct system. Since the cystic duct is a narrow channel only small calculi can traverse it and reach the common duct. The common duct has a wider lumen especially in the supraduodenal segment and the calculi can move freely. When there is an obstructive factor to the outflow of bile, the calculi will grow and may reach a considerable size, far greater than any calculus which could have traversed the cystic duct.

The supraduodenal segment of the common duct is relatively unsupported by surrounding structures and can dilate considerably between the layers of the lesser omentum. The pancreatic segment of the duct, however, is surrounded by glandular tissue and dilatation is less readily accomplished. The opening at the ampulla of Vater is narrow and it is here that many calculi passing down the duct become impacted. Where impaction has occurred at the ampullary or supra-ampullary segments of the duct, the surrounding glandular tissue becomes the site of inflammation and when explored at operation may closely simulate a carcinoma at the head of the pancreas.

44

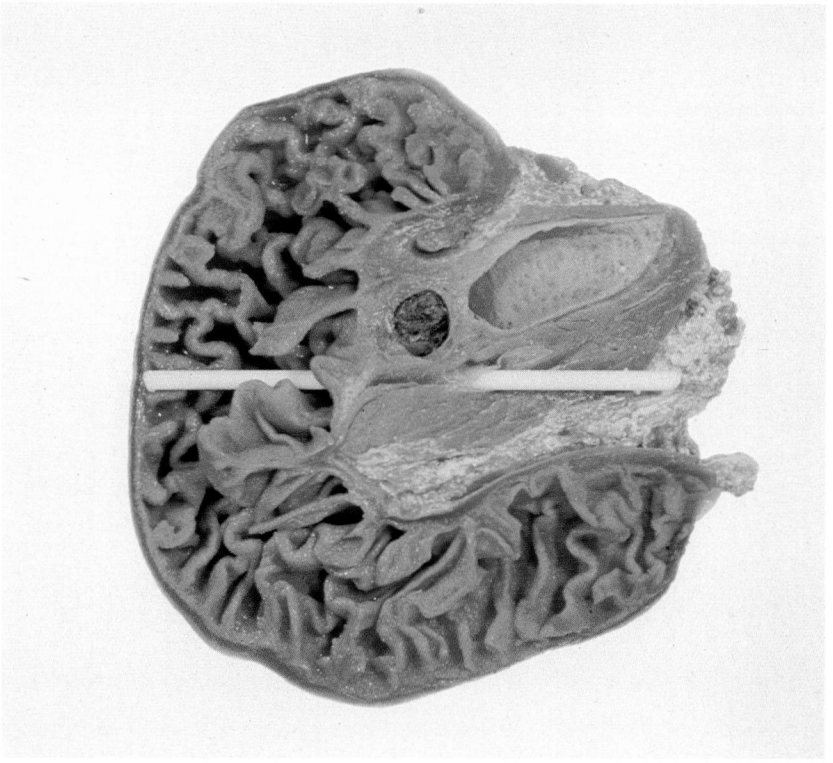

44 From an adult. Half of a longitudinal section of the duodenum showing the presence of a calculus in the common bile duct which is impacted at the ampulla of Vater.

A white glass rod indicates the pancreatic duct.

G.C.4496

The presence of a calculus in the common duct is suggested by the following features and the incidence of these findings is shown:

Indications	Choledocholithiasis(%)
Previous jaundice	34
Abnormal liver function	45
Multiple small stones	17
Dilated cystic duct 5 to 10 mm	31
10+mm	68
Dilated common duct 10 to 15 mm	22
15+ mm	73
Indurated pancreas	28

Digital examination of the common duct at operation is not reliable, because 25% of duct calculi are missed. Therefore operative cholangiography is necessary.

Cholangitis

The presence of obstruction encourages the multiplication of bacteria which may have descended from the infected gallbladder, the liver, or from the intestine following fistula formation.

Macroscopically the duct is thickened and the usual 'bluish' bile cannot be seen. The duct may look inflamed and feel thick. On aspirating or opening it the bile may be purulent. Spread of infection may lead to cholangiohepatitis and later abscess formation or septicaemia. Clinically, this is suggested by Charcot's triad of intermittent pain, intermittent fever and intermittent jaundice.

45 From a male aged 70 years who developed jaundice 3 weeks before death. Clinical examination showed the liver and gallbladder to be enlarged and tender. The cause of death was right sided cardiac failure.

The illustration demonstrates the presence of a calculus impacted at the ampulla of Vater causing dilatation of the common bile duct which can be seen immediately above the pylorus. The cut surface of the liver shows fibrosis of the portal tracts.

Microscopically grey rings of fibrosis were present around dilated small bile ducts. Portal tracts could be seen to link together. This is evidence of commencing cirrhosis and therefore meant that the biliary obstruction had been present for some time.

45

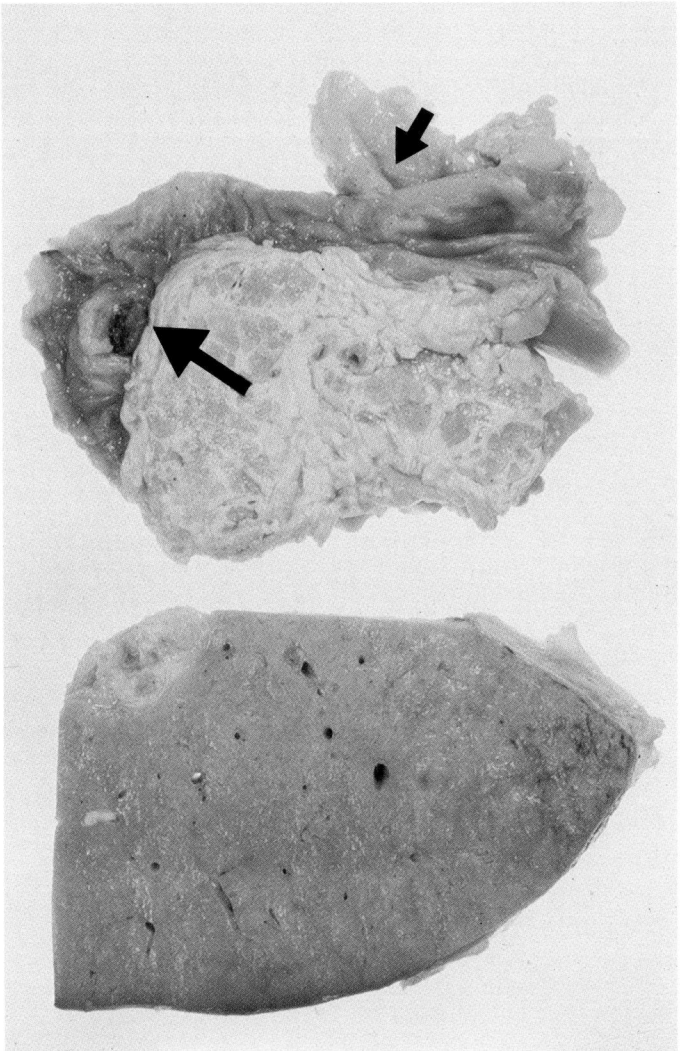

G.C.15087

Calculus migration and obstruction

Obstructive jaundice

A calculus may remain in the common duct causing either intermittent or persistent jaundice due to obstruction especially at the lower end of the common duct where it most frequently becomes impacted. The patient presents with a history of biliary colic followed by jaundice.

Other causes of obstructive jaundice attributed to calculus include:
1 Pressure on the common duct due to a stone in the outlet of the gallbladder.
2 An enlarged gallbladder.
3 Oedema of the duct wall and surrounding tissues.

Stricture of the common duct is also a cause of obstruction. This may arise as the result of the trauma occasioned by a calculus which may have been passed earlier. This causes progressive jaundice. Stricture may be a frequent complication of operation, the duct having been traumatised either at operation or followed drainage. The duct may also have been divided necessitating repair or it may have been included in a ligature.

Cirrhosis

Prolonged obstruction of the common duct, either intermittent or continuous, aggravated by infection leads to damage to the liver and consequent cirrhosis.

The clinical features are diagnostic and the liver function tests reveal both obstruction and cellular damage. Macroscopically the liver is enlarged in the early stages but later becomes contracted. The surface is nodular and paler.

The microscopic changes are characteristic.

Pancreatitis

A calculus may impact at the lower end of duct distal to the junction of the common bile and pancreatic ducts resulting in back flow of infected bile into the pancreatic duct system. This may result in acute pancreatitis.

The clinical features suggest a history of gallstone but the patients appear more seriously ill and have a significantly raised serum amylase. Surgical opinion is that gallstone pancreatitis should be treated like acute cholecystitis by early operation.

The macroscopic appearance at operation varies according to the severity of the pancreatitis. There is free intraperitoneal fluid, high in enzyme content, areas of fat necrosis. enlargement of the pancreas, oedema and, on occasions, areas of necrosis. The proximal common duct is dilated and the changes of cholecystitis are seen. Pancreatitis is described fully in Section 17.

Biliary fistula

The fixed gallstone whether in the gallbladder, the cystic duct or in the common duct causes ulceration and surrounding inflammation. Neighbouring organs become adherent and the calculus, by deep erosion, creates a fistulous opening most commonly to the duodenum, stomach or small intestine. The calculus may then pass through the fistula and enter the intestine. The calculus may be passed per rectum or may lead to gallstone ileus. Occasionally the calculus enters the general peritoneal cavity and an abscess forms around it. The abscess and calculus may then discharge through the abdominal wall or may erode into the pleural cavity or even the lung with possible expectoration of the calculus or extrusion when the empyema is drained.

Gallstone ileus

In addition to those calculi which enter the alimentary canal through a fistulous formation some calculi pass through the sphincter of Oddi and enter the duo-denum. These may pass per rectum without causing symptoms or may aggregate faecal content onto their surface and cause obstruction (gallstone ileus) usually in the lower ileum. The diagnosis is indicated by a previous history of dyspepsia and possibly biliary colic.

Radiological examination may show the presence of an obvious gallstone. Gas may also be found radio-logically in the biliary duct.

47

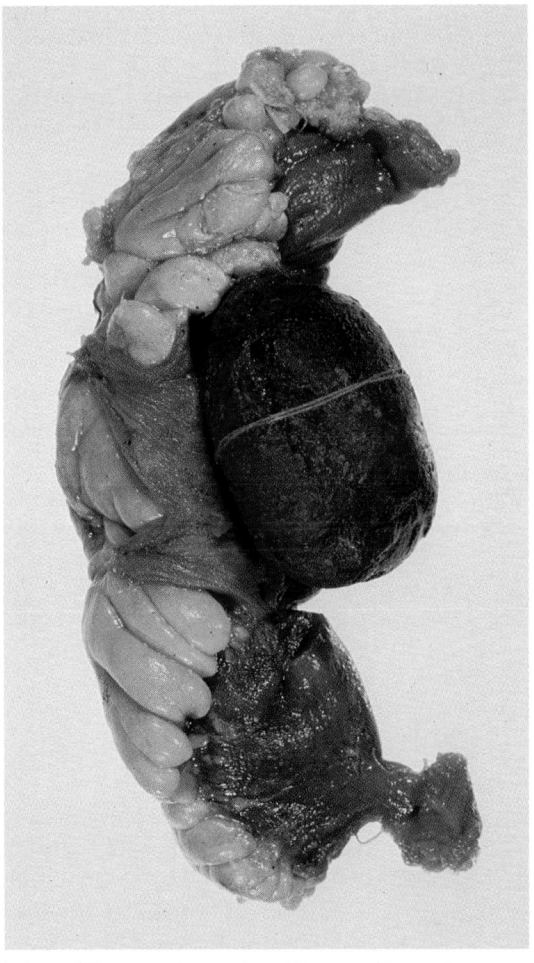

46

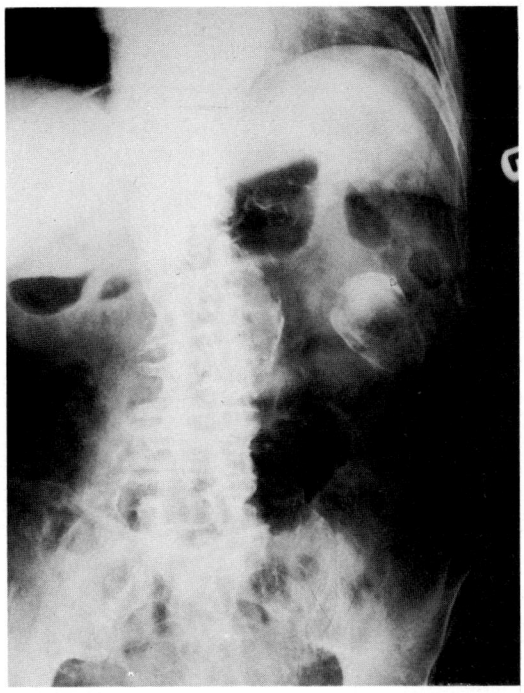

46 Supine film showing a large calcified gallstone which at operation was found lodged in the upper jejunum causing 'gallstone ileus'. The calculus was successfully milked back into the stomach and removed through a gastrotomy.

47 Illustration of gallstone ileus from a female aged 88 years. At operation a segment of gut was resected.

The specimen was opened to illustrate the interior and disclose the gallstone. There is considerable submucous haemorrhage and commencing ulceration. The gallstone is of the mixed variety.

Bile peritonitis

The escape of bile into the peritoneal cavity may be the result of perforation either of the gallbladder or of the ducts. Rupture may occur in a thin walled gallbladder especially at points of weakness such as a dilated Rokitansky sinus or a diverticulum. Rupture also occurs if an impacted calculus has caused erosion of the wall.

Perforations may seal over rapidly and be difficult to identify at operation. A post-operative hazard is the slipping of a ligature on the stump of the cystic duct following cholecystectomy. The bile which escapes into the peritoneal cavity causes peritoneal inflammation with effusion. The irritant factors are the bile salts. The degree of reaction depends upon the bile salt content of the escaping fluid but the reactive peritoneal effusion rapidly reduces the intensity of the irritant. The condition may be localised or diffuse. Spontaneous recovery can occur if the collection of bile is small and localised but if larger, aspiration or drainage is required. If the bile is infected the lesion carries a high mortality with evidence of profound toxicity and shock.

Bile peritonitis should be distinguished from biliary ascites occurring in association with common duct obstruction, jaundice, and in malignant disease of the liver.

Course of disease

The histological changes of cholecystitis are irreversible but the imbalance of the bile constituents can be reversed by the intake of drugs such as Cheno-deoxycholic or Urso-deoxycholic acid. This permits solution of the cholesterol part of the calculi but is only effective on small stones mainly made up of cholesterol. Small amounts of calcium may be left which break up and pass down the cystic duct. Such dissolution may take many months (even where the stones are small and not formed of calcium). Those drugs have side effects, such as diarrhoea, that require control with cholestyramine. Cessation of therapy results in a reversal to an abnormal ratio of bile contents and to further stone production.

Patients are therefore doomed to recurrent attacks of gallbladder obstruction which at best may settle with dietary restrictions, antispasmodics and analgesics. The obstruction may become complete giving rise to either a mucocoele or an empyema of the gallbladder. Alternatively, the stone may pass into the common bile duct with obstructive jaundice, cholangitis, pancreatitis or septicaemia. In any series of patients coming to operation, 20% will have stones in the common bile duct and the incidence is doubled when the operation is for an acute episode of pain. Recurrent episodes may damage the ducts with stricture formation, the liver with cirrhotic change and the pancreas with inflammation, fibrosis and duct stricture.

The mortality rate following cholecystectomy alone can be less than 0.5%, and, when the duct is opened this increases to a mortality rate of 2%. These figures reflect the results in expert hands, and the national rate in any country is considerably in excess of this. Mortality increases over the age of 45 years, and there seems little justification in postponing surgery in the younger patient.

Gallbladder – Miscellaneous lesions

Foreign bodies

Occasionally foreign bodies such as silk sutures or catheters are left in the bile ducts leading to precipitation of bile salts in which they become encrusted. In tropical countries occasionally an ascaris ascends along the common duct causing intermittent obstruction.

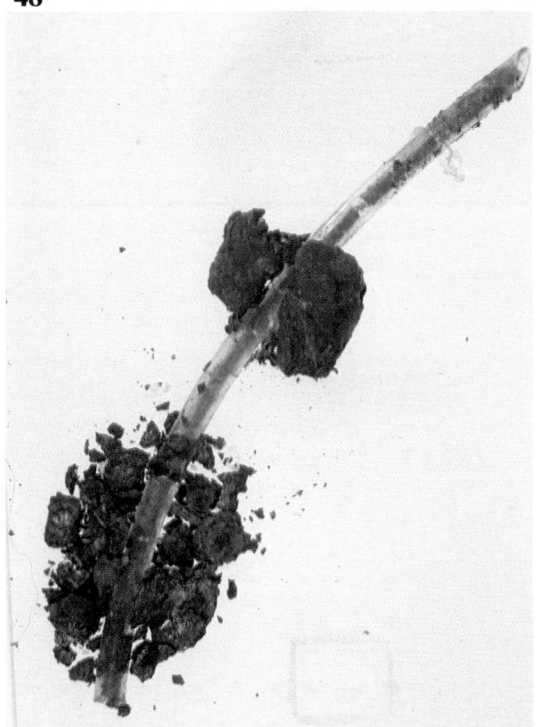

48 The patient, an adult male, was originally operated on for intermittent jaundice and at operation a lesion of the hepatic duct believed to be possibly malignant was found. A polythene tube was inserted to secure bile flow. After an interval of improvement recurrent attacks of jaundice necessitated further operation when the polythene tube was found to be lodged in the lower part of the common duct. The tube has become encrusted on its surface and in its lumen with bile salts.

Torsion

When the gallbladder possesses a mesentery it is unduly mobile and can undergo rotation. This leads to the occlusion of the cystic duct and occlusion of the blood supply to the viscus. The rotation may be partial or complete. Clinically the condition presents as acute cholecystitis or acute appendicitis. It requires urgent operative intervention since gangrene of the gallbladder may occur rapidly after rotation and in such cases the mortality is high. In 50% of cases torsion occurs in a gallbladder which is the seat of calculus formation. In such cases unduly severe contractions of the gallbladder may have been a precipitating factor.

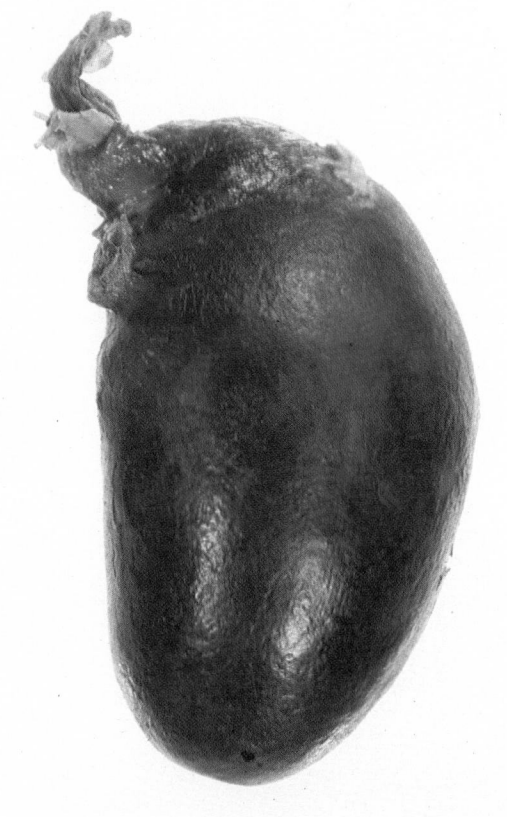

49 This specimen from a boy aged 12 years occurred in a gallbladder in which no calculi were present. The gallbladder was attached to the liver only by a thin fold of peritoneum, the cystic duct and the cystic artery, and a complete 360° rotation clockwise had occurred. At operation the gallbladder was enlarged, gangrenous and distended, with blood-stained fluid.

A.A. Gunn

467

Neoplasms of the gallbladder, bile ducts and ampulla of Vater share many features in common and it is therefore convenient to consider these tumours together.

Incidence

Benign tumours of the gallbladder and bile ducts (papilloma and adenoma) are extremely rare. Carcinomas of the gallbladder and of the bile ducts are well recognised but uncommon lesions and occur in almost equal numbers in the two sites. Tumours arising in the bile ducts cause early obstruction leading to jaundice and the diagnosis is established while the tumour is still small. In most cases there is no biliary infection and the gallbladder may be dilated as well as the ducts (Courvoisier).

Site

Of tumours arising in the bile ducts approximately half are found in the common bile duct and a quarter in the hepatic ducts. Tumours at the lower end of the bile duct present special difficulties since they may arise from the lining of the duct, the mucosa of the duodenum or the parenchymal cells of the pancreas. The number arising from duct epithelium is less than that in other segments of the duct.

Age

Maximal incidence 60–65 years.

Sex

Gallbladder carcinoma M:F – 1:3 or 4
Bile ducts carcinoma M:F – 2:1

Pathology

Tumours of the gallbladder, bile ducts and of the ampulla are all of comparable character and only vary according to the site at which they arise.

Histologically the tumours are adenocarcinomas with varying degrees of differentiation and infiltration and irregular acinar formation with cubical or low columnar cells. Mucin is present in variable degree (both intra-cellular and intra-acinar) and a colloid or mucoid carcinoma may arise. In the gallbladder papillary forms occur. A degree of stromal reaction may, or may not, be marked. These features are illustrated in the following specimens.

Gallbladder

The tumour is most commonly an adenocarcinoma and the wall of the gall-bladder becomes thickened and rigid (70%). See **8** of this section. In approximately 30% of cases the tumour is a papillary type of carcinoma. The concurrent presence of calculi is very common and these may be responsible for surface necrosis and ulceration.

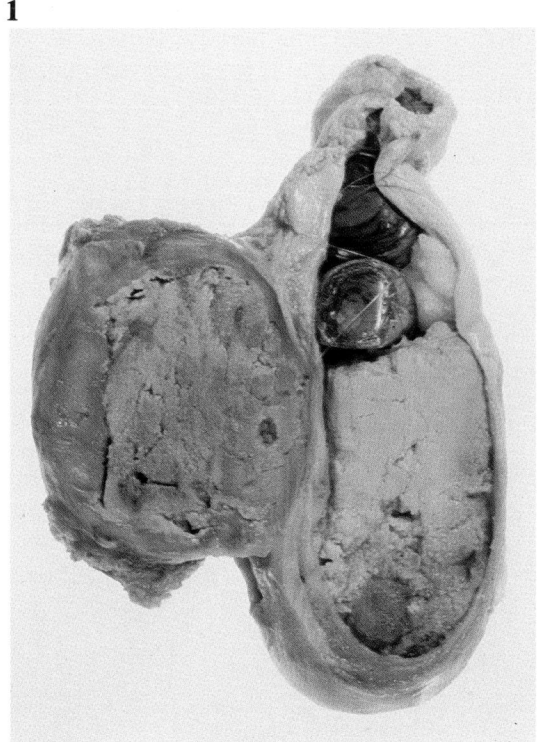

1 From a female aged 70 years. This patient presented features indicative of cholelithiasis and operative intervention was undertaken.

The opened gallbladder is slightly distended, the fundus and adjacent half is filled with a greyish-white soft tissue mass and the rest of the cavity is filled with dark calculi of moderate size. A calculus of rather lighter colour is impacted at the commencement of the cystic duct. The gallbladder wall is not thickened and there is little evidence of pericholecystitis. To one side the gallbladder shows the presence of a tumour the surface of which is nodular. The tumour on section shows a marginal zone of grey-brown homogeneous material around a more necrotic looking centre in which are a few small haemorrhages.

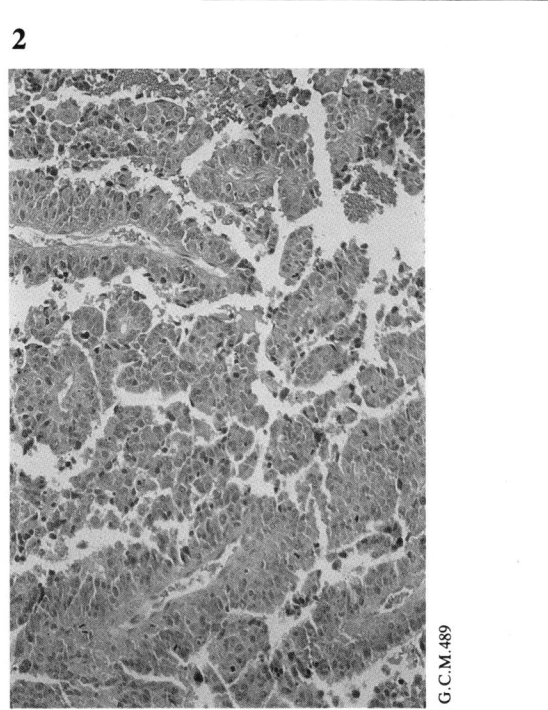

2 Gallbladder – carcinoma. (From another case.) A well differentiated tumour with a villous papillary pattern. *(H&E ×125)*

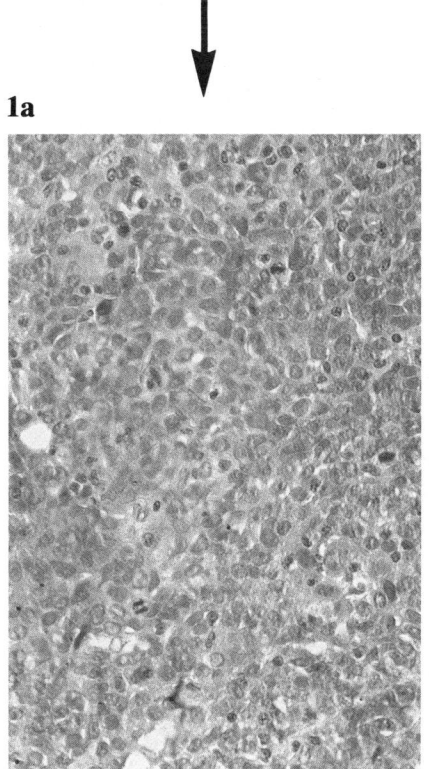

1a Gallbladder – carcinoma. Mitotic activity was high in this poorly differentiated tumour composed of solid masses of closely packed cells. *(H&E ×312.5)*

Bile duct

An infiltrating lesion invading the wall of the duct and causing early stenosis. Growth is slow and the tumour frequently appears to remain localised. It is held that tumours of the bile ducts are commoner where fluke infestation and suppurative cholangitis occurs.

3

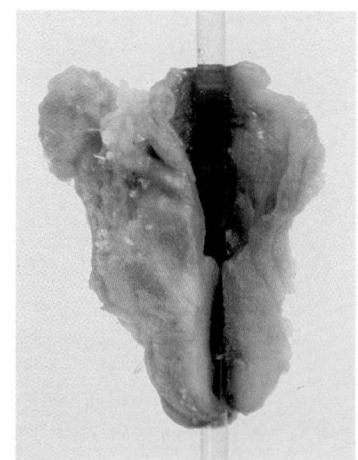

G.C.13672

3 From a male aged 54 years. This patient was admitted with a four week history of obstructive jaundice. No previous illness. Laparotomy showed distended biliary tree due to tumour in retropancreatic part of the common bile duct. The bile duct was resected without damage to the pancreas and continuity restored by choledochoduodenostomy. A tumour encircles the common duct and involves the cystic duct. Where the duct wall has been sectioned the tumour presents as a whitish, fleshy mass. A narrow rod has been inserted into the lumen of the tumour. Proximally the common duct appears to be dilated.

Histologically the tumour was an adenocarcinoma.

4

G.C.X.993

4 Percutaneous transhepatic cholangiogram. Obstruction at the porta by tumour.

5

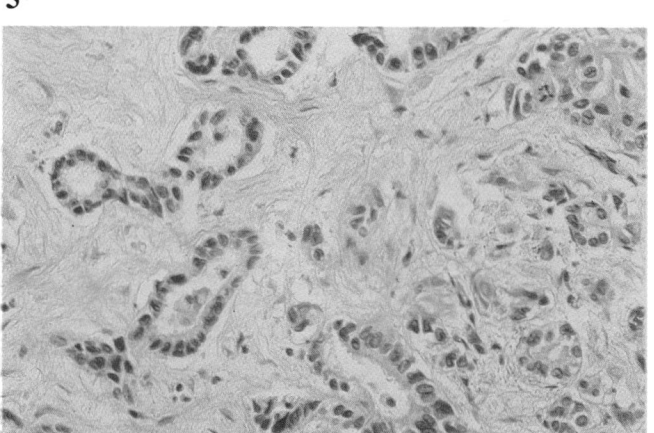

G.C.15175

5 Bile duct – carcinoma. A well differentiated adenocarcinoma with considerable fibrosis. *(H&E × 250)*

The scirrhous type of adenocarcinoma is more frequently seen in lesions of the common duct but is also found in tumours arising in the gallbladder.

Ampulla of Vater

Tumours at the ampulla of Vater may arise from the epithelium of the common bile duct or the duodenal mucosa. They present as an ulcer projecting into the lumen of the duodenum, often polypoid and are a source of early occult bleeding into the gut. These tumours show limited invasion and metastasise to the hilar nodes. Jaundice occurs relatively early.

These tumours are closely simulated by neoplasms originating in the pancreas. The latter show a greater degree of invasiveness, the onset of jaundice is later and the prognosis much more grave. The differential diagnosis from chronic pancreatitis or an impacted calculus may be difficult clinically.

The diagnosis can be made by endoscopic examination with catheterisation of the duct.

6

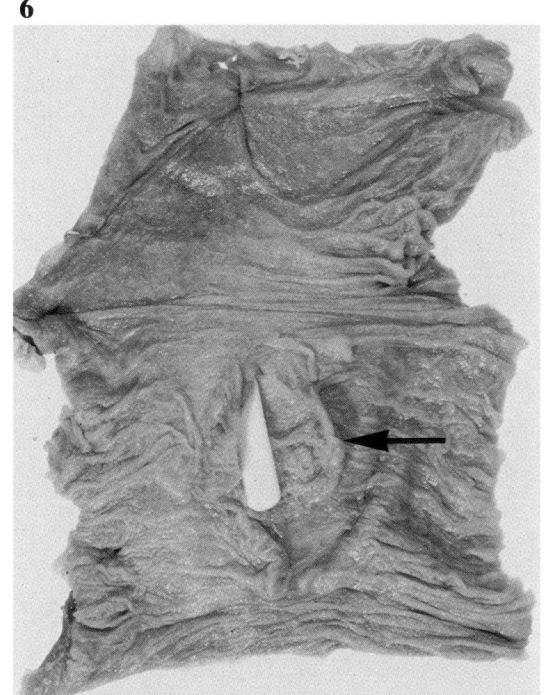

G.C.10498

6 From a female aged 38 years who presented with a 4 month history of loss of weight and a 2 month history of progressive, painless, greenish jaundice. On examination the liver was enlarged and the gallbladder distended.

At operation a tumour at the ampulla of Vater was palpable. There was no evidence of extension of the disease locally or to lymph nodes.

In the specimen the duodenum has been opened on its convex border and the illustration is that of the interior. The duodenal papilla is enlarged to form a cylindrical mass about 2cm in diameter. The surface is covered with normal mucosa except in the region of the orifice where there is an excavated ulcer. A segment has been removed and reveals the ampulla distended by tumour tissue. A white rod indicates the opening of the common bile duct which is much enlarged.

6a Ampulla of Vater – carcinoma. A less well-differentiated invasive portion of the same tumour.
(*H&E ×100*)

6a

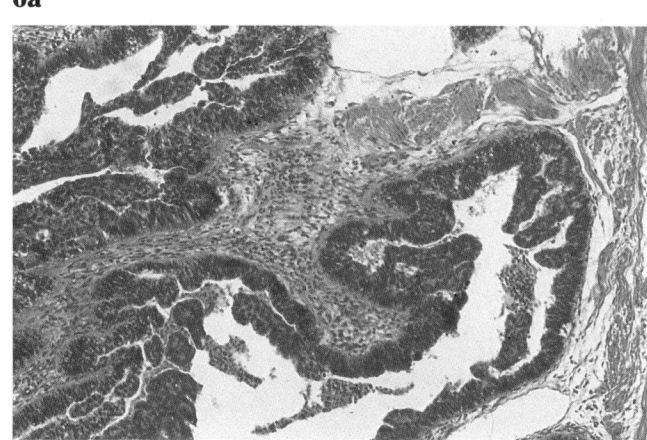

Spread

1   Direct spread to the liver is common and presents as an ingrowth into the adjacent liver tissue. It is noted that this spread is usually limited in extent and is confined to the right lobe of the liver.

Direct spread into adjacent stomach, duodenum or colon occurs and may lead to the formation of fistulae.

2   Carcinoma arising in the gallbladder shows lymphatic spread via the cystic node then upwards to the hiatal node and downwards to the pancreatoduodenal group. Lymphatic spread is found in approximately 1 in 4 of cases.

3   Vascular spread is usually unimportant or infrequent. Early haematogenous spread appears to be relatively infrequent. Widespread haematogenous spread may occur at a late stage of the disease.

7

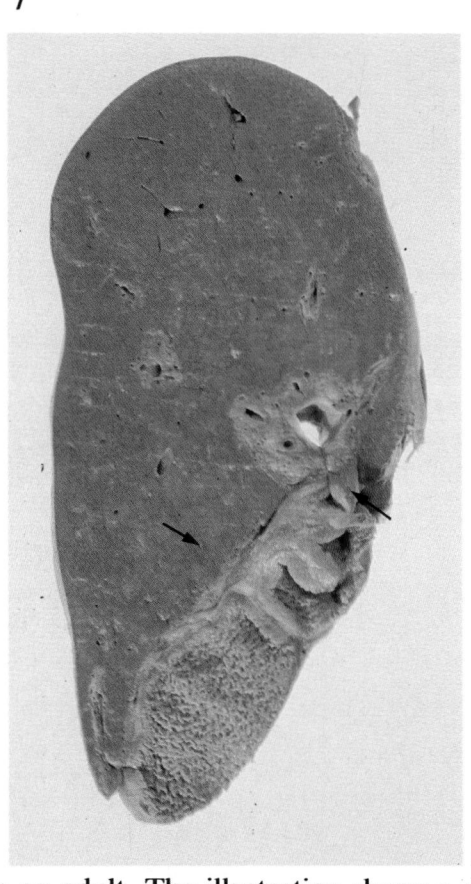

G.C.4625

8

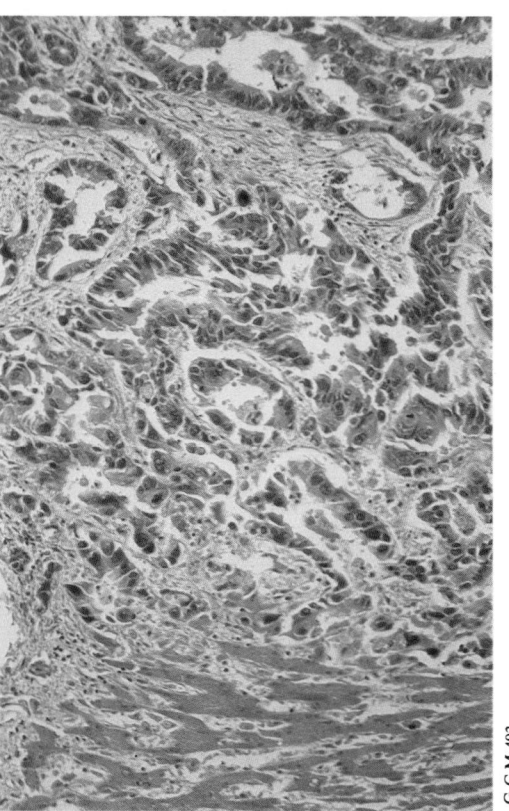

G.C.M.493

7   From an adult. The illustration shows a carcinoma of the hepatic duct with invasion of the adjacent liver tissue. The hepatic duct is occluded by tumour. Towards the fossa for the gallbladder the parenchyma is mottled by white carcinomatous areas which tend to coalesce. The other intra-hepatic ducts are dilated. The gallbladder and cystic duct show no abnormality.

8   Gallbladder – carcinoma (from another case). Adenocarcinoma invading liver. *(H&E ×150)*

Complications

Empyema of the gallbladder is the result of superimposed infection. This is comparable to the empyema that occurs as the result of an impacted calculus.

Squamous carcinoma

Squamous carcinoma of the gallbladder is a well recognised entity but is a rare and controversial lesion. In 10% of adenocarcinomas of the gallbladder areas of squamoid change are found. This 'metaplastic change' occurs in the tumour and the theory that there is a pre-existing innocent metaplasia of the gallbladder mucosa resulting from irritation by a calculus is a phenomenon seriously questioned by many authorities.

9a

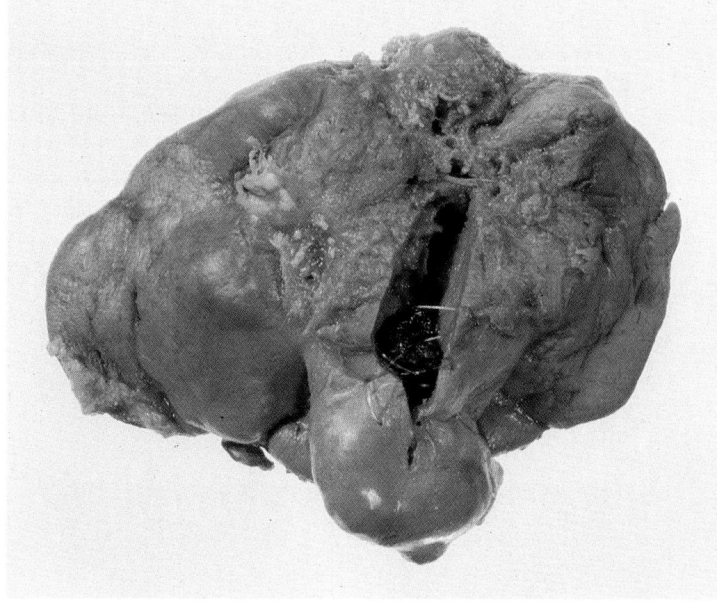

G.C.10522

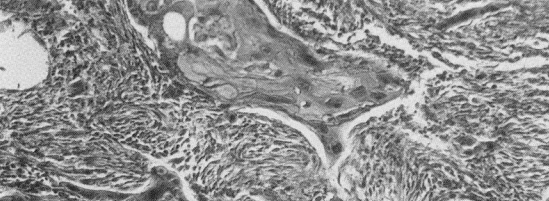

9 Gallbladder – squamous carcinoma. This well differentiated tumour has formed cell nests and caused marked fibrosis. *(H&E ×125)*

9a From a female aged 76 years. Vague history of dyspepsia and flatulence for many years. A palpable swelling was noted below the right costal margin.

At operation a tumour at the margin of the liver was disclosed. This was firmly adherent to the transverse colon and first part of the duodenum. The primary site of the tumour was difficult to ascertain but the disease was strictly limited and a wide resection of the adherent parts was undertaken. On dissection of the specimen the primary lesion was found to be a carcinoma of the fundus of the gallbladder in which numerous calculi were found. The illustration is that of the thickened fundus of the gallbladder projecting from the liver magin.

Ninety per cent of cases of carcinoma of the gallbladder show evidence of cholecystitis or the presence of calculi. The relationship of carcinoma to either of these lesions is disputed. It has been held that the calculi cause changes in the mucosa that may be metaplastic especially squamoid, or neoplastic. Having regard to the frequency with which calculi are present in the gallbladders of individuals without carcinoma but who are in the same age period as those with carcinoma mere coincidence can be assumed. Further the presence of a carcinoma may provide a nidus for the formation of calculi or cause disturbance of the secretion. All suggest that a relationship to the calculi may be that of a sequel to rather than the cause of the tumour.

A.I.S. Macpherson

A majority of lesions of the bile ducts are associated with obstruction to the outflow of bile and this results in:

1 Dilatation of the ducts proximal to the obstruction.
2 Jaundice (obstructive) if the common bile duct or both hepatic ducts are involved.
3 Infection of the stagnant bile leading to ascending cholangitis.
4 Multiple liver abscesses or secondary biliary cirrhosis.

Diagnosis

The presence of dilated bile ducts may be demonstrated *in vivo* by ultrasonography, by radiography after injecting water-soluble contrast medium directly into the dilated intrahepatic ducts (percutaneous transhepatic cholangiography) or in some cases by endoscopic retrograde cholangiopancreatography (ERCP).

1

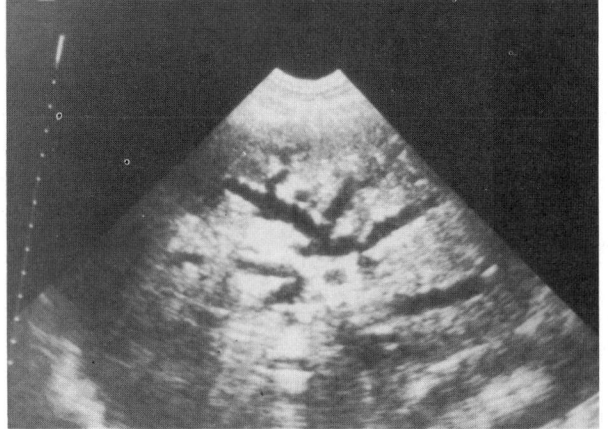

1 Longitudinal ultrasound scan of liver and right kidney. The bile ducts are dilated.

2

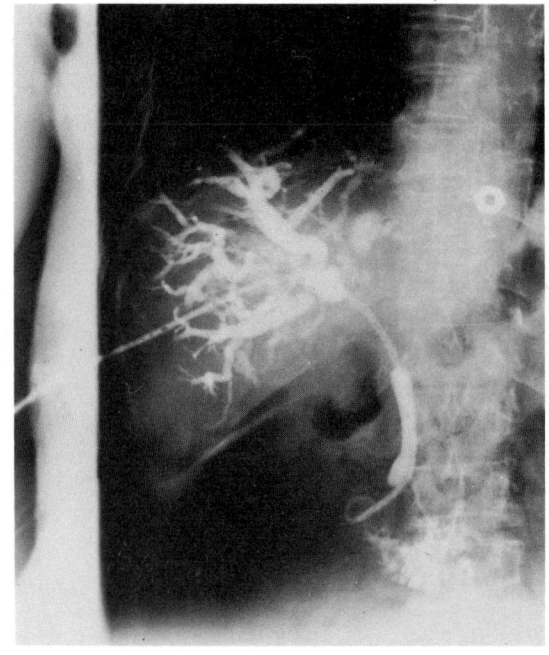

2 Percutaneous bile duct drainage and catheter bypass of portal tumour following percutaneous cholangiography to show the dilated ducts.

Lesions which cause obstruction to the flow of bile from the liver to the duodenum may be classified as:

1	Congenital	Atresia of the ducts
		Choledochal cyst
2	Intrinsic	Impacted biliary calculus
		Parasites and flukes
3	Lesions in the wall	Stricture
		Sclerosing cholangitis
		Neoplasm
4	Extrinsic lesions	Neoplasm
		Inflammation

Atresia – choledochal cyst

Prolonged neonatal jaundice may be due to atresia of the bile ducts (60%), or neonatal hepatitis. Atresia may be extrahepatic, intrahepatic or both and is commoner in Japan than in Western countries.

The aetiology is unknown but experimentally produced obstruction of the bile ducts can lead to a similar pathological picture in the liver. If untreated liver cirrhosis follows with all its usual complications. Males and females are equally affected.

Microscopically bile duct proliferation and portal fibrosis are the features of intrahepatic atresia. Bile plugs in the canalicular bile ducts are a feature of extrahepatic atresia.

Choledochal cystic dilatation of the common bile duct may occur with or without biliary atresia. Jaundice may occur at different times.

1 Neonatal jaundice if there is associated biliary atresia.
2 Jaundice of later onset, usually intermittent, due to inadequate emptying of the cystic common bile duct leading to cholangitis. Atresia is not present.

In both types hepatitis develops depending on the degree and duration of obstruction, and cholangitis.

The anatomical types of atresia are various but the continuity of the hepatic, common bile duct or alimentary connections remains the vital factor in prognosis. Ascending cholangitis is a common complication. Polycystic kidneys and hepatocellular carcinoma uncommonly occur with biliary atresia.

Ch.C = Choledochal cyst

GB = Gallbladder

Panc = Pancreas

3

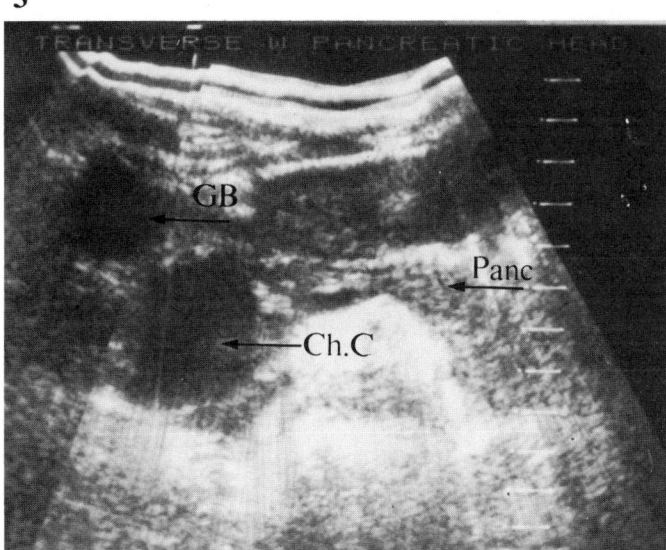

G.C.X.82

3   Transverse ultrasound scan showing gallbladder, choledochal cyst and pancreas.

4

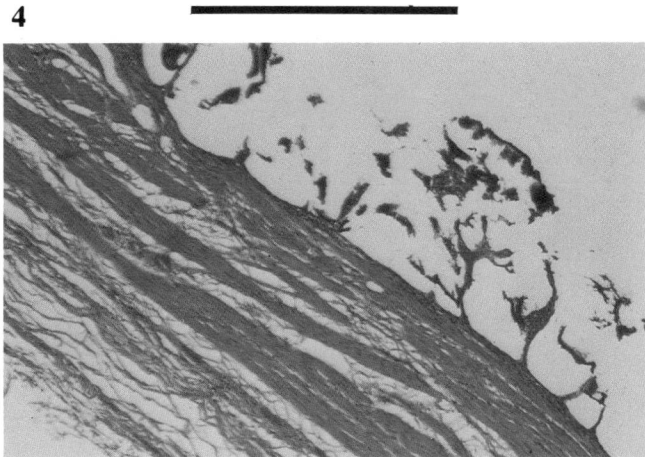

G.C.M.1010

4   Microscopic structure of the wall of a choledochal cyst. Note the loosely attached but fragmented epithelium and the underlying muscular layer.

4a

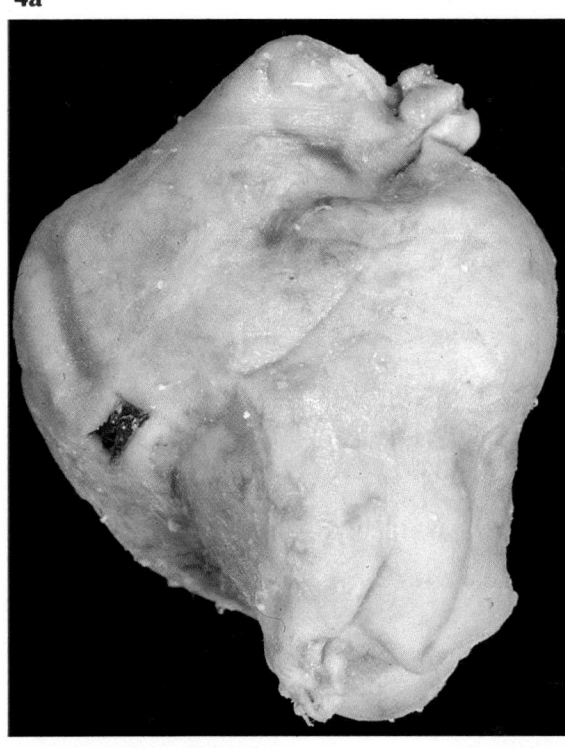

G.C.14333

4a   A 10-month-old male child presented with jaundice and severe vomiting. There was a large right sided abdominal mass. Laparotomy revealed a large choledochal cyst. A dilated common hepatic duct and gallbladder were attached to its upper aspect. A normal common bile duct joined the lower part to the duodenum. As jaundice was minimal it appeared that these structures communicated with the cyst and allowed some bile drainage. The cyst was excised and hepatic duct joined to duodenum. The patient was alive and well 20 years later.

Calculus

Secondary duct calculi

Calculi in the bile ducts are usually secondary to gallbladder disease. It is held that calculi are present in the common duct in approximately 10 to 15% of cholecystectomies.

A small calculus may (and often does) pass into the duodenum or may remain in the common duct and gradually grow by accretion until it becomes impacted at the lower end. Such impaction may be continuous, leading to progressive obstructive jaundice, or intermittent, the sphincteric contraction which holds the calculus relaxing and allowing it to drop back into the dilated common duct. Recurrent or persistent impaction leads to dilatation of the proximal bile ducts, stagnation of bile, infection usually from the already infected gallbladder, obstructive jaundice and fever due to cholangitis. A gallstone passed into the duodenum may, in the course of its passage through the small intestine, grow by accretion of 'faecal' material to such an extent that it impacts in the lower ileum – 'gallstone ileus'.

Primary duct calculi

Stone formation is less common within the hepatic or common duct where there has been stagnation, dilatation and infection. These calculi are comparable in composition to stones in the gallbladder. Pure pigment stones also form in the common duct and are seen in association with haemolytic jaundice and are also reported in patients with recurrent malaria.

5

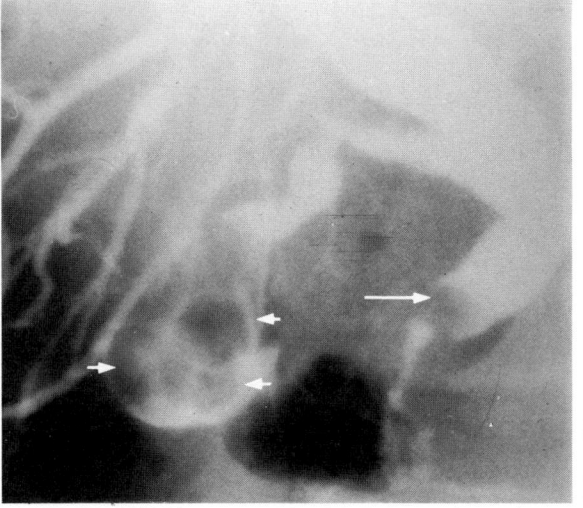

G.C.X.1009

5 Percutaneous transhepatic cholangiogram showing an obstructing calculus in the lower end of the common bile duct with dilatation of the common hepatic and bile ducts and multiple calculi in the gallbladder.

6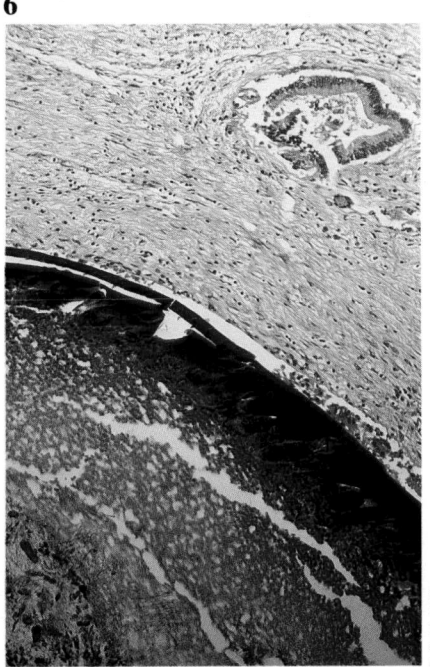

7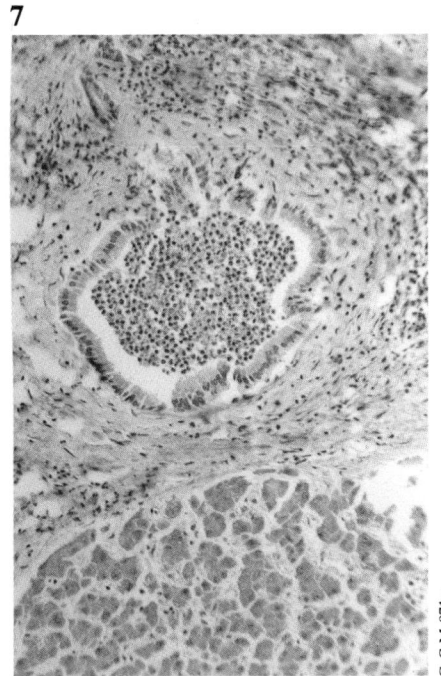

8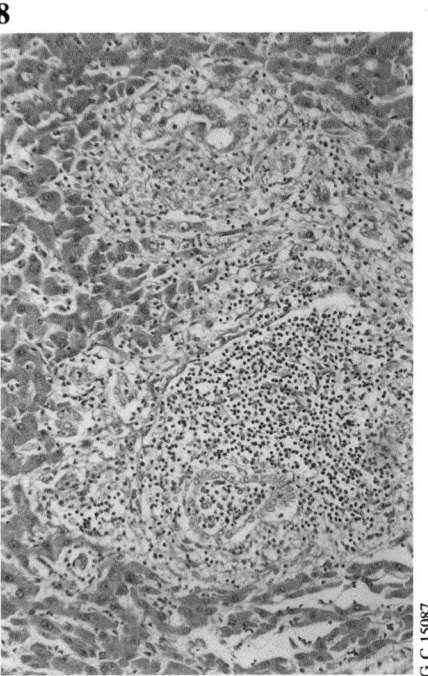

G.C.M.1002

G.C.M.871a

G.C.15087

6 Common bile duct – obstructing calculus. Part of a calculus which has obstructed the duct and has caused portal erosion of the epithelium and chronic inflammation in its wall. Bile pigment forms the outer layers but cholesterol crystals can be seen centrally. *(H&E ×100)*

7 Liver – obstructive cholangitis. A bile duct within a portal tract is distended by inflammatory cells. *(H&E ×125)*

8 Liver – obstructive cholangitis due to stone in ampulla of Vater. The portal tracts are heavily infiltrated by polymorphs, plasma cells and lymphocytes. The bile duct epithelium is hyperplastic and there is some fibrosis. *(H&E ×125)*

Parasites

In parts of the world where they are endemic, parasites may enter and obstruct (generally partially) the bile ducts. The round worm *(Ascaris lumbricoides)* may invade the common duct from the duodenum and a hydatid cyst may rupture and discharge its contents into an intrahepatic duct. Liver flukes *(Clonorchis sinensis* and *Fasciola hepatica)* can also invade the bile ducts, probably through the liver substance.

Clonorchis sinensis stimulates an adenomatous reaction in the mucosa which may undergo malignant change.

9

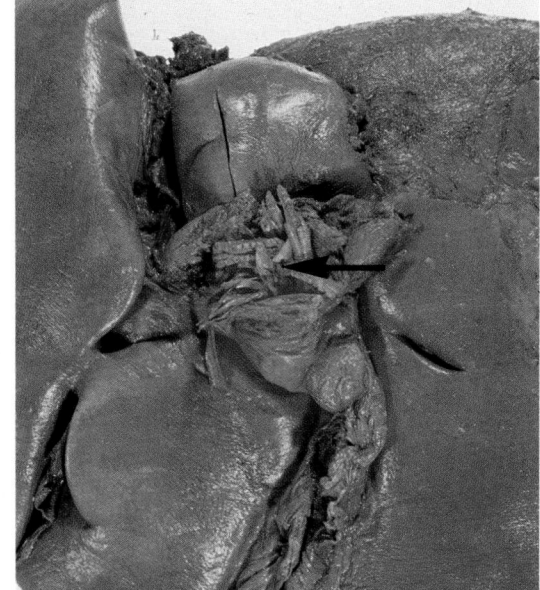

G.C.503

9 *Ascaris lumbricoides* impacted in the common duct.

A.I.S. Macpherson

477

Oriental cholangiohepatitis
(recurrent pyogenic cholangitis)

This is a distinctive form of cholangitis which occurs amongst the Chinese and shows a particular geographical range. The maximum incidence is in the south-east coastal area of China but extends as far north as Japan and as far south as Singapore. Major studies of this lesion have been undertaken in Hong Kong.

Aetiology

The aetiology of the condition is obscure and diverse views have been advanced:
1   A primary liver lesion most probably a clonorchis infestation.
2   An ascending infection from the intestine.
3   Arising as a portal pyaemia which leads to a hepatitis followed by a descending infection of the bile ducts.

The view that this disease is attributable to clonorchis infestation largely rests upon the fact that it is essentially limited to those areas where clonorchis infestation is common. Proof of the relationship is lacking. In many instances there is no evidence of the fluke or its ova in the content of the affected common duct. This can be explained by assuming that when an acute infection occurs the ova and the parasites may be destroyed.

It has been suggested that the clonorchis causes an irritation of the bile ducts with epithelial changes within the liver but that the worm itself does not play a direct part in the disease.

10

Incidence

10 The sex incidence is equal and the accompanying graph shows the age incidence.

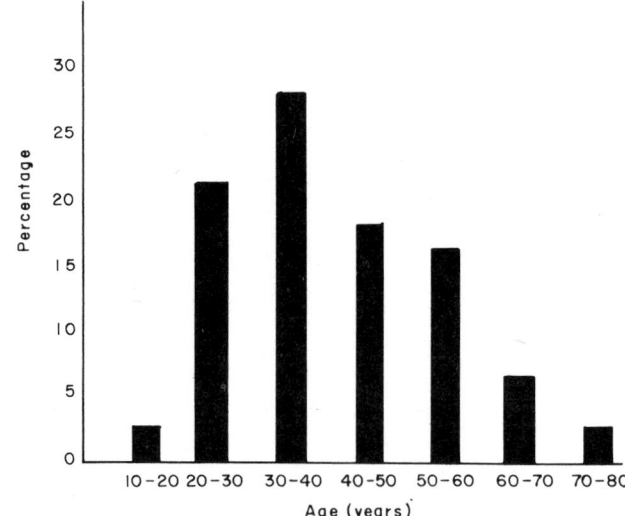

Pathology

A recurrent disease. During the acute phase the liver is enlarged and the surface covered with filmy avascular adhesions. On the cut surface dilated hepatic ducts are often seen, forming cyst-like areas which contain bile pigment, calculi and mucus. True abscess formation may occur.

The gallbladder is distended, thin walled and contains

Stones present in 80% of cases	
Calcium	0.5%
Cholesterol	20.2%
Bilirubin	79.3%

A portal pyaemia is frequently demonstrated at the time of operation. *E. coli* and *Enterococcus* have been recovered both from the portal vein and the bile ducts. Other organisms have also been found in smaller numbers.

pus. The common duct is grossly dilated and may contain pigment calculi. Typically it is filled with dark sludge (mud). A stone can be found causing either incomplete or complete blockage at the sphincter of Oddi. Stricture formation of ducts within the liver is an occasional finding. The acute stage is characterised clinically by pyrexia, marked toxaemia and jaundice.

Bile culture		
	Acute	Remission
Number of cases	60	120
Number of positive cultures	57	108
Percentage	95	90

11

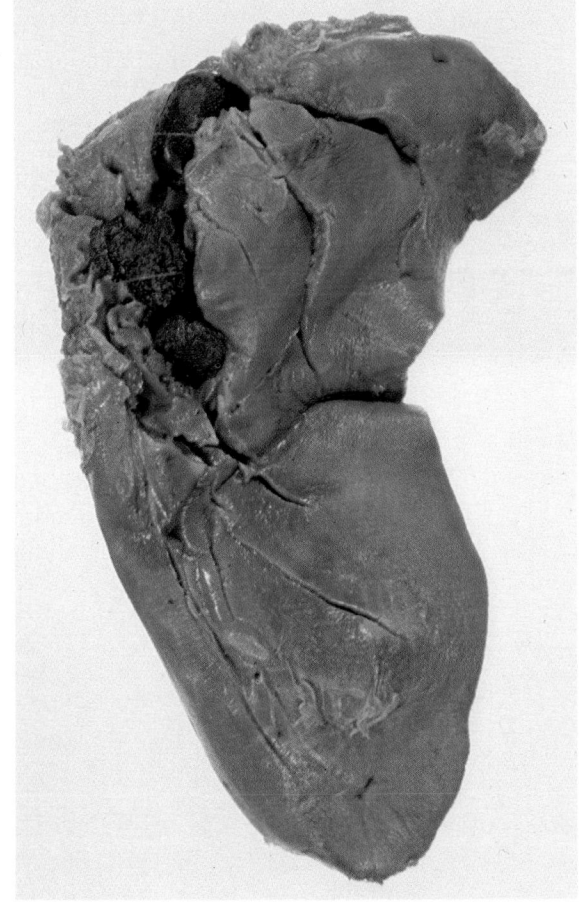

G.C.14029

11 From a female aged 59 years. Recurrent attacks of jaundice, fever and upper abdominal pain for 3 years. Operation disclosed that calculi were present in the left hepatic duct which necessitated resection of the left lobe of the liver in addition to common duct drainage.

Mortality

In a Hong Kong survey of 276 cases 31 patients died, a mortality of 11%.

G.B.Ong

Stricture

The most common cause of stricture formation in the biliary tract is operative mishap. This arises from a failure to secure full exposure and identification of the ducts and blood vessels leading to traumatisation, division or ligature of the common bile duct in mistake for the cystic duct.

Injury to the common duct may also occur when a probe is passed along the duct to ascertain the presence or absence of a calculus and goes through its wall.

Stricture can occur following ulceration by an impacted calculus.

After injury the obstruction to the flow of bile may be immediate or gradual. There is great dilatation of the bile ducts proximal to the obstruction and infection of the stagnant bile leads to recurrent attacks of ascending cholangitis. The wall of the duct becomes thickened by the deposition of fibrous tissue to form a circumferential ring.

12

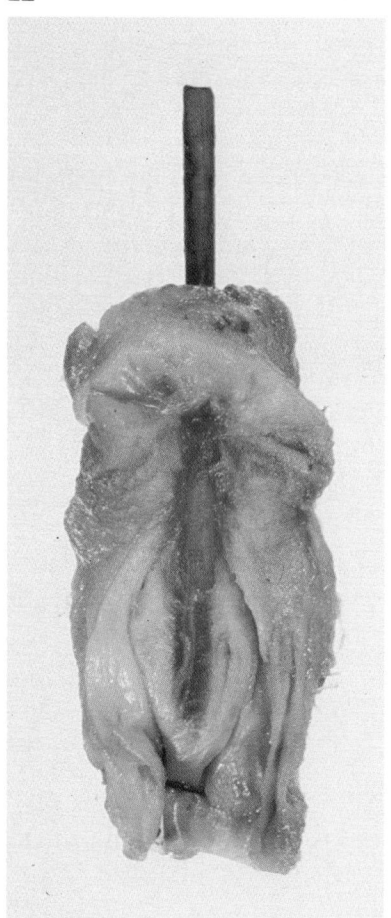

12 From a female aged 60 years. At cholecystectomy in 1959 it was found that there was no cystic duct, the gallbladder draining directly into the common duct which was inadvertently divided and repaired by an end-to-end anastomosis.

In 1962 she developed jaundice and fever. At operation a stricture of the common duct was found and resected. Note the narrowing of the lumen and the gross thickening of the duct wall.

G.C.13603

Sclerosing cholangitis

The aetiology of this uncommon condition is unknown. It causes diffuse narrowing of the intra- and extra-hepatic bile ducts and may be associated with other gastro-enterological diseases, e.g. ulcerative colitis. The walls of the bile ducts are diffusely thickened by chronic inflammatory tissue and the lumen is narrowed, but the mucosa is generally intact. Cholangiography by ERCP or at operation demonstrates irregularity of the common duct and 'beading' of the intra-hepatic ducts due to multiple strictures.

13

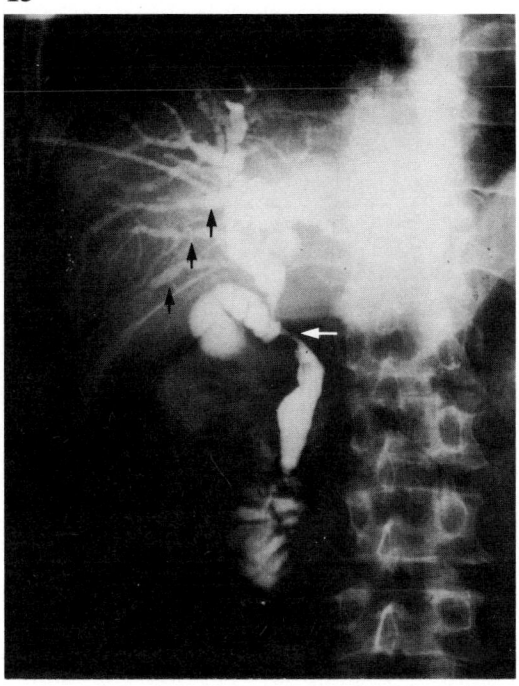

13 Bile duct – sclerosing cholangitis.

Neoplasms

See Section 16/2 U.

Extrinsic lesions

Extrinsic lesions involving the bile ducts occur in the intra-pancreatic segment and at the porta hepatis. At the lower end the duct may be invaded or compressed by lesions of the head of the pancreas, especially carcinoma and at the upper end by enlargement of lymph nodes in the porta hepatis due to lymphoma, chronic inflammation or metastases from gastric or pancreatic carcinoma. Inflammation in the hepato-renal recess, particularly post-operative infection, may lead to fibrosis and scarring around the bile ducts with consequent narrowing and the sequellae of an obstructive lesion.

A.I.S. Macpherson

481

The pancreas is an exocrine gland assisting in the digestion of food and an endocrine gland secreting a variety of hormones which control a number of important physiological functions. The endocrine functions are dependent on the activity of the cells of the islets of Langerhans – minute structures scattered throughout the pancreatic parenchyma.

Development

The pancreas develops as two buds, one from the dorsal and one from the ventral aspect of the primitive duodenum. The ventral bud divides, one part forming the biliary system and the liver, and the other the main pancreatic duct in the head of the pancreas.

During rotation of the duodenum the dorsal and ventral rudiments are brought together and fuse. The dorsal bud gives rise to most of the gland and only the uncinate process and infero-posterior portion of the head are formed from the ventral bud.

The main duct of the pancreas is formed from the short duct of the ventral bud and most of the duct of the dorsal bud the proximal part of which usually persists as the accessory duct.

1

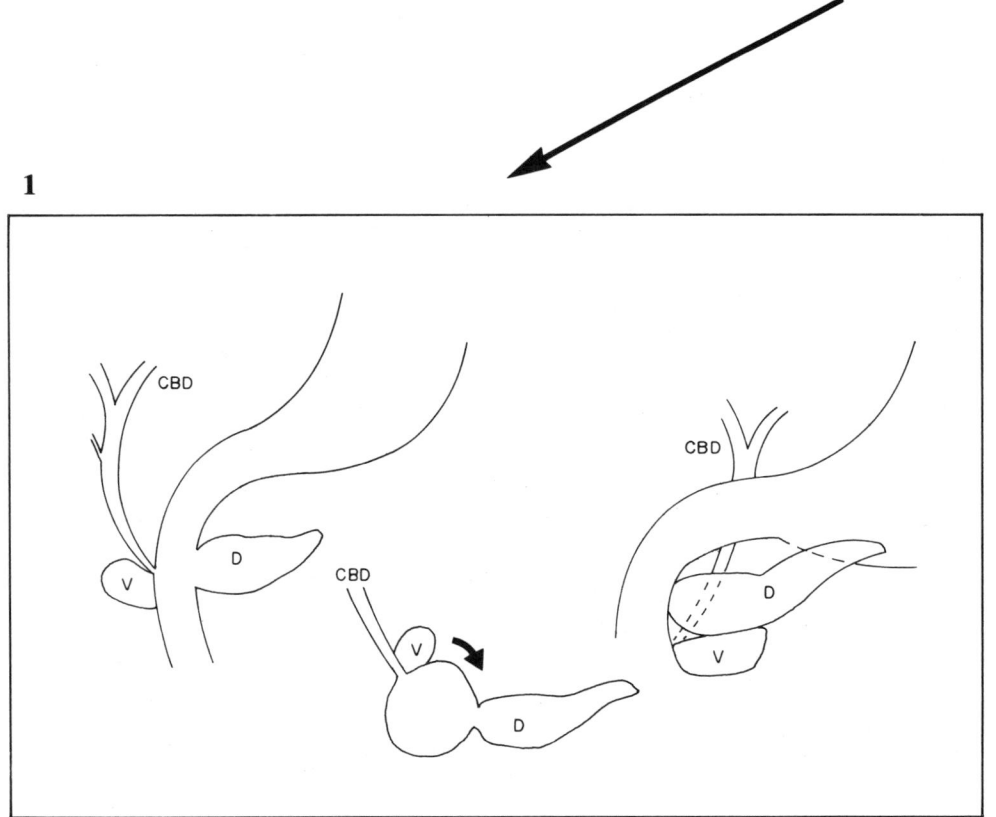

CBD = Common bile duct
V   = Ventral pancreas
D   = Dorsal pancreas

Annular pancreas

Annular pancreas is a rare congenital abnormality in which a ring of pancreatic tissue encircles the duodenum often constricting it. It is usually due to a maldevelopment of the ventral pancreatic bud which fails to migrate and join the dorsal bud in the normal way. A major pancreatic duct is often found in the annular tissue and care must be taken to avoid its transection in patients with duodenal stenosis since a pancreatic fistula will almost certainly result.

Anatomy

The organ is divided into the head, neck, body and tail. The position of the head, clasped by the first three parts of the duodenum, is relatively constant. The body and tail may occupy a variety of positions with corresponding alteration of the course of the duct. The body and tail may vary from the transverse with the common appearance of a relatively straight duct to the curved in which the duct has a sigmoid shape. Other variations demonstrate an L-shaped or an inverted V duct.

2

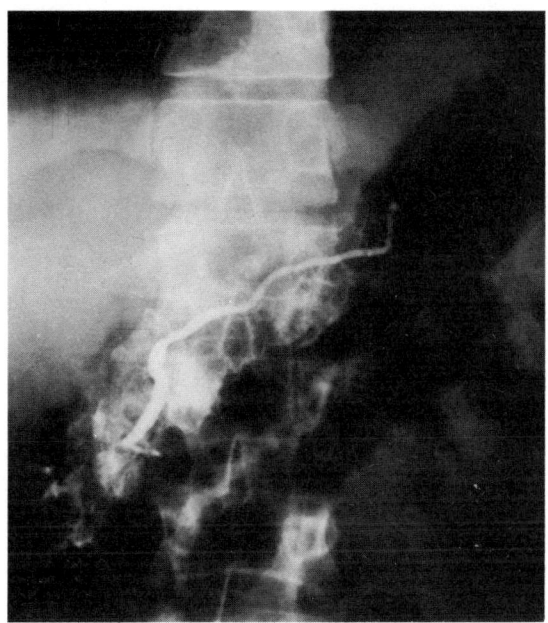

G.C.X.1029

2 Pancreatogram showing normal position of the pancreatic duct extending obliquely across the upper abdomen.

3

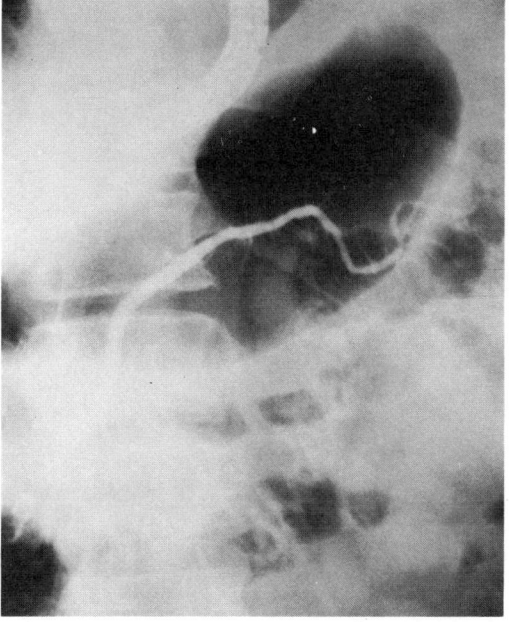

G.C.X.1030

3 An example of normal pancreatic duct taking a more horizontal course towards the left with an S-shaped curve.

The main pancreatic duct (of Wirsung) traverses the whole length of the pancreas and in 90% of patients it joins the common bile duct to form a common channel entering the duodenum at the ampulla of Vater. The position of the ampulla is variable and although it usually lies on the medial wall of the second part of the duodenum at about its mid-point, it may be found throughout the second part or even in the upper wall of the third part or, more rarely, in the first part (see Section 16/2).

The ampulla produces a weak spot in the wall of the duodenum through which diverticula may develop. The smaller pancreatic duct (of Santorini) enters the duodenum above the ampulla. It usually communicates with the main duct so that, if the latter is obstructed, pancreatic secretions may still enter the duodenum.

Histology

The pancreas has a lobular structure each individual lobule being drained by a short slender duct. The arterial supply of the head comes from the pancreatico-duodenal arteries while the body and tail are nourished mainly by branches from the splenic artery which lies in intimate contact with the gland along its upper border.

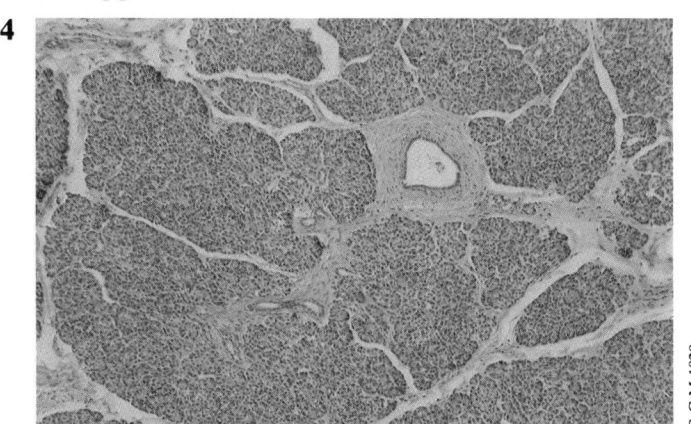

4 Normal pancreas showing lobules with one inter-lobular duct and several small intralobular ducts. *(H&E ×62.5)*

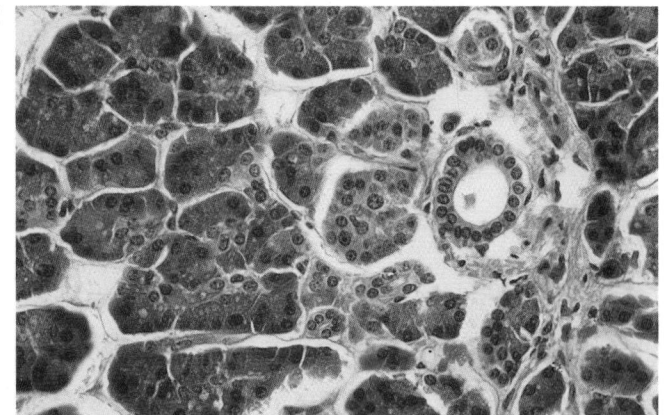

5 Normal pancreas showing acinar cells with eosinophilic zymogen granules. Alongside the intralobular duct there is a small islet of Langerhans. *(H&E ×312.5)*

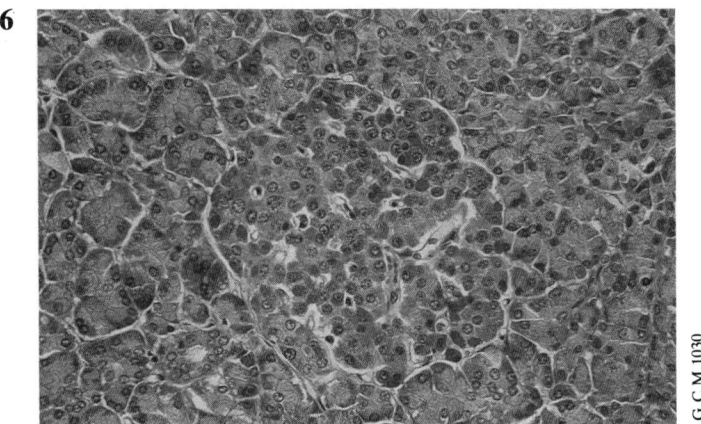

6 Normal pancreas. Centrally there is an islet of Langerhans. Gomori's stain differentiates between the blue staining ß cells and the bright ∝ red cells. *(Chrome alum, haematoxylin, phloxine ×250)*

Heterotopic pancreas

Accessory or heterotopic pancreatic tissue may be found in any part of the wall of the duodenum and even in the stomach, jejunum or outside the gastro-intestinal tract. It forms a discrete nodule which is usually submucosal but may lie within the gut wall or the sub-serosa. It may be the site of a tumour of pancreatic or islet cell type.

7 Specimen from a partial gastrectomy carried out for a duodenal ulcer. Situated immediately inferior to the first part of the duodenum and partly in its wall is a small circular mass paler in colour than the mucosa. Sections show this to be aberrant pancreatic tissue with the presence of islets.

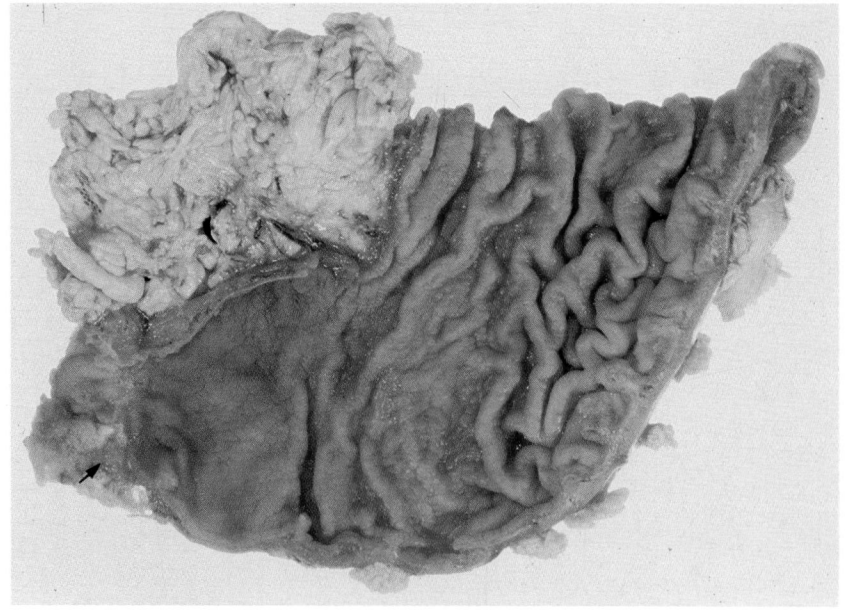

Exocrine function

The great bulk of the pancreas is an exocrine gland secreting a digestive juice which passes into the second part of the duodenum and mixes with the food as it leaves the stomach. It secretes approximately 1500 ml of alkaline juice per day. Its main enzymes are amylase, lipase, and a group of proteolytic enzymes such as trypsin and chymotrypsin which are secreted in an inactive form. Secretion is stimulated partly by the intestinal hormones secretin and cholecystokinin and partly by reflex mechanisms.

The pancreas is an important digestive organ and complete loss of its secretions, as following total pancreatectomy or in very severe chronic pancreatitis, results in malabsorption particularly of fat but also of protein (see Section 15 A).

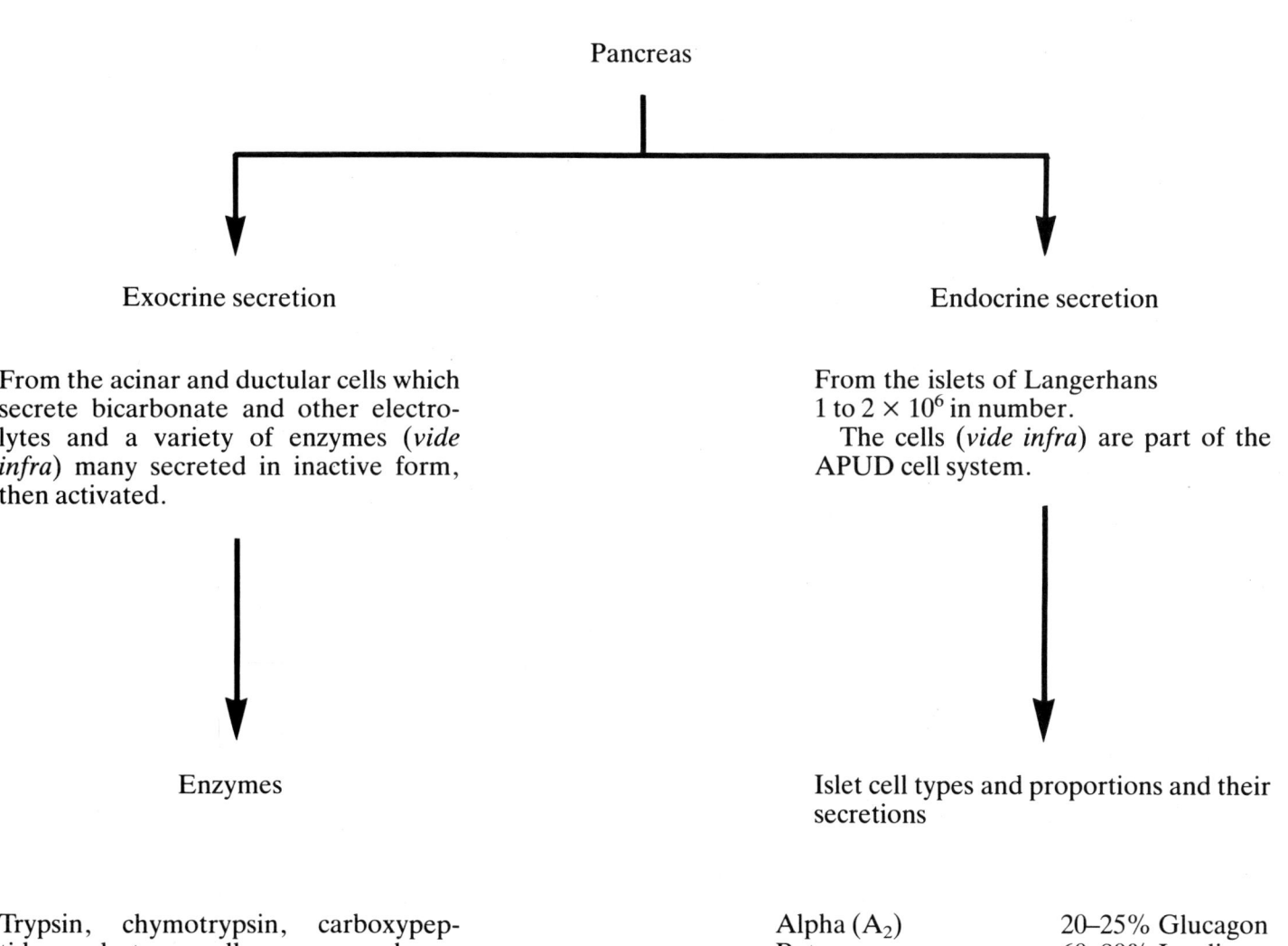

Pancreas

Exocrine secretion

From the acinar and ductular cells which secrete bicarbonate and other electrolytes and a variety of enzymes (*vide infra*) many secreted in inactive form, then activated.

Enzymes

Trypsin, chymotrypsin, carboxypeptidase, elastase, collagenase, nuclease, amylase, lipase, phospholipase, cholesterol esterase.

Endocrine secretion

From the islets of Langerhans 1 to 2×10^6 in number.

The cells (*vide infra*) are part of the APUD cell system.

Islet cell types and proportions and their secretions

Alpha (A_2)	20–25%	Glucagon
Beta	60–80%	Insulin
Delta (A_1)	10–15%	Somatostatin
D cell		Pancreatic polypeptide
Cell type unknown		Vasoactive intestinal peptide

A.C.B. Dean

Pancreatitis is classified as either acute, acute relapsing, chronic or chronic relapsing. In spite of the similarity in their aetiology, these are not different manifestations of a single clinical entity and acute or acute relapsing pancreatitis does not progress to chronic pancreatitis.

Acute pancreatitis

Aetiology

Acute pancreatitis is an acute inflammatory reaction in the pancreas and surrounding tissues in the form of autodigestion induced by the release of active pancreatic enzymes from damaged pancreatic cells. There are many hypotheses as to the mechanism involved including bile and duodenal juice reflux, pancreatic duct obstruction, infection both bacterial and viral, and vascular obstruction and ischaemia. Evidence both clinical and experimental has been given in support of each of these factors. It is also possible, however, that the process starts as a primary intracellular derangement.

In Britain the main aetiological factors are biliary disease and alcohol. Other factors are hyperparathyroidism, hyperlipidaemia, trauma both accidental and surgical, viral (mumps) and drug induced (corticosteroids). Pancreatitis is a rare complication of corticosteroid therapy. Now an increasing number of cases are being seen following endoscopic retrograde cholangiopancreatography or translumbar aortography.

Pathology

The pathological picture varies widely from the relatively mild changes found characteristically in acute relapsing pancreatitis to the most severe changes in acute haemorrhagic pancreatitis where there may be extensive subcapsular haemorrhage and considerable necrosis of pancreatic tissue. In these severe cases the mortality is high, varying in different series from 30 to 60%. The classical picture in acute pancreatitis of moderate severity, however, is a swollen oedematous gland with inflammation and oedema of the surrounding tissues and areas of fat necrosis in the intra-abdominal fat. If the patient recovers, the pancreas regains a remarkably normal appearance with normal exocrine and endocrine function so that malabsorption and diabetes do not occur.

1

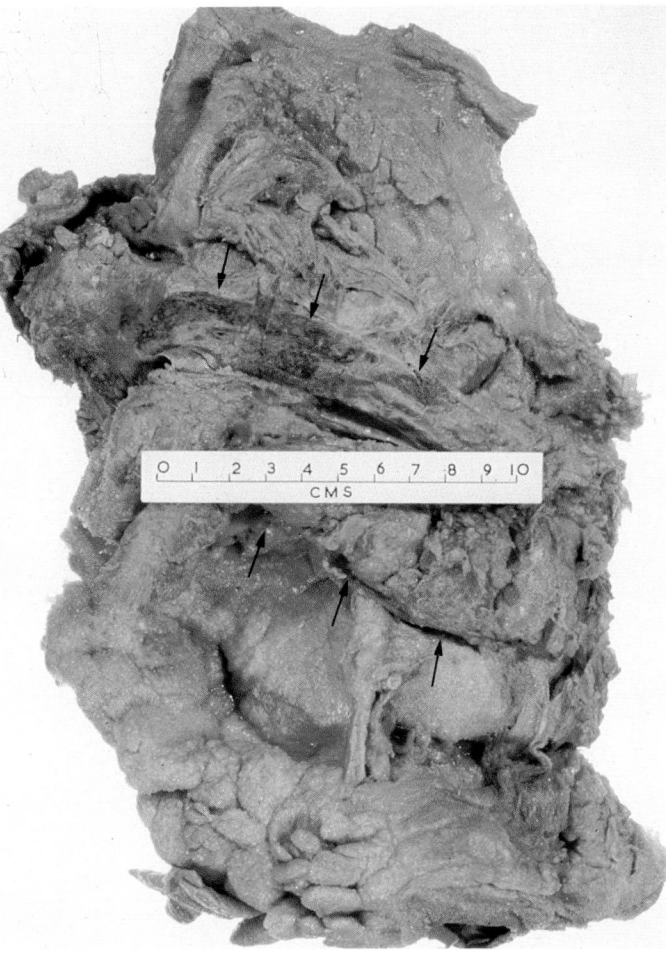

G.C.4539

1 From a female aged 49 years. This obese patient was admitted as an acute abdominal emergency simulating intestinal obstruction. At operation extensive fat necrosis was found. The pancreas was noted to be enlarged, hard and haemorrhagic.

The specimen shows the classical features of enlargement, oedema and areas of fat necrosis. The arrows indicate the pancreas which has been split longitudinally showing haemorrhage in the head.

Histology

3

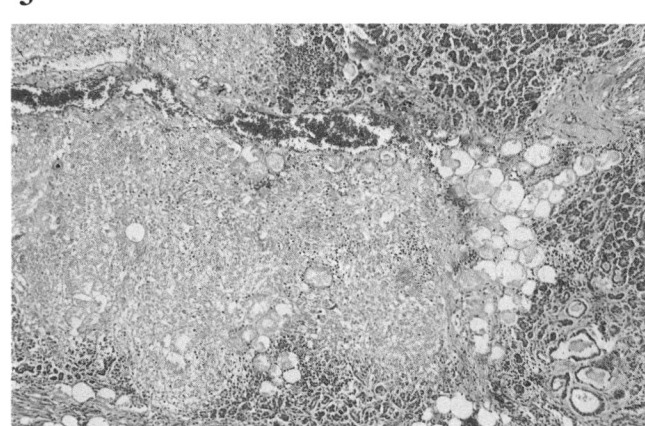

G.C.M.1024

3 Acute pancreatitis. Much of the pancreatic tissue and fat in this section is necrotic and structureless. Haemorrhage occurs when the walls of the engorged blood vessels are weakened. *(H&E × 50)*

2

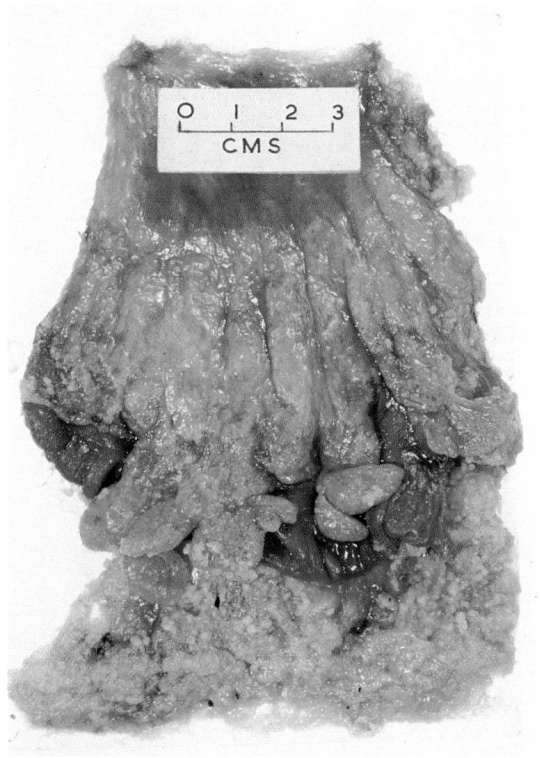

G.C.9538

2 Omentum from an adult who died from acute haemorrhagic pancreatitis. Haemorrhage into the swollen oedematous omentum has occurred in several places.

The characteristic opaque chalky appearance of fat necrosis is well shown in the inferior portion.

487

Acute pancreatitis (*Continued*)

Complications

The mortality and morbidity of acute pancreatitis are largely due to the onset of complications. Severe hypovolaemia may occur in the early stages due to the massive exudation of fluid comparable to that seen in severe scalding and sometimes referred to as the pancreatic burn. This may lead to shock and renal failure.

Pseudocyst

The formation of a pseudocyst arises as the result of inflammation to the pancreatic parenchyma. There is an outpouring of fluid into the lesser sac and if the epiploic foramen becomes occluded the fluid collection may assume massive proportions. The fluid within the cyst is rich in amylase. Smaller pseudocysts arise close to the pancreas and indicate that the original leakage of fluid from the pancreas was limited.

The pseudocyst produces little in the way of symptoms unless it becomes large enough to compress neighbouring organs particularly the stomach which is displaced forwards, upwards and to the left producing nausea, anorexia and epigastric fullness and discomfort. If exposed by operation such a cyst will be seen to bulge forwards through the gastrocolic and gastrohepatic mesenteries.

Pseudocysts may regress spontaneously or alternatively progressively increase in size necessitating operative intervention.

If the pseudocyst is operated on early in its development, severe bleeding from the acutely inflamed wall is a common complication. It is usual to wait for 6 weeks to see if operative intervention is indicated. If surgery is necessary before then because of progressive enlargement, external drainage is preferred as it minimises the risk of haemorrhage but it may result in a persistent fistula. The best treatment for a pseudocyst after 6 weeks is anastomosis of the cyst to either the stomach or a loop of jejunum. The pseudocyst drains into the gastro-intestinal tract and the anastomosis eventually disappears when the defect in the pancreatic duct heals and the secretions drain by the normal route.

4

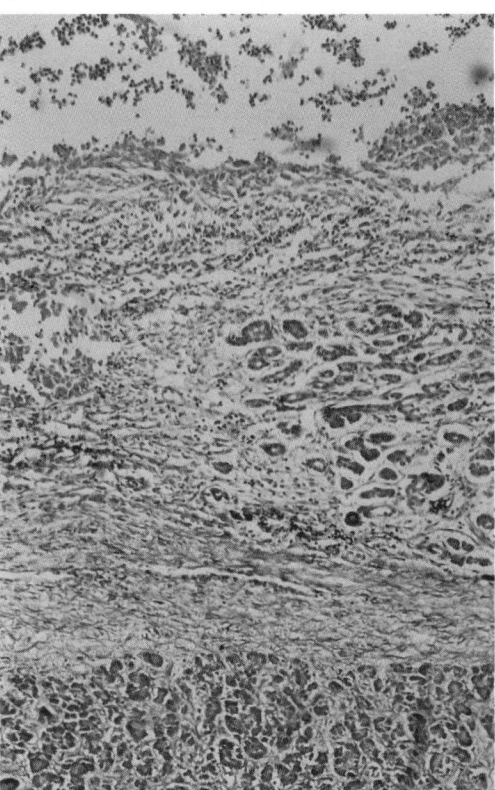

G.C.15132

4 Pseudocyst of pancreas. The cyst contains necrotic debris and inflammatory exudate. A wall of atrophic and fibrotic pancreas heavily infiltrated by chronic inflammatory cells separates the lumen from the adjacent pancreas. (*H&E* × 97.5)

488

Pseudocyst formation may also arise:
1 Following trauma to the pancreas.
2 In association with leakage from a peptic ulcer of the posterior wall.
3 Polyserositis.
4 Healed tuberculous peritonitis.

Pseudocysts must be differentiated from:
Simple cysts lined by columnar mucin-secreting epithelium.
Congenital cyst disease.
Dermoid cysts.
Benign cystadenoma $\left.\right\}$ *vide infra*
Cystadenocarcinoma
Parasitic cysts (e.g. hydatid disease).

Pancreatic abscess

Pancreatic abscess is a serious complication usually occurring within a few days of the onset of an acute episode. The entry of organisms into an area of damaged pancreatic tissue leads to the formation of an abscess in or close to the pancreas. If the abscess is not drained the mortality rate is virtually 100%.

Respiratory complications

Respiratory complications may occur, particularly the shock lung syndrome and pleural effusion. In cases of severe haemorrhagic pancreatitis, a consumptive coagulopathy may develop together with diabetic coma, hypocalcaemia and confusion.

Ascites

Pancreatic ascites is an uncommon complication and is due to excessive exudation of fluid rich in pancreatic enzymes into the peritoneal cavity.

Chronic pancreatitis

In chronic pancreatitis the inflammation in the gland is low grade and prolonged. It may be almost continuous or, in chronic relapsing pancreatitis, it may run an intermittent course.

Aetiology

Alcohol is the most important aetiological factor and is exacerbated by malnutrition. Biliary disease and hyperlipidaemia are also factors.

Pathology

Progressive destruction of the parenchyma with fibrosis dominates the histological picture. The gland becomes firm and the main duct system characteristically shows alternating fibrous strictures and a saccular dilatation. In some patients the strictures predominate and much of the duct system may be stenosed. In others the fibrosis is mainly in the terminal part of the main ducts and there is extensive dilatation.

5

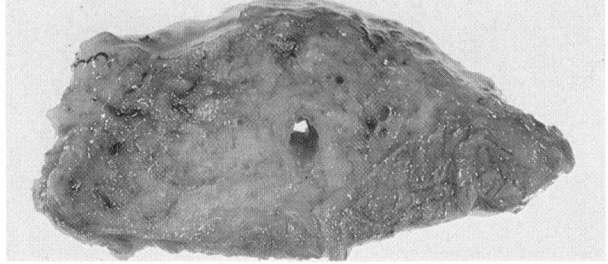

G.C.14342

5 This complete transection of the tail of the pancreas well demonstrates the essential changes of acute pancreatitis. It shows atrophy. The loss of pancreatic parenchyma is occurring secondary to the chronic inflammatory process. The dilated pancreatic duct can be seen in cross-section. Its wall exhibits dense fibrosis. In this case the inflammation occurred secondary to duct obstruction. These changes may lead to a gross reduction in size. The histological features are demonstrated on the page opposite (**8**).

6

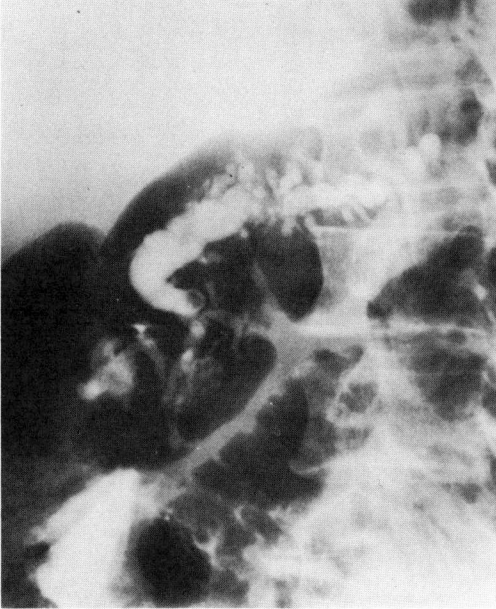

G.C.X.1031

6 Pancreatogram in a case of chronic pancreatitis. The pancreatic duct is markedly dilated.

Microscopical appearances

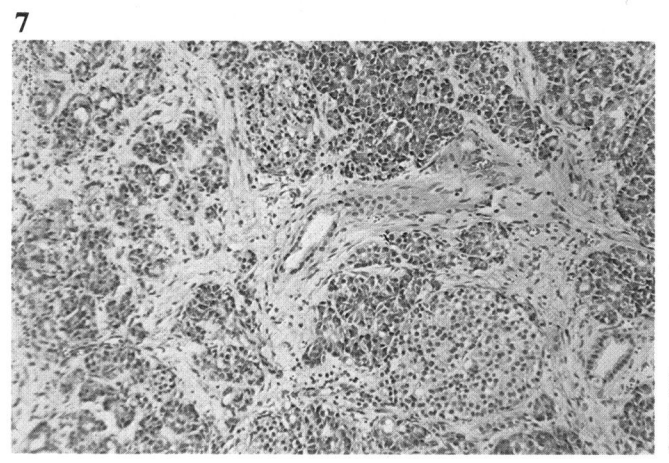

7 Chronic pancreatitis. In this field of relatively mild chronic pancreatitis there is some loss of acinar tissue and of zymogenic cells. Fibrosis has thickened the stroma. The islet appears normal. *(H&E × 100)*

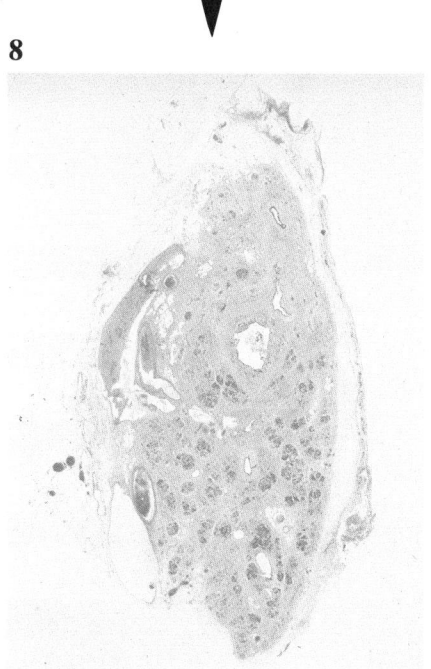

8 A cross-section of the pancreas **(5)** showing advanced chronic pancreatitis. The ducts are dilated and only small foci of dark-staining acinar and islet tissue survive amid the extensive fibrosis. *(H&E × 3.75)*

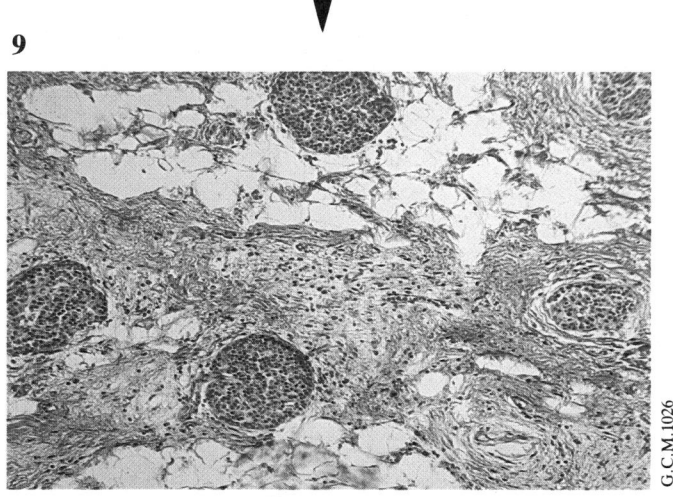

9 Chronic pancreatitis. In this field of advanced disease, the acinar component has been replaced by fibrous tissue. Islets survive and are unusually prominent in the atrophic pancreas. *(H&E × 100)*

Chronic pancreatitis (*Continued*)

Plugs form in the dilated ducts and these may calcify forming pancreatic calculi visible on X-rays as 'pancreatic calcification'. It was originally believed that calcification occurred in the pancreatic parenchyma but is now realised that this is uncommon and that the appearance of calcification is usually due to multiple small calculi throughout a dilated duct system.

10

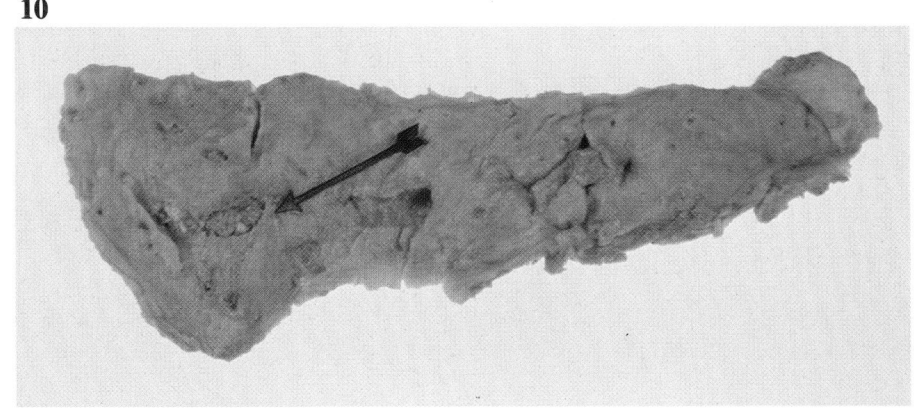

G.C.11405

10 This specimen obtained at post mortem consists of a coronal section of pancreas showing lithiasis. The pancreas is shrunken and pale.

On the cut surface the duct is seen to be dilated and in the portions which lie in the head and body amorphous white chalky deposits are present. The parenchyma is atrophic and there is excess of fibrous tissue.

11

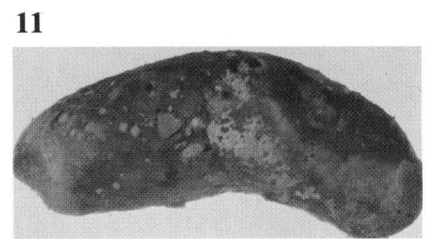

G.C.6234

11 This calculus 2.5 cm in length was removed post mortem from a stout florid multipara aged 76 years who had vague symptoms of indigestion, frequent epigastric pain and recurrent slight jaundice.

For some years she was thought to be suffering from gallstones but post mortem examination disclosed a normal gallbladder. The concretion was movable within the pancreatic duct which was somewhat dilated.

12

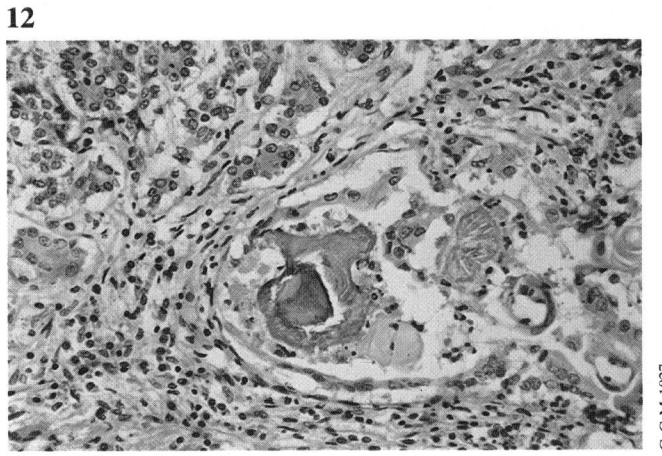

G.C.M.1027

12 Chronic pancreatitis in a patient with alcoholic cirrhosis.

Microcalculi resulting from calcification of inspissated secretion in ducts have resulted in debasement of duct epithelium and chronic inflammation in and around the duct. (*H&E* × *250*)

Progress of disease

The disease is characterised by severe pain and by progressive loss of both exocrine and endocrine function until the patient develops malabsorption and diabetes. The pain is due mainly to distension of the obstructed duct system. It may be relieved by procedures such as the Puestow's operation which drains the dilated ducts into a Roux loop of jejunum. Eventually when most of the pancreatic tissue has been destroyed the pain decreases since there is no longer sufficient secretion to distend the ducts. The condition has 'burnt itself out'. Pancreatic abscess and pseudocyst can occur but are much less common than in acute pancreatitis.

Other lesions

Mucoviscidosis (fibrocystic disease)

This is one manifestation of a hereditary congenital abnormality of mucous secretion which affects all mucous secreting glands. Viscid mucus obstructs the pancreatic ducts with distension and some alveolar rupture. The result is an early pancreatitis and subsequent fibrosis. Although the steatorrhoea and malabsorption secondary to the pancreatic changes can be evident at a very early age they are usually associated with and often overshadowed by the other manifestations of the disease such as the bronchiolitis.

Rupture

Rupture of the pancreas may result from stab wounds or from severe direct non-penetrating violence to the abdomen the pancreas being crushed against the vertebral column. The injury is frequently associated with multiple involvement of other viscera and major vessels and consequently shock and haemorrhage are prominent features. The injury to the pancreas may be in the nature of bruising, partial rupture with haemorrhage or complete division.

Incidence – In the United Kingdom a high proportion of cases of rupture of the pancreas is attributable to road accidents.

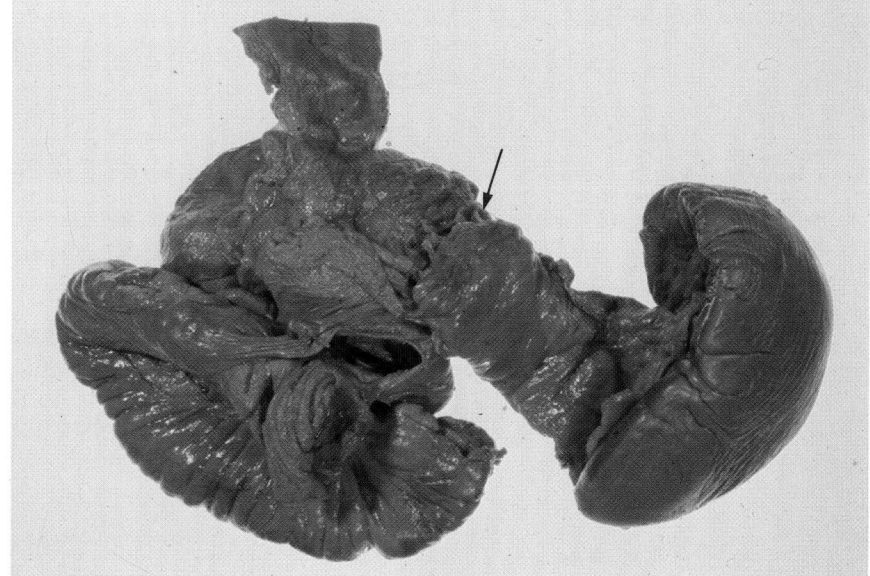

13

13 Traumatic rupture of the pancreas from a child aged 4 years.

G.C.3838

A.C.B. Dean

493

Exocrine tumours

Tumours of the pancreas often present an indefinite clinical picture and diagnosis is accordingly difficult except when the common bile duct becomes obstructed. Barium meal examination and ultrasonography are helpful in the recognition of these deep seated tumours. Not infrequently it is only when the lesion has reached an advanced stage and there is a palpable mass that the condition is recognised.

Alternatively, the presence of metastases may give rise to the presenting symptoms and signs.

The exocrine tumours fall into two groups, those which are cystic and may be benign or malignant, and the solid infiltrating adenocarcinoma. The location of the tumour may be in the head, body or tail of the pancreas. Where the tumour lies in the head of the pancreas it may distort the contour of the duodenum, compress, occlude or infiltrate the common duct or simulate a carcinoma of the ampulla of Vater.

Cystadenoma

This tumour occurs much more frequently in women (M:F – 1:8) and most often in the sixth and seventh decades. It presents as a lobulated mass growing in the substance or apparently from the surface of any part of the pancreas. The stomach is displaced forwards and depending on the location of the tumour, upwards or to the right. The duodenum may also show distortion. The cysts contain clear mucin but this may be discoloured by intra-cystic bleeding. Some are so large that they become palpable.

1

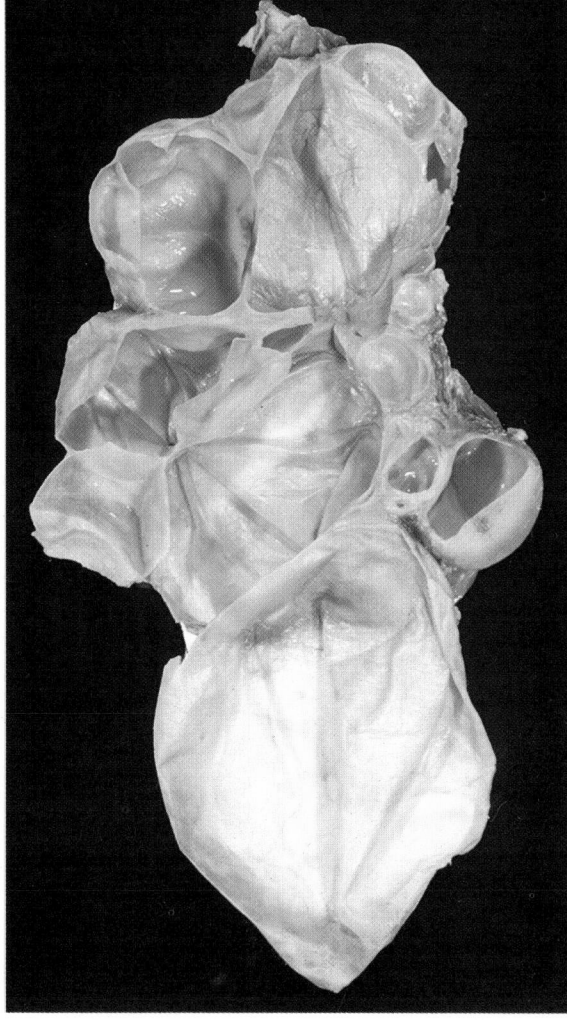

1 A female aged 37 years developed a palpable mass extending from the costal margin to below and to the left of the umbilicus. It was attached to the neck of the pancreas by a narrow pedicle and was resected.

G.C.9576

Most cystadenomas are small. They contain small cysts which are lined by low columnar epithelium separated by a stroma which radiates out from a central core and may show abundant mucoid material or even calcification.

2

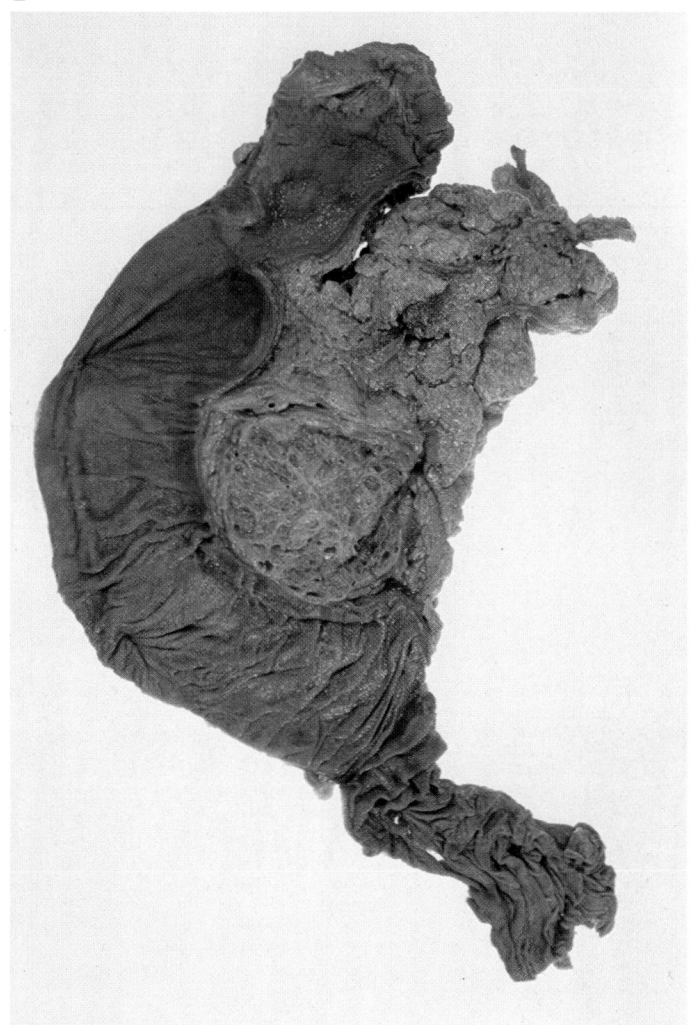

G.C.10897

2 From a female aged 57 years. This patient was admitted to hospital as a case of biliary colic and at operation stones were found in the gallbladder, but in addition a mass, apparently simple, was found in the head of the pancreas. A cholecystgastrostomy was performed followed one month later by a standard duodenopancreatectomy. The patient made an uneventful recovery.

The illustration shows a round tumour approximately 4cm in diameter in the head of the pancreas. It is closely adherent to the first and second parts of the duodenum. Around half its circumference it appears to have a very definite capsule, and in no part is there any evidence of invasion of adjacent tissues.

The cut surface of the tumour shows the presence of numerous cysts of varying but limited size, some containing blood. The cysts are separated by fine fibrous septa which give the impression that they run towards a central nidus.

2a

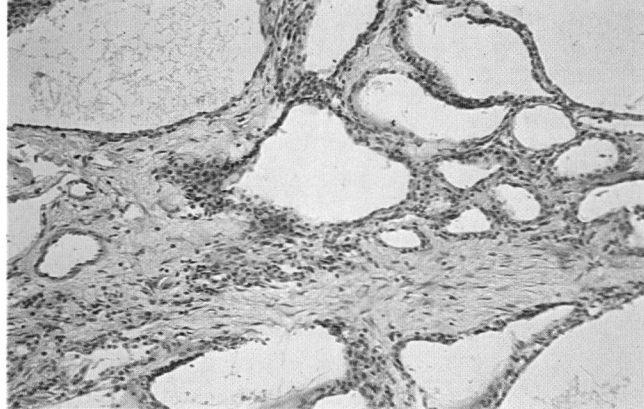

2a Pancreas – cystadenoma.
The tumour is formed by innumerable locules lined by mucin-secreting epithelium usually in a single layer. In smaller locules the epithelium is cubical or columnar but in larger locules it becomes flattened due to pressure.
(H&E ×125)

Exocrine tumours *(Continued)*

Cystadenoma *(Continued)*

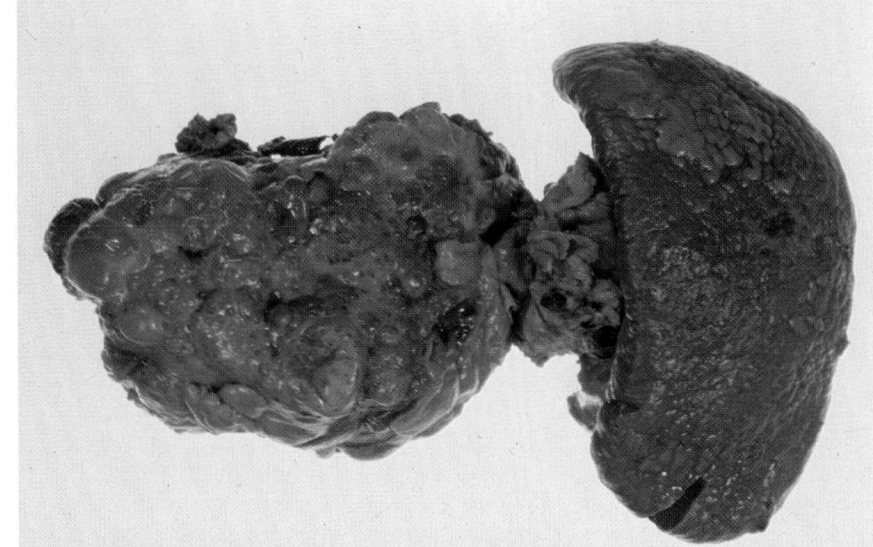

Lobulated anterior surface of the tumour.

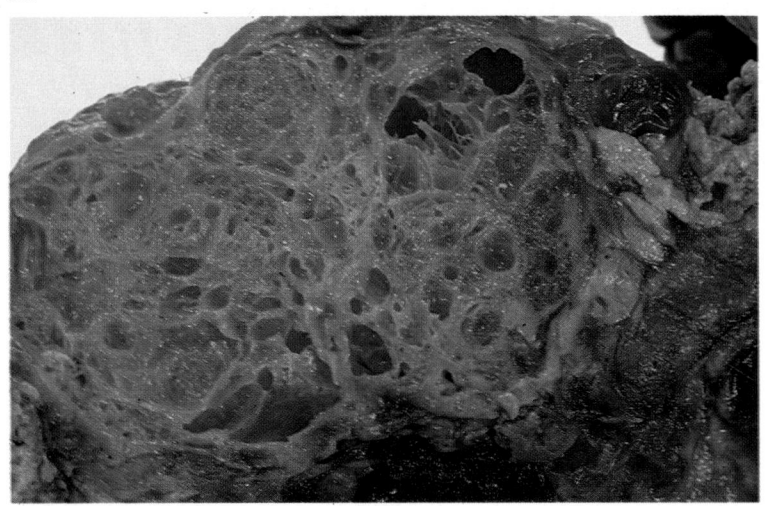

Cut surface of posterior aspect of tumour.

3 and **3a**   From a male aged 73 years. There was a 2 month history of epigastric discomfort and a sense of fullness after meals and lasting for 1 to 2 hours. Clinically no abnormality was found. Barium meal showed a deformity of the posterior wall of the stomach suggestive of an extrinsic lesion, probably a retroperitoneal mass either in the tail of the pancreas or kidney. At laparotomy a cystic tumour mass was found in the tail of the pancreas and was removed together with the spleen.

The tumour, measuring 7 × 5 × 3cm, was located in the body and tail of the pancreas and projected forwards as a lobulated mass. Its surface consists of innumerable small translucent cystic masses some of them purple as a result of haemorrhage. On the cut surface numerous microcystic translucent areas are separated by fibrous septa from larger cysts. The tumour has separated readily from adjacent structures – its margins are well defined indicating its benign character.

Histologically the cysts were lined with a single layer of cuboidal or flattened cubical epithelium. There was no evidence of mitotic activity or of malignancy. Except in its location this tumour is comparable in all respects to the previous illustration.

Cystadenocarcinoma

The frequency of malignant change in cystadenoma is not known but is probably small. The tumours are large and multilocular but with an increased proportion of solid tissue. Spread is at first local by invasion through the capsule and later to the regional lymph nodes. Intra-cystic haemorrhage is common and may lead to pressure on the vasa brevia or the splenic vein. Age and sex incidence is similar to cystadenoma.

The histological appearances are those of a well-differentiated adenocarcinoma with heaping and thickening of the epithelial lining of the cysts.

4

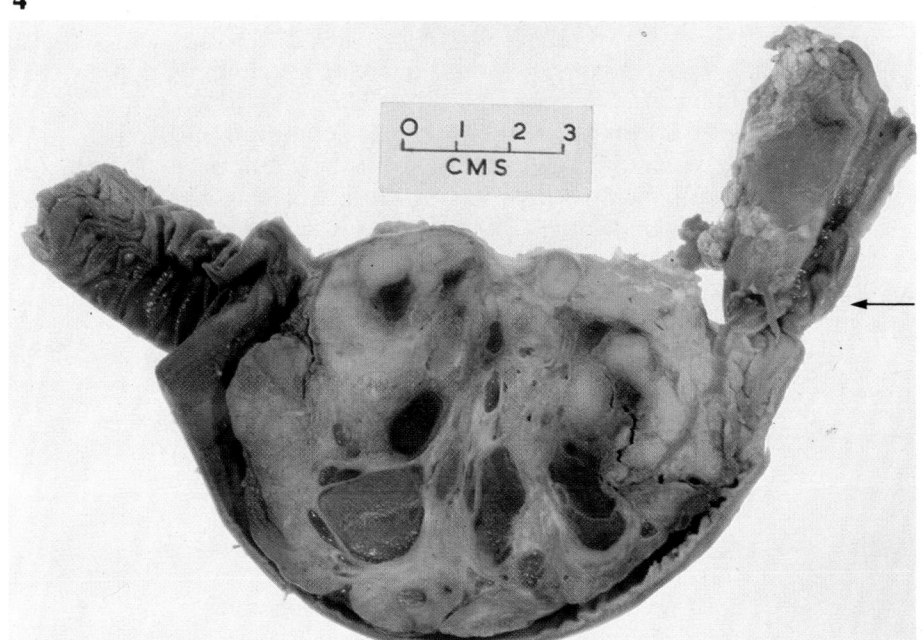

4 From a male aged 56 years. Three month history of deteriorating health associated with obvious anaemia.

Barium meal showed gross widening of the duodenal loop.

The specimen viewed from the back consists of the pylorus (arrow) and first, second and third parts of the duodenum, and the head of the pancreas invaded by a lobulated tumour compressing the duodenum.

On section the tumour is seen to consist of dense white masses containing several cysts. The tumour is reasonably well defined but is clearly malignant.

5

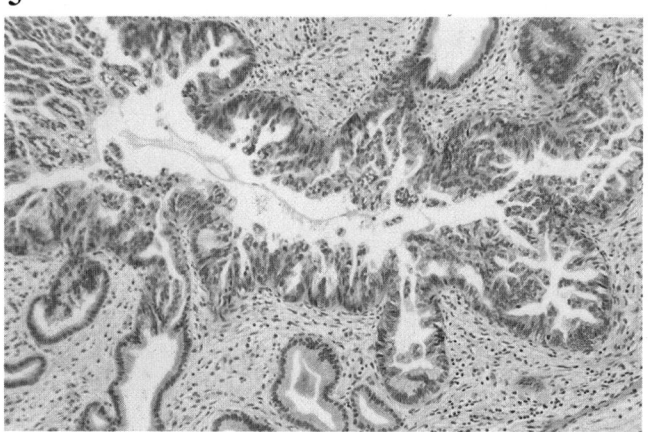

5 Pancreas – cystadenocarcinoma. The epithelium lining the cysts is papillary and hyperchromatic and invades the surrounding stroma. *(H&E ×100)*

497

Exocrine tumours *(Continued)*

Adenocarcinoma

Adenocarcinoma of the pancreas is a common tumour and its incidence is increasing. In the U.S.A. it is now commoner than carcinoma of the stomach and is the fourth commonest cause of death from cancer. It occurs about twice as frequently in the head as in the body and tail. It spreads early mainly by lymphatic and perineural spread but blood-borne metastases are also common. Microscopic foci of tumour may be found in other parts of the pancreas due either to local spread or to multifocal origin of tumour. The prognosis is bad even after radical surgery.

The tumour presents as a hard, indefinite infiltrating mass with an irregular margin. Mucoid changes may occur. It may be difficult to differentiate from chronic pancreatitis or tumours of the lower end of the common duct or ampulla of Vater. Pancreatic duct obstruction and proximal dilatation are common and may contribute to the patient's pain or may produce chronic pancreatitis. Compression of the common bile duct leads to obstructive jaundice, and invasion of the splenic or portal veins to blood spread to the liver and elsewhere, sometimes causing unusual presenting symptoms. The onset of diabetes or deterioration of pre-existing diabetes may be a feature. Rarely thrombophlebitis may be associated. In the absence of jaundice diagnosis is difficult but may be assisted by ultrasonography, CAT scan or by selective angiography of the coeliac and superior mesenteric arteries.

6

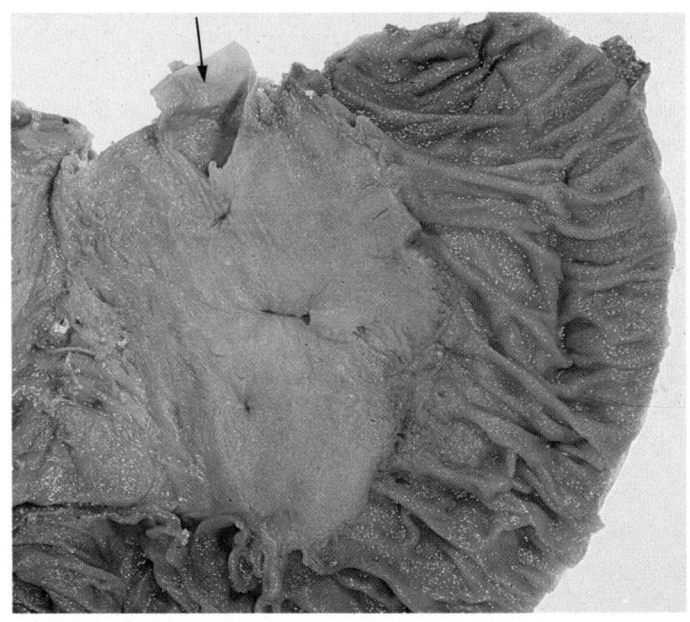

G.C.10199

6 Tumour of head of pancreas causing bile duct obstruction – posterior view of bisected specimen.

Tumour infiltrates the head of the pancreas diffusely. A greatly dilated common bile duct can be seen entering the upper margin of the tumour.

From a male aged 35 years. Two month history of loss of appetite and progressively increasing painless jaundice. On exploratory laparotomy a tumour in the head of the pancreas was resected together with a portion of the common duct, the pyloric end of the stomach, the duodenum, and part of the jejunum.

The head of the pancreas is enlarged and almost completely replaced by whitish, partly bile-stained, ill defined tumour. It has ulcerated through the duodenal wall over an area measuring 3 cm. Slightly above this area there are nodular outgrowths from the main tumour mass which extend to and involve the muscular coats of the duodenum. The common duct is dilated and as it passes through the tumour, appears to be completely occluded.

Microscopic features

Most pancreatic carcinomas appear to arise from duct epithelium. Thus well-differentiated tumours are formed by columnar hyperchromatic epithelium arranged in ductular pattern often with papillary ingrowths. In some instances epithelium of these ductular structures is so well-differentiated that it is difficult to distinguish from the hyperplastic ductular epithelium sometimes seen in chronic pancreatitis. In other cases dedifferentiation can be marked. In all cases fibrosis and atrophy of surrounding pancreas are common. In a proportion of pancreatic carcinomas the tumours appear to arise from acinar tissue. They have a solid lobular pattern and have the staining affinities of the tissues from which they arise.

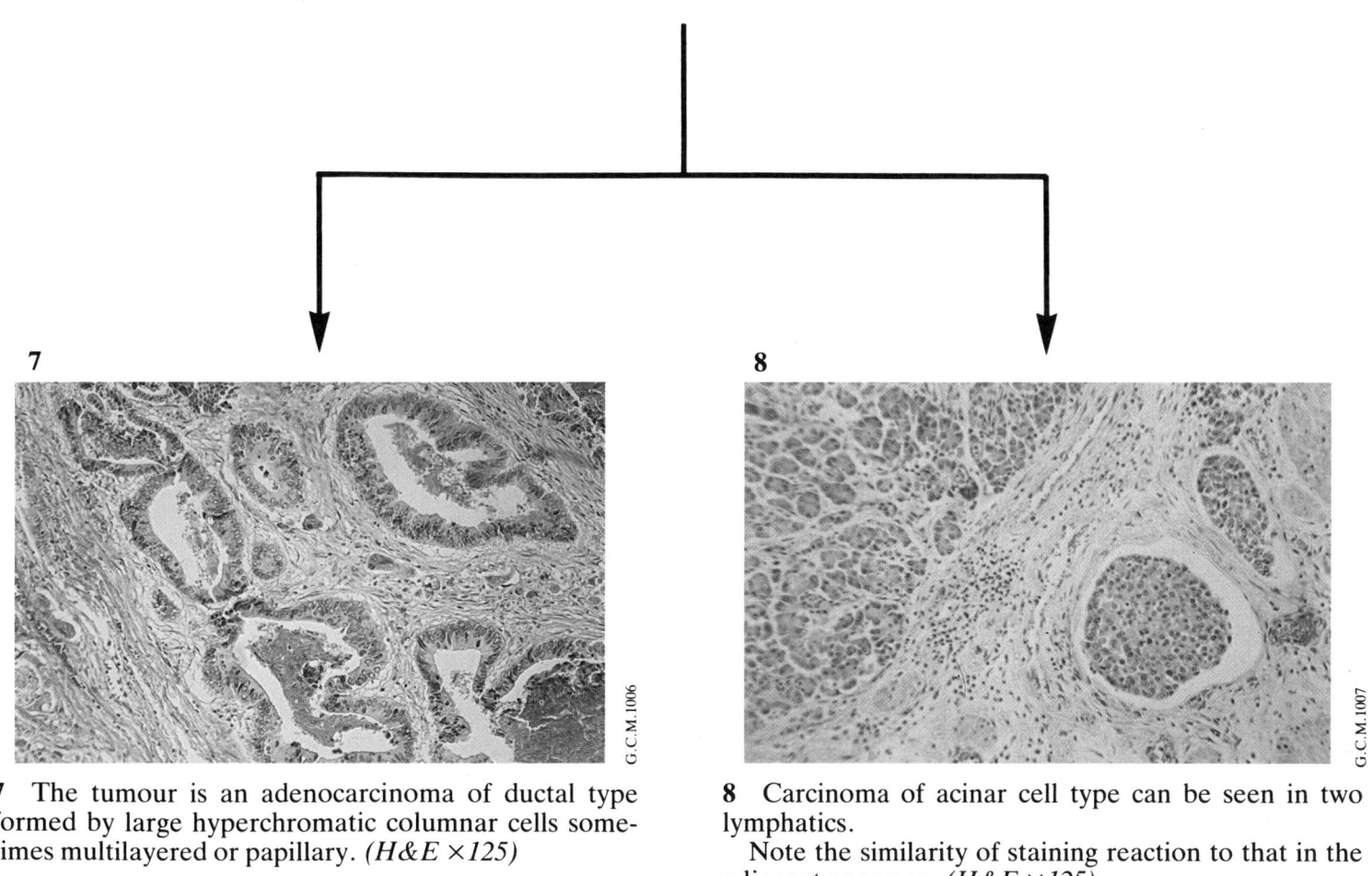

7 The tumour is an adenocarcinoma of ductal type formed by large hyperchromatic columnar cells sometimes multilayered or papillary. *(H&E ×125)*

8 Carcinoma of acinar cell type can be seen in two lymphatics.
Note the similarity of staining reaction to that in the adjacent pancreas. *(H&E ×125)*

Carcinoma of the ampulla of Vater

Note is made in Section 16/2U that carcinoma of the pancreas may produce a lesion located close to and involving the ampulla of Vater and this has to be differentiated from tumours arising in the common bile duct or from the duodenal mucosa.

Exocrine tumours *(Continued)*

Adenocarcinoma *(Continued)*

Obstructive jaundice

The development of progressive jaundice in an elderly patient is the typical picture of carcinoma at the head of the pancreas. Although the jaundice is classically described as painless, vague upper abdominal pain is common and may be severe and felt also in the back.

Illustrative case

9

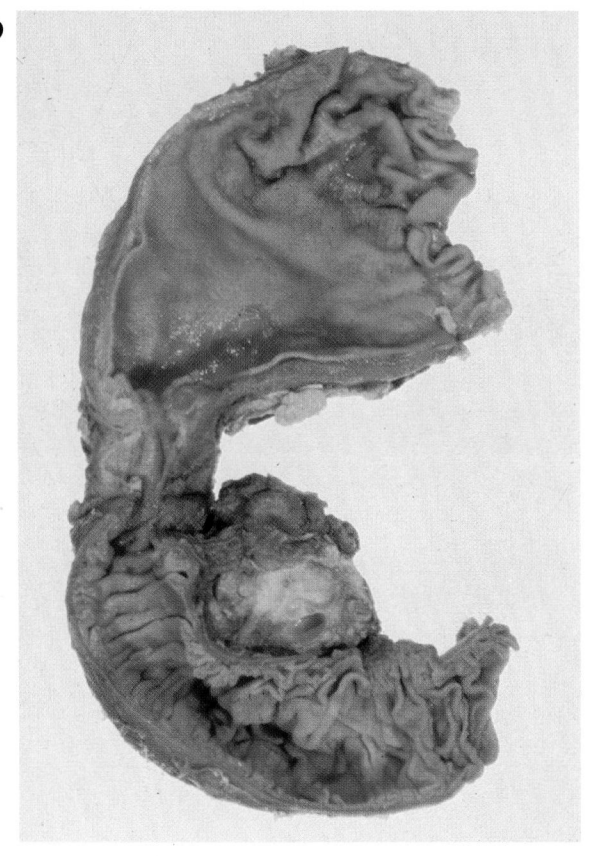

G.C.13910

9a

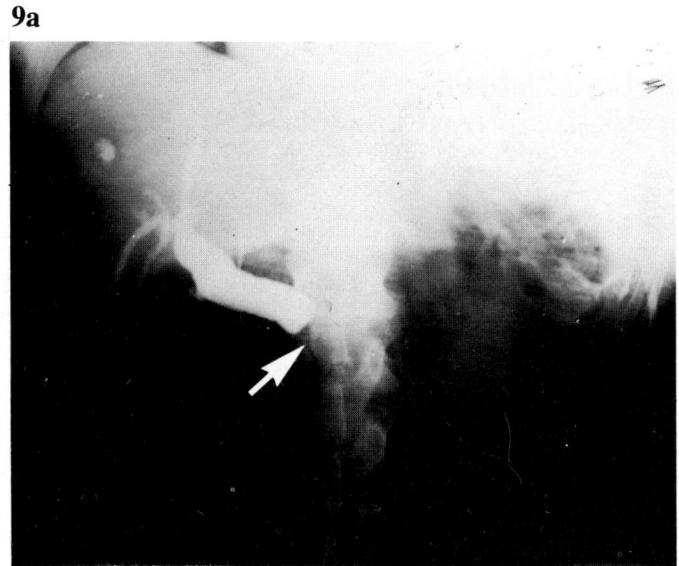

9 From a female aged 62 years. Progressive jaundice had developed over a period of 2 weeks associated with epigastric pain, anorexia and nausea. She had noticed that the urine had been very dark and the stools had been pale, greasy and foul smelling. Clinical examination of the abdomen showed only slight enlargement of the liver. Percutaneous transhepatic cholangiography disclosed a complete occlusion of the common bile duct.

The operative specimen shows a small rounded and lobulated tumour in the head of the pancreas. On section the tumour consists of white fleshy material containing a number of small cysts. The tumour showed lobular invasion to the surrounding tissue. A probe passed into the ampulla could not be passed into the bile duct.

The histological appearances were those of an adenocarcinoma derived from the duct epithelium.

Radiology

10

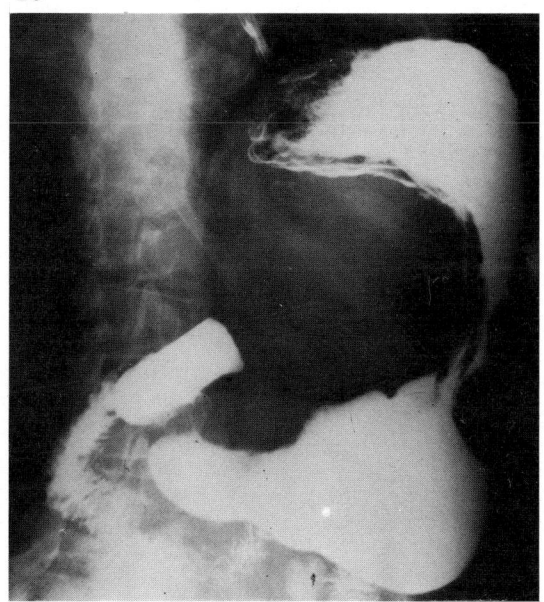

G.C.X.93

10 Barium meal demonstrates displacement of the stomach to the left and forward by cystadenoma of the tail of the pancreas.

11

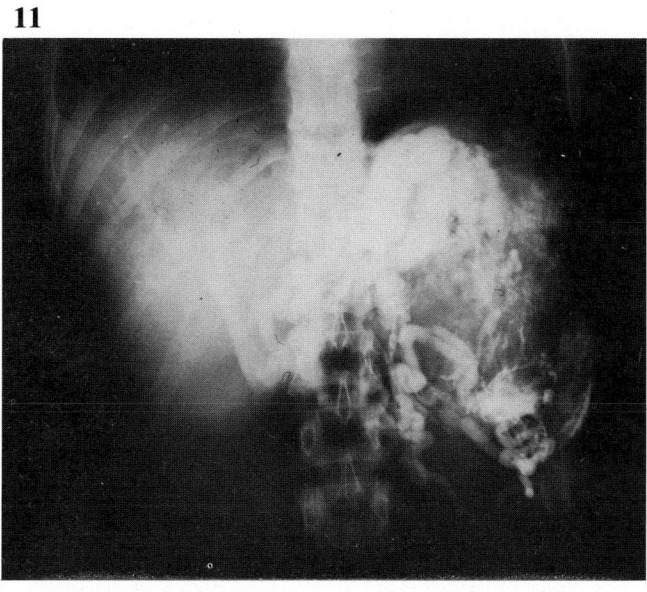

G.C.X.91

11 Adenoma of body of pancreas. Obstruction of the splenic vein with resulting varices demonstrated by splenic venography.

12

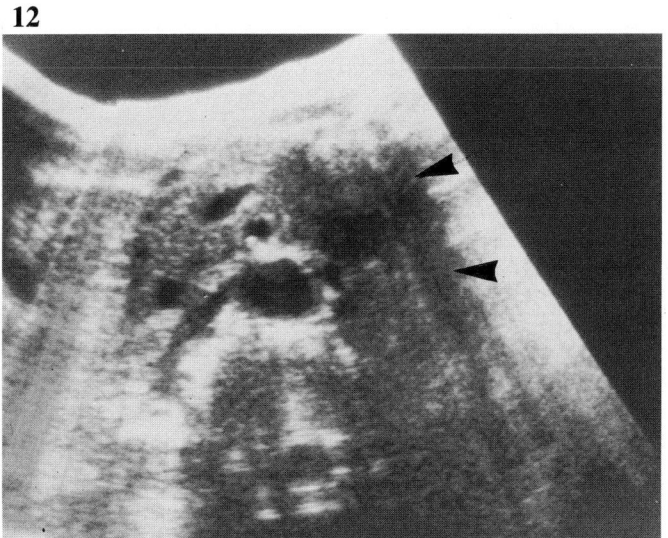

G.C.X.1042

12 Transverse ultrasound demonstrates a hetero-echoic mass in the body and tail of the pancreas.

13

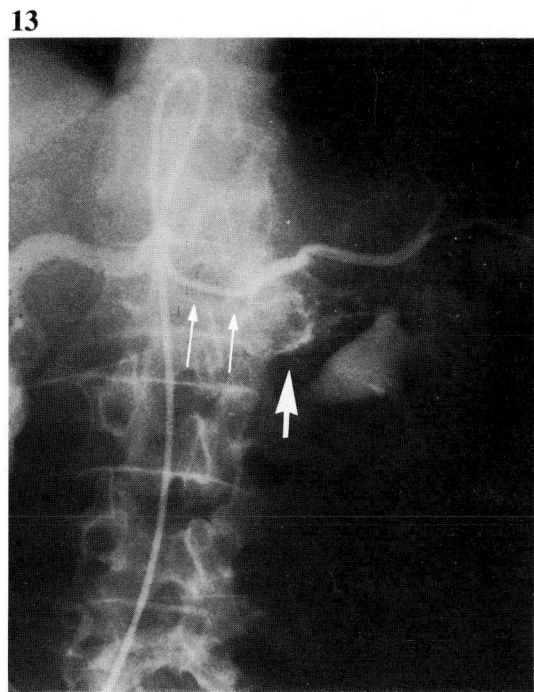

G.C.X.1042

13 Selective angiography showing encasing of the proximal 4cm of the splenic artery by a pancreatic carcinoma with a tumour blush due to the neoplastic circulation.

Endocrine tumours

Endocrine tumours occur in the islet cells of the pancreas and belong to the group known as APUDOMAS. The majority of these tumours are small and frequently multiple. They may be discovered incidentally at post mortem or exposed at operation. They are identified as small circumscribed nodules and in size mostly vary between 1 and 2 cm in diameter. They may be found in any part of the pancreas but the majority are located in the tail. Most islet cell adenomas of the pancreas irrespective of their differing hormonal effects have similar characteristic histological patterns. They are composed of winding ribbons of columnar epithelial cells set in a stroma which may be markedly hyaline. Occasional groups of tumour cells may resemble hyperplastic islets although the differentiation into ∝ and ß cells is lacking

The tumours may be either benign or malignant and do not possess a capsule. It is characteristic of the malignant tumour that it grows rapidly and metastasises especially to the liver. The differentiation between the benign and malignant forms of tumour on microscopical examination presents great difficulties and the physiological effects of the tumour are important in arriving at a diagnosis.

These tumours may secrete excessive quantities of the normal hormone produced by their cells of origin or secrete one or more hormones not normally produced by the cells from which the tumour originated but which are characteristically produced by other APUD cells. In the latter case, as well as the ectopic hormones, the normal hormone of the cell of origin may also be secreted.

Type of islet cell	Tumour	Hormone selected	Clinical features
Delta (A_1)	*Gastrinoma	Gastrin	Zollinger Ellison syndrome (a) Severe peptic ulceration (b) Marked hyperchlorhydria (c) Increased serum gastrin levels (3 to 3000 times normal)
	Somatostatinoma	Somatostatin	—
Beta	Insulinoma	Insulin	– Patients show Whipple's triad: (a) Fasting hypoglycaemia (b) Blood sugar level less than 50 mg% (2.8 mm/litre) (c) Symptomatic relief following I.V. glucose. Serum insulin levels inappropriately elevated.
Alpha (A_2)	Glucagonoma	Glucagon	(a) Weight loss (b) Diabetes (c) Diarrhoea (d) Anaemia (e) Migrating erythema
D_1	Pancreatic polypeptidoma	Pancreatic polypeptide	—
**	Vipoma	VIP	WDHA syndrome (a) Watery diarrhoea (b) Hypokalaemia (c) Achlorhydria
**	Carcinoid (very small percentage found in pancreas)	Amines (5 HT) Peptides Kallikrein Motilin Substance P ? Prostaglandins	(a) Flushing (b) Diarrhoea (c) Abdominal cramps
**	Carcinoma of islet cells	ACTH → Cortisol	Severe forms of Cushing's syndrome

*Gastrin is not normally produced by adult pancreas. **Cell type not determined.

Gastrinoma

This tumour is associated with the clinical condition known as the Zollinger–Ellison syndrome. It presents as single or multiple adenomas of the D cells of the islets of Langerhans. Usually found in the pancreas, the adenoma can occasionally arise in other sites (from the G cells of the stomach, in the hilum of the spleen or in the duodenum). It secretes considerable quantities of the hormone gastrin, a hormone not normally produced by the islet cells of the adult pancreas, to the extent that the fasting serum gastrin levels have been shown by radioimmunoassay to be elevated to between 500 and 1000 pg/ml (normal is 30–150 pg/ml). The pathophysiological effects are an increase in the parietal cell mass to approximately six times the normal with hypertrophy of the gastric rugae and an enormous output of acid and pepsin from the stomach. The mucosal folds in the small intestine are increased and there is peptic ulceration (which may be single or multiple) classically in the distal duodenum and jejunum, although gastric and oesophageal ulceration may also occur. Steatorrhoea may be present in some patients. The increased acidity in the upper intestine inactivates pancreatic lipase and precipitates the bile salts, hence proper micelle formation cannot occur with consequent impaired fat digestion and absorption. The Zollinger–Ellison syndrome should be suspected where the basal acid output is greater than 15 mm/hour and the $\frac{\text{Basal acid output}}{\text{Maximal acid output}} \times 100$ is greater than 60%. The gastrin secreted by the adenoma may stimulate the parietal cell mass to near maximal limits, even under basal conditions, so that administered gastrin (Pentagastrin) usually has little additional effect on acid output.

14

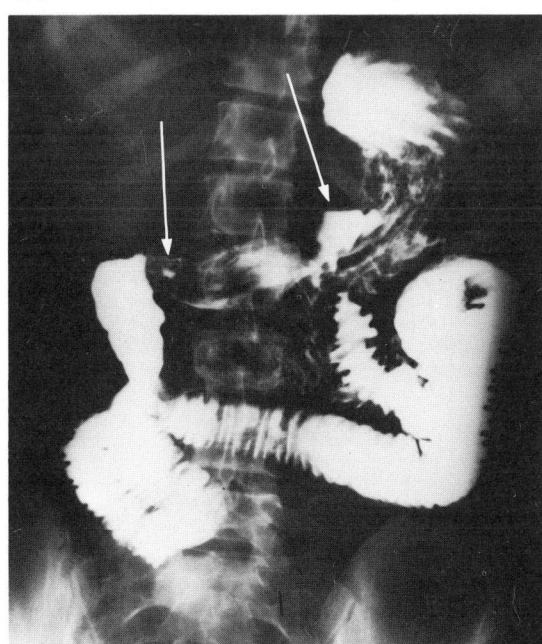

14 When the patient was 22 years old she suffered from recurrent peptic ulceration caused by a non-specific islet cell tumour with metastases – Zollinger–Ellison syndrome. The diagnosis was confirmed at laparotomy. The patient was re-examined 3 years later for continuing symptoms and a barium meal showed a lesser curve gastric ulcer and a pre-pyloric ulcer. There was also irregular narrowing of the third and fourth parts of the duodenum due to compression from a pancreatic tumour. One week later a total gastrectomy was performed and the operation confirmed the presence of a tumour in the pancreas and secondaries in the liver.

The patient made an immediate recovery but died three years later with widespread metastases.

15

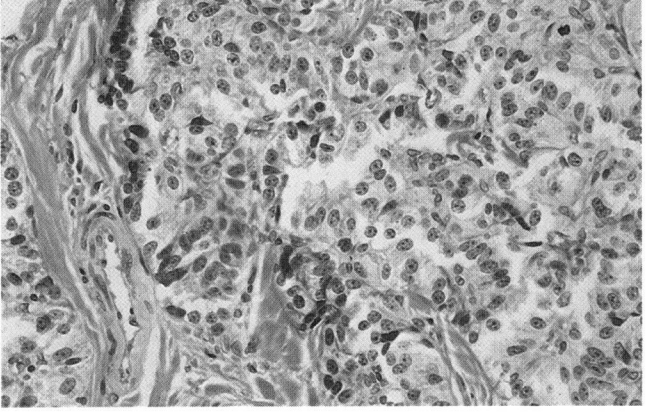

15 Pancreas – gastrin-secreting islet adenoma. This particular tumour is only moderately well-differentiated and shows some variation in nuclear size. (*H&E ×250*)

Insulinoma

An insulinoma is a tumour of the B cells of the islets of Langerhans of the pancreas and its effects are mediated through excessive and autonomous insulin secretion, not inhibited by a fall in the blood glucose level. The serum insulin concentration is inappropriately elevated with a consequent increased uptake and utilisation of glucose by the tissues while in the liver glycogen synthesis is stimulated and gluconeogenesis depressed. These effects lead to a fall in the blood glucose level.

Patients with this tumour display signs of intermittent hypoglycaemia including confusion, irritability, and even loss of consciousness with epileptiform convulsions. These may be mistaken for neurological or psychiatric disorders. Since hypoglycaemia is a potent stimulus to sympathetic discharge and adrenal catecholamine secretion there may be tremors, sweating and palpitations. Exercise, because of an increased peripheral uptake of glucose can exacerbate the development of the hypoglycaemia but it is also prone to occur in the fasting state, especially in the early morning.

With time the attacks increase in frequency and severity and because neurones depend on glucose for their metabolism there may be permanent cerebral neuronal damage.

The diagnosis is usually made by the demonstration of Whipple's triad:

1   Symptoms produced by fasting.
2   A blood sugar level less than 50 mg % (2.8 mm/litre).
3   Symptomatic relief following ingestion of food, or intravenous glucose.

Benign insulinoma

In 10% of cases there is more than one tumour but multiple adenomas are uncommon. Single adenomas of 0.5 cm diameter or more can usually be palpated if the pancreas is mobilised but multiple adenomas are usually of microscopic size.

16

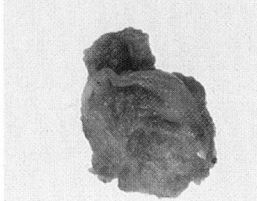

G.C.10346

16   From a male aged 24 years with a history of three attacks of unconsciousness over a period of 9 months. He was admitted to hospital on the third occasion and exhibited abnormal neurological signs.

Biochemical studies demonstrated the features indicative of a pancreatic islet cell tumour and at operation a 1 cm single nodule was discovered in the head of the pancreas. The tumour was excised and the patient made a good recovery and 2 months later the blood sugar was found to be normal.

The tumour was identified at operation by careful palpation and by its slightly purple colour.

17

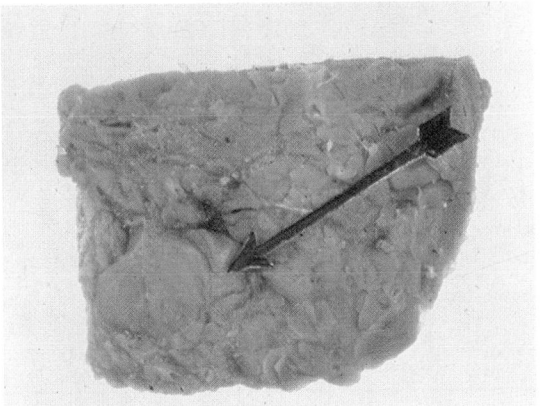

17 This second example of an insulinoma differs from the previous one in that it is larger and lies in the tail of the pancreas. It was rounded and well circumscribed and measured 1.25 cm in diameter. The tumour was yellowish-white and firm.

Microscopic features

18

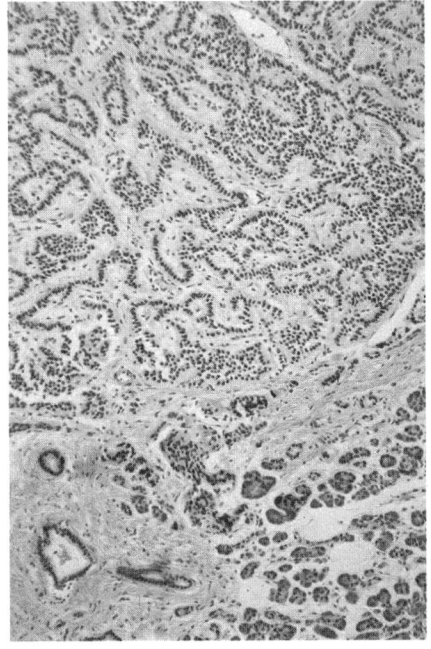

19

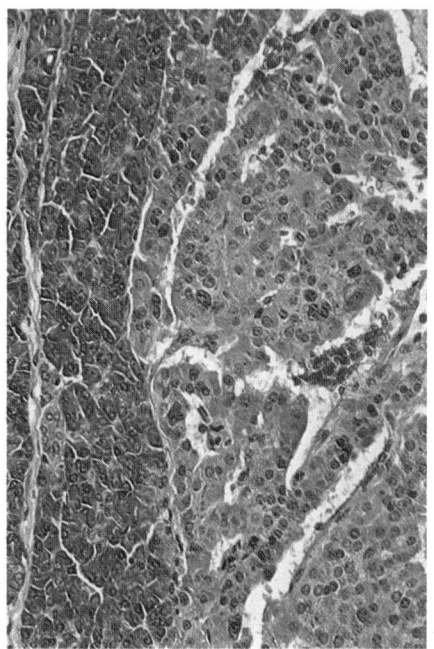

20

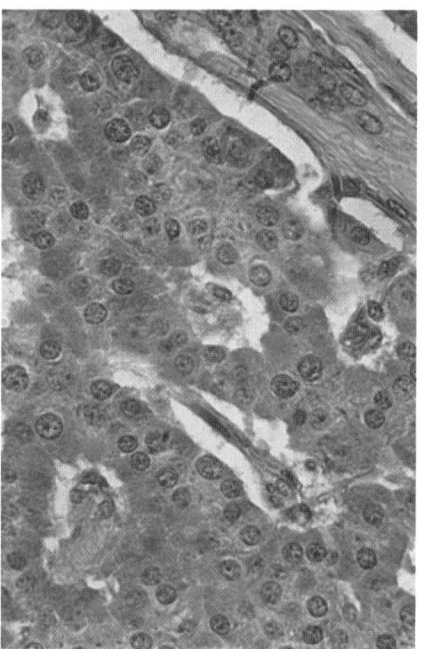

18 Pancreas – insulin-secreting adenoma. A peripheral portion of the adenoma with adjacent pancreas. The tumour is composed of columnar epithelium usually arranged in a single layer in winding columns. There is some stromal hyalinisation. *(H&E ×112.5)*

19 Pancreas – insulin-secreting islet adenoma. Part of an islet adenoma with adjacent acinar tissue (left) stained by Gomori's method to demonstrate the blue-staining secretory granules in the adenoma. Apart from the absence of other cells there is a resemblance to normal islet tissue. *(Chrome alum, haematoxylin, phloxine ×250)*

20 Pancreas – insulin-secreting islet adenoma. A higher power view of the same tumour. *(Chrome alum, haematoxylin, phloxine ×500)*

Insulinoma – malignant

It may be difficult on histological examination to be certain whether an islet cell tumour is benign or malignant. Fortunately most are benign but metastasis or infiltration of adjoining tissues proclaim about 10% of insulinomas to be malignant.

21

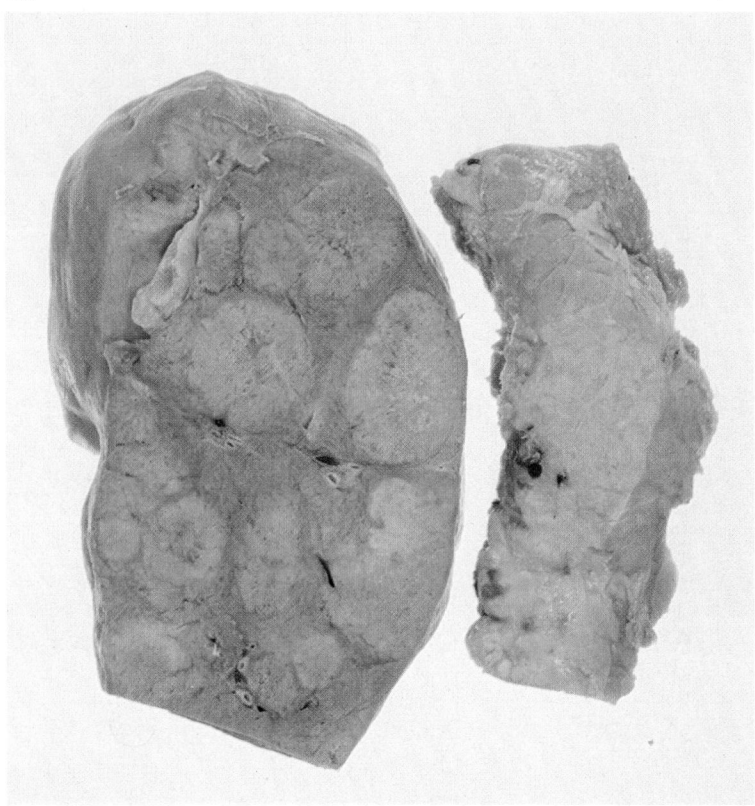

G.C.15058

21 From a male aged 72 years. This patient was admitted to hospital and after investigation the diagnosis of an insulin-secreting tumour of the pancreas was made. At post mortem examination an islet cell carcinoma of the pancreas with liver metastases was found.

21a

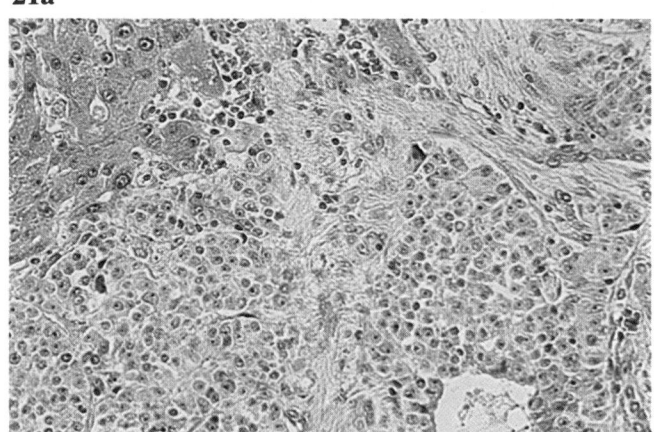

21a A section of the liver shown above illustrates the invasion of liver parenchyma by islet cell carcinoma. Despite the obvious malignancy the tumour cells are fairly uniform and no mitotic figures can be seen in this field. *(H&E ×250)*

Islet tumour – other types

Insulinomas and gastrinomas are the islet cell tumours which most commonly produce recognised clinical syndromes. Islet cell tumours can produce a variety of additional hormonal disturbances (*vide supra*) but some are apparently unaccompanied by endocrine disturbances either because they are non-functional or because their effects are not recognised during life.

22

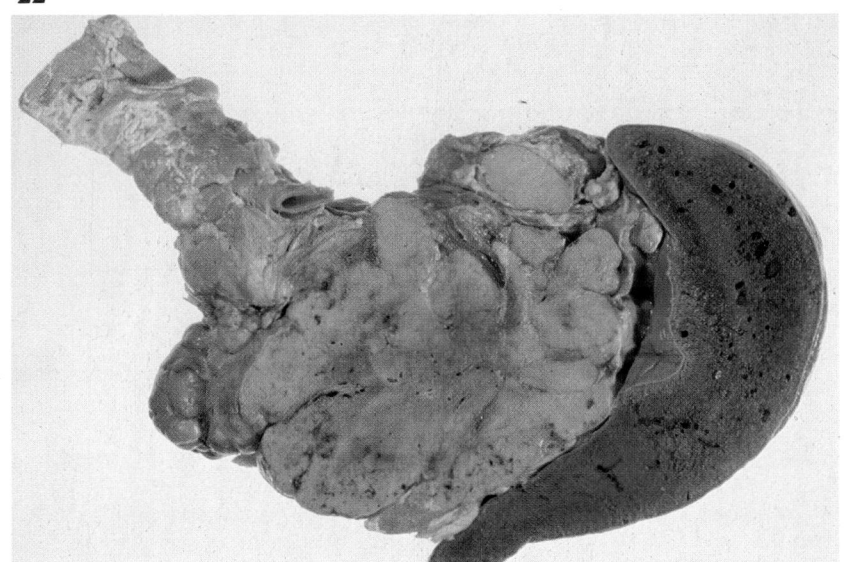

G.C.15037

22 The tumour illustrated is a post mortem specimen of the tail of the pancreas and spleen from a female aged 63 years who took soluble aspirin for rheumatism and died from massive haemorrhage arising in acute gastric erosions. The duodenum was scarred but was not actively ulcerated.

The lobulated tumour arose in the tail of the pancreas and measured 14 × 9 × 8cm. Solitary metastatic nodules were found in the liver and in the second lumbar vertebra. Despite its size, the tumour had the characteristic microscopic structure of an islet cell tumour.

22a

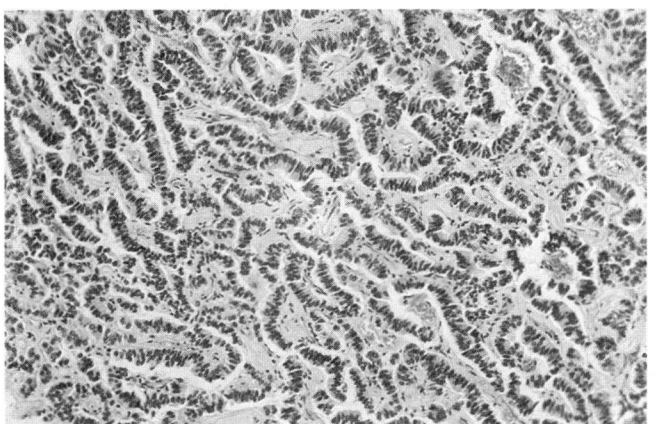

22a Pancreas – malignant islet cell tumour. This portion of the carcinoma shows the characteristic histological pattern of an islet cell tumour.
(Alcian green, phloxine, tartrazine ×100)

22b

22b Pancreas – malignant islet cell tumour. Another portion of the same tumour showing dedifferentiation with loss of polarity and some nuclear pleomorphism.
(H&E ×300)

A.C.B. Dean

Spleen

Anatomy

The spleen is derived from condensations of mesoderm in the dorsal meso-gastrium which coalesce to form a single organ consisting of white and red pulp enclosed in a fibrous capsule. Failure to coalesce results in the formation of *accessory spleens* (spleniculi), most often found in the gastrosplenic ligament or along the upper border of the pancreas or in the adjacent greater omentum. The normal spleen is very constant in size throughout life weighing 100 to 150 g. It is attached to the posterior abdominal wall by the lienorenal ligament between the leaves of which lie the splenic artery and vein and the tail of the pancreas.

Blood supply

The splenic artery is a branch of the coeliac axis. It runs a sinuous course laterally along the upper border of the pancreas and gives off branches to this organ. Before it reaches the hilum of the spleen it gives off the short gastric arteries to the fundal region of the stomach. Thereafter it divides and subdivides in the hilum and substance of the spleen to form end-arteries to the pulp.

The splenic vein is formed from the union of two or more tributaries in the splenic hilum where it lies posterior to the artery. It runs medially behind the body of the pancreas and joins the superior mesenteric vein to form the portal vein. It receives the inferior mesenteric vein shortly before it terminates and numerous small veins from the pancreas.

Circulation through spleen

1

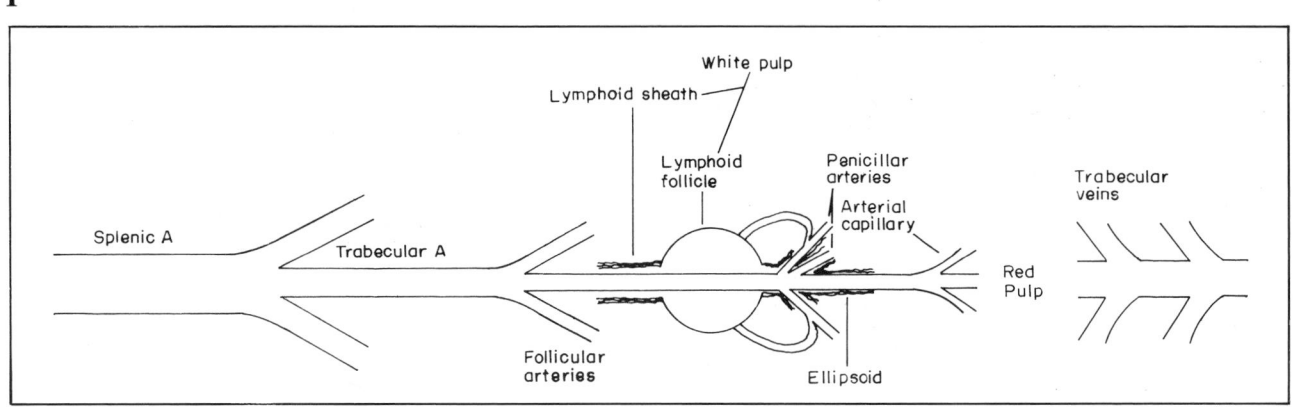

Structure

The white pulp

The white pulp is composed of lymphoid tissue which forms a sheath around the intrasplenic branches of the splenic artery. This sheath is expanded in places to form the Malpighian bodies (lymphoid follicles) and is continued around the arterial capillaries where it is called an ellipsoid. The function of the white pulp is the same as lymphoid tissue elsewhere but it is particularly concerned with the formation of antibodies to blood-borne antigens. The function of the ellipsoids appears to be essentially phagocytic, separating particulate matter at an early stage as it enters the spleen.

The white pulp and its relationship to the intrasplenic arterial circulation is depicted in **1** opposite.

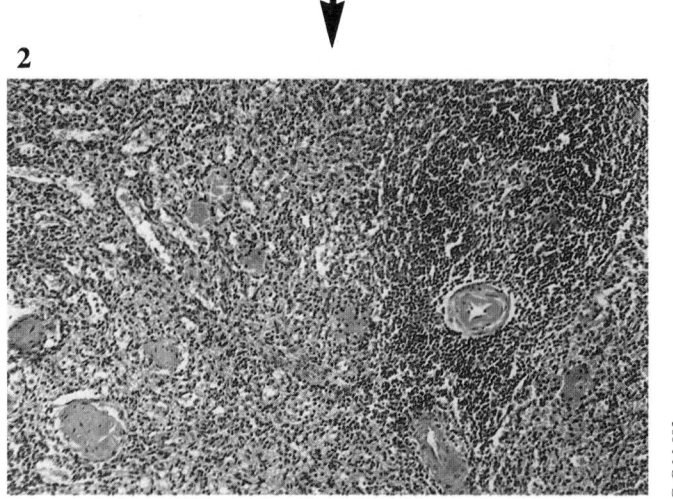

2 Normal spleen. Darkly stained lymphocytes of the Malpighian body surround an arteriole and contrast with the red pulp. A few trabeculae can be seen end on. *(H&E ×100)*

Infection

Present evidence is that the spleen helps to combat systemic infection in three ways:

1 Filtration from the blood stream and phagocytosis of particulate matter and bacteria, especially those with a capsule, e.g. pneumococcus.

2 Production of antibodies particularly IgM. This function has especial importance in children in whom antibody production elsewhere in the body is much less developed than in adult life. Splenectomy should therefore be avoided before the age of 10 years except in the most compelling circumstances.

3 Production of Tuftsin, a tetra-peptide which is necessary for efficient phagocytosis.

Structure *(Continued)*

The red pulp

The red pulp consists of a network of sinuses interposed between the arteries and the veins and separated from each other by pulp spaces lined by the mesenchymal cells which form the cords of Billroth. Amongst these cells are macrophages, lymphocytes, reticular cells and plasma cells. Slow flow of blood through the pulp spaces permits prolonged and intimate contact between the phagocyte cells and the constituents of the blood and foreign particles such as blood-borne bacteria, parasites, macroglobulins and tumour cells. The flow is particularly slow if the red blood cells are abnormal in shape, e.g. spherocytes or sickle cells, or are coated with antibody as in auto-immune haemolytic anaemia when the coated erythrocytes are rapaciously engulfed by the macrophages. The volume of erythrocytes sequestrated in the pulp spaces can be measured by labelling with Cr^{51} and is called the Spleen Pool.

Circulation through red pulp (intermediate circulation)

3

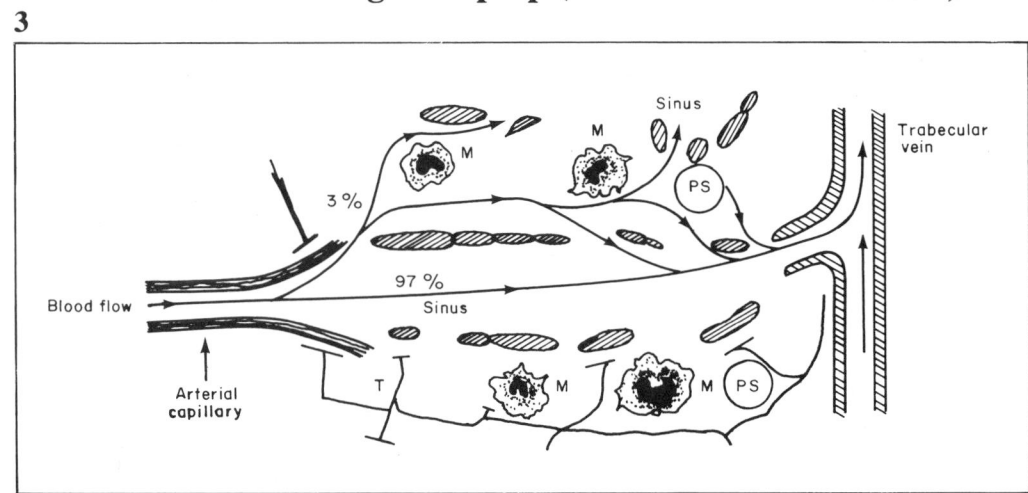

M = Macrophage
T = Trabecular network
PS = Pulp spaces in cords of Billroth

4

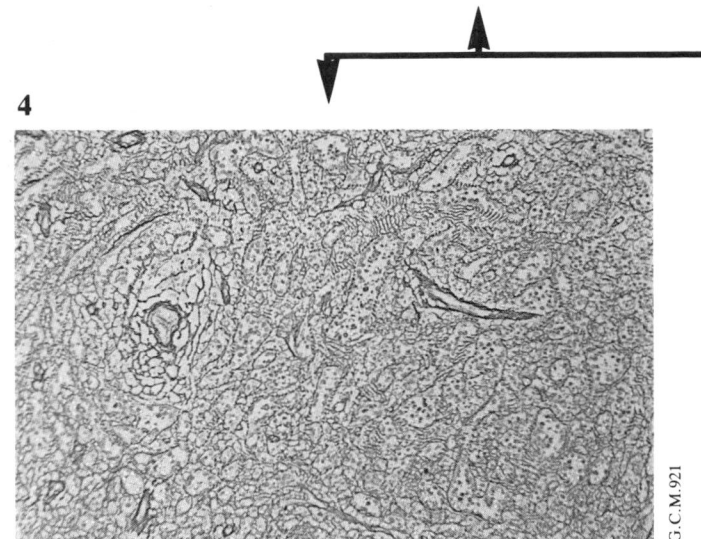

5

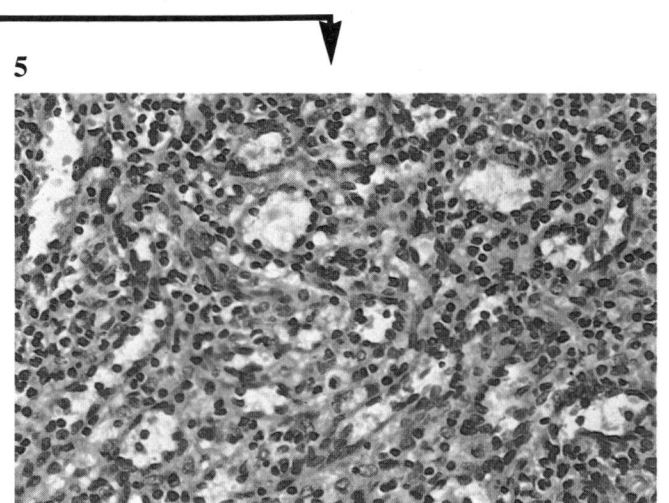

4 Splenic reticulin. The venous sinusoids are delineated by the pronounced transverse bands of reticulin. Between them lie the cellular cords of Billroth. *(Slidders' Reticulin ×125)*

5 Spleen. The venous sinusoids are lined by endothelial cells. *(H&E ×312.5)*

Splenomegaly

In health the spleen should not be palpable. Enlargement of the spleen causes it to project downwards, forwards and to the right from beneath the left costal margin. If the spleen can be felt, it is at least three times the normal size or is displaced anteriorly by a cyst or other retroperitoneal swelling which may be detectable by ultrasound or computerised axial tomography (CAT) scanning. In addition to variation in size, the consistence of the enlarged spleen differs in different diseases. In acute systemic infections the enlargement is slight and the substance of the spleen soft and friable. Hyperplasia of the reticuloendothelial tissues or malignant proliferation of lymphoreticular cells gives rise to a firm swelling which preserves the outline of the spleen so that the anterior border with its notch can be defined clinically. Splenomegaly is usually associated with adverse effects on the blood, leucopaenia, thrombocytopaenia and anaemia, which are together called hypersplenism, and if these are serious they can be relieved only by splenectomy. However, not all of the many causes of splenic enlargement are of direct interest to the surgeon.

Causes of splenomegaly

1. Lympho-reticular hyperplasia
   (a) Acute and
       generally transient
   (b) Chronic
   - Bacteraemia
   - Typhoid fever
   - Infective mononucleosis
   - Kala-azar
   - Malaria
   - Tropical splenomegaly syndrome
   (c) Chronic with granuloma
       formation
   - Tuberculosis*
   - Sarcoidosis*
   - Brucellosis

2. Congestion of the pulp spaces
   - Congenital haemolytic anaemia*
   - Acquired (including auto-immune) haemolytic anaemia*
   - Polycythaemia vera
   - Pernicious anaemia

3. Congestion of the venous sinuses
   - Congestive cardiac failure
   - Portal hypertension*

4. Lympho-proliferative diseases
   - Hodgkin's lymphoma*
   - Non-Hodgkin's lymphoma*
   - Lymphatic leukaemia

5. Myeloproliferative diseases
   - Myeloid leukaemia*
   - Myeloid metaplasia (Myelofibrosis)*

6. Cysts

7. Tumours
   - Benign – haemangioma*
            – hamartoma*
   - Malignant – haemangiosarcoma*
               – lymphoma*
               – metastases*

8. Diseases of connective tissue
   - Disseminated lupus erythematosus
   - Polyarteritis nodosa*
   - Rheumatoid arthritis (Felty's syndrome)*

9. Infiltration
   - Amyloidosis*
   - Lipoid storage diseases, e.g. Gaucher's

*Indicates a condition of special surgical importance which is discussed further.

Lympho-reticular hyperplasia

Lympho-reticular hyperplasia is a reactive phenomenon occurring in systemic infections, with consequent increased lymphocyte and macrophage activity, or infectious mononucleosis leading to moderate soft enlargement which disappears as the primary disease subsides.

Chronic infection

Chronic infections may be tropical or granulomatous. Tropical infections are protozoal (malaria, kala-azar) or idiopathic in which no cause is demonstrable but a response to anti-malarial treatment often occurs. In these diseases the spleen can be very greatly enlarged.

The granulomas include tuberculosis and sarcoidosis. Tuberculosis of the spleen may be miliary or consist of numerous larger caseating foci which may coalesce to form one or more large 'tuberculomas'.

In sarcoidosis the characteristic lesion is discrete non-caseating 'tubercles' which can be observed by the naked eye but in which acid and alcohol fast bacilli cannot be demonstrated.

6

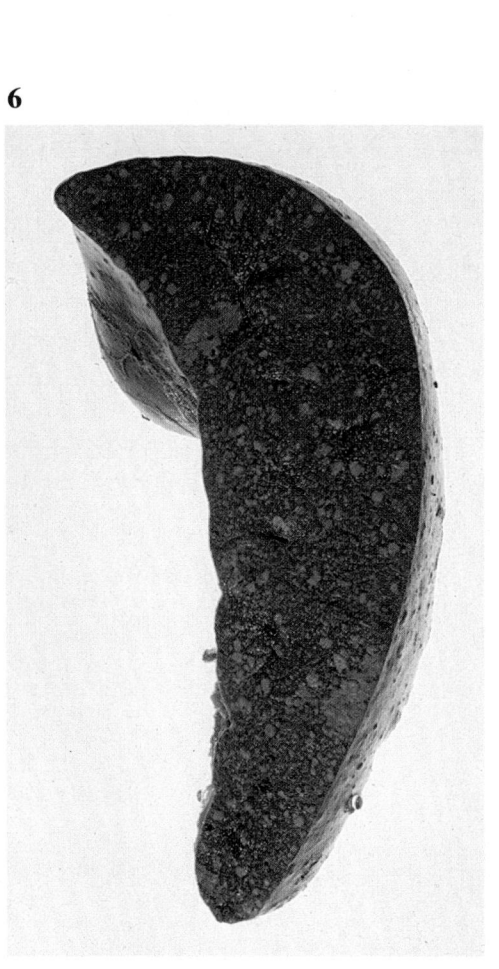

G.C.7436

6 From an adult in whom the spleen, the liver and the kidneys were similarly affected.

The spleen is enlarged and on its surface subcapsular tubercles were obvious. On section multiple tubercles are present diffusely scattered throughout the splenic pulp. Some are fused together forming conglomerates.

7

G.C.M.922

7 Miliary tuberculosis. The coalescing miliary tubercles contain multi-nucleated giant cells surrounded by caseating tissue. *(H&E ×125)*

8

G.C.M.923

8 Caseous nodule. This part of a structureless caseous nodule is separated from splenic pulp by a zone of chronic inflammation and fibrosis. *(H&E ×62.5)*

Congestion of the pulp spaces

9 Congestion of the spaces in the red pulp due to the sequestration of abnormal red blood cells is characteristic of haemolytic anaemia both congenital and auto-immune. The spleen is firm but compressible, the capsule smooth and the red pulp deep red. The cords of Billroth are congested with red blood corpuscles and phagocytosis of the abnormal cells by macrophages can be seen.

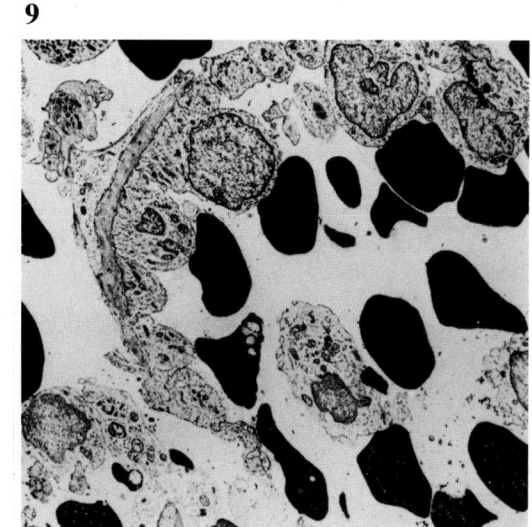

Congestion of the venous sinuses

Congestion of the venous sinuses arises if the pressure in the portal vein is elevated. It is commonplace in severe congestive cardiac failure but is seen in its most severe form in portal hypertension when the spleen is enlarged, firm, beefy on cut section and characteristically shows flecks which are the scars of old haemorrhage into the pulp (see Section 16/1 O).

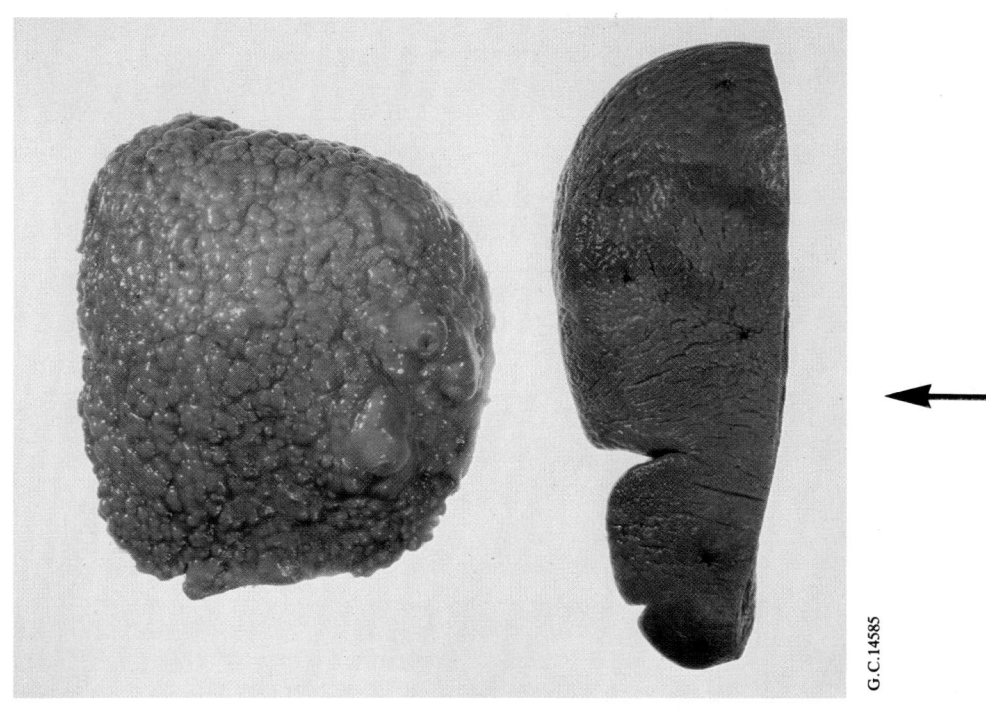

10 From a male aged 45 years who died following an oesophageal haemorrhage. An example of splenomegaly associated with marked post-necrotic cirrhosis. Note the nodular surface of the liver and its shrunken appearance.

The spleen demonstrates the changes already noted. It was five times the normal weight and the wrinkling of its surface suggests that it was probably even larger before the oesophageal haemorrhage. The normal weight ratio of the liver to the spleen is 10:1 but in advanced cirrhosis the spleen may attain equality.

Lymphoproliferative diseases

Hodgkin's disease

This group includes lymphoma (both Hodgkin's and non-Hodgkin's) and lymphatic leukaemia. The spleen may be greatly enlarged but with the exception of giant follicular lymphoma the gross appearances are not characteristic. In Hodgkin's disease Reed–Sternberg giant cells, proliferation of reticular cells and lymphocytes may be found, but in the late cases the lymphocytes are greatly reduced in number (lymphocyte depletion).

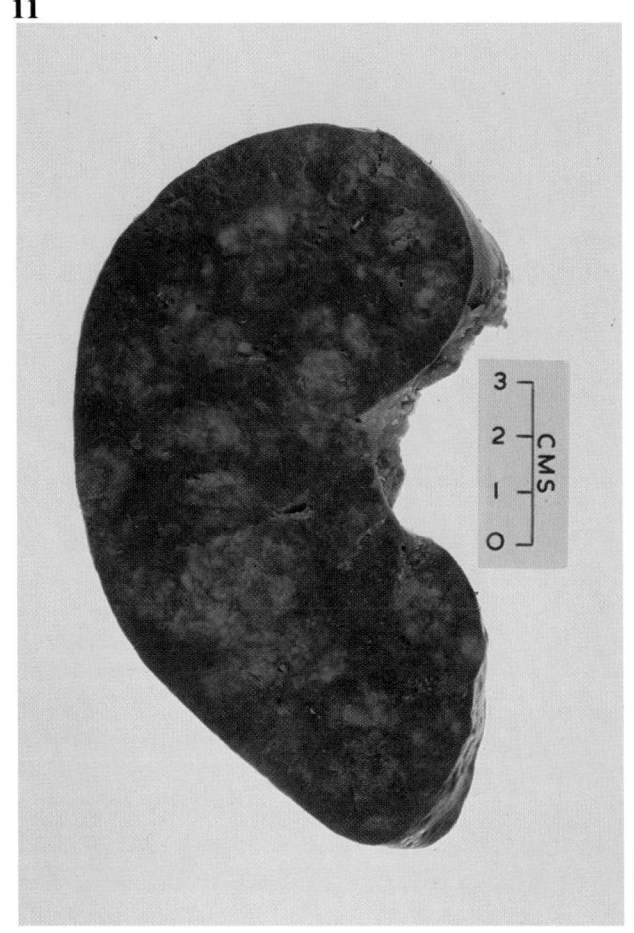

11 The spleen is enlarged and shows many foci of pale tissue typical of advanced Hodgkin's disease.

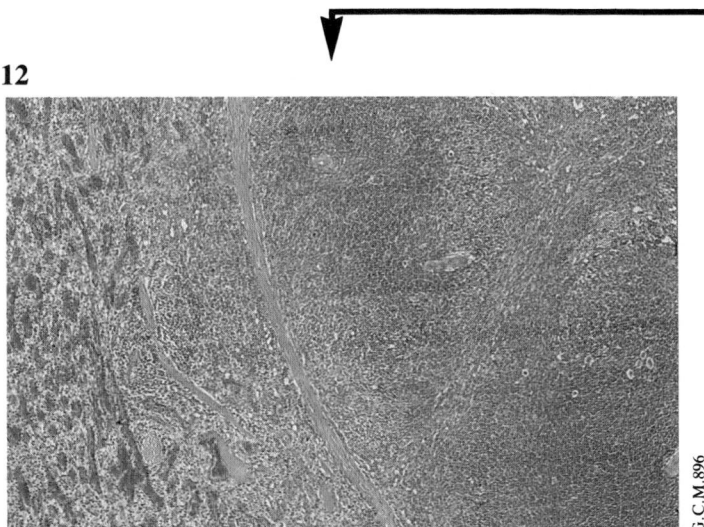

12 Spleen – Hodgkin's disease. Peripheral portion of infiltrate still retaining some follicular pattern. The surrounding red pulp is compressed. *(H&E ×50)*

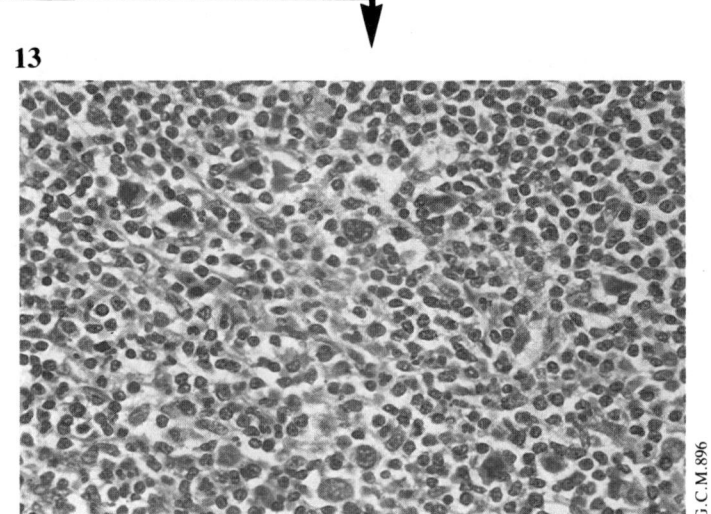

13 Same case. Reed–Sternberg giant cells are present amongst the neoplastic lymphoid cells. *(H&E ×400)*

Reticulosarcoma

Reticulosarcoma (reticulum cell sarcoma) is a term formerly applied to a malignant large cell lymphoma and characterised by firm splenic enlargement with reticulin formation.

15

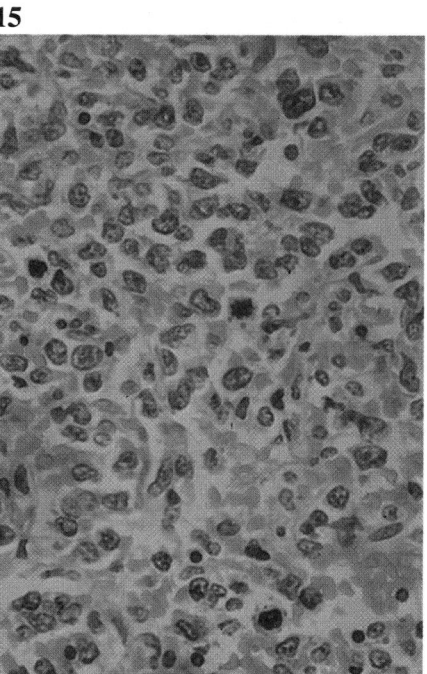

15 Spleen – reticulosarcoma. Large neoplastic reticulum cells predominate, and several are in mitosis. *(H&E ×500)*

14

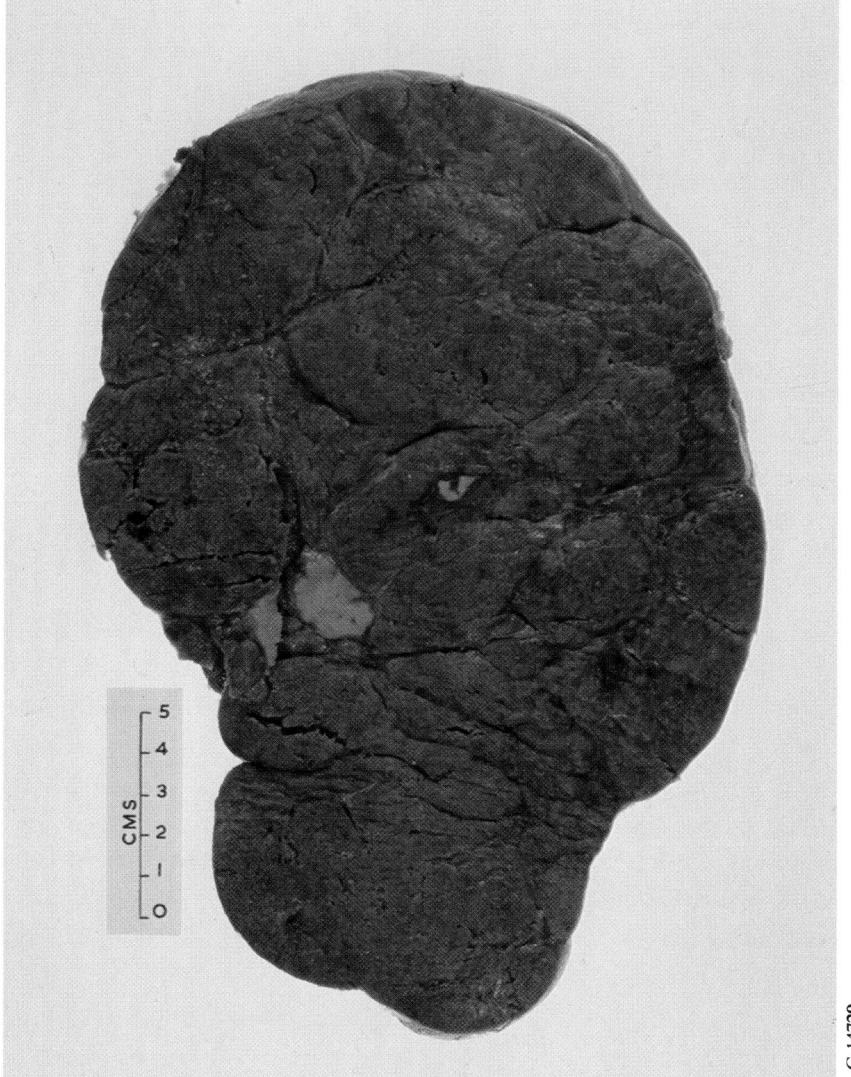

14 The spleen is greatly enlarged and both the capsule and the cut surface show nodularity. Several infarcts are present on the cut surface varying from about 3 cm in diameter to a few millimetres.

In recent years the classification of lymphomas has been and still is undergoing modification as a result of immunological studies including cell surface labelling techniques and of concepts based upon maturation of undifferentiated cells towards T and B lymphoid cells.

Myeloproliferative disease

Myeloid metaplasia

When bone marrow is replaced by fibrosis or by tumour its haematopoietic function is diminished or lost and this function may then be assumed by the spleen. This is strikingly seen in myelofibrosis where the spleen becomes greatly enlarged due to myeloid metaplasia. However, the blood cells so formed, especially the red cells, are often abnormal and may be rapidly haemolysed in the spleen. Splenectomy is sometimes necessary but may be disastrous if the spleen is also the main site of granulocyte and platelet formation.

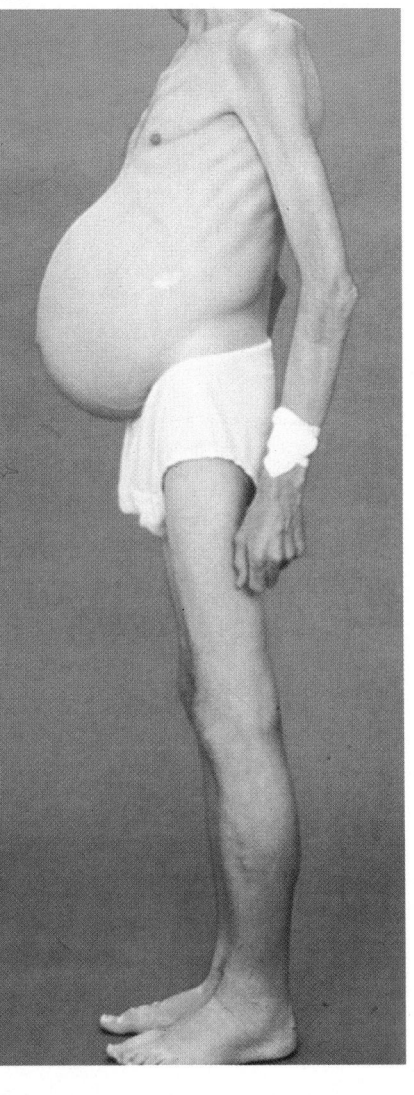

16

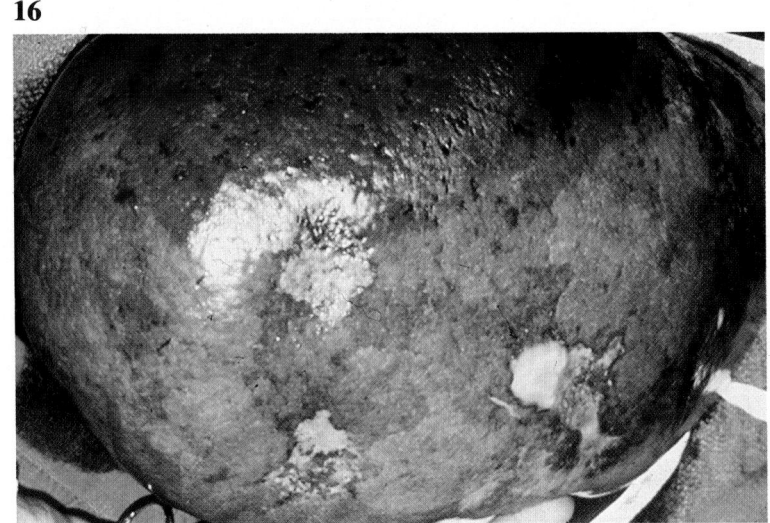

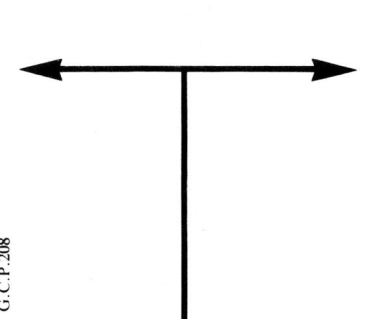

16 Male aged 53 years. Five year history of anaemia and increasing splenomegaly. When the patient was first seen the spleen was found to fill the left half of the abdomen. Blood count Hb 5 to 8g, WBC 3000 to 4000/mm³ with many primitive cells, platelets 200 000–240 000/mm³. Marrow showed many bizarre and primitive cells, megakaryocytes and excess reticulin. Spleen pool 0.724 litre. The clinical diagnosis was myelofibrosis. Because transfusions were needed every 2 to 3 weeks splenectomy was performed. The spleen weighed 5.237 kg (normal weight 0.15 kg) and showed myeloid metaplasia and many infarcts. The liver also showed extra-medullary haematopoiesis and diffuse intracellular haemosiderin.

17

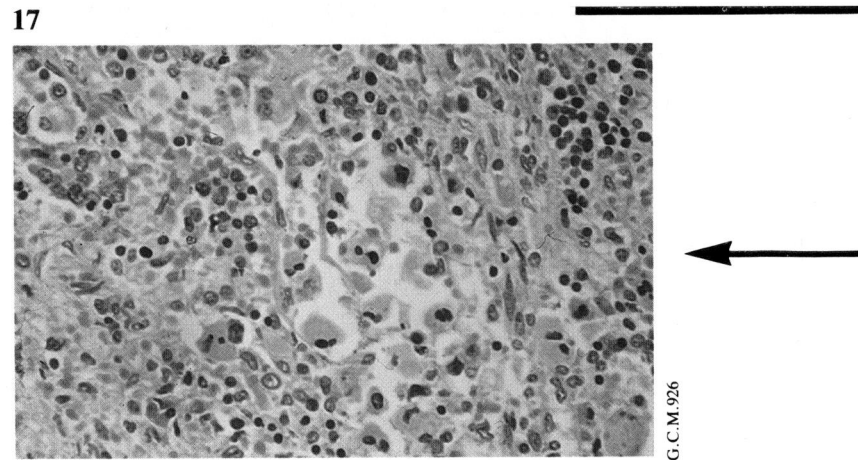

17 Spleen – haematopoiesis in a case of myelofibrosis. Centrally there are numerous immature megakaryocytes. A cluster of nucleated red cells can also be seen (top right). *(H&E ×375)*

Myeloid leukaemia

In chronic myeloid leukaemia, the white pulp is replaced and the architecture obscured by masses of myeloid cells.

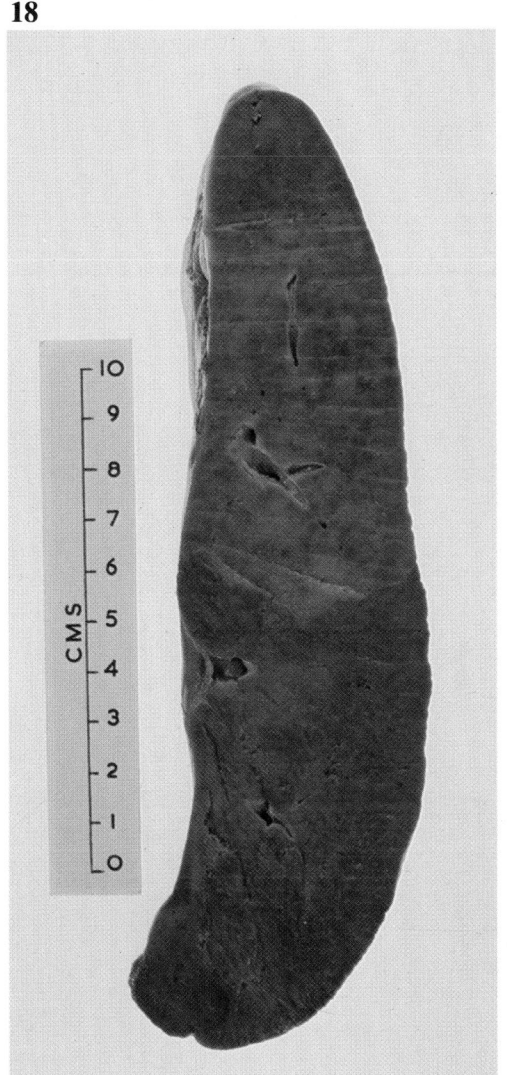

18 Spleen – myeloid leukaemia. The spleen is much enlarged and its capsule free from perisplenitis. The cut surface shows the pallor of the splenic pulp which is mottled with yellow patches due to accumulation of leucocytes. The trabeculae are not in evidence. The diagnosis, established by blood examination, was confirmed on section of the spleen.

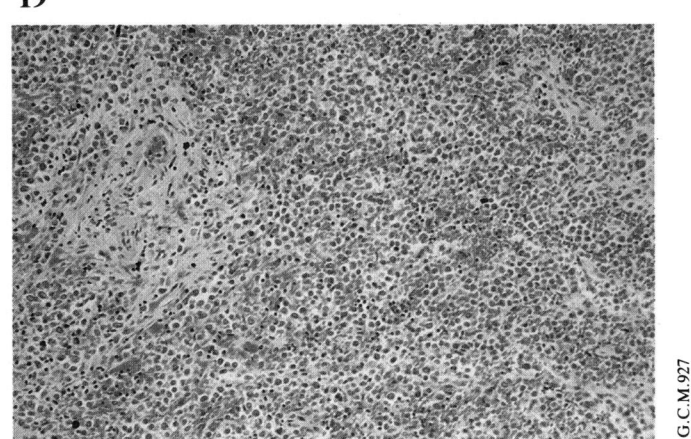

19 Spleen – myeloid leukaemia. The red pulp is massively invaded by cells of the myeloid series and the Malpighian bodies are inconspicuous. *(H&E ×125)*

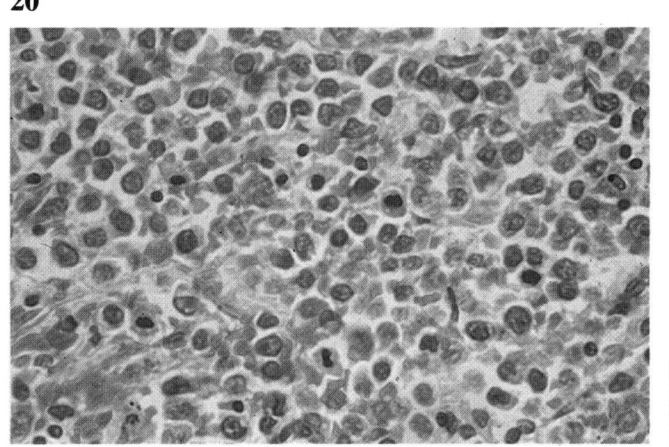

20 Same case. Myeloblasts, some in mitosis, predominate in the leukaemic infiltrate. *(H&E ×500)*

517

Cysts

Cysts of the spleen are rare. They can be classified as degenerative, congenital, parasitic or neoplastic. The most frequently encountered is the degenerative cyst (75%).

Degenerative

Degenerative cysts result from the liquefaction of a haemorrhage (either spontaneous or following minor trauma) into the pulp with surrounding necrosis. The cyst wall is fibrous and often calcified and the contents are dark brown. Occasionally if it is subcapsular it may rupture and when the trauma is not remembered the term 'spontaneous rupture' is sometimes applied.

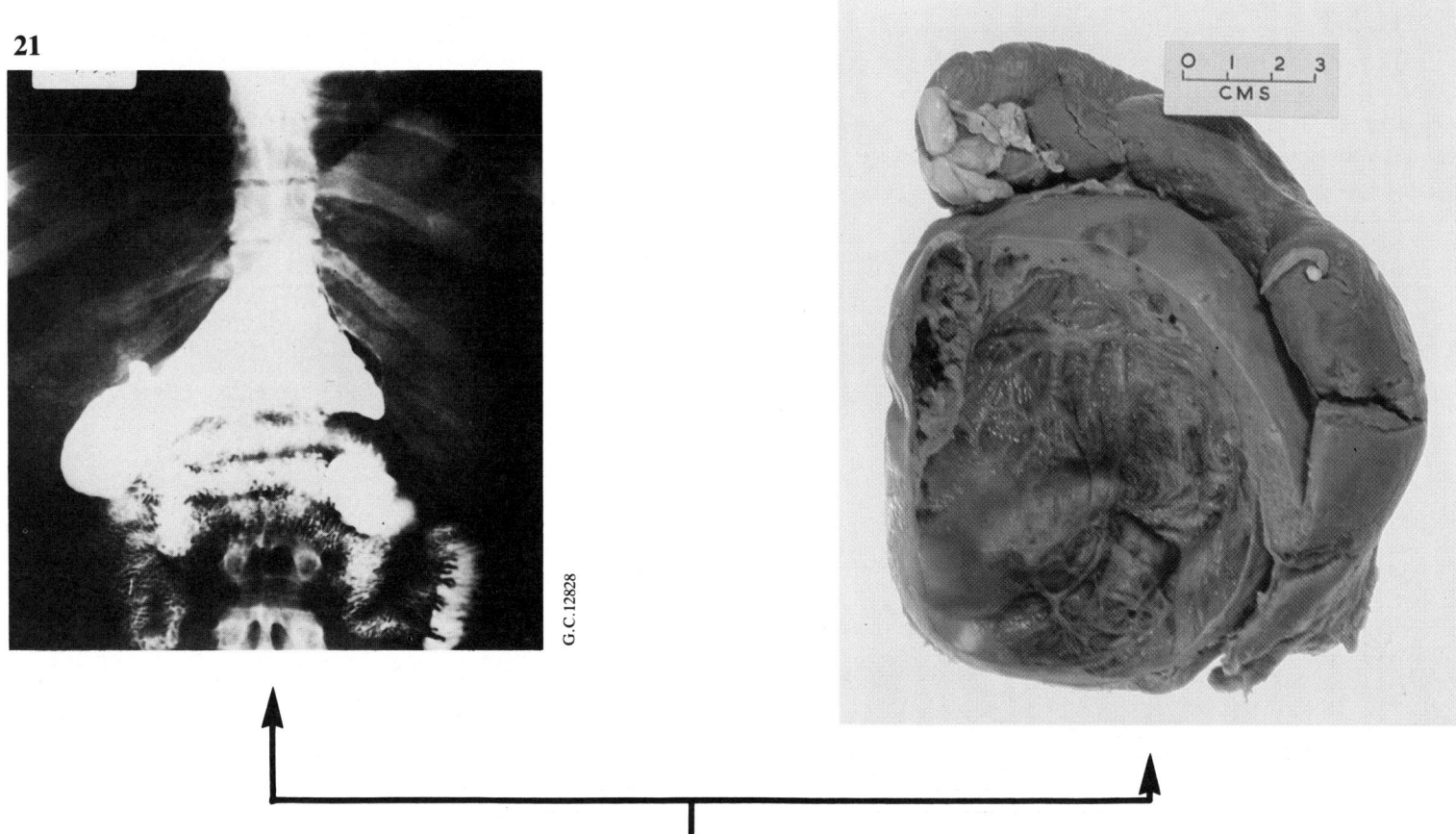

21 and 21a From a female aged 22 years who complained of pain in the left loin and at the left shoulder tip. Preliminary radiological examination demonstrated elevation of the left diaphragm and downward displacement of the left kidney. A barium meal demonstrated displacement of the stomach by a probable splenic mass. On examination of the specimen removed at operation a large subcapsular haematoma on the medial aspect of the spleen was observed. The external aspect is smooth but internally the haematoma shows a trabeculated wall which is partly translucent.

Microscopically the area sectioned showed part of the haematoma with fresh and coagulated blood and fibrin deposit. The wall of the haematoma shows a lining of macrophages with cholesterin crystals in foci – an indication of some duration of haemorrhage. There is no evidence of tumour.

22

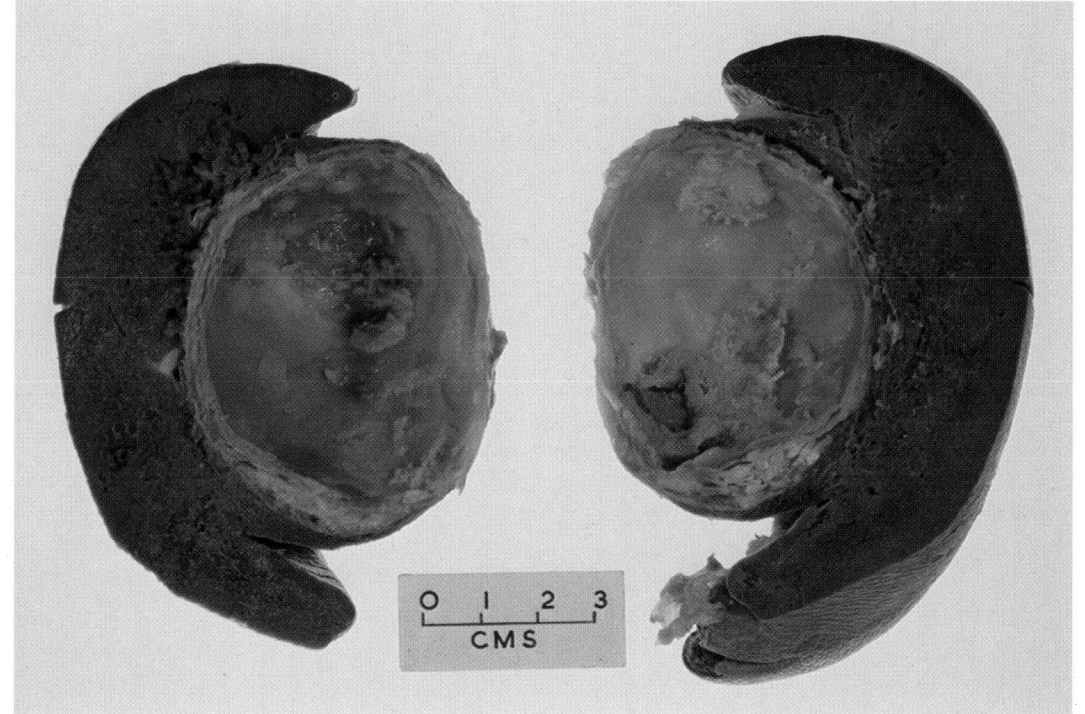

22 The patient, a female aged 52 years, was a hemiplegic. She developed episodic attacks of pain in the left lower chest and upper abdomen. These attacks were of considerable severity and on investigation in hospital a large calcified cyst suspected of being splenic was discovered. There is an ovoid cyst lying at the hilum of the spleen.

On the cut surface the cyst appears to have arisen within the substance of the spleen. A small covering of splenic tissue extends over the upper and lower poles of the cyst but medially the cyst wall appears to be without any such splenic tissue. The wall of the cyst is wholly calcified and contained an ochre coloured fluid with much debris some of which remains adherent to the inner lining of the specimen.

23

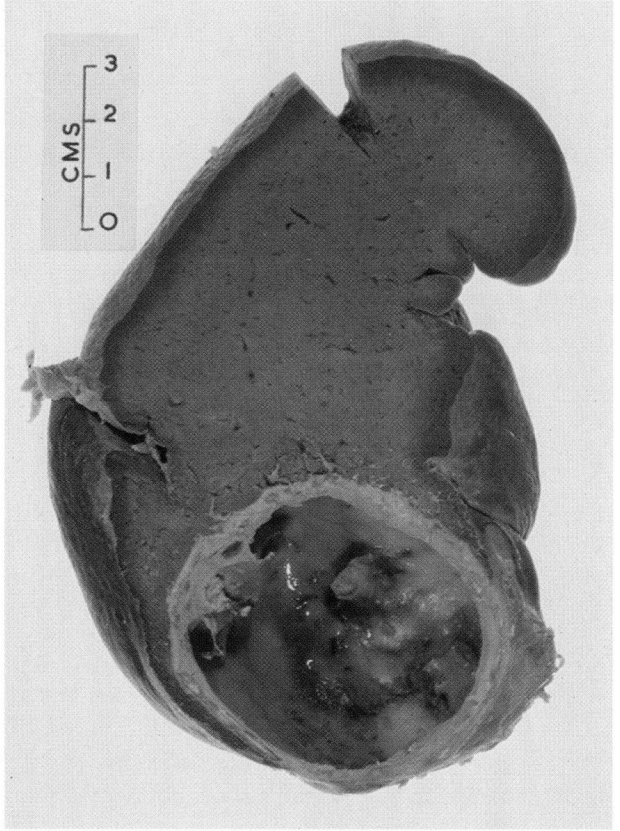

23 From a 21-year-old Indian. Vague upper abdominal pain of 2 or 3 months duration. A straight X-ray demonstrated a calcified cyst in the lower part of the spleen. No history of trauma or malaria.

The spleen is enlarged. At the lower pole there is a calcified cyst. In contradistinction to the other specimens illustrated this specimen demonstrates a cyst in the substance of the organ. In the other specimens the cysts are hilar and subcapsular.

Cysts *(Continued)*

Congenital

Congenital cysts are due to a defect in the aggregation of the mesodermal islands which fuse to form the anatomical spleen in the embryo. Two types are described:
1 A single cyst which may grow to a considerable size, usually lying posterior to the spleen and expanding it to cap the cyst like a beret. It is usually discovered in young persons. The wall is formed by fibrous tissue lined by flattened cells which may resemble endothelium and the content is usually pultaceous material. Sometimes the lining cells are epithelioid and very occasionally there may be hair or teeth within the cyst (dermoid cyst).
2 Small, multiple cysts scattered throughout the spleen are very rare. The origin of these cysts is uncertain. They have been described as lymphangiomatous and have been reported in association with polycystic disease of the liver and kidney.

24

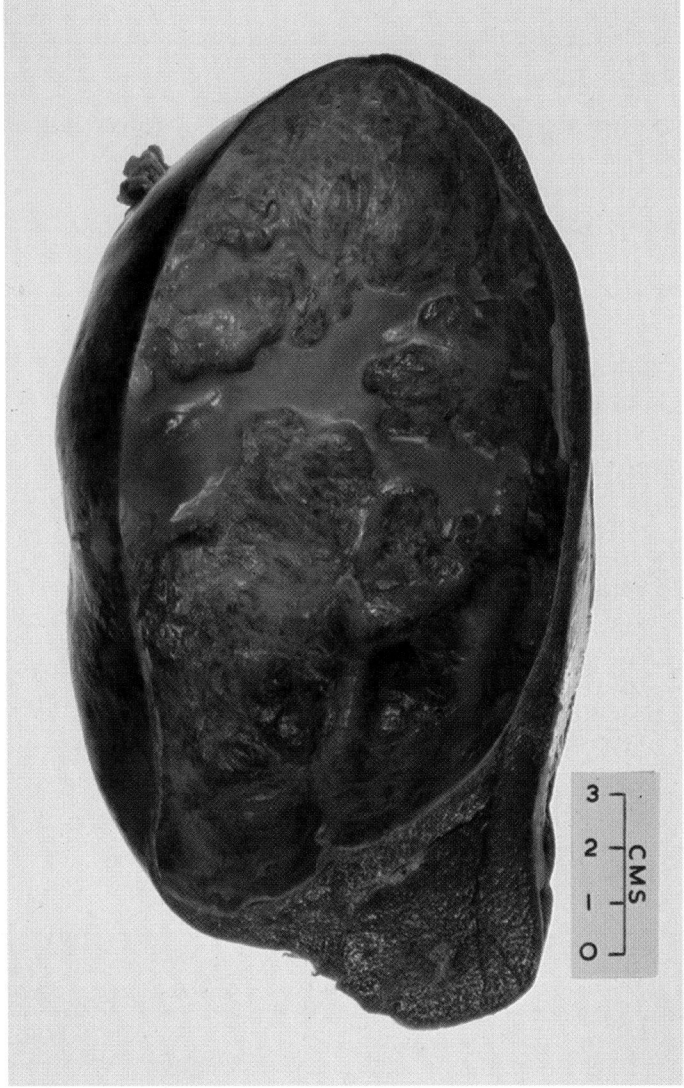

24 From a nullipara aged 18 years. This large swelling which was impacted in the pelvis possessed a long pedicle 20 cm in length which ran upwards carrying the blood supply to the spleen. The spleen forms a projection 6.5 cm broad and 3.8 cm in depth at one extremity of the cyst and a thin layer of splenic pulp passes more than half way along the cut margin of the wall of the cyst. Superficially the cyst is smooth and congested but fibrous and comparatively avascular around the attachment of a long strand of omentum. On its inner surface many branching fibrous trabeculae are present and areas of hard gelatinous-looking fibrin containing in many places plaques of calcareous deposits. Microscopically sections from the thicker part of the wall show characteristic splenic structure of Malpighian bodies, trabeculae and pulp. There is some fibrosis apparent in the trabeculae and in the pulp and in parts of the fibrous tissue there is calcification. The cyst wall is thin and fibrous.

G.C.8531

Parasitic

The commonest parasitic cyst is the hydatid cyst caused by *Echinococcus granulosus* but it is much rarer in the spleen than in the liver or lung. The cyst comprises the usual fibrous ectocyst and the inner germinal membrane or endocyst from which the brood capsules develop and where the scolices of future tape worms grow. The cyst wall may calcify which is usually accepted as a sign of quiescence, or it may rupture with dissemination of daughter cysts in the peritoneal cavity.

25

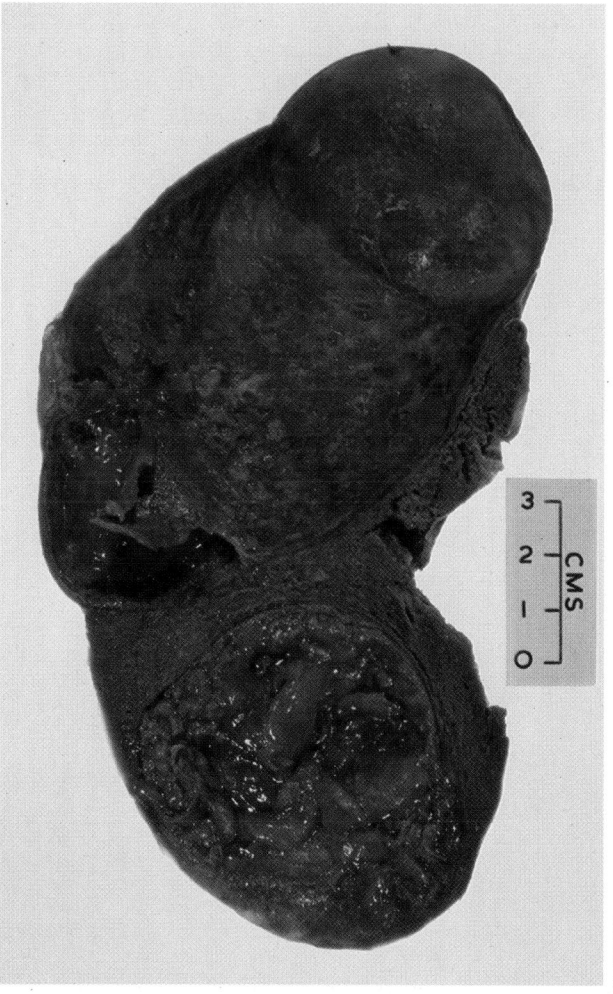

25 A portion of spleen showing echinococcal (hydatid) cysts. From a male aged 49 years.

The portion of spleen includes two large cysts which are visible on the serous aspect and occupy the greater portion of the spleen. There are numerous adhesions over the surface and what splenic tissue remains appears fibrotic.

Microscopic examination showed the characteristic features of hydatid disease. There were neither scolices nor hooklets in the cysts examined.

Ultrasound examination

Examination by ultasound is a technique whereby tumours, cysts and ruptures of the spleen may be demonstrated.

26

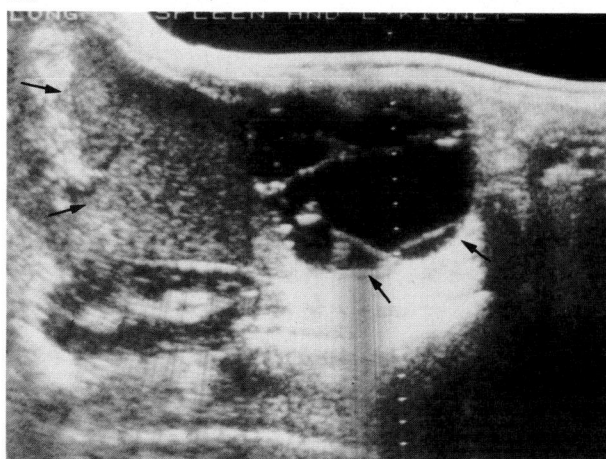

26 Ultrasound examination showing an enlarged spleen with a multiloculated cystic subcapsular collection at its lower pole. The spleen, which was removed at operation, is illustrated.

26a

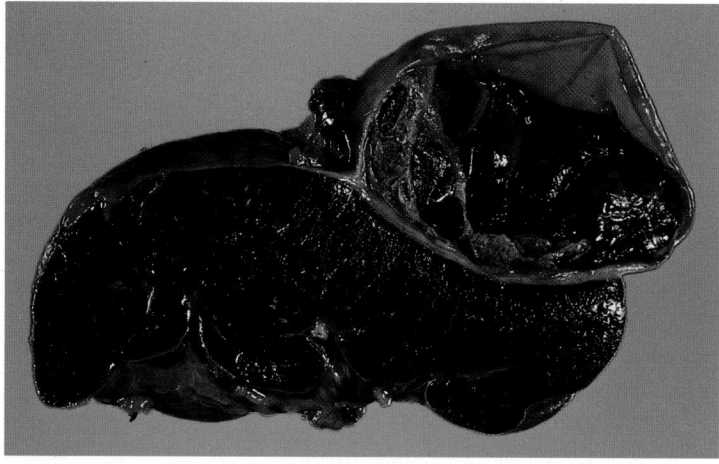

26a The spleen weighed 550 g. The spleen measured 13 × 7 × 10 cm. There is a large subcapsular cyst on the convex aspect near the lower pole. On cross section the cyst is filled with blood and is lined by a ragged membranous material. Histologically the diagnosis of hereditary spherocytosis was confirmed.

Tumours

Tumours of the lymphoma and myeloma groups have already been described. Other splenic tumours are rare, the commonest being the haemangioma.

Haemangioma

Haemangiomas of the spleen may be capillary or cavernous in type. They have been described as 'tumours' but the majority are essentially hamartomatous malformations. Occasionally they are found incidentally at autopsy as small, single or multiple nodules. Rarely diffuse involvement of the whole spleen causes a degree of splenomegaly which demands surgical intervention either because of its size or the risk of rupture. Occasionally comparable lesions are found concurrently in the liver.

Malignant blood vascular tumours are rare and may occur as solitary tumours confined to the spleen or as part of a more widespread process involving liver and other organs including the lungs.

Metastatic tumours

The incidence of metastases in the spleen is uncommon when compared with that in other organs such as the liver and bone marrow which are also rich in reticuloendothelial cells. It has been postulated that the high lymphoid content of the spleen results in an environment inimical to the proliferation of tumour cells unless there is a breakdown in the immune system.

27

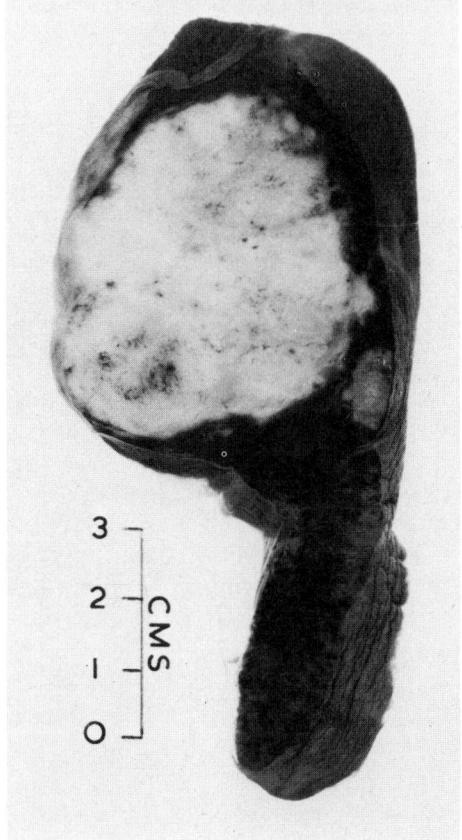

27 From a female who had a mastectomy for carcinoma of the breast. When she died some years later a large solitary metastasis was found in the spleen.

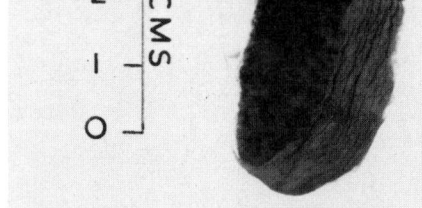

G.C.P.209

Diseases of connective tissues

Polyarteritis nodosa

Polyarteritis nodosa is a generalised disease affecting the medium and smaller arteries. There is destruction of the media and thrombosis may result. Occasionally evidence of this disease is seen in the spleen and may lead to infarction.

28

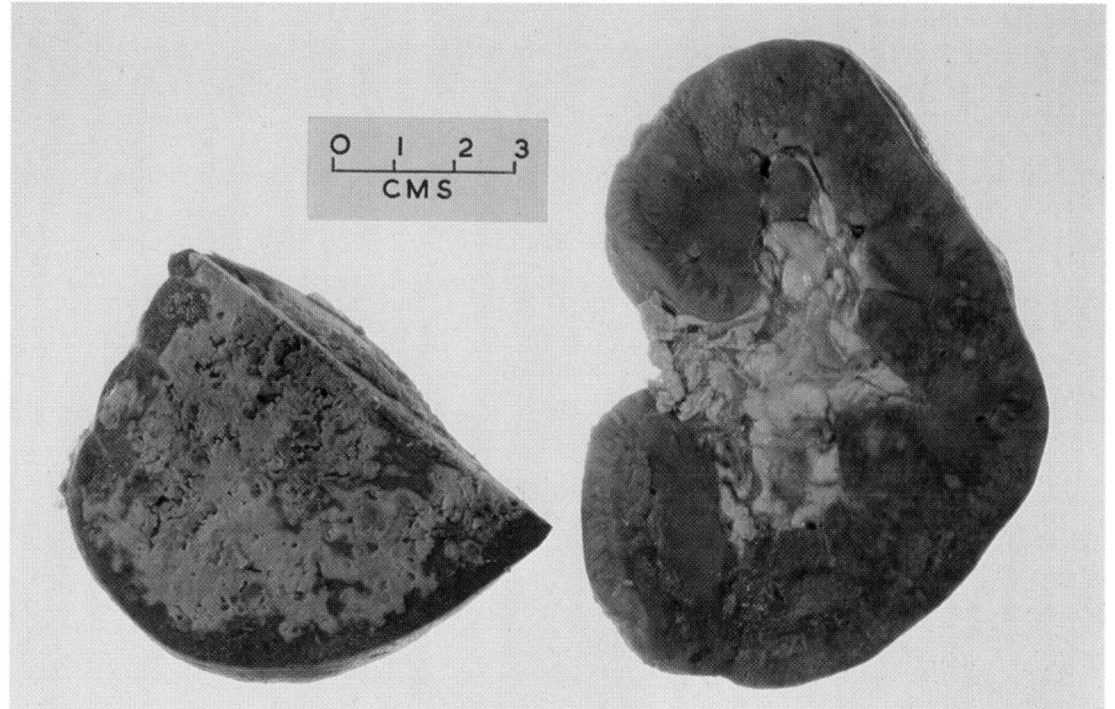

G.C.14793

28 From a male aged 52 years. Three year history of illness terminating with cardiac failure. At post mortem examination evidence of widespread polyarteritis nodosa was found.

The illustration shows specimens of the spleen and kidney in both of which there is evidence of infarction. This is much more marked in the spleen than in the kidney.

Felty's syndrome

The occurrence of splenomegaly and hypersplenism in rheumatoid arthritis is called Felty's syndrome. Anaemia is constant, partly due to haemolysis but more so to the combination of an increased splenic pool and a raised plasma volume. Granulocytopaenia is invariable and is usually severe (less than $2000/mm^3$). This is often associated with the occurrence of septic ulcers or other infections. Electron-microscopy of the spleen shows that the macrophages are actively destroying the granulocytes. Increase of lymphoid tissue and plasma cells suggests enhanced antibody formation. The splenic enlargement is due to a combination of pulp congestion and reticulo-endothelial hyperplasia. The consistence of the spleen is firm but compressible and the cut surface has no distinctive features. In about half of the cases the liver may show lymphoid infiltration of the portal tracts or even diffuse fibrosis.

Infiltration

Amyloidosis

The spleen is frequently affected in amyloidosis and there is usually involvement of other organs. The spleen is moderately enlarged and firm. Early changes are subendothelial deposits of amyloid in the walls of smaller blood vessels. In more advanced cases the distribution may be focal, mainly in the Malpighian bodies, giving rise to the so-called 'sago spleen'; or it may be diffuse with confluent patches of amyloid replacing large areas of both the red and the white pulp. The nature of amyloid is still uncertain, but it appears to be a protein-polysaccharide complex which is deposited when abnormal lympho-reticular function is associated with prolonged antigenic stimulus.

Amyloidosis in the spleen, as elsewhere, may be primary or secondary. The latter is far more common and is encountered secondary to a number of chronic diseases, e.g. tuberculosis, osteomyelitis, Hodgkin's disease, rheumatoid arthritis and leprosy.

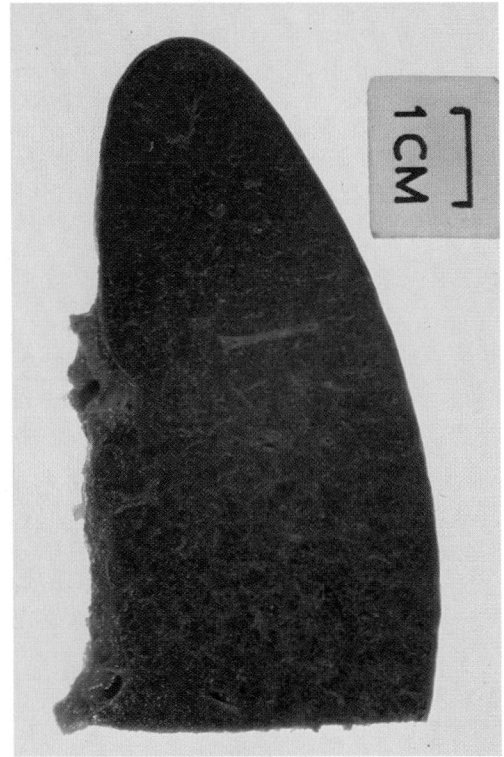

G.C.14809

29 From a female. Upper darker portion of spleen treated by Lugol's iodine to demonstrate the presence of amyloid. The distribution of the amyloid in the substance of the spleen is partly diffuse and partly focal. The sharp outline is indicative of the firm character of the spleen.

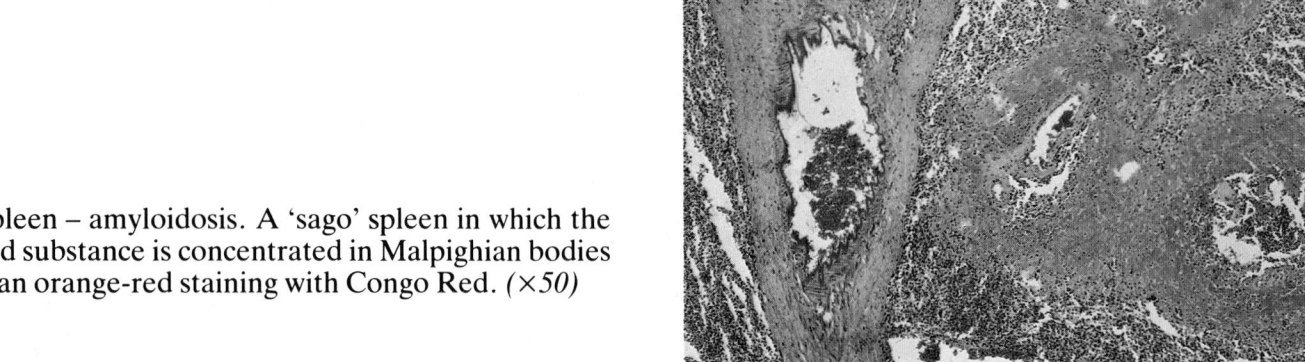

G.C.M.895

30 Spleen – amyloidosis. A 'sago' spleen in which the amyloid substance is concentrated in Malpighian bodies giving an orange-red staining with Congo Red. (×50)

Idiopathic thrombocytopenic purpura (ITP)

Two forms of thrombocytopenic purpura occur, primary and secondary. In primary purpura the spleen is not enlarged. In secondary purpura splenomegaly is usually present but it is not invariable. The other important diagnostic difference is the presence of large numbers of megakaryocytes in the marrow in ITP and their deficiency or absence in secondary purpura.

In ITP the platelet count is low and the platelet survival time is greatly diminished. Antibodies to platelets can be demonstrated. Sequestration and destruction of other antibody coated platelets occur in the spleen and, as the disease progresses, in the liver. On light microscopy the germinal centres of the Malpighian bodies are seen to be enlarged indicating immunological reactivity and on electron-microscopy ingested remnants of lipid-rich cell membranes, probably platelets, are present in digestive vacuoles in the macrophages.

Present evidence suggests that the disease has clearly an immunological basis.

31

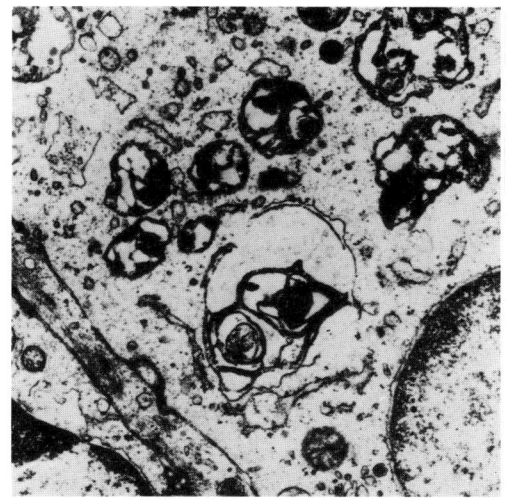

G.C.M.928

31 Macrophage showing a digestive vacuole containing myelin figures, the lipid-rich remnants of all membranes, probably platelets. *(EM × 32000)*

Infarction

32

Occlusion of the main trunk of the artery in the splenic hilum may cause massive infarction. Embolic occlusion of end-arteries leads to small pale infarcts in the pulp. These lesser infarcts may present as subcapsular pale triangular areas as illustrated. The surface of the area is depressed.

Infected (septic) emboli cause infarction followed by abscess formation.

32 Post mortem finding from an adult.

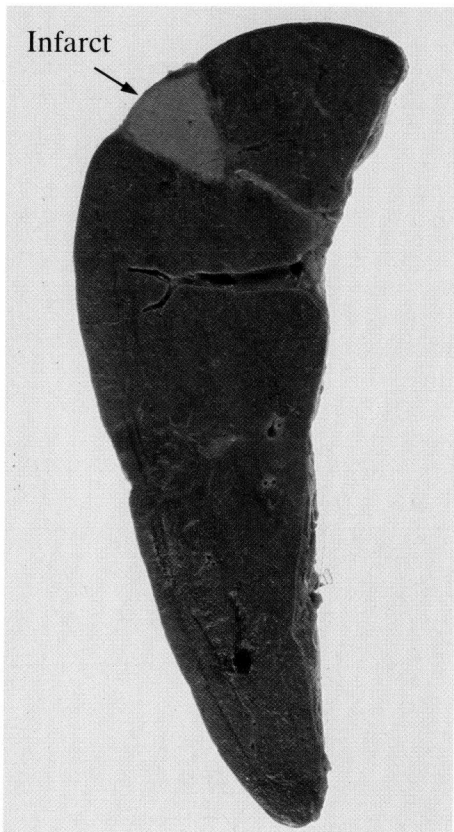

Infarct

G.C.9531

Rupture

Rupture of the normal spleen may result from:

(a) a blow over the lower posterior chest wall causing splitting of the convex diaphragmatic surface of the spleen. Bleeding from this type of injury is not usually profuse initially but tends to recur. Arbitrarily, if it recurs within 48 hours of injury the rupture is termed Biphasic; if more than 48 hours, Delayed.

(b) severe more widespread injury leading to multiple visceral ruptures and generally gross damage with consequent severe haemorrhage from avulsion of major arteries.

The enlarged diseased spleen is frequently excessively friable and rupture may result from minor and often ill-recollected trauma. This is true when splenomegaly is due to mononucleosis or typhoid fever. In tropical countries the enlarged malarial spleen is likewise excessively friable.

33

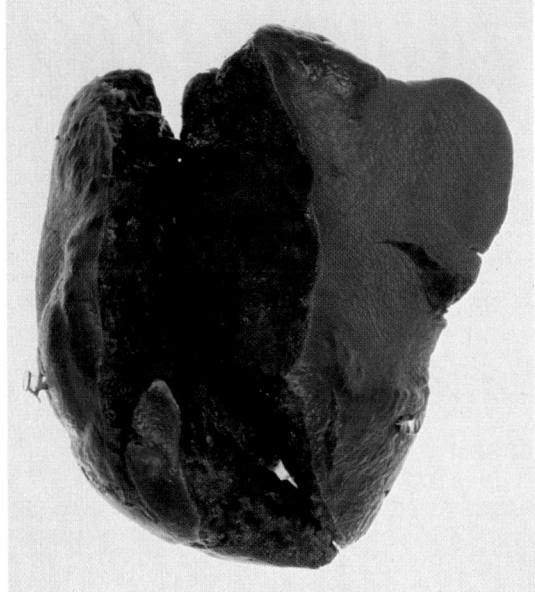

G.C.7713

33a

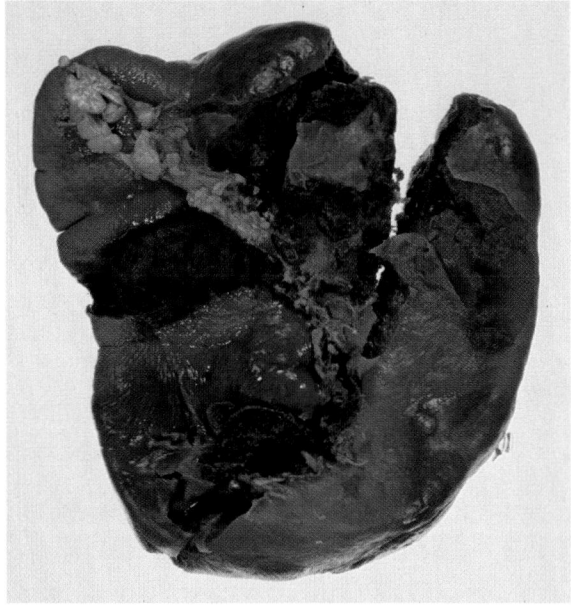

33 and 33a From an adult male who was involved in a motor traffic accident. He was struck on the left side of the lower chest by the radiator of the car. Rupture of the spleen was diagnosed. Splenectomy was followed by recovery.

The diaphragmatic surface of the spleen is crossed obliquely by an irregular laceration which is continuous with a wider laceration on the visceral surface. A deep laceration notches the superior border and continues on the visceral surface. Both lacerations extend into the hilum.

34

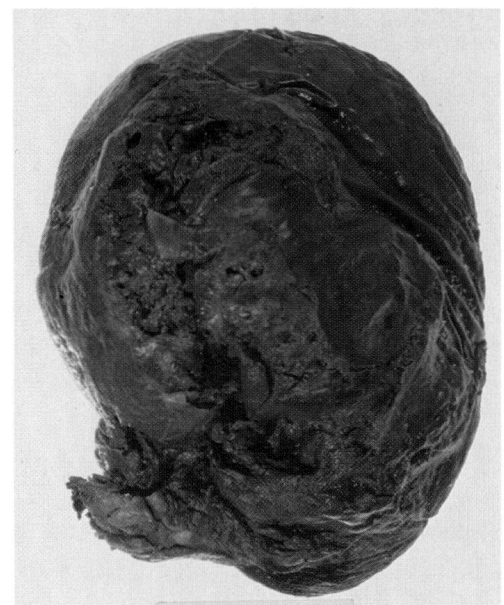

G.C.7799

Rupture of the spleen by penetrating injury often through the left lower chest, e.g. stab wounds or gunshot wounds. Usually there is injury to other organs as well and in gunshot wounds there is gross disruption of the spleen.

34 War wound 1915. The spleen is grossly lacerated by a missile which penetrated the superior diaphragmatic surface, traversed the substance of the spleen and partially detached the lienorenal ligament.

A.I.S. Macpherson

Homicidal rupture

In the practice of Chinese 'boxing' (koon thow), the equivalent of Japanese karate, a major technique is jabbing blows with the fully extended fingers. Such blows are designed to disable or to kill.

An atlas has been published to illustrate the especially vulnerable areas of the body amongst which is shown a point below the left costal margin. The spleen can thus be injured and is especially vulnerable if enlarged. As a method of murder the victim is usually attacked in a crowded place and is being hustled by accomplices when the blow is struck. The assailant disappears in the crowd and the serious nature of the assault may not become apparent to the victim for some time.

35

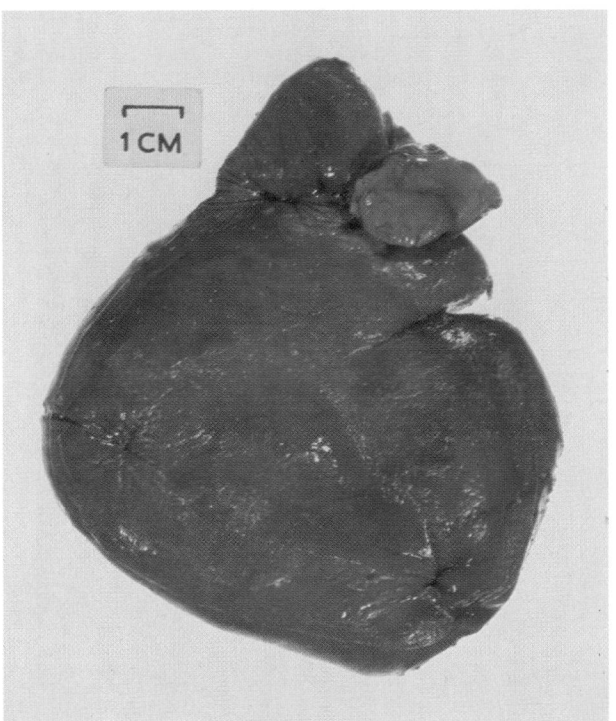

35a

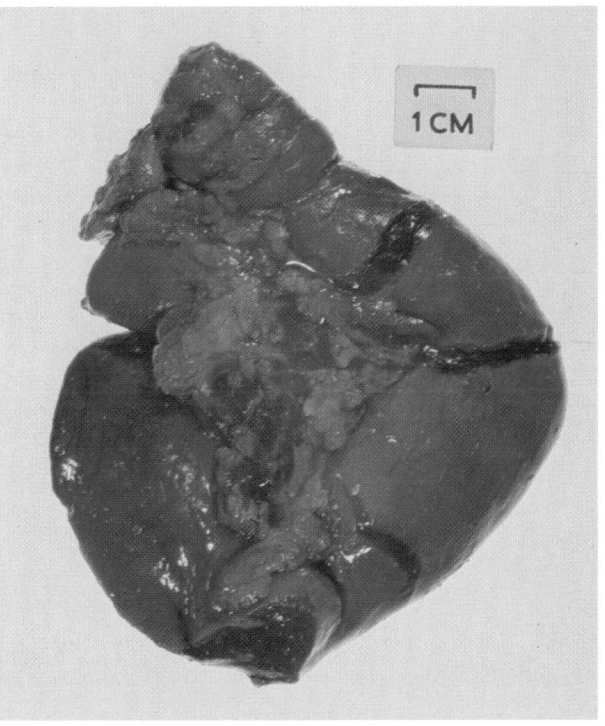

35 From a middle-aged Chinese male who was found lying doubled up in pain after a fracas had dispersed. On admission to hospital the abdomen was rigid. There was a suspicion of free fluid in the peritoneal cavity. A small bruise was present over the left costal margin in the left hypochondrium. Successful splenectomy was carried out.

35a The spleen was normal in size, shape and texture showing no signs of previous disease. On its costo-diaphragmatic surface was a double indentation corresponding to the tips of the attacker's fingers (**35**). The surface was not torn. Radiating from the hilum were a series of linear ruptures reaching right up to the edge of the spleen from which bleeding occurred (**35a**). It would appear that the inward pressure on the dia-phragmatic surface has caused a bursting from within outwards at the hilum.

Specimen by courtesy of the Department of Forensic Medicine, University of Edinburgh.

Yeoh Bok Choon

Aneurysm of the splenic artery

The development of a splenic aneurysm has been shown to occur in association with portal hypertension and splenomegaly, in atherosclerosis and has also been described as a sequel to subacute bacterial endo-carditis. The explanation of the occurrence of aneurysm most commonly in women and particularly its relationship to pregnancy remains unsolved. Splenic aneurysms have also been shown to occur in association with aneurysms of the cerebral vascular system which suggests a possible congenital defect.

Incidence

In contradistinction to other aneurysms those of the splenic artery are commoner in women and frequently are first recognised during pregnancy. The total number of cases reported in the literature is small but in one series of 190 cases 127 were female (67%) and 58 were in the child bearing age period. When the aneurysm was diagnosed 31 patients were pregnant. Many splenic aneurysms give no symptoms and are found incidentally. The common initial manifestation is rupture of the aneurysm, presenting as an acute abdominal catastrophe.

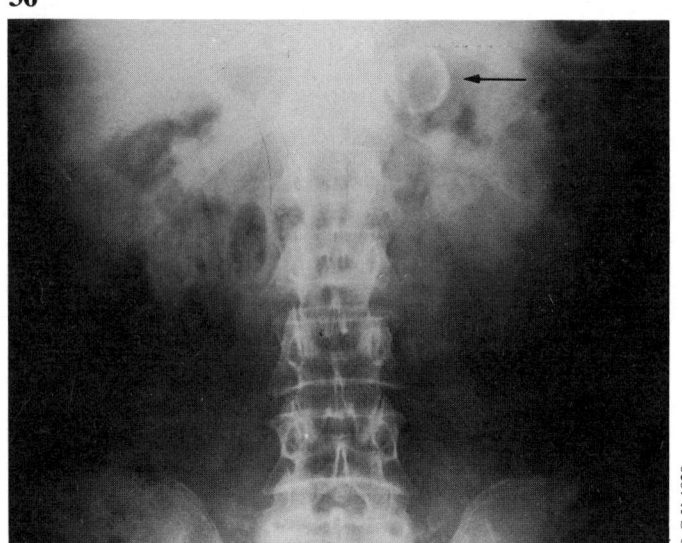

36 Calcified splenic artery aneurysm.

G.C.X.1028

37 From a female aged 62 years who lived in Shetland. In 1940 a hydatid cyst of the right lung was excised. In 1961, following two haematemeses she was admitted to hospital for investigation. The significant points in the clinical examination were a large Caput Medusae, splenomegaly and a bruit over the epigastrium. Radiological examination disclosed varices in the lower oesophagus and a calcified circular shadow in the left hypochondrium which was recognised as a splenic aneurysm. Hepatic function was normal. At operation there were splenomegaly and three aneurysms in the splenic artery. The spleen, together with that portion of the splenic artery on which the aneurysms were located, was removed and a lienorenal anastomosis performed. The liver showed no gross abnormality. The fresh specimen removed at operation is illustrated. The patient made a good recovery surviving the operation for 9 years and eventually died of a cerebral haemorrhage.

The aneurysm develops in the main trunk of the splenic artery and approximately one third of the lesions are multiple. The aneurysm is eccentric being located on the convexity of the normal spirals of the splenic artery. Sclerotic changes are common and there may be calcification. Adhesions to adjacent parts are frequent. Intra-splenic aneurysms have also been described in association with aneurysm at the hilum. The common factors in these cases have been portal hypertension and previous intra-splenic injection.

Atherosclerosis

The majority of splenic aneurysms are degenerative and associated with either generalised or focal atherosclerosis. Fragmentation of the internal elastic lamina and degeneration of the media occur particularly at the convexity of the bends in the splenic artery and may progress to calcification. In some instances the changes appear to be limited to the splenic artery suggesting that they are secondary to a local factor and not to systemic disease.

38

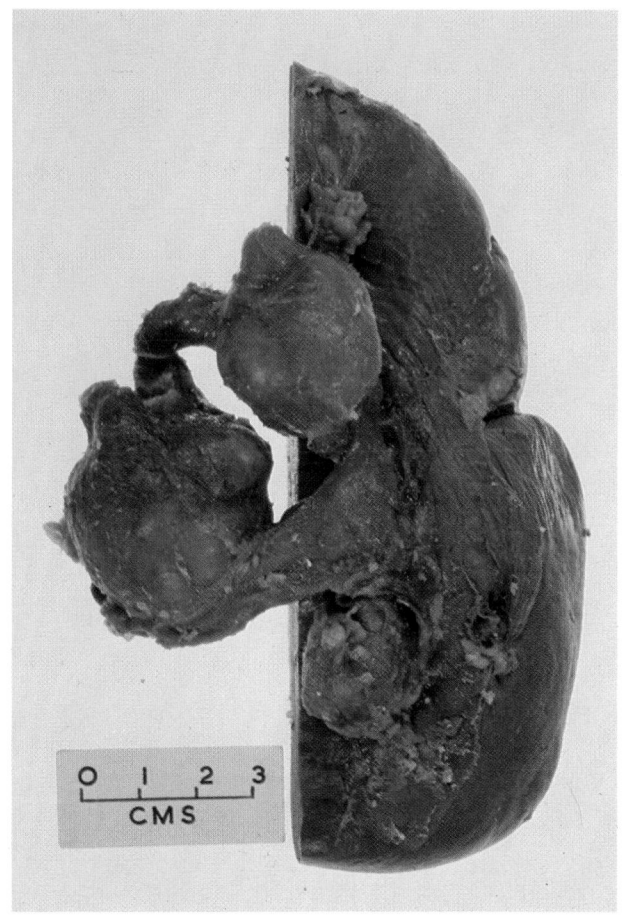

38 From a female aged 41 years. Long history of general ill health and weakness. Investigations were indicative of hepatic cirrhosis associated with hypersplenism in the form of a thrombocytopaenia. Some years previously she had suffered from a subarachnoid haemorrhage due to rupture of an aneurysm of her anterior cerebral artery. At operation for the removal of the spleen she was found to have a small cirrhotic liver. The spleen was enlarged but the outstanding finding was the presence of three aneurysms.

Complications

Rupture of the aneurysm occurs in approximately half of cases and is the initial clinical feature. Typically there is a preliminary non-fatal haemorrhage followed 6 or 7 days later by a fatal haemorrhage. Bleeding occurs into the lesser sac or into the retroperitoneal space.

A.I.S. Macpherson

The growth of endometrial masses in the subserosa and muscularis of the intestine is a common occurrence but rarely causes symptoms. Two explanations of this lesion are advanced:

1   Shed endometrial cells are projected by reflux action along the Fallopian tubes and are discharged into the peritoneal cavity to become attached to the serosal surface of adjacent intestine.

2   The uterus develops from the paramesonephric (Müllerian) ducts which arise from the wall of the coelomic cavity. The peritoneum has a similar embryological origin. It is suggested that by metaplasia of the serosa cell tissue comparable with the endometrium may be formed.

Deposits of endometrial tissue are most commonly found in the lower abdomen and pelvis. The small intestine may be affected but more commonly the sigmoid colon and rectum are involved. It is not an uncommon incidental finding in operative specimens of the large intestine which have been resected for other diseases.

1

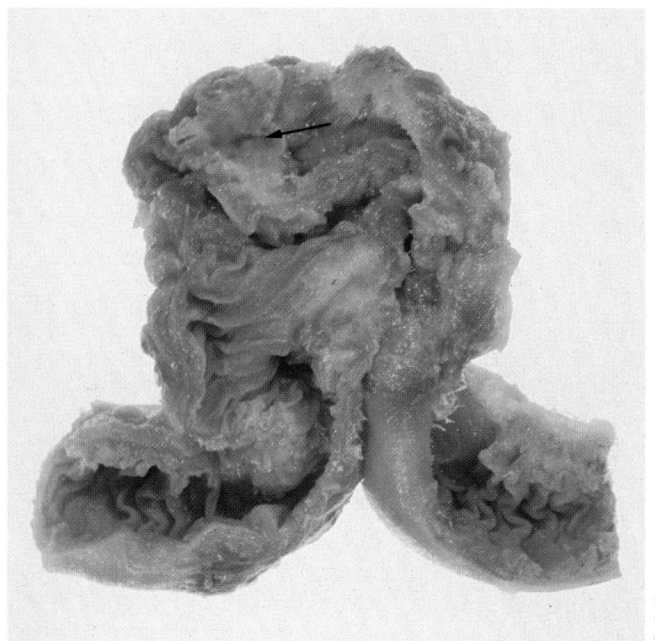

G.C.13481

1   From a female aged 29 years who had experienced pain in the right iliac fossa for 4 months. A few days before laparotomy the pain recurred and signs of intestinal obstruction developed.

At operation loops of terminal ileum, which were bound together by fibrous adhesions, were resected. In the resected bowel there were points of constriction. At each site a central area a few millimetres in diameter, reddish-brown or stained by haemosiderin, was surrounded by dense fibrous tissue.

Endometriomas of the colon and rectum are usually fairly small firm tumours which lie in the subserous and muscular coats of the bowel and which sometimes reach the sub-mucosa. The lesion may project into the lumen of the bowel as a polypoid mass but this is always covered by intact colonic or rectal mucosa. Rectal bleeding is uncommon in this condition and usually occurs because of vascular congestion of the overlying mucosa rather than because of ulceration. Large bowel endometriomas tend to be somewhat indurated. This is due to hypertrophied smooth muscle and fibrosis which develop around the endometrial tissue following repeated haemorrhage.

Endometriosis may also involve the large bowel in the form of multiple small nodules on the peritoneal surface and it may give rise to plaques of indurated tissue in the pouch of Douglas. Ectopic endometrial tissue may invade and infiltrate both the rectum and vagina and may be massive enough to cause rectal obstruction. It may produce rectal bleeding because of the associated congestion of the rectal mucosa and it may penetrate through the vaginal wall producing dark blue haemorrhagic polypoid masses which cause vaginal bleeding.

Occasionally the uterus, posterior vaginal fornix and rectum may be bound together by a mass of endometriomatous tissue which can sometimes simulate a secondary carcinomatous deposit.

1a

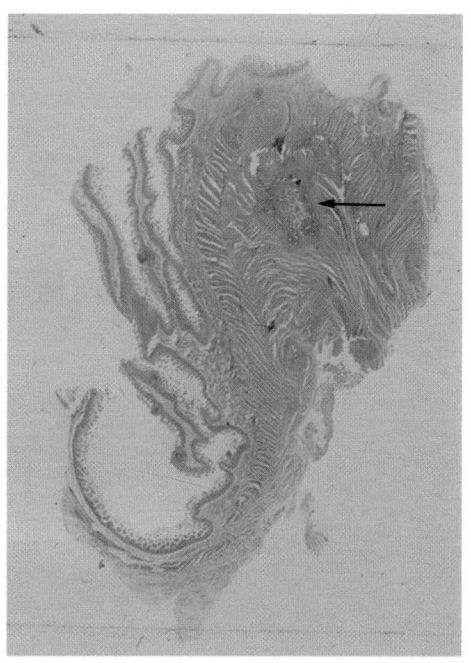

G.C.13481

1b

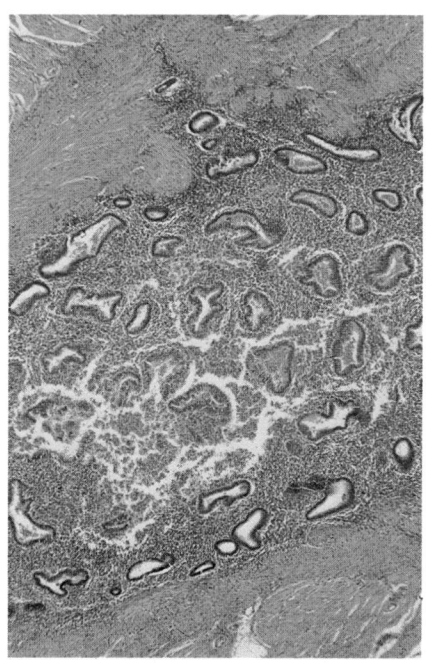

G.C.13481

1a Ileum – endometriosis. A section of the ileum at a point of constriction.

Reaction to the focus of endometrium has resulted in fibrosis, kinking and hypertrophy of muscularis. *(H&E × 4.5)*

1b Ileum – endometriosis. Higher power of same section showing the stromal and epithelial components of the endometrium – some haemorrhage. *(H&E × 40)*

2

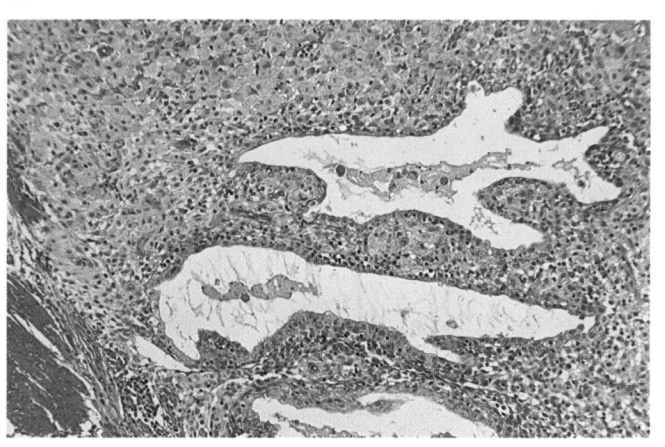

G.C.M.818

2 Appendix – endometriosis. In the appendicular muscularis pale swollen decidual cells surround the endometrial glands. *(H&E × 100)*

I.F. MacLaren

531

Infection may reach the peritoneal cavity in three ways:

1 From the exterior by wounding, at a surgical operation or through the Fallopian tube.
2 From the alimentary tract or one of its derivatives. The most frequent cause is acute appendicitis, but it may follow many acute intra-abdominal conditions such as a perforated peptic ulcer, acute pancreatitis or mesenteric thrombosis.
3 From the blood stream. Rarely as in acute pneumococcal peritonitis, the infection may be blood-borne from a distant site.

Peritonitis always begins locally. It may remain localised or may spread and become diffuse. The early pathological changes include a local hyperaemia, with loss of the normal peritoneal sheen, associated with the deposition of a thin layer of fibrin. The affected areas become sticky and the adjacent surfaces, parietal and visceral, become adherent, thereby localising the infection. The extent and nature of the local inflammatory response varies with the infecting organism.

Peritonitis which remains localised from its onset or which becomes limited as a result of adhesion formation tends to be localised to a specific anatomical area.

1 Local – At the site of the initial perforation or inoculation.
2 Pelvic – The infection which is generally secondary to a perforated appendicitis, diverticulitis or salpingitis becomes localised by the adhesion of loops of small or large intestine and the omentum and the consequent isolation of the pouch of Douglas or the rectovesical space from the peritoneal cavity. The tendency is for the abscess to point into the rectum or the vagina and to discharge spontaneously.
3 Subphrenic – The localisation of intraperitoneal infection between the diaphragm and the liver on the right side and the diaphragm and the stomach on the left is known as a subphrenic abscess and commonly follows a perforated peptic ulcer or a perforated gallbladder. There are six anatomical compartments in this area, two intraperitoneal and one extraperitoneal on each side. These are anatomical features which are fully described in text books of anatomy. The abscess may contain only pus or pus and gas combined, the latter with a detectable fluid level. The tendency in the case of a subphrenic abscess is for progression, initially with extension of the inflammatory process through the diaphragm to produce an associated pleural effusion and basal consolidation but ultimately the abscess bursts into the pleural cavity with consequent empyema or broncho-pleural fistula.

Subphrenic abscess

1

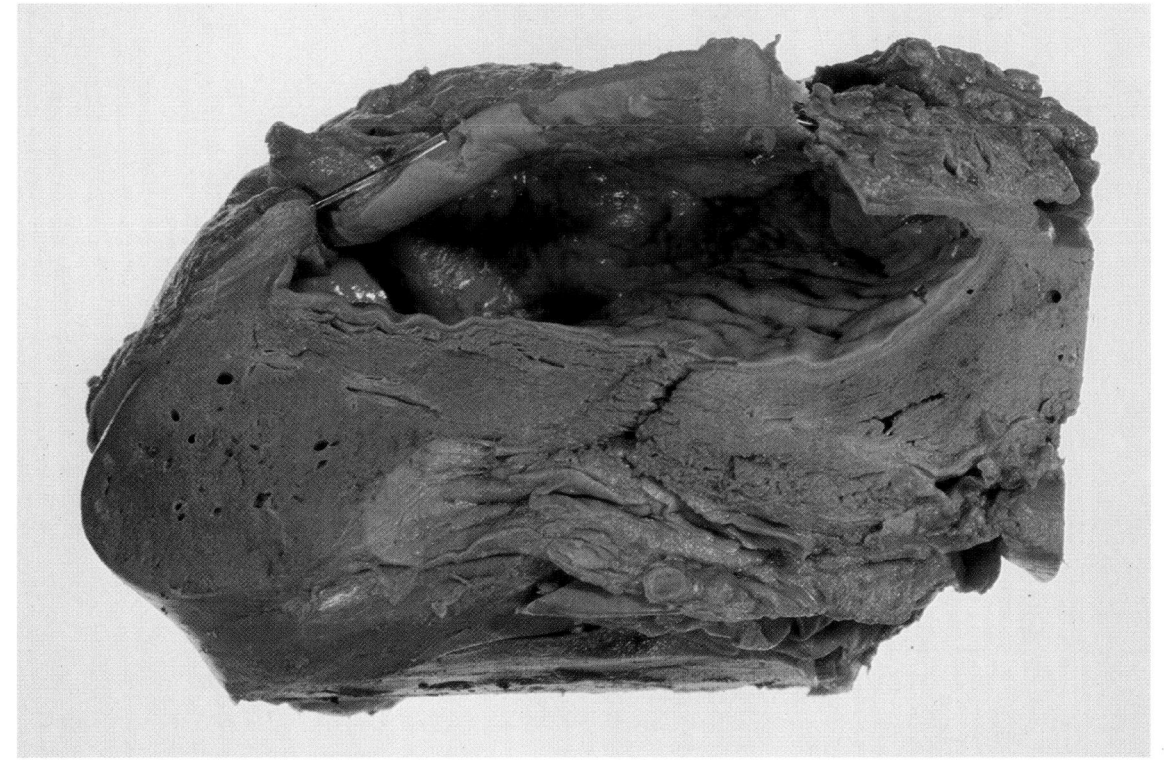

1 Posterior half of liver. Between the liver and the diaphragm is a subphrenic abscess where the surface of the liver is hollowed and the parenchyma compressed. The internal surface of the abscess is corrugated and rough from flakes of fibrinous deposit.

The abscess lies below the right half of the diaphragm and probably originated from a perforated ulcer.

2

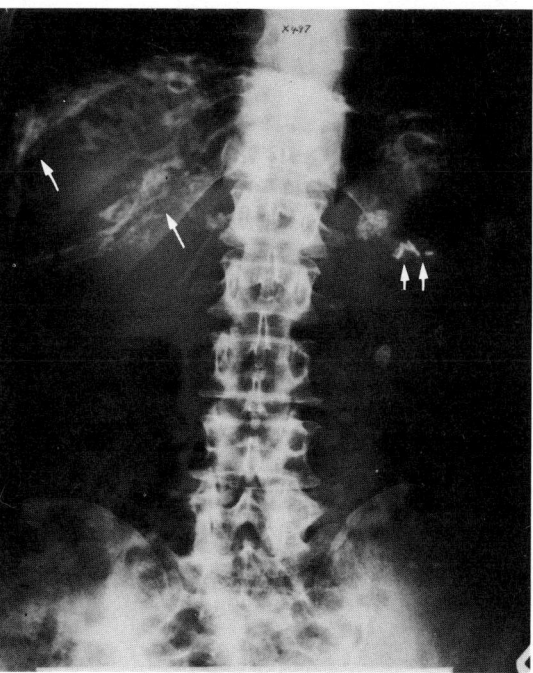

2 The X-ray shows extensive subphrenic calcification due to an old and healed subphrenic abscess. The condition may have been pyogenic following operation (gastrectomy). The metallic clips are in the stump of the stomach and were used for closure. Two calculi are present in the left kidney.

533

Tumours arising primarily in retroperitoneal connective tissues form a rare but varied group and were first described by Morgagni in 1761. The term 'retroperitoneal tumour' is generally understood to exclude neoplasms of organs in, or impinging on, the retroperitoneal space – such as kidneys, adrenal glands, pancreas and those arising from bone. Secondary tumours are also excluded. Neoplasms arising from lymphoid tissue are recorded in a later section. Lipomatous tumours are the commonest of the group. Tumours of neural origin or plain muscle are slightly less frequent. Tumours of vascular origin are still less common. Rhabdomyosarcomas and fibrosarcomas have been reported as rare findings.

1

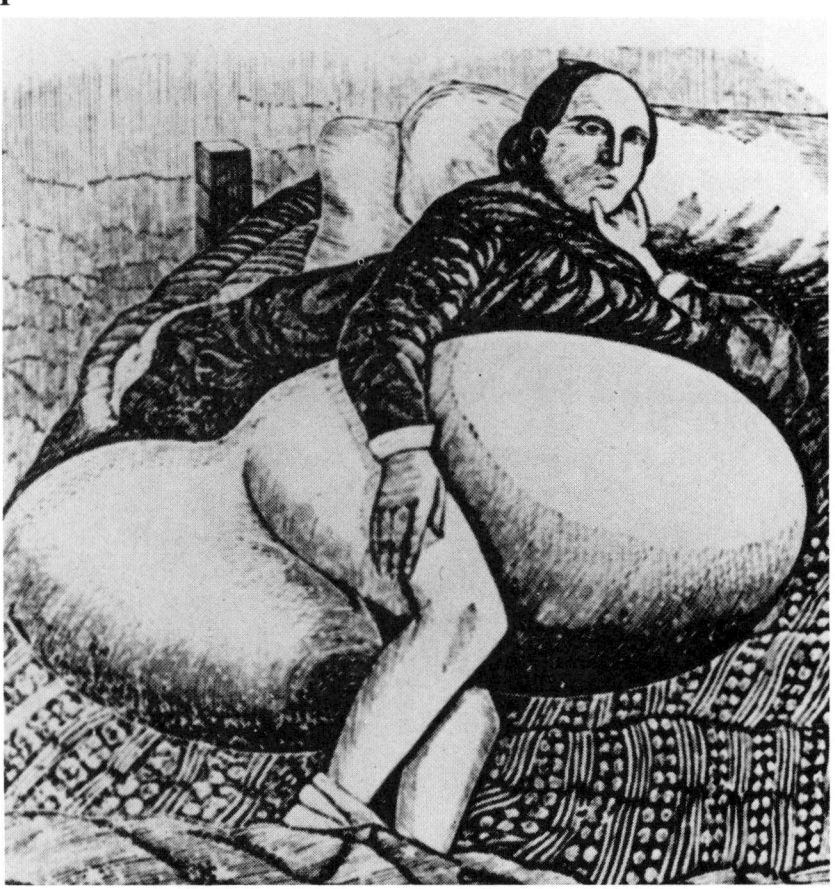

G.C.P.218

1 This case was described by Delamater in 1859 and illustrates the enormous size to which a retroperitoneal tumour can grow.

The patient was a female weighing 269 lb. and the tumour was a 'lipoma' which weighed 179 lb.

The retroperitoneal space refers to the loose areolar tissue behind the peritoneum of the posterior abdominal wall. It extends from the level of the twelfth rib above to the lumbo-sacral joint and iliac crest inferiorly and is traversed by the main blood vessels, the ureters, renal and gonadal vessels. It contains much lymphatic and nervous tissue. This areolar space is potentially large and allows primary and metastatic tumours to expand grossly in size before signs and symptoms appear. Symptoms are usually related to the displacement of organs or to the development of a large mass.

Liposarcoma

In early accounts the tumour was regarded as a simple lipoma but these tumours recur and metastasize and with full examination reveal areas of sarcomatous character. This is the retroperitoneal tumour possessing the greatest potential of growth and is illustrated in Delamater's case (see **1**).

Middle-aged patients with a female preponderance.

2

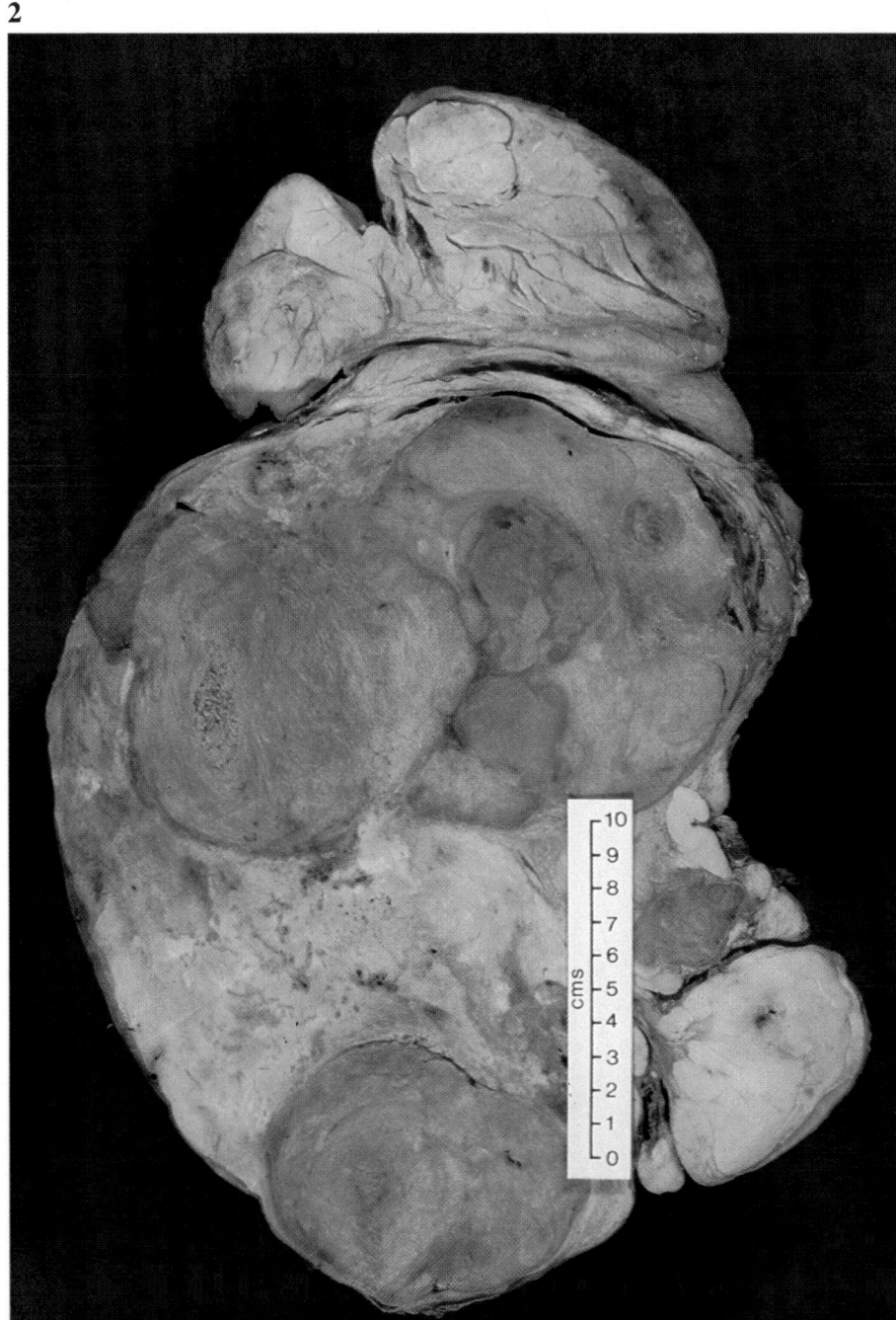

G.C.10209

2 From a male aged 40 years who had a large, soft tumour in the right abdomen. At operation the proximal colon was displaced downwards and to the left by the tumour mass. The tumour weighed 18 lb. and measures 39 × 22 cm. A further operation was carried out for a residual mass. The patient died 12 days later.

This case illustrates the difficulty of ensuring that the whole tumour mass is removed. At first operation isolated lobules readily escape detection.

Liposarcoma *(Continued)*

Pathology

The commonest origin of these tumours is in the perirenal fat but comparable neoplasms may arise in other retroperitoneal areas, in the mesentery or in the appendices epiploicae. The tumour may form a well defined single lobulated mass or may consist of a main tumour with numerous satellite lobules. This is illustrated in the first specimen (**2**). The tumour may be essentially lipomatous or may be largely myxomatous – intermediate types occur.

These tumours may attain an enormous size but characteristically, while organs may be displaced, they are not invaded, e.g. in perirenal lipomas the kidney is not involved and retains full function. The typical picture is of lobulated, defined growths of varied appearance and consistency, ranging from masses of yellow fat to tumours of greyish-white, harder or mucoid structure. The cut surface is usually yellow with mucoid, haemorrhagic or necrotic areas.

Histology

The tumour consists of well-differentiated fatty tissue usually more cellular than normal. Myxomatous tissue is found in the majority of cases and, in some, may form the major component of the tumour (**3**). Sometimes highly anaplastic areas may be found with monstrous multinucleated and vacuolated cells and atypical mitotic figures. This suggests that a more correct name for these tumours should be lipomyxosarcoma. The degree of pleomorphism and the frequency of mitoses varies in different areas of the neoplasm. When found, such areas are regarded as evidence of sarcomatous change (**4**).

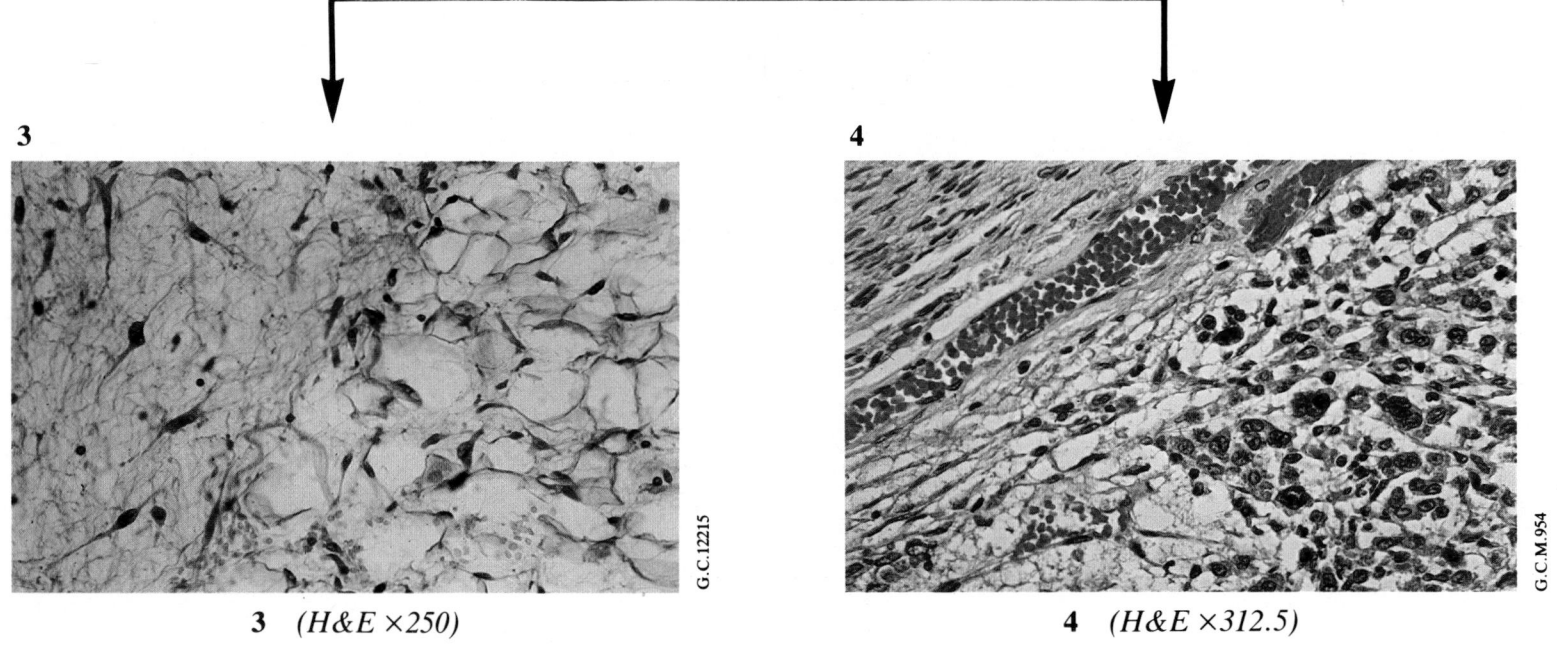

3   *(H&E ×250)*   **4**   *(H&E ×312.5)*

Spread

Local recurrence after removal is common even when the tumour has apparently been defined and easy to enucleate. The tendency of the tumour to form satellite lipomas probably explains this. Growth is slow but progressive. Distant metastases are rare. It is said that the more myxomatous types show some response to irradiation.

Lipomatosis

This is a variant in which the tumour growth appears to occur synchronously in the retroperitoneal fat, the mesentery, and the taeniae coli. To this lesion the term 'lipomatosis' is applied and indicates that the tumour is multicentric in origin and not a single focus with spread.

The histological picture is the same as in the single tumour and its behaviour is similar.

5

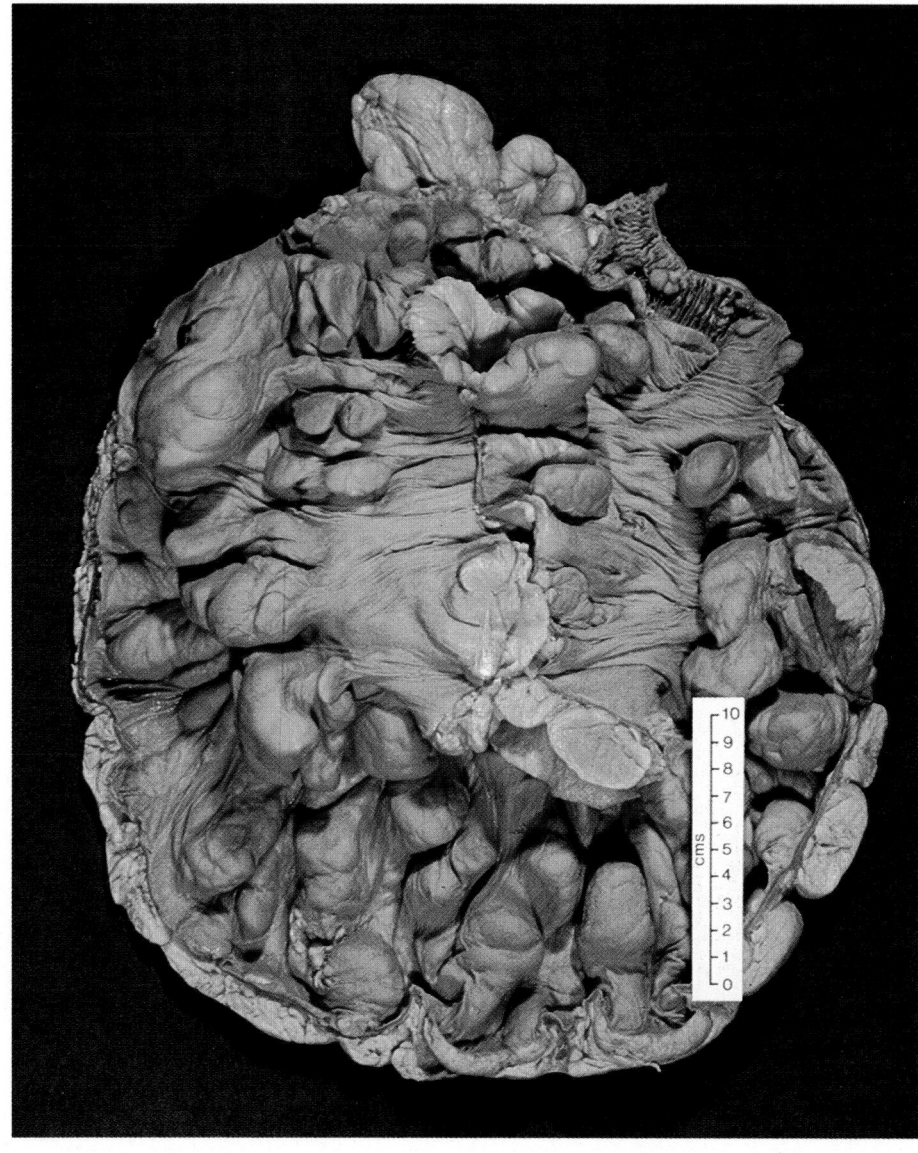

5 From a male aged 36 years. No clinical details are available. At operation the condition of lipomatosis was disclosed. The specimen consists of the terminal 1.5 metres of the ileum and its mesentery. The intestine has been laid open. The lesion consists of a large number of lipomatous masses, some in the mesentery, others affecting the ileum and in these instances the tumour may be either submucosal or subserosal. The lumen of the ileum has been grossly distended. On the cut surface the mucosa is flattened and the rugae are stretched, and in comparison with the size of the distended bowel appear to be flattened and fewer in number than normal. Where the tumours have been cut across the fatty nature of the tissue is clearly visible.

Leiomyoma

The tumour, which occurs equally in the sexes, is rare in young persons. Both simple and malignant forms occur. Growth is slow but the tumour, if malignant, becomes fixed to surrounding parts and later haematogenous metastases occur. The illustrated specimen demonstrates the main features.

6

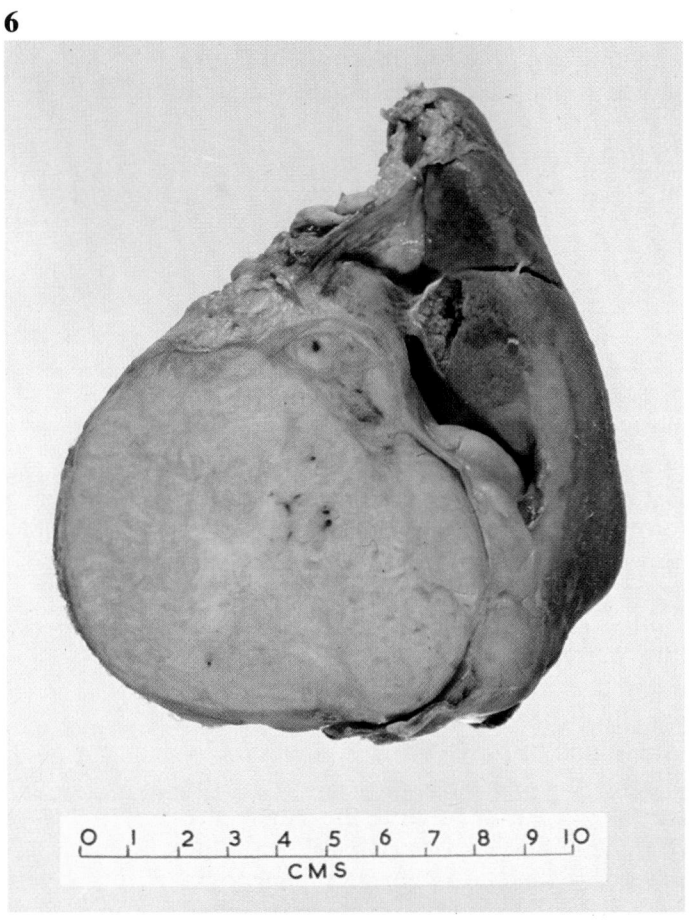

6 From a female aged 74 years. Lying apparently in the gastro-lienal ligament, is a large bosselated tumour. The definition of the tumour is distinct and sharp and this is most clearly seen on the cut surface. It lies in close approximation to the hilum and medial surface of the spleen. The main mass of the tumour is roughly spherical or ovoid but a number of small satellite masses are clearly seen representing local extension of the tumour. The cut surface shows a homogeneous white fleshy appearance with some few areas only irregularly scattered where the tissue appears to be more translucent.

Histology

7

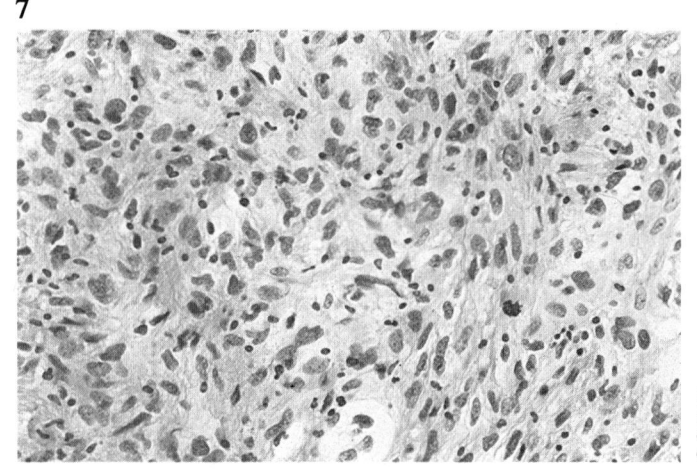

7 In this leiomyosarcoma there is still some suggestion of spindle cells being arranged in bands, but the regularity of pattern and the cellular uniformity seen in leiomyomas have been lost. The nuclei are enlarged, pleomorphic and show mitotic activity whilst the cellular arrangement tends to be haphazard. *(H&E ×250)*

Nerve sheath tumours

In the retroperitoneal space neurilemmomas and neurofibromas are occasionally found and in this situation frequently attain a considerable size. The tumours may show only the characteristics of either type or be mixed. Other features of neurofibromatosis are commonly associated.

8

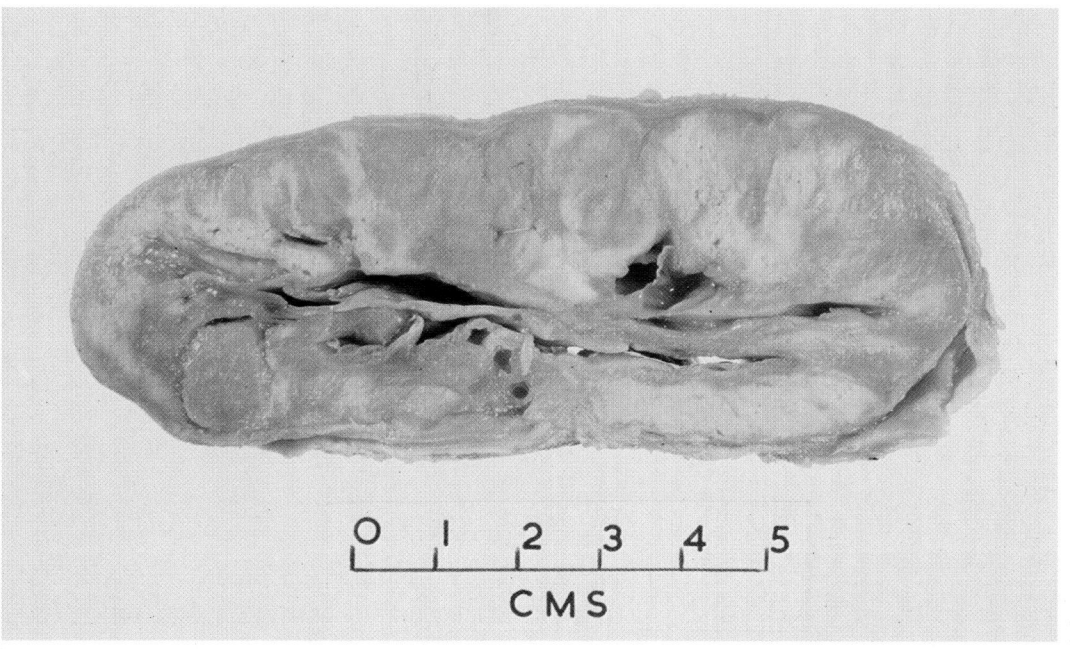

8 This specimen exhibits the typical features of retroperitoneal neurilemmoma. The tumour was an elongated mass measuring 11 × 4.5 cm. The tumour is smooth in outline and the cut surface demonstrates the presence of an area of central softening, but the main bulk of the tumour is white and fleshy with little evidence of fasciculation. Histologically the tumour is a neurilemmoma.

Where the tumour is a neurofibroma it may be less well defined, is adherent to surrounding tissues, is less likely to show central softening but there will be more prominent fasciculation of the cut surface. Both types of tumour are commonly related to the nerves from which they originate.

Nerve cell tumours

Neuroblastomas and ganglioneuromas also arise in the retroperitoneal space. These tumours are more fully discussed in a later section.

Haemangiopericytoma

This very uncommon retroperitoneal tumour of vascular origin was first described in 1942 but similar neoplasms have been described in many parts of the body.

Pathology

A slow growing tumour, usually well defined, which may reach considerable size. The tumour is usually pigmented – a brownish yellow. In 10 to 20% of cases it is clearly invasive.

9

G.C.13414

9 From a female aged 56 years. A chance finding at operation carried out for a femoral hernia. The tumour is a lobulated mass with a translucent capsule through which cystic areas can be seen. In some of these cysts haemorrhage has occurred. There are fissures running between the lobules one of which has been sectioned showing this to be a solid, fleshy tumour of yellowish-white colour and with evidence of invasion of the capsule (arrow). There is one lobule which is whiter and more solid in character and would almost appear to be the one from which the tumour has arisen. The other lobules seen are darker in colour and have a more translucent appearance which suggests that they are semi-cystic in character. There are also areas of haemorrhage in these lobules.

Histology

The characteristic feature of the lesion is the presence of blood spaces surrounded by pericytes. The precise nature and origin of these pericytes are controversial. The tumour consists of a rich network of capillaries lined by normal endothelium and surrounded by single or multi-layered pale cells with prominent vesicular nuclei. In very solid areas the vessels may be difficult to identify but reticulin silver stains will outline the vessels and show individual cells to be surrounded by a basket of reticulin fibres. In other areas the vessels may show dilatation towards cyst formation. It has been stated that 'it is usually impossible to predict the likelihood of malignant behaviour on the basis of microscopy'.

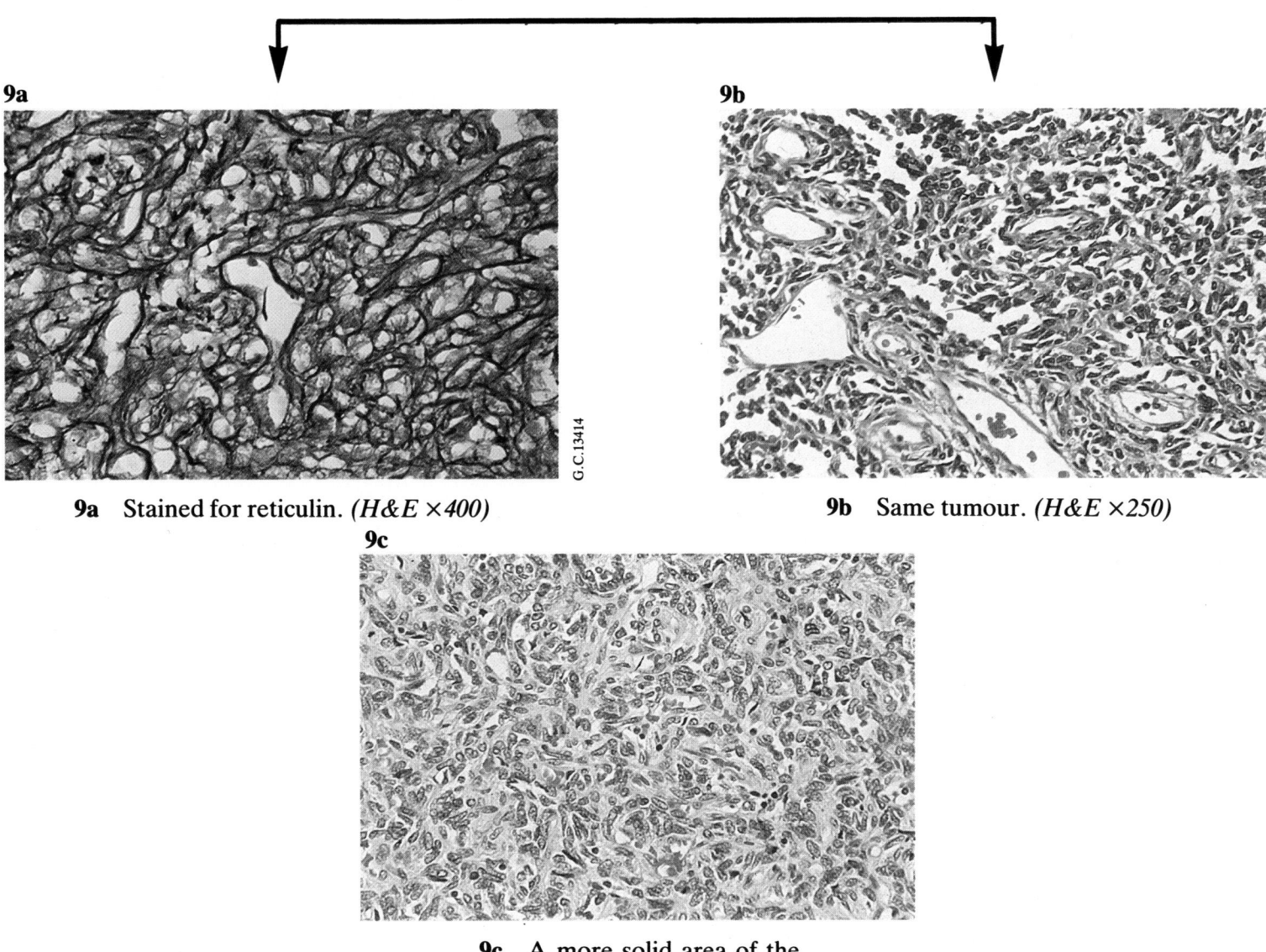

9a   Stained for reticulin. *(H&E ×400)*

9b   Same tumour. *(H&E ×250)*

9c   A more solid area of the same tumour. *(H&E ×250)*

Spread

Growth is usually slow and expansive but there is infiltration at the edge.
Satellite nodules or metastases by the blood stream occur in 11 to 20%.

J. Cook

Malignant mesothelioma

A very rare tumour occurring mostly in men aged 50 to 69 years who have had an occupational exposure to asbestos. Clinically over half the patients present with ascites. The tumour may form nodular masses or plaques, or may show diffuse peritoneal thickening. Two cell types predominate in the tumour:
1   Cells varying in their appearance from the cubical cells of hyperplastic mesothelium to poorly differentiated cells difficult to differentiate from the malignant epithelial cells of carcinoma ('epithelial' type).
2   Spindle-shaped or fusiform cells with elongated or ovoid nuclei. Differentiation varies and some cells in poorly differentiated areas have giant nuclei ('sarcomatoid' type).

Histology

The histological appearances of the tumours vary according to the proportions of 'epithelial' and 'sarcomatoid' elements. The majority are predominantly 'epithelial' and most of the remainder are mixed 'epithelial' and 'sarcomatoid'.

The 'epithelium' may mass in solid sheets of cells or form tubular or papillary structures. Poorly differentiated tumours resemble carcinomas but secrete different mucins. Strong PAS staining of the cells rules out mesothelioma.

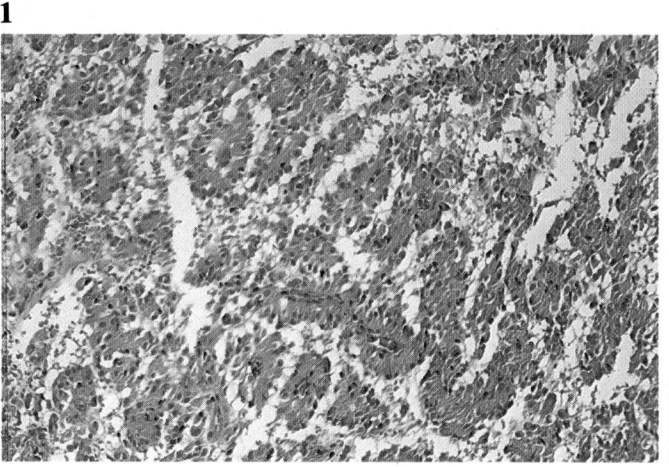

1   Peritoneum – mesothelioma. The tumour is composed of elongated 'epithelial' type cells arranged on a sparse vascular stroma to form delicate papillary processes. *(H&E ×125)*

Spread

Spread is mainly by local invasion but metastases by lymph or blood stream occurs late in the disease.

Secondary carcinoma

Involvement of the peritoneal cavity is common in all forms of malignancy occurring in the alimentary tract. The secondary tumours may be single or multiple often resulting from diffuse lymphatic permeation or diffuse free dissemination throughout the cavity especially when, for example, a carcinoma has penetrated all coats of the bowel and has reached the peritoneal surface. The appearances show variation. Sometimes the metastases are solid nodules, but in other instances there is a large mucoid element. The appearances may suggest a primary mesothelioma but the diagnosis must ultimately depend upon microscopic examination. These tumours may be associated with ascites.

Granuloma

Certain granulomatous conditions may result in lesions which simulate tumour formation from which they have to be differentiated.

In addition to the granulomas arising from bacterial infection, there are granulomatous conditions which are caused by the introduction of foreign substances such as talc or starch at the time of operation. These are derived usually from the surgeon's gloves and in the past, talc has been the major culprit. They provoke a chronic inflammation which results in formation of granulomatous nodules resembling tubercles or carcinomatous seedlings on the peritoneum, and in the development of adhesions which eventually become densely fibrous.

Microscopically there is a chronic inflammatory reaction with striking formation of multinucleated giant cells particularly in the case of talc. When the condition is suspected the histological sections are best viewed in polarised light. Talc is brilliantly birefringent, and starch gives rise to the characteristic Maltese cross birefringence.

Uncommonly a similar reaction may be caused by a variety of substances introduced into or rupturing into the peritoneal cavity and recently a particularly acute form of granuloma with eosinophilic reaction to the cellulose of disposable gowns has been described.

N. Maclean

Index

Forthcoming volumes in the series

Volume 2
Lesions of the Head and Neck, Skin, Endocrine system and Breast

Head and Neck
Anomalies of the skull, face and mouth.
Infections of the face and neck.
Tumours of the skull, jaws, mouth and pharynx.

Skin
Neoplasms.

Endocrine system
Thyroid, adrenal, parathyroid and pituitary.

Breast

Volume 3
Genitourinary system

Congenital and acquired lesions including tumours of the renal tract. This covers the surgical pathology of the kidney, ureters and bladder. Lesions of the male genital tract including diseases of the prostate and testis. Female genital tract. The major lesions of the uterus, ovaries and fallopian tubes.

Volume 4
Cardiovascular system

This includes a study of lesions of the heart both congenital and acquired, and the vascular and lymphatic systems.
Respiratory system. The major lesions of the bronchus, lungs and pleura.
Lesions of the mediastinum.

Volume 5
Orthopaedic lesions

This covers the major lesions both congenital and acquired of bones and joints.